NCLEX-PN®

A Study Guide for Practical Nursing

Fourth Edition

JoAnn Zerwekh, EdD, RN, FNP

Executive Director
Nursing Education Consultants
Nevis, Minnesota

Nursing Faculty
University of Phoenix, Online Campus
Phoenix, Arizona

Jo Carol Claborn, MS, RN, CNS

Executive Director
Nursing Education Consultants
Dallas, Texas

Nursing Education Consultants
Midlothian, Texas

Production: Gingerbread Press
Cover Design: Tim Fennell

✦

✦

Printed in the United States of America
Nursing Education Consultants
P.O. Box 465
Ingram, Texas 78025
1-800-933-7277
ISBN 1-892155-05-2, 4th Edition, 2003
Library of Congress Catalog Card Number: 2002114073

✦

Any procedure or practice described in this book should be applied by the health-care practitioner under appropriate supervision in accordance with professional standards of care used with regard to the unique circumstances that apply in each practice situation. Care has been taken to confirm the accuracy of information presented and to describe generally accepted practices. However, the authors, editors, and publisher cannot accept any responsibility for errors or omissions or for consequences from application of the information in this book and make no warranty, express or implied, with respect to the contents of this book.

The authors and publisher have exerted every effort to ensure that drug selection and dosage set forth in this text are in accord with current recommendations and practice at the time of publication. However, in view of the ongoing research, changes in government regulations, and the constant flow of information relating to drug therapy and drug reactions, the reader is urged to check the package insert of each drug for any change in indications and dosage and for added warnings and precautions. This is particularly important when the recommended agent is a new or infrequently used drug.

This book is written to be used as a review book for the NCLEX-PN®. It is not intended for use as a primary resource for procedures, treatments, medications or to serve as a complete textbook for nursing care.
Copies of this book may be obtained directly from *Nursing Education Consultants.*

Last Digit is the Print Number: 6 5 4 3 2 1

To our daughters
Ashley, Jaelyn, and Kimberley
You make us proud with all your accomplishments
We love you dearly

Preface

This 4th edition of ***NCLEX-PN®: A Study Guide for Practical Nursing*** presents updated information specifically designed to assist you in preparing for the National Council Licensure Examination for Practical Nurses (NCLEX-PN®). While offering a systematic, logical review of essential content, this text emphasizes the integrated approach to nursing practice that the NCLEX-PN® is designed to test. This book's primary purpose is to assist you to thoroughly review facts, principles, and applications of the nursing process. It should alleviate many of the concerns you may have about what, how, and when to study.

We have spent a great deal of time studying the NCLEX-PN® test format and have incorporated this information into this book. In our review courses which we have taught across the country, we have identified specific student needs and put it all together so that you can be successful on the NCLEX-PN®. We have study questions at the end of each chapter to check your reading and study, in addition to the practice test at the end of the book and the computer disk.

For today's visually oriented students, we have designed graphics that highlight important information.

NCLEX Alert identifies what we feel are frequently tested concepts that we have interpreted from the PN Job Task Analysis from the National Council State Boards of Nursing, Inc.

NCLEX ALERT: Identifies critical information that is part of the NCLEX-PN Test Plan.

Geriatric Priority: *identified priorities of nursing care that are important in the care of the elder client.*

NURSING PRIORITY: *Identifies priority nursing concepts of care that are associated with a disease or condition.*

Pedantic Priority: *Identifies priorities of nursing care that are important considerations in the care of infants and children*

Disease conditions are easily located:

Disease Conditions

Information on self care can be found under nursing interventions:

Self-Care

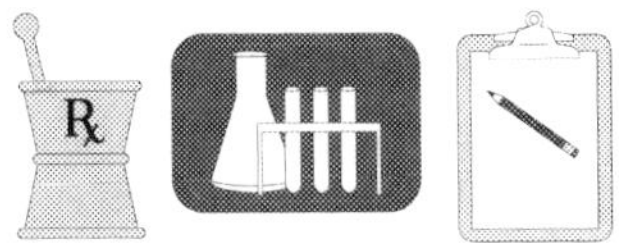

Appendices highlight medications, diagnostic, and nursing procedures in each chapter.

- Discussion of principles of effective test taking and testing strategies
- Test questions with answers and rationale for testing practice
- Current information on NCLEX-PN®.

The comments from our review course participants on our third edition have helped to shape the development of this fourth edition. We hope this text will prove even more beneficial to nursing faculty, students, and graduate nurses.

JoAnn Zerwekh

Jo Carol Claborn

Acknowledgments

We wish to express our appreciation to our children — Tyler and Ashley Zerwekh, Mike Brown, Kimberley Aultman, and Jaelyn Conway for their continuing support as their mothers wrote, rewrote, and put together the fourth edition of this review book. To our parents, Charles Graham and Hazel Cooper, who continue to provide steadfast, loving support in all that we do. To Lucy Claborn, who continues to amaze us with her youth and vitality. To Robert and Tom, thank you for your tolerance, love, and willingness to continue to share in our hectic professional lives.

The revision of a book offers the opportunity to be responsive to nursing faculty and students who have utilized the book. We appreciate their comments and suggestions for the production of this fourth edition. It is a privilege to express an appreciation to the individuals who assisted us in the technical preparation and production of this fourth edition. Our sincere appreciation to:

- Elaine Nokes, our administrative assistant, who keeps everything organized and running smoothly for our business;
- C.J. Miller, RN, BSN, for the creative characters that introduce each chapter;
- Robert Zerwekh, PhD, for developing the software testing program;
- All the staff at Gingerbread Press, Inc. for their persistence and patience in working with us on the production and printing;
- James Halfast for his assistance in typesetting and rescuing us when Corel Ventura™ "hiccoughed;"
- Tim Fennel for creating and producing the cover design — your ideas and design continually amaze us!

Contributors

Sharon Decker, MS, RN
Texas Tech University
Health Science Center
Lubbock, Texas

Tom Gaglione, RN, MN
Nursing Education Consultants
Nevis, Minnesota

Alice B. Pappas, PhD, RN
Baylor University School of Nursing
Dallas, Texas

Susan Priest, RN, MSN, CNS
Alvin Community College
Alvin, Texas

Cathy Rosser, RN, MSN
University of Texas at Tyler, Texas

Linda Stevenson, PhD, RN
Baylor University School of Nursing
Dallas, Texas

Joanna Barnes, RN, MSN
Grayson County College
Denison, Texas

Mary Ann Yantis, PhD, RN
Baylor University School of Nursing
Dallas, Texas

Table of Contents

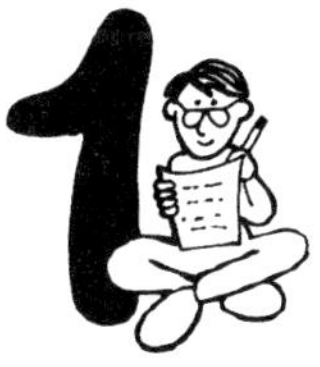

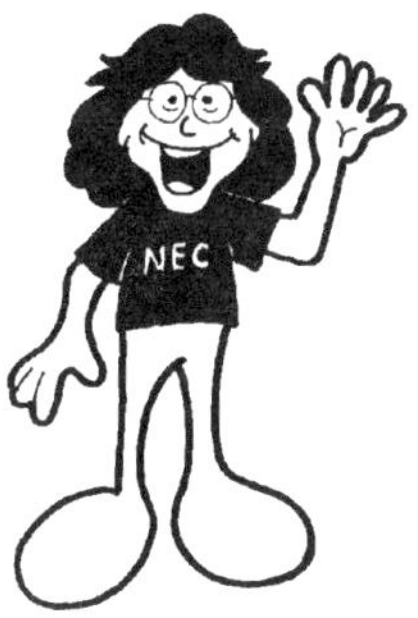

Introduction and NCLEX-PN™ Testing Strategies

The National Council of State Boards of Nursing (NCSBN) is responsible for the development of the NCLEX-PN™. The NCSBN was established by the state boards of nursing as the national credentialing organization for nursing. The National Council is composed of members from all of the respective state boards of nursing. The NCLEX-PN™ is used by all of the states to determine entry into nursing practice as a practical nurse. Each state is responsible for the testing requirements, retesting procedures, and entry into practice within that state. Every state requires the same competency level or passing standard on NCLEX, there is no variation in passing standards from state to state.

Test Plan

The test plan is based on research done by the National Council every 3 years. The purpose of the research is to determine the activities of practical nurses within a year of completing school and the NCLEX-PN. This research indicates that the majority of graduate nurses are working in an acute care environment and are responsible for caring for adult clients.[1] The exam consists of questions that are designed to test the candidate's ability to apply the nursing process and to determine appropriate nursing responses and interventions in order to provide safe nursing care. The framework of the test plan reflects two components: the nursing process and areas of client needs.

Phases of the Nursing Process

Each question is based on the nursing process and all questions reflect some type of nursing decision or action. All of the questions in the test bank are categorized according to the nursing process. See Table 1.1 for commonly used terms that are incorporated into a question to designate levels of the nursing process. You have had the nursing process since the beginning of school, there is nothing new about the nursing process on NCLEX. The process must go in order - data collection, planning, implementation, and evaluation. You must have adequate data before you can proceed with the process. Frequently questions will be based on obtaining critical assessment data; other questions will present the assessment data in the stem of the question. It is important to keep the steps of the nursing process in mind when critically evaluating an NCLEX question.

Areas of Client Needs

The areas of client needs reflect an integrated approach to the testing content. There are no predetermined number of questions or percentage of questions that reflect medical surgical nursing, pediatrics, obstetrics, etc.

The areas of client needs are:

A. Safe Effective Care and environment -
   1. Coordinated Care - 6-12%
   2. Safety and Infection Control 7-13%

B. Health Promotion and Maintenance
   3. Growth and Development - 4-10%
   4. Prevention and Early Detection of disease - 4-10%

C. Psychological Integrity
   5. Coping and Adaptation - 6-12%
   6. Psychosocial Adaptation - 4-10%

D. Physiological Integrity.
   7. Basic Care and Comfort - 10-16%
   8. Pharmacological Therapies- 5-11%
   9. Reduction of Risk Potential - 11-17%
   10. Physiological Adaptation - 13-19%

The National Council Detailed Test Plan for the NCLEX-PN™ Examination may be obtained from the National Council of State Boards of Nursing, Inc. (www.ncsbn.org).[1]

NCLEX questions are based on critical thinking concepts, which will demonstrate your ability to make decisions and solve problems. NCLEX questions are not fact, recall, or memory level questions. Nurses who have taken the NCLEX will be the first to tell you that the questions are not like anything you had on nursing school examinations. The questions and answers have been thoroughly researched and have been tested prior to your examination. This is what is call a "standardized exam." The standardization is important because the NCLEX is used nationwide to determine entry level into practice. This means that regional differences in nursing care will not be a component of the exam. All of the questions have been designed according to the client needs as reflected on the test plan, then researched and documented as entry level nursing behaviors for practical nurses. What was new information in the last month's journal will not be immediately reflected on the NCLEX.

Table 1-1: DESCRIPTORS FOR STEPS OF THE NURSING PROCESS

Data Collection	Planning	Implementation	Evaluation
assess	include	implement	evaluate
determine	plan	teach	monitor
observe	generate	give	question
collect	arrange	administer	repeat
recognize	formulate	document	re-establish
monitor	short-term goal is...	inform	consider
find	long-term goal is...	encourage	
gather	patient outcome is...	advise	
describe		explain	
		provide	

NCLEX ALERT: *The NCLEX-PN is a test that requires application of nursing concepts and principles across the life span.*

Throughout this book are NCLEX-Alerts that call your attention to areas that have been identified on the test plan or test blueprint. Pay attention to this information and think about how this concept or principle can apply to different types of clients.

NURSING PRIORITY: *This is critical information to consider in order to care for a specific client safely.*

Another characteristic of this book is the Nursing Priorities. As conditions are discussed, the nursing priorities call your attention to critical information regarding a client with specific conditions being presented.

What is Computer Adaptive Testing (CAT)?

Computer adaptive testing allows for a test to be generated according to each candidate's needs. As a candidate progresses through questions, the computer will select the next question to be presented in order to provide an opportunity to demonstrate competence. The NCELX-PN™ is graded in a different manner from conventional school exams. It is not based on the number of questions answered correctly, but rather the level of competency. The pass/fail is determined by the competence level based on the level of difficulty of the questions presented.

When each candidate begins their test, a test bank of questions will be loaded into the computer. Different candidates will receive different sets of questions, but the pool of questions will be based on the same test plan. For example, standard precautions is a critical element of the test plan. There are lots of situations and clients where this concept can be tested. You may receive an obstetrical client, someone else a respiratory client, and still someone else a newborn client.

The questions to be presented are determined by your response to the previous question. When you get a question correct, you will get a harder question the next time. The more of the harder questions you answer correctly, the closer you are to passing. You cannot skip questions, or go back to previously answered questions. As you progress through the exam, it is interactively assembled as you go. As long as you answer the questions correctly, you will get a harder question. When you answer a question incorrectly, the computer will select an easier question. The really easy questions are often below the level of competency.

Taking the NCLEX

When you begin taking your NCLEX, there will be a tutorial to help you get started and to make sure you understand how to use the computer. You will have a maximum of 5 hours to complete the examination. You can take two breaks during the testing period.

Your examination will stop when one of the following occurs:

1. You have answered 85 questions and demonstrated minimum competency, or a lack of minimum competency.

2. You have completed the maximum number of 205 questions.

3. You have been testing for 5 hours.

You will receive somewhere between 85-205 questions. The number of questions on your NCLEX is not indicative of your level of competency. A lot of candidates who complete all 205 questions will have demonstrated a level of minimum competency and therefore pass NCLEX. You will use a mouse to select your answers, so your don't have to worry about different computer function keys. There will also be an onscreen calculator to use for your math problems. If you have any problems with the environment or with the equipment, there will be someone there to assist you.

When you receive your Candidate Bulletin from the National Council, read it carefully. This will provide you with a lot of information that will give you direction and answer some of the questions you may still have regarding the NCLEX.

Successful Test Taking on NCLEX

NCLEX ALERT: *You must practice testing skills for them to become part of your testing abilities. Practice test-taking is necessary if you are going to be able to fully utilize these skills on the NCLEX-PN™.*

The ability to take an examination is a skill that is developed through practice and experience. Being able to take an examination effectively is almost as important as the basic knowledge required to answer the questions correctly. Everyone has taken an examination only to find in the review of the exam that questions were missed due to poor testing skills. Nursing education provides the graduate with a comprehensive base of knowledge; how you, the graduate, utilize this knowledge will determine your success on the examination.

The NCLEX-PN™ is designed to evaluate minimum levels of competency for entry level practical nursing. The exam is not testing your total knowledge, your knowledge of specialty areas, or any degree of professionalism. It is designed to test whether you have an adequate knowledge base in order to practice nursing safely. On NCLEX, the questions are described as being based on clinical situations common in nursing; uncommon situations are not emphasized. NCLEX questions are not fact, recall, or memory level questions, they are questions you are going to have to "critically think" about to answer.

Practice testing is an excellent method of studying for NCLEX. However, you have to use the results to determine if there are areas of content you need to review, or if you are missing questions due to poor testing strategies.

NCLEX Testing Strategies

The NCLEX questions are different from those you have had in school. One of the biggest problems graduates encounter is that there appears to be two or more correct answers. Sometimes you may feel that you want more information. You have got to answer the question as it is presented, no one is going to clarify or answer any questions you may have about the question. Presented here is information that is critical for you to consider when evaluating and answering NCLEX questions.

✎ **The NCLEX Hospital** - What a great place to work! On the NCLEX, all of your clients are being cared for in the NCLEX Hospital. Questions ask for nursing care and decisions based on a situation where everything you need to care for the client in the best possible way is available to you. *NCLEX questions are based on textbook practices, not on the real world.* Clients are going to respond just like the nursing textbooks indicate they will. If you have had a lot of clinical experience, you may find yourself thinking that you cannot do something because you do not have adequate staff, or equipment, or it just is not "realistic" to do it that way. It is in the NCLEX Hospital. This approach is necessary since this is a nationally standardized examination.

✎ **Calling the Doctor (or anyone else)** -This is an exam on nursing care, evaluate the question carefully and see what nursing action needs to be taken before consulting or calling someone else. This includes charge nurse, social workers, respiratory therapist, hospital chaplain, as well as the doctor. After carefully evaluating the question, if the client's condition is such that you cannot do anything to resolve the problem, or immediately assist the client, then calling the charge nurse or the doctor may be the best answer. Frequently, there is a nursing action to be taken before contacting anyone.

✎ **Doctor's Orders** - You can assume that you have a doctor's order to provide the nursing care in the options presented to you. If the questions asks for administration of a specific medication for the client's problem, then consider that you have an order for it. If a question is asking whether or not you need a doctor's order for an action, it will be stated as such in the stem of the question. For example, the question may request a dependent or independent nursing action.

✎ **Focus on the client** - Look for answers that focus on the client. Wrong choices would be those that focus on maintaining hospital rules and policy or dealing with equipment. Evaluate the status of the client first, then deal with the equipment problems or concerns.

✎ **Laboratory Values** - It is important to know the normal lab values for the most common laboratory tests. It is also important to know what to anticipate the lab values to indicate when a client's condition is improving or when it is getting worse. A guideline here is

Table 1-2: IMPORTANT LAB VALUES

Know These Lab Values:	
Potassium	Prothrombin time
Glucose (blood sugar)	Partial thromboplastin time
Complete Blood Count (CBC)	Arterial blood gas (ABG's)
Hemoglobin	Oxygen (PO2)
Hematocrit	Carbon dioxide (PCO2)
Platelets	pH (acid or alkaline)
White cell count	Bicarbonate (HCO3)
Creatinine	Bicarbonate (HCO3)
Blood urea nitrogen (BUN)	Specific gravity of urine

Review the normal values, significance of an increase or decrease, and the specific nursing actions in the respective chapters. Specific values and nursing implications may be found in the appendix of each of the respective chapters.

to consider lab values and abnormal lab values that will influence the delivery of nursing care. Check Table 1-2 for examples of commonly utilized laboratory tests. For example, when a client's blood sugar is 50mg, and he is awake and alert, you are going to find a complex carbohydrate to feed him. If a client has a Hgb of 8.5, you don't want him doing any unnecessary physical activities, and you will need to keep him warm.

✎ **Positions** - There are numerous areas on the test plan that can incorporate positioning a client. If the positioning appears in the stem or the question, then you need to consider if the position is for comfort, for treatment, or to prevent a complication. Evaluate the question - what is it you want to accomplish with the position, and why is it important for this client?

Sometimes the position appears in the options. Consider if positioning is important to the care of this client. For example, the semi-Fowlers position is very important to a client who is having difficulty breathing, the supine position or low-Fowlers may be the position of comfort for a client postoperatively. Determine why you are placing a client in a specific position and then determine if this is priority in planning or intervention. Check Appendix 3.1 for a further description of positions.

Management of Client Care

Don't panic with management questions. As the role of the practical nurse has expanded, this is an area that has been increasingly important over the past few years. There are licensed practical/vocational nurses (LVN/LPN), and unlicensed assistive personnel (UAP), or patient care attendants (PCA) to supervise and direct in the provision of safe nursing care. Frequently, this is information you had in class, but did not have the opportunity to apply the principles in the clinical setting. If you will pay attention to some of the rules of supervision, you should be able to answer these questions. Pay attention to whom you are assigning the care or nursing activity - is it to another LVN/LPN, or is it to a less qualified, unlicensed person (UAP/PCA)?

✎ **Don't assign data collection, evaluation, or nursing judgment to an unlicensed person** - These are levels of the nursing process that must be done by a licensed nurse.

✎ **Watch teaching assignments** - This is an area that is most often the responsibility of the registered nurse, but may be incorporated into the PN exam as specific instructions from the registered nurse.

✎ **Keep in mind the NCLEX Hospital** - You will have all of the time, equipment, and assistance you need. The client in the question is the only client you have to be concerned about. Your focus is on the client or clients in the question - don't worry about what is happening on the rest of the unit, or what you think the rest of your client assignment may involve.

✎ **Determine your most stable client** - The one who has the most predictable outcome and is *least* likely to have abrupt changes in his condition that would require nursing judgments. These are the clients you can possibly assign some of their nursing care activities to someone else. When determining the most stable clients, Maslow should also be considered. Very carefully consider any clients with respiratory compromise, they are most likely the clients where you will want to focus your nursing care.

✎ **Identify your priority client** - This is the client who is *most likely* to experience harm, or ill effects if he is not taken care of first. Priority clients would include those with respiratory compromise, those whose condition is unstable or changing. It is not unusual for

NCLEX to give you a typical nursing care assignment and ask you what you should do first, or who you should care for first. You will need to identify your most unstable client, see him first and/or determine what needs to be done now for this client.

✎ **Assign tasks that have specific guidelines** - Those tasks that have specific guidelines that are unchanging and are utilized in the care of a stable client may be assigned to an unlicensed person. Bathing, collecting urine sample, feeding, oral hygiene, and ambulating are just a few examples of these activities. Be careful to work through each option and eliminate the incorrect ones, so you are left with the right answer.

Establishing Nursing Priorities

Almost all nurses will tell you that the NCLEX is full of priority questions. These questions may be worded as: "what is the priority nursing action," "what is the first nursing action," "what is the best nursing action." In other words, the NCLEX wants to know if you can establish what is the most important action for you to take to care for a client in the situation presented. This is frequently where three or four of the options are correct, however one of options needs to be done prior to the others presented. This is where some critical thinking is needed. There are three areas to consider when determining priority nursing actions - Maslow, the nursing process, and client safety.

✎ **Maslow Hierarchy of Needs** - And you thought this was just for fundamentals! *Always consider Maslow and that physiological needs come first.* When evaluating options identify those that are physiological and psychosocial, most often one of the physiological needs will be the correct answer. You have to take care of a client's physical needs before you can take care of his psychosocial or teaching needs. Also remember the ABC's - airway, breathing, and circulation as the critical physiological needs - and at the base of Maslow. But be cautious, don't always jump on the airway as the best answer - sometimes the client does not have an airway problem! Maslow's needs also apply to the psychosocial questions, take care of physical needs first, than focus on the psychosocial needs. (See the section in this chapter regarding answering psychosocial questions)

✎ **Nursing Process** - The first step in the nursing process is data collection. This is frequently the first nursing action as well. Data collection must be done in order to determine what nursing implementation actions are appropriate. Go back to Table 1-1 for words that indicate levels of the nursing process. If the client data is provided in the stem of the question, then consider Maslow when selecting the best nursing action.

✎ **Safety Issues** - This may include situations in the hospital or home. The first issue to consider is meeting basic needs of survival - oxygen, nutrition, elimination. Reducing environmental hazards is also a concern. This could be prevention of falls, accidents, or medication errors. The environmental safety would also include prevention of spread of diseases, this may include how to avoid contagious diseases, importance of immunizations, or even activities such as hand washing. When critically evaluating questions that involve a client's safety and there are multiple options that appear to be correct - determine what activity will be of most benefit to the client, or what will cause the least harm to the client.

STRATEGIES TO EVALUATE MULTIPLE-CHOICE QUESTIONS

These are testing strategies that will help you during school, as well as on NCLEX. Start practicing them now, and you will increase your testing scores in school as well as being one more step closer toward success on NCLEX.

Question Characteristics

The majority of questions on the NCLEX, as well as your nursing school exams, are multiple choice. This is a type of testing that is most familiar to you.

1. Read the question carefully before ever looking or considering the options. If you glance through the options you may pick up key words that will affect the way you perceive the question and you will try to predict a right answer.

This will prevent you from formulating an opinion about the answer before you have read the question. On a paper and pencil test, just cover the answers with your hand or a notecard. If you practice this before NCLEX, then when you take the exam on the computer you will be able to carefully evaluate the question before looking at the answer options.

2. Do not read extra meaning into the question. The question is asking for specific information. If it appears to be simple "common sense," then assume it is simple. Do not look for a hidden meaning in a question. (Don't make the client any sicker then he already is!)

Example: A bronchoscopy was performed on a client at 7 am. He returns to his room and the nurse plans to assist the client with his AM care. The client refuses the care. What is the best nursing action?

① Encourage the client to take a warm shower to increase respiratory humidification.

② Perform all of his AM care to decrease the risk of overexertion.

③ Postpone the AM care until client is more comfortable and can participate.

④ Cancel all of the AM care since it is not necessary to perform after a bronchoscopy.

The correct answer is # 3. The question is asking for a nursing judgment regarding AM care. Do not read into the question and make it more difficult by trying to put in information relating to respiratory care.

3. Read the stem correctly. Make sure you understand exactly what information the question is asking. Watch for words that provide direction to the question - "the client would need further teaching," "indicates the client understands the preoperative teaching, medication administration ...", "contraindicated," "the client should avoid." Try rewording the question to better understand what it is asking.

These words or phrases change the direction of the question. It may help to rephrase the question in your own words in order to better understand what information is being requested.

Example: A client had a cardiac catheterization using the left femoral artery. During the first few hours after the procedure, what nursing intervention would be most important to identify one of the most common complications?

① Check his temperature and pulse every hour.

② Elevate the head of the bed 90 degrees.

③ Cough, turn, and deep breath every hour.

④ Check the femoral and pedal pulses every hour.

Rephrase the question: the client had a cardiac catheterization - what are the most common complications? Hematoma at injection site, dysrhythmias, and emboli. Which of these answers reflect observation, or data collection for these complications? The temperature has nothing to do with the complications. Turn cough and deep breath will be done after the first few hours post-test. Elevating the head of the bed may be contraindicated due to location of injection site, only one left that reflects a common complication is checking the pedal pulse to determine if there is a hematoma developing.

4. Watch where your client is in the disease process or condition he is experiencing. Examples of this are terms, such as "immediately postoperatively," "the first post operative day," "experienced a myocardial infarction this am."

Example: A mother who is three days postpartum comes into the clinic complaining of soreness and fullness in her breasts. She wants to stop breast feeding until her breasts begin to feel better. What is the best nursing action?

Rewording - What is happening to the mother 3 days postpartum. Think about when milk begins to fill the breast, and what would happen if she quit breast feeding now?

① Demonstrate how to apply a breast binder to decrease the discomfort.

② Agree with the client, she should stop breast feeding until she is more comfortable.

③ Explain the breast discomfort is normal and will subside as the infant begins to nurse.

④ Suggest that she decrease her fluid intake for 24 hours in order to decrease milk production.

Think about where the client is 3 days post partum and what is important for her to do to establish breast feeding and to decrease discomfort during this particular period of time. It would be a different situation if she was feeling discomfort, and she had been successfully breast feeding for 3-4 months. The correct answer is #3.

5. Identify the step of the nursing process being tested. Remember, you must have adequate assessment data before you can continue. Identify the steps of the nursing process for each option - then look for the data collection. Look for key words that can assist you in determining what type of information is being tested. (see Table 1-1)

Example: An elderly client from a residential facility is brought into the emergency room. There are numerous bruises and abrasions in various stages of healing on the client's face and arms. The attendant from the residential facility explains that the elderly client fell down. What is the priority nursing action?

① Call the residential facility and ask for an incident report.

② Put ice on the bruises and cover the abrasions with Vaseline gauze.

③ Notify the charge nurse.

④ Determine the extent of injuries.

The correct answer is #4, to determine or assess the extent of injuries. The stem of the question did not present adequate enough information on which to make a nursing judgment. Options #1, #2, and #3 relate to nursing actions that would be done after the injuries have been adequately evaluated.

6. Before considering the options, think about the characteristics of this condition and critical nursing concepts. What are the nursing priorities in caring for a client with this condition/procedure/medication/problem?

Example: An obese client is 3 days post colon resection. He has been complaining of abdominal tenderness and during the dressing change you observe a loop of bowel protruding through the incision. What is the best nursing action?

Think about post operative care of an abdominal surgery client and what are the common discomforts and problems an obese client might encounter? Don't look at the options - think.... Is this a common complication in clients who are obese, what are specific nursing implications when this occurs, any specific safety issues here, is there a nursing action you can do to take care of the problem? If you are unsure, go back and reassess the question. Now progress to the options:

① With a sterile glove, manually replace the intestine through the incisional area.

② Place a sterile saline soaked dressing over the wound and notify the charge nurse.

③ Irrigate the wound with normal saline and apply a sterile dressing.

④ Cover the wound with a sterile saline dressing and apply an abdominal binder.

In this question, option #2 is correct. A critical issue here is do not attempt to replace the intestine through the incision.

7. Don't focus on predicting a right answer! Frequently, the answer you want is not going to be an option! Keep in mind the characteristics and concepts of nursing care for a client with the condition or problem in the situation presented.

Example: A client has an ulcer (2 in x 2 in) on his right calf that is draining purulent fluid. The vital signs are P-114, R-22, T-102°. Which order will the nurse implement first?

Reword the question: The client has an infection in the ulcer on his leg, his temperature is up, so is his pulse - this is a normal response to infection. What nursing actions do I need to do first?

① Administer Cefazolin (Ancef), 1gm, PO q6h.

② Schedule blood cultures x 2, 20 minutes apart and from different venipuncture sites.

③ Apply polysporin (Bacitracin) ointment topically to leg ulcer TID.

④ Administer acetaminophen (Tylenol), 650 mg suppository, q4h for temp > 101.8° F.

Consider #1 - This is an antibiotic that will begin to fight the infection.

Consider #2 - This is important to do in order to identify the causative bacteria. Cultures must be done prior to starting the antibiotic. This is more important now than #1.

Consider #3 - This is treating the infection topically - it will cause a decrease in the bacteria, still need to get the blood cultures first - eliminate this option.

Consider #4 - This is treating the symptoms, not the cause of the problem, not as important as #2, eliminate this option.

All of these options are feasible for treating this client, however obtaining the blood culture is the most important. If you had approached this question with a specific answer in mind (give an antibiotic), you would have found that answer, however it would have been wrong.

8. Evaluate all of the options in a systematic manner. After you understand the question, read all of the options carefully. Remember, distracters are plausible to the situation and are designed to "distract" you from the correct answer. *NCLEX Style* - all of the options may be correct, but one is the best answer.

Example: A client has just returned to his room from the recovery room following a lumbar laminectomy. The nurse is planning care to prevent complications in the immediate postoperative period. What is an important nursing action?

① Monitor vital signs every four hours.

② Have him turn, cough, and deep breathe.

③ Evaluate every two hours for urinary retention.

④ Determine when he last had a bowel movement.

In evaluating the options, all are plausible for the situation. However, consider that this is the client's operative day, and the question is asking for complications the client might encounter in the immediate post operative period. Distracters #1, #2, #4 are general nursing measures for any surgical client. #1 the vital signs are not frequent enough. #2 is okay and should be done, #4 should be done, but at a later time. #3 is something that is a common problem in the immediate postoperative period for a laminectomy client.

9. As you read the options, eliminate those you know are not correct. This will help narrow the field of choice. When you select an answer or eliminate an option, you should have a specific reason for doing so.

Example: An elderly client is admitted with a diagnosis of cataracts. What information would the nurse find in the data collection for this client?

① Enlarged pupil. (No, the size of the pupil is not associated with cataracts.)

② Itching and burning of the eyelids. (No, these symptoms suggest an infection.)

③ Diminished visual acuity. (Yes, a change in the ability of the client to see clearly due to the opacity of the lens occurs with a cataract.)

④ Eye pain. (No, this does not occur with cataracts.)

After systematically evaluating each of the options, #3 is the best answer.

10. Identify similarities in the options. Frequently the options will contain similar information but one will be different. The different one may be the correct answer.

Example: A client is on a high protein, low residue diet. What foods would best meet the requirements for this diet?

① Roast beef, slice of white bread.

② Fried chicken, green peas.

③ Broiled fish, green beans.

④ Cottage cheese, tomatoes

Distracters #2, #3, and #4 all contain a vegetable that has a peeling and is high residue. The correct answer is #1, for both high protein and low residue. NCLEX does not focus on recipes that contain a mixture of foods that you wonder just how they made that dish. There are no special characteristics to the food, if it has a special characteristic it will be stated ("low sodium," or "low fat"). Also consider the method of food preparation - the NCLEX hospital dietary department does not fry a lot of foods.

11. Select the most comprehensive answer. All of the options may be correct, but one may include the other three options or need to be considered first.

Example: The nurse is planning to teach a diabetic client about his condition. Prior to the teaching, what is important for the nurse to evaluate?

① Required dietary modifications.

② Understanding of the exchange list.

③ Ability to administer insulin.

④ Present understanding of diabetes.

Options #1, #2, and #3 are certainly important considerations in diabetic education. However, they cannot be initiated until the nurse evaluates the client's knowledge of his or her disease state. When two options appear to say the same thing, just in different words, then look for another answer. Options #1 and #2 both refer to the client's understanding of nutrition.

12. After you have selected an answer, reread the question. Does the answer you chose give the information the question is asking for? Sometimes the options are correct but do not give the information the question is asking for.

Example: An elderly client had a thoracotomy. He is three days post-op with a temperature of 102° F. He is complaining of severe chest pain, and his cough is productive with thick yellow mucus. What measures should the nurse take to decrease the client's chest pain?

① Encourage deep breathing and coughing.

② Teach him to take short, shallow breaths.

③ Support the incisional area with a pillow while he coughs.

④ Administer an analgesic and encourage him to remain in bed.

The question is asking for nursing measures to decrease chest pain. Option #1 is correct for the situation but would increase his chest pain. Option #2 will increase his pulmonary congestion. Option #4 will decrease his pain but will increase his congestion. Therefore, the correct answer is #3. After evaluating all of the distracters, the one that answers the question correctly, based on the situation, is #3. Always recheck your answer to make sure it provides the information requested.

13. Multiple-multiple-choice questions are not utilized on the examination. However, you will find questions in which the options contain several items to consider. After you are sure you understand what information the question is requesting, evaluate each part of the option. Is it appropriate to what the question is asking? If an option contains one incorrect item, the entire option is incorrect. All of the items listed in the option must be correct if it is to be the answer to the question.

Example: The nurse is evaluating an elderly client who is at high risk for developing shock. Which nursing observations would be are critical to monitor?

① BP 180/92, pulse 60, respirations 24.

② Pulse 98, BP 170/88, oriented.

③ Respirations 28, pulse 64, confused.

④ BP 98/60, pulse 120, lethargic.

In a methodical evaluation of the items in the options, you can eliminate options. #1 - BP is too high, pulse too low. #2 BP is still high. #3 pulse is too low, therefore #4 is correct. BP is down; pulse is rapid; and client is experiencing change in level of consciousness. These are critical elements in determining adequacy of cardiac output.

14. Multiple-choice mathematical computations will be included in the exam. Mathematical computations may include calculations of IM, PO, sub-q dosages; and conversion of units of measurement. You should be able to apply the appropriate formula to the situation. Some of the questions may call for two computations, as in a dosage question for which you must convert all items to one unit of measurement before calculating the dosage.

Example: The doctor has ordered ampicillin 250 mg IM. Available is ampicillin 1 gm in 5 cc. How many cc would you administer?

① 0.25 cc

② 1 cc

③ 1.25 cc

④ 1.5 cc

First, you must convert milligrams and grams to the same unit of measurement. There are 1000mg in 5cc, therefore there are 200mg per cc. Memorize the formulas necessary to calculate the information. Frequently these questions will contain options that are similar, making guessing hazardous. Correct answer is option #3.

THERAPEUTIC NURSING PROCESS: PRINCIPLES OF COMMUNICATION

Throughout the examination, there will be questions requiring utilization of the principles of therapeutic communication. In therapeutic communication questions, don't assume the client is being manipulative, or is in control of how he feels. Psychosocial problems or mental health problems are most often not under the conscious control of the client.

NCLEX ALERT: *Listening to a client's concerns and assessing a client's and family's response to illness are two primary areas of the psychosocial component.*

✦ **Situations requiring utilization of therapeutic communication are not always centered around a psychiatric client.** Frequently, these questions are centered around the hospitalized client who is experiencing stress and anxiety. Anticipate questions relating to therapeutic communication in the care of clients experiencing stress and anxiety as a result of their physiological problems. These areas could be reflected in a question that involves an obstetrical client, parents of a hospitalized child, and or the cancer client

✦ **Look for responses that focus on the concerns of the client.** Do not focus on the concerns of the nurse, hospital, or of the physician.

✦ **Watch for responses that are open-ended and encourage the client to express how he feels.** Focus on responses that encourage the client to describe how he/she feels. Clients frequently experience difficulty in expressing their feelings. These responses are frequently open-ended statements by the nurse.

✦ **Eliminate responses that are not honest and direct.** In order to build trust and promote a positive relationship, it is important to be honest with the client. Telling the client "don't worry," or "everything is going to be all right,"or "your doctor knows best" will be wrong answers.

✦ **Look for responses that indicate an acceptance of the client.** Regardless of whether his views or moral values agree with yours, you should respect and accept them. This is not the time to tell the alcoholic that he should quit drinking.

✦ **Be careful about responses that give opinions or advice on the client's situation.** Don't assume an authoritarian position. You should not insist that the client follow your advice.

✦ **Do not select responses that block further interaction.** These are frequently presented as closed statements, or encourage a yes or no answer from the client. "Did your family visit today," "How are you feeling about what happened?"

✦ **Don't tell the client how he should or should not feel.** Look for responses that encourage the client to describe how he feels, responses that reflect, restate, or paraphrase feelings expressed.

✦ **Don't ask "why" a client feels the way they do.** Frequently if they understood why they felt the way they do, they would be able to do something about it. The most common answer when a nurse asks a client why he feels this way is "I don't know" and that does not help anyone.

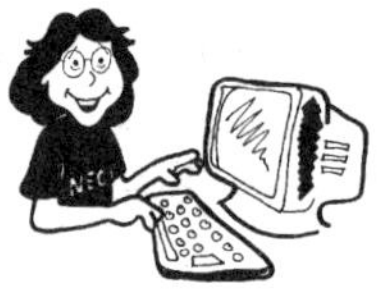

- **Do not use coercion to achieve a desired response.** Don't tell them they can't have their lunch until they get out of bed, or bribe a child to take his medicine by promising him candy.
- **See examples of therapeutic and non-therapeutic communication in Chapter 6, Table 6-1.**

Testing Tips for Success

- **Do not indiscriminately change answers.** If you decide to change an answer, you should have a specific reason for doing so. Sometimes you do remember information and realize you answered the question incorrectly. Frequently, students "talk themselves out" of the correct answer and change it to the incorrect one. On NCLEX, once the question leaves the screen, you cannot access it again.
- **Watch your timing. Do not spend too much time on one question.** It is very important you practice your timing on the sample exams. Watch timing on computer testing. The NCLEX will allow a total of 5 hours to complete the examination. You can plan for about a minute a question. Some questions you will answer quicker, others may take some time. Don't spend more than 2 minutes on a question. If you don't have a good direction for the right answer in 2 minutes, then you probably don't know the answer. Pick the best one you can and move on. (Remember - you are not supposed to know all of the right answers.)
- **Remember the NCLEX is a nursing competency examination, and the correct answer will focus on nursing knowledge and the provision of nursing care.** It does not focus on medical management or making a medical diagnosis.
- **Eliminate distracters that assume the client "would not understand," or "is ignorant" of the situation, or those distractions that "protect them from worry."** For example, "The client should not be told she has cancer because it would upset her too much."
- **There is no pattern of correct answers.** The exam is compiled by a computer, and the position of the correct answers is selected at random. So, don't believe those who say to pick answer #3, when you are guessing.

STUDY HABITS

- **Study effectively**

  Use memory aids, mind mapping, and mnemonics. Memory aids and mind mapping are tools that assist in drawing associations from other ideas with the use of visual images (see Figure 1-1). Mnemonics are words, phrases, or other techniques to help you remember information. Images, pictures, and mnemonics will stay with you longer than just reading the information.

  Develop 3x5 cards with critical information. Don't overload the card, put a statement or question on one side, and answers or follow up information on the other side. For example, on one side you might put "low potassium," on the back side you would put the values. Another card might be "nursing care for hypokalemia," on the back list the nursing care. These cards are much easier for you to carry than the load of books or notes. When you have developed your set of cards with priority information, trade them with a friend and see what is on their cards. These can be used whenever you have only 15-20 minutes of quick study time. Take about 20 cards with you to soccer practice, doctor's office, or anywhere you are going to have to sit and wait for a few minutes. This is quick, easy, and very effective.

  Plan your study time when you are most receptive to learning. Don't wait until the end of the day when you finish everything else. It is difficult to get up at 6am, work all day, deal with family activities, and finally get some study time at 10pm.

  Set a schedule - Let everyone know the schedule. Don't expect your family to leave you alone while you study - this is frequently too much to ask of children and spouse. Go to the library, nursing school, someone's house where there are no disturbances.

  Start planning your review and study about 2-3 months prior to the NCLEX. Do not wait until you get out of school or until the week before the exam to start reviewing. Even if you are/were an "A" student, you need to review.

- **Set a study goal.**

  Decide on a study method.

  Divide the review material into segments.

  Prioritize the segments; review first the areas in which you feel you are deficient and/or weak.

  Identify areas which will require additional review in the review book and/or in a basic nursing textbook.

  Establish a realistic schedule and follow it. Planning for 8 hours of studying on your day off does not work. Instead, plan for 2-4 hours each day, and maybe 4 hours on your days off

  Plan on achieving your study goal several days prior to the examination.

✦ **Group study.**

Keep the group limited to four or five people.

Group members should be mature and serious about studying.

The group should agree on the planned study schedule.

If the group makes you anxious or you do not feel it meets your study needs, do not continue to participate.

✦ **Testing practice.**

Include the testing practice in your schedule.

Plan for answering one question per minute. This will allow you to evaluate the pace of the exam and keep you on target with your timing as your practice answering test questions.

Try to answer the questions as if you were taking the real exam. Do not answer a question and go look up the right answer. If you have 45 minutes to practice testing, set aside 30 questions. Go through and answer the 30 questions in about 30 minutes, then review the answers for the next 15 minutes.

Utilize the testing strategies in the comprehensive practice test in the back of this book and on the computer disk.

Evaluate the practice exam for problem areas.
a. Testing skills.
b. Knowledge base.

Evaluate the questions you answer incorrectly. Review the rationale for the right answer and understand why you missed it - was it a testing skill or did you not know the information?.

Utilize the questions at a later point to review the information again.

There is a CD-Rom with additional practice questions in the back of the book. The more questions you practice, the better you will be able to implement your testing strategies.

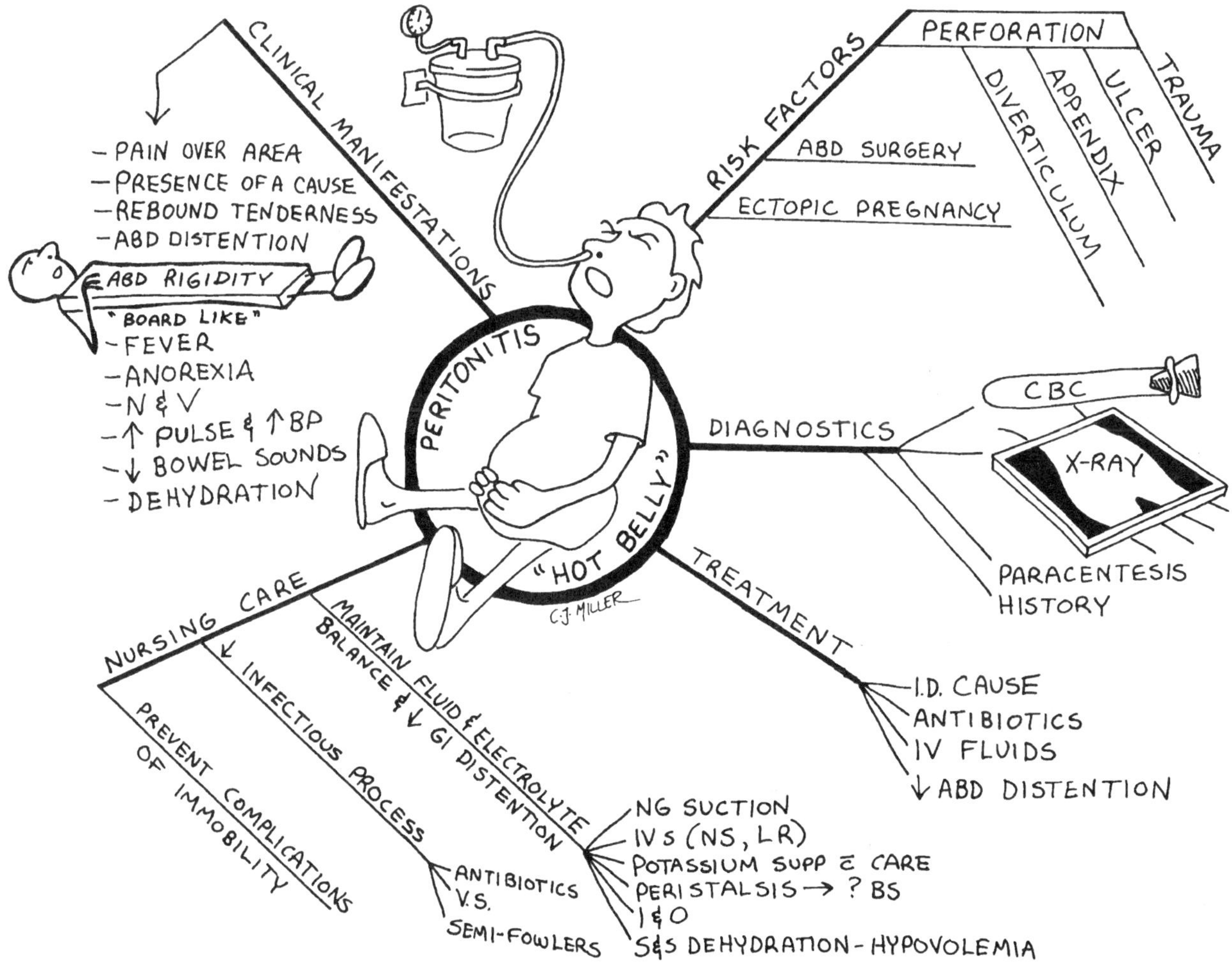

Figure 1-1: Peritonitis "Hot Belly"
Reprinted with permission: Zerwekh, J., Claborn, J., & Miller, C. (2000): *Memory Notebook of Nursing* Vol 1, 2nd ed, Ingram, TX: Nursing Education Consultants Publishing, Inc., pg. 85.

DECREASE ANXIETY

Your activities the day of the examination strongly influence your level of anxiety. By carefully planning ahead, you will be able to eliminate some anxiety-provoking situations.

- ✦ Visit the examination site prior to the day of the exam. Evaluate travel time, parking, and time to get to the designated area. Get an early start to allow extra time.
- ✦ If you have to travel a significant distance to the examination site, try and spend the night in the immediate vicinity. Don't cram 4 or 5 people in one room. Each of you needs your own bed!
- ✦ Do something pleasant the evening prior to the examination. This is not the time to "cram."
- ✦ Anxiety is contagious. If those around you are extremely anxious, avoid contact with them prior to the examination.
- ✦ Carefully evaluate if you want to go to the testing site with anyone else. If they finish before you do, it will put increased pressure on you to hurry up and finish - you don't need that!
- ✦ Make your meal before the test a light healthy one.
- ✦ Avoid eating highly spiced or different foods. This is not the time for a gastrointestinal upset.
- ✦ Wear comfortable clothes. This is not a good time to wear tight clothing or new shoes.
- ✦ Wear clothing of moderate weight. It is difficult to control the temperature to keep everyone comfortable. Take a sweater or wear clothes that can be removed if you get too warm.
- ✦ Wear soft-soled shoes; this decreases the noise in the testing area.
- ✦ Make sure you have the "Authorization to Test" papers that are required to gain admission to the exam site.
- ✦ Do not take study material to the exam site. You cannot take it into the exam area, and it is too late to study.
- ✦ If you wear reading glasses, be sure to take them with you to the testing center.
- ✦ Do not panic when you encounter a clinical situation you have not heard of. Use good test-taking strategies, select an answer, and continue. Remember, you are not going to know all of the right answers.

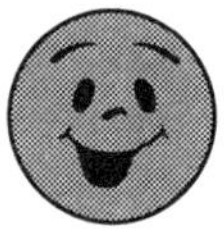

- ✦ Reaffirm to yourself that you know the material. It is not time for any self-defeating behavior or self-talk.
- ✦ **YOU WILL PASS!!** Build your confidence by visualizing yourself in 6 months working in the area you desire. Create that mental picture of where you want to be and who you want to be- an LPN/LVN. Use your past successes to bring positive energy and "vibes" to your NCLEX exam.
- ✦ **WE KNOW YOU CAN DO IT!**

1. Smith, June E., et al. (2001). *Linking the NCLEX-PN National Licensure Examination to Practice: 2000 Practice analysis of Newly Licensed Practical/vocational Nurses in the U.S.*, Chicago: National Council of State Boards of Nursing, Inc.

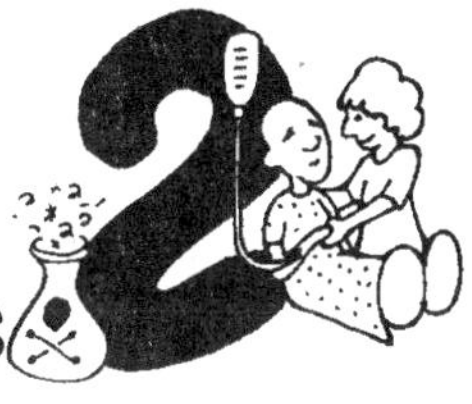

Health Implications Across the Lifespan

GROWTH AND DEVELOPMENT

NCLEX ALERT: *Provide physical care appropriate to developmental level (e.g., newborn, child, older adult, etc.)*

A. Physical Development. (Table 2-1)

B. Psychosocial development is predictable and is observed to occur in a pattern across the years.

C. Nursing care for clients should be planned according to their developmental age, not their chronological age.

Dietary Considerations Throughout the Life Span

NCLEX ALERT: *Use measures to improve client's nutritional status, (e.g., small feedings, preferred foods, ethnic foods, etc.).*

Infant

1. Growth.
   a. Birth weight doubles in 4 months.
   b. Birth weight triples at 1 year.
   c. Infant gains only another 4-6 lbs. until 2 years old.
   Example: Birth weight $7\frac{1}{2}$ lbs.; at 4 months 14 lbs.; another $7\frac{1}{2}$ lbs. will be added in the next 8 months.
   d. A newborn infant will lose weight for the first few days, but should not lose more than 10% of its birth weight or take longer than 10-14 days to regain it.
   e. Newborn has a higher fluid requirement in relation to body size than the adult.
2. Diet.
   a. Ideal food is breast milk, because it is nutritionally superior to alternatives.
   b. Cereal is usually the first solid food given at 6 months; infants less allergic to rice cereal; then offer oats, barley and wheat in this order.
   c. The order of introduction of food is cereal, fruits, vegetables, and meats.
   d. Before adding another food wait 4-7 days to ensure no allergic or adverse reaction has occurred due to new food item.
   e. Milk intake should not exceed 1 qt. daily to prevent refusal of other foods.
   f. Introduce fruit juices when introducing use of the cup around 6-9 months.

Pediatric Priority: *Infants should not be given honey until after the first birthday.*

3. Nursing Implications.
   a. Newborns cannot swallow voluntarily until 10-12 weeks of age.
   b. Extrusion reflex (pushing food out of mouth with tongue) lasts until 4 months.
   c. Usual progression of food: texture is strained to mashed to minced to chopped to cut table foods.
   d. Increase the use of small sized finger foods as pincer grasp develops (9 months).
   e. Texture of food becomes increasingly important from 6 months to 1 year, but the food must be easily dissolved, (e.g., crackers or zwieback).

Pediatric Priority: *Raw carrots, celery, popcorn, nuts, and hard candies should be postponed until the toddler stage for safety.*

Toddler

1. Growth - steady increases.
2. Diet.
   a. Needs 16 oz. of milk daily; more than 24 oz. can lead to milk anemia (peak incidence at 18 months).
   b. Good rule in food selection is one tart, one mild, and one crisp.
   c. Prefers finger foods, (e.g., raw vegetables).
   d. Tends to refuse casseroles, salads, and mixed dishes.
3. Nursing Implications.
   a. Struggle for autonomy may be manifested by refusal of food, mealtime negativism, and ritualism.
   b. Bribery and rewards for eating should be avoided.
   c. Don't mix food on plate.

Table 2-1: GROWTH AND DEVELOPMENT

Birth – 4 months	Consistently gains weight (5-7 oz per week) Posterior fontanel closes Responds to sounds and begins vocalizing Gains head control → lifts chest → rolls over one way Smiles responsively → smiles when spoken to	Teething may begin Coordination progresses from jerky movement to grasping objects Provide toys that increase hand-eye coordination
4-9 months	Doubles birth weight (gains 3-5 oz per week) Teething begins with lower incisors Sits with support Turns over both directions Begins crawling	Reaches for objects and grasps them Begins "stranger anxiety" Begins vocalizing with single consonants Provide brightly colored toys that are easy to grasp Enjoys noisemakers and mirrors, plays pat-a-cake
9-12 months	Birth weight triples Head and chest circumference is equal Anterior fontanel begins to close Teething - has 6-8 teeth Sits alone → moves from prone to sitting position Crawling → pulling up → walks holding onto furniture	May stand alone Has developed crude to fine pincer grasp Transfers objects from one hand to another Recognizes own name Enjoys playing alone (solitary) Explores objects by putting them in the mouth.
Toddler (12 - 24 months)	50% of height at 2 years Exaggerated lumbar curve Mobile – walks/runs/jumps Walks up and down stairs-one foot at time. Begins using eating utensils Obeys simple commands Begins to develop vocabulary	Speech becomes understandable Thumbsucking may be at peak Solitary play at 12 months, parallel play at 18 months Beginning to develop bladder and bowel control Attention seeking behavior – temper tantrums Enjoys activities that provide mobility – riding vehicles, wagons, pull toys
Preschool (3-5 years)	Birth length doubles at 4 years Coordination continues to improve Rides tricycle, throws a ball Walks stairs with alternating feet	Begins self care abilities Knows own name Good verbalization – talks about activities Plays "dress up", cars, dolls, grooming aids
School Age (6-10 years)	Growth spurts begin Increasingly active Very concerned with body image Need for conformity – rules and ritual	Increasing importance of peer groups Plays with groups of same sex Competes for attention
Adolescence (11 -17 years)	Beginning and completing puberty Girls maturing earlier than boys Very conscious of changes in body Rapid growth	Move from concrete to abstract thinking Increased independence Strong peer group association Increased interest in opposite sex
Young Adult (18-30 years)	Physical maturity Full mental capacity Assumes responsibility for own learning Adult relationship with parents	Launches career Selects a mate, begins own family Begins involvement in community
Adult (30-60 years)	Physiological processes begin slow decline Cognitive skills peak Creativity at maximum Increase in community involvement Increase in concern for future of society	Family tasks Assist children to responsible adulthood Role reversal with aging parents Defines role of grandparenting
Older Adult (60 + years)	Decline of physiological status Demineralization of bones ↓ Cardiac output ↓ Respiratory vital capacity ↓ Glomerular filtration rate ↓ Serum albumin ↓ Glucose tolerance	Maintains reasoning ability and abstract thinking Thinking slows Restructure in family roles Retirement Reorganization of activities Continues with community involvement and politics

Preschooler

1. Growth.
   a. Growth rate slows and appetite decreases.
   b. Activity level and nutrient need remain high.
2. Diet.
   a. Food jags are common; may refuse to eat anything except one food at each meal.
   b. Continues to refuse casseroles and mixed food items.
   c. Finger foods remain popular.
3. Nursing Implications.
   a. Children should not have to be made to clean their plates. If sufficient amounts are not eaten during mealtimes, then eliminate snacks.
   b. Recognize that refusing to eat is a way to attract attention.

School age

1. Growth.
   a. Growth is slow and steady.
   b. Food intake gradually increases while energy needs per unit of body weight decline.
   c. Yearly gain of 3-5 kg. in weight and 6 cm. in height, ending with a growth spurt in puberty
2. Diet.
   a. Food intake is more varied.
   b. They enjoy most foods, with vegetables being least favorite.
3. Nursing Implications.
   a. After-school snacks are popular; encourage fruits, raw vegetable sticks, and peanut butter sandwiches.
   b. Child learns good table manners from imitating parents.
   c. Promote good health habits, (e.g., regular exercise; weight control is a balance between physical activity and food intake), routine dental check-ups for dental caries.

Adolescent

1. Growth.
   a. Rapid growth rates and maturation changes make children vulnerable to nutritional deficiencies.
   b. Girl's peak growth occurs between $10\frac{1}{4}$ and $13\frac{1}{2}$ years of age.
   c. Boy's peak growth occurs between $11\frac{3}{4}$ and $14\frac{1}{2}$ years of age. Energy needs are highest in boys between 15-18 years of age, when muscle mass is greatest.
2. Diet.
   a. Diets in general are deficient in calcium and Vitamin C.
   b. Six out of ten girls eat only 2/3 of the nutrients required. Girls tend to be deficient in iron, while boys tend to be deficient in thiamine as well.

Adult

1. Growth.
   a. Body fat as proportion to body weight age 20-80 increases 35%.
   b. Plasma volume age 20-80 decreases by 8%.
   c. Lean body mass and total body water age 20-80 decreases by 17%.
2. Diet.
   a. Energy requirements decrease with age.
   Example: 55-year-old man requires 2400 kcal; at age 76 requires only 2050 kcal.
   Example: 55-year-old woman requires 1800 kcal at age 76 only requires 1600 kcal.
   b. Improved financial status during middle adulthood increases intake of rich foods and frequency of dining out.
   c. Obesity gradually becomes a problem as a sedentary lifestyle develops.

> ***Geriatric Priority:*** *Usually it takes more time for an older person to eat and early satiety is reached. Encourage frequent small feedings, rather than 3 meals. Providing liquid supplements is beneficial.*

3. Nursing Implications.
   a. Adherence to a prudent diet pattern.
   b. Promotion and continued maintenance of a regular exercise program.
   c. Reduce sodium intake to 3-6 gm. daily.
   d. Reduce serum cholesterol level to below 200 mg/dl, with HDL level above 35mg/dl.

Older adult

1. Diet.
   a. Encourage a diet low in fat, high in fiber, iron, Vitamin C, thiamine with adequate sources of calcium.
   b. If confined to bedrest, the elderly need fluid intakes as high as 3-4 L/day to prevent kidney

Box 2-1: Elderly Care Focus
Age- Related Factors Influencing Geriatric Care

Frequent absence of social and financial support
Example: diseased spouse, inadequate income from pension

Presence of significant concurrent illness
Example: dementia, COPD, CHF, depression, diabetes

Altered pain perception
Example: increased incidence of referred pain.

Impaired homeostatic mechanisms
Example: increased problems with dehydration, incontinence, impaired defecation, altered immune status.

Impaired mobility
Example: dependent on walkers, need for bed transferring, use of transportation, may have Parkinsonism, degenerative joint disease

Increased frequency of adverse reactions to drugs

Impaired equilibrium, resulting in falls

NCLEX ALERT: *Provide care that meets the special needs of the older client.*

c. stones, providing they have no fluid restrictions, (e.g., CHF).

d. Since the older adult often has impaired renal function, *excessive* protein intake should be avoided.

2. Nursing Implications.
   a. Income is usually fixed; may have less money to spend on food.
   b. Food shopping and transportation may be a problem due to physical disability.
   c. Alteration in taste and reduced digestive function occurs.
   d. Often need to wear dentures.
   e. Constipation is a chronic problem; encourage fluids and high fiber diet.

Geriatric Priority: *The older adult may intentionally restrict fluids because of nocturia or stress incontinence.*

   f. Loneliness and depression are often associated with poor appetite.

Nutritional Assessment

A. Assess nutritional needs.

B. Client profile—age, sex, height, weight, socioeconomic status, culture.

C. Nutritional status—food habits, observe for physical signs indicative of nutritional status.

Figure 2-1: Food Pyramid

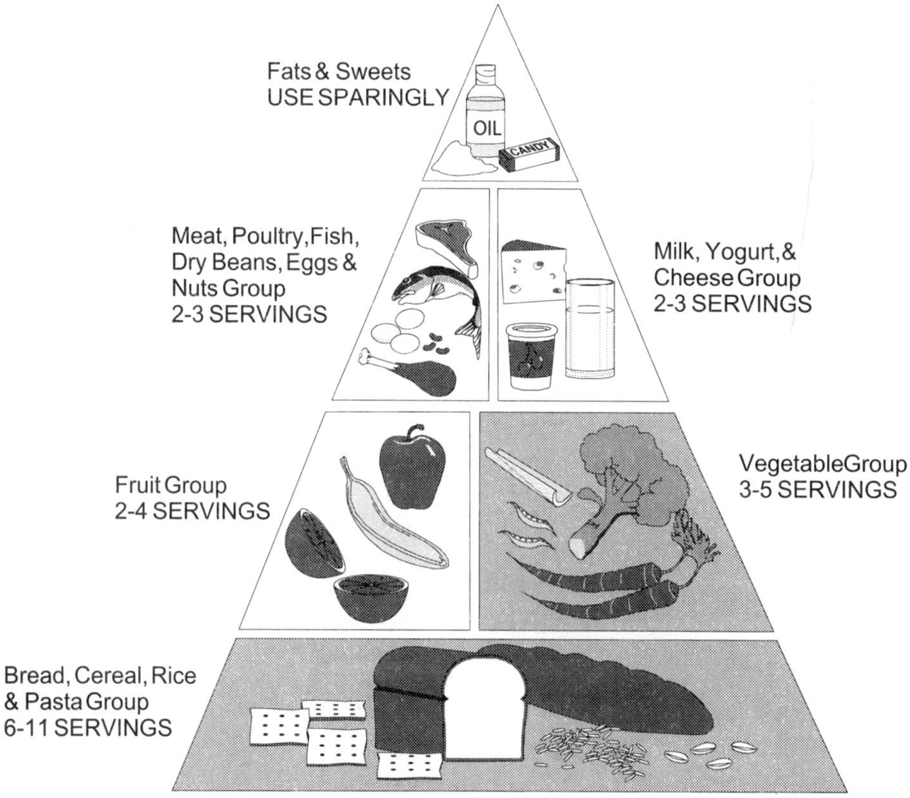

The Food Pyramid emphasizes foods from the five food groups shown in the three lower sections of the pyramid.

Each of these food groups provides some, but not all, of the nutrients you need.

Foods in one group can't replace those in another.

No one food group is more important than another - for good health, you need them all.

D. Determine disease or pathophysiologic process.

E. Be alert to high-risk patients—overweight, underweight, congenital anomalies of G.I. tract, surgery of G.I. tract, problem with ingestion, digestion, absorption, and patients on IV therapy for 10 days or more.

NCLEX ALERT: *Evaluate a client's nutritional status (e.g., diet history, laboratory work, skin turgor).*

Diet Therapy for High-Level Wellness

A. Food pyramid (See Figure 2-1).

B. Prudent diet.

1. Increased amounts of fruits, vegetables, and grains.
2. Reduced amounts of animal fats, cholesterol, refined sugar, salt, and alcohol.
3. Adaptations to the Food Pyramid.
   a. Meat—increase amounts of fish, chicken, turkey, and veal; also increase use of legumes, nuts, and seeds as a source of protein; limit egg yolks to 2 or 3 weekly, including those used in cooking.
   b. Milk—use low-fat dairy products.
   c. Fruits and Vegetables—increase total intake.
   d. Grains, Breads, and Cereals—select whole grain products and starches as source of carbohydrates.

THERAPEUTIC MEAL PLANS

❑ **A therapeutic meal plan or prescription diet is a modification of an individual's normal nutritional needs based on the pathophysiologic disease process. See Table 2-2.**

NCLEX ALERT: *Identify client's ability to eat (chew, swallow)*

CHILDHOOD DISEASES

Varicella (Chicken pox)

Characteristics

1. An acute viral disease characterized by a maculopapular rash with vesicular scabs in multiple stages of healing.
2. Incubation period: 2 to 3 weeks; usually 13 to 17 days.
3. Transmission: direct contact, airborne droplets, and contaminated objects.
4. Communicability: One day prior to lesions, and approximately 6 days after initial outbreak of lesions.

Data Collection

1. Malaise and extreme pruritus.
2. Rash appears profusely on trunk and sparse on extremities. Begins as a macule and progresses to papule, vesicle, and then crusts.
3. .All three stages usually are present in varying degrees at one time.
4. Complications: secondary infection may lead to sepsis, abscess, cellulitis, or Reye's syndrome.

Nursing Intervention

1. Preventive - varicella immunization (Table 2-3).
2. Skin care to decrease itching.
   a. Topical calamine lotion or Benadryl and/or other antihistamine.
   b. Cool baths with bactericidal soaps.
   c. Paste of baking soda on lesions.
3. Keep fingernails of child short; apply mittens to infants prn.
4. Isolate until all vesicles have crusted.
5. Avoid use of aspirin.

Parotitis (Mumps)

Characteristics

1. An acute viral disease characterized by tenderness and swelling of one or both of the parotid glands and the salivary glands.
2. Incubation period: 14 to 21 days.
3. Transmission: direct contact and droplet.
4. Communicability: one week before swelling and immediately after swelling begins.

Data Collection

1. Headache, fever, malaise.
2. Swelling of salivary glands leading to difficulty in swallowing, earache.
3. Complications:
   a. Post-infectious encephalitis.
   b. Meningoencephalitis.
   c. Orchitis, epididymitis.

Nursing Intervention

1. Preventive - mumps, measles, and rubella (MMR) immunization (Table 2-3).

Table 2-2: THERAPEUTIC MEAL PLANS

Diet	Purpose/ Use	Foods Allowed	Foods Restricted
Clear Liquid	To begin introduction of food after removal of N/G tube or after GI surgery	Liquids that are clear.	Milk products, juice with pulp, any solid food.
Full Liquid	To begin introduction of food , used after removal of N/G tube or after GI surgery	Any food that is liquid at room temperature	Any solid food
Soft Diet	To progress diet as tolerated, should be easy to chew, and swallow.	Soft, tender foods easy to swallow and digest	Highly seasoned foods, whole grains, fruits, vegetables, nuts, fried foods.
Mechanical Soft Diet	To assist clients who cannot chew effectively	Soft foods easy to chew and to swallow.	Tough foods that are difficult to swallow
Bland Diet	To eliminate foods irritating to the digestive system. Used in clients after GI surgery, peptic ulcer disease, GI inflammatory problems.	Milk, custards, refined cereals, creamed soups, potatoes (baked or broiled). All foods are white – no bright colored food.	Highly seasoned or strong flavored foods. Tea, colas, coffee, fruits, whole grains, raw fruit
Low Residue Diet	Decrease fiber or stool in GI tract. Acute episodes of enteritis, diverticulitis, diarrhea, after GI surgery	Clear liquids, meats, fats, eggs, refined cereals, white bread, peeled white potatoes, small amount milk.	Cheeses, whole grains, raw fruits and vegetables, foods that are high carbohydrate are usually high in residue and fiber.
High Residue Diet	Prevent constipation and acute diverticulitis	Raw fruits and vegetables, whole grains; high carbohydrate foods are high in residue and fiber.	Undigestible fibers – celery, whole corn; seeds such as sesame and poppy, foods with small seeds.
Lactose Free Diet	Used for lactose intolerance	Non milk products, yogurt	Milk and milk products, processed foods may have dried milk as filler.
PKU Diet	To control intake of phenylalanine, an essential acid Affected children cannot metabolize it.	Specially prepared infant formula if not breastfed. Vegetables, fruits, juices, some cereals, and breads. May allow 20-30mg phenylalanine per kg body weight to maintain normal growth needs.	Most high protein foods – meat and dairy products are significantly reduced.
Low Fat/Low Cholesterol Diet	Gall bladder spasms, increased cholesterol, or malabsorption of fat	Skimmed or low fat milk, fruits, vegetables, breads, cereals, reduced amount of red meat.	Egg yolks, whole milk, fried foods, processed cheese, shrimp, avocados.
Low Sodium Diet	Reduce sodium intake to decrease body retention of fluids. Especially in cardiac and or hypertensive clients.	Salt free preparations, fresh fruits, vegetables with no added salt.	Processed foods, smoked or salted meats, prepared foods, frozen/canned vegetables
High Potassium Diet	Clients on diuretics and/or digitalis; replaces lost potassium	Dried fruits, fruit juices, fresh fruits - bananas, apricots, grapefruit, oranges, and tomatoes	No specific restrictions
Renal Diet	Control potassium (K), sodium (Na) and protein in clients with renal problems.	High biologic protein (limited intake) – eggs, milk, meat; decreased Na products, and decreased K (cabbage, peas, cucumbers are low K).	High potassium foods, high sodium foods (processed foods), salt substitutes with high potassium
Low Purine	To decrease serum levels of uric acid. Gout, kidney stones	Vegetables, fruits, cereals, eggs, fat free milk, cottage cheese.	Glandular meats, fish poultry, nuts, beans, oatmeal, whole wheat, cauliflower.
Acid Ash Alkaline Ash	Used to prevent formation of renal stones by promoting acid urine.	Meats, cereals, eggs, corn, cranberries, prunes, plums	Fruits, vegetables, limited intake of milk.

2. Bed rest until swelling subsides.
3. Fluids and soft bland food.
4. Orchitis - warm or cold pack for relief of discomfort, light support to scrotum.
5. Hot or cold compresses to swollen neck area to decrease discomfort.

Rubeola (Measles, Hard measles, Red measles)

Characteristics

1. An acute viral disease.
2. Incubation: 10 to 21 days.
3. Transmission: respiratory droplet and direct contact with contaminated articles from infected person.
4. Communicability: 4 days before the appearance of the rash to 5 days after the rash.

Data Collection

1. Fever, malaise, and symptoms of a cold.
2. Koplik's spots - small, irregular red spots noticed on the buccal mucosa opposite the molars; usually appear two days prior to rash.
3. Maculopapular rash begins on face and gradually spreads downward.
4. Photophobia, bronchitis.
5. Complications: otitis media, pneumonia, laryngotracheitis, and encephalitis.

Nursing Intervention

1. Preventive - MMR immunization (See Table 2-3).
2. Bedrest until fever subsides.
3. Dim lights to decrease photophobia.
4. Tepid baths and lotion to relieve itching.
5. Force fluids to decrease dehydration as temperature may spike to 104°.

Table 2-3: RECOMMENDED CHILDHOOD IMMUNIZATION SCHEDULE — 2002
The shaded areas indicate the acceptable ages for the immunizations.

Vaccine	Birth	1 mos	2 mos	4 mos	6 mos	12 mos	15 mos	18 mos	4-6 yrs	11-12 yrs	14-18 yrs
Hepatitis B*	Hep B-#1	Hep B-#2			Hep B-#3						
Diphtheria, tetanus, pertussis*			DTaP	DTaP	DTaP	DTaP			DTaP	Td	
H.influenzae type b*			Hib	Hib	Hib	Hib					
Polio*			IPV	IPV	IPV				IPV		
Pneumococcal			PCV	PCV	PCV						
Measles, mumps, rubella*						MMR			MMR		
Varicella zoster virus vaccine*						Var				Var	

Source: Adapted from the Centers for Disease Control and Prevention, Advisory Committee on Immunization Practices (ACIP), Recommended childhood immunization schedule, United States, www.cdc.gov/nip/recs/child-schedule.

NCLEX ALERT: *Evaluate client's immunization status.*

6. Collect data for symptoms of complications.

Rubella (German Measles, Three-Day Measles)

Characteristics

1. An acute, mild, systemic viral disease that produces a distinctive three-day rash and lymphadenopathy.
2. Incubation: 14 to 21 days.
3. Transmission: direct contact, air droplets, and transplacentally (in congenital rubella).
4. Communicability: approximately 1 week prior to rash to about 5 days after rash began.

Data Collection

1. Low-grade fever, headache, malaise, and symptoms of a cold.
2. Rash first appears on face and spreads down to neck, arms, trunk, and then legs.
3. Diagnostics: rubella antibody titer; persistent titer of 1:8 usually indicates immunity.
4. Complications: teratogenic effect on fetus.

Nursing Intervention

1. Primarily symptomatic; bedrest until fever subsides.
2. Preventable - Immunization (Table 2-3)

Roseola Infantum (Exanthem Subitum)

Characteristics

1. A common, acute, benign viral infection usually occurring in infants and young children (ages 6 months to 3 years) which is characterized by a sudden onset of high temperature followed by a rash.
2. Incubation period: usually 5-15 days.
3. Transmission: unknown, probably airborne.
4. Communicability: unknown.

Data Collection

1. Sudden onset of high temperature (104° - 105° F).
2. As fever drops, abrupt appearance of a maculopapular, non-pruritic rash which blanches or fades under pressure.

Nursing Intervention

1. Symptomatic - tepid baths, offer fluids frequently, cool clothing.
2. Incubation period: 7 to 14 days.
3. Transmission: probably air or droplet.
4. Communicability: uncertain, symptomatic outbreaks usually subside within 1 to 2 months after onset of rash.

Fifth's Disease

Data Collection

1. A common benign viral infection which occurs without fever and is characterized by a "slapped cheek" rash appearance.
2. Incubaton period usually 4-14 days.
3. Transmission: probably respiratory.
4. Complications: self-limited arthritis and arthralgia.

Nursing Intervention

1. Primarily symptomatic treatment.
2. Child is not isolated; may attend school.

Diphtheria

Characteristics

1. An acute, highly contagious d infection caused by the *Corynebacterium diphtheriae* - resembles the common cold. Primarily affects the upper respiratory tract.
2. Incubation period: usually 2 to 6 days.
3. Transmission: air droplets or contaminated articles.
4. Communicability: greatest during mild respiratory infection prior to paroxysms of coughing.
5. Preventive - DPT immunization (see table 2-3).

Pertussis (Whopping Cough)

Characteristics

1. An acute inflammation of the respiratory tract caused by the *Bordetella pertussis*, which occurs in all ages but is most severe in children under 2 years of age.
2. Incubation period: 5 to 21 days, average is 10 days.
3. Transmission: air droplet.
4. Communicability: greatest before the onset of paroxysms of coughing.
5. Preventive - DPT immunization (See Table 2-3).

Tetanus (Lockjaw)

Characteristics

1. An acute, very serious, potentially fatal disease characterized by muscle spasms and convulsions due to the anaerobic gram-positive bacillus, *Clostridium tetani*.
2. Incubation period: generally from 4 to 20 days; however, may be as long as six weeks; average is 10 days.
3. Transmission: through a puncture wound that is contaminated by soil, dust or excreta that contains *Clostridium tetani*, or by way of burns and minor wounds, (e.g., infection of the umbilicus of a newborn).
4. Preventive.
   a. Careful cleansing and debridement of wounds.
   b. Immunization - DPT (See Table 2-3).
   c. Stress importance of maintaining active immunization with a booster dose of tetanus toxoid every 10 years.

Poliomyelitis (Polio, Infantile Paralysis)

Characteristics

1. An acute, contagious disease affecting the central nervous system.
2. Transmission: direct person-to-person contact, fecal-oral and nasopharyngeal secretions.
3. Communicability: virus in throat for one week after onset, in feces intermittently for 4-6 weeks.

Data Collection

1. Initial symptoms are similar to non-paralytic poliomyelitis with asymmetrical weakness of various muscles, loss of superficial and deep tendon reflexes.
2. Extent of paralysis depends on the level of the spinal cord motor lesion which can be either cervical, thoracic, or lumbar.
3. Complications: permanent paralysis, respiratory arrest, and kidney stones due to immobility.

Nursing Intervention

1. Preventive - inactivated polio immunization (IPVe) (See Table 2-3).
2. Complete bed rest during acute phase.
3. Maintain respiratory status.
4. Physical therapy to prevent muscle wasting.
5. Positioning to prevent contractures.

Scarlet Fever (Scarlatina)

Characteristics

1. Group A *beta-hemolytic* streptococcal infection that occurs most commonly in children ages 2 to 10; often follows acute streptopharyngitis, impetigo, or even a superficial wound infection.
2. Incubation period: range of 1 to 7 days.
3. Transmission: direct person-to-person contact with oral, nasal or contaminated articles.
4. Communicability: 10 days or the course of the clinical illness.

Data Collection

1. Sudden onset of fever - 103° F.
2. Sore throat, nausea, vomiting, and strawberry tongue.
3. Diffuse, fine erythematous rash that blanches on pressure and resembles a sunburn with goosebumps.
4. Desquamation of the skin usually begins by the end of the first week.
5. Diagnostics: history of a recent streptococcal infection, positive antistreptolysin O (ASO titer), and a positive throat culture of group A *beta-hemolytic* streptococci.
6. Complications: otitis media, rheumatic fever, and glomerulonephritis.

Nursing Intervention

1. Respiratory isolation, until 24 hours after antibiotics are started.
2. Administration of a full course of penicillin (or erythromycin in penicillin-sensitive children).
3. Administration of antipyretics to control fever and anesthetic throat sprays or gargles to relieve sore throat.
4. Encourage fluids to prevent dehydration during febrile phase.

Infectious Mononucleosis (Kissing Disease)

Characteristics

1. An acute, self-limiting infectious disease caused by the Epstein-Barr virus (EBV); member of the herpes group viruses, occurring most often among young persons between the ages of 12 and 25 years of age.
2. Incubation period: 2 to 6 weeks.

3. Transmission: direct intimate contact; probably oralpharyngeal route.
4. Communicability: unknown.

Data Collection

1. Onset of symptoms occurs any time 10 days to 6 weeks following exposure - may be acute or insidious.
2. Malaise, sore throat, fever with generalized lymphadenopathy.
3. Diagnostic: Increase in WBC, positive mono spot test.
4. Complications: hepatic involvement, otitis media, in severe cases may have cardiac and neurologic involvement.

Nursing Intervention

1. Encourage rest and provide comfort measures to alleviate symptoms of sore throat and fever.
2. Provide adequate nutrition - soft foods and plenty of fluids.
3. Penicillin is prescribed for the sore throat to prevent secondary beta-hemolytic strep infections.

CANCER

Characteristics of Cancer

❑ **Cancer must be regarded as a group of disease entities with different causes, manifestations, treatment, and prognoses. The basic disease process begins when normal cells undergo change and begin to reproduce in an abnormal manner.**

Major Dysfunction in the Cell

A. Cellular proliferation - cancer cells divide in an indiscriminate, unregulated manner.

B. There is a loss of contact inhibition. The cells have no regard for cellular boundaries; normal cells respect boundaries and do not invade adjacent areas or organs.

C. Tumors (neoplasm).

1. Benign - encapsulated neoplasm that remains localized in the tissue of origin.
   a. Exerts pressure on surrounding organs.
   b. Will decrease blood supply to the normal tissue.
2. Malignant - non-encapsulated neoplasm that invades surrounding tissue. Depends on the stage of the neoplasm as to whether or not metastasis or spread to distant body parts has occurred. There are four primary mechanisms by which the metastasis spreads.

Table 2-4: CANCER'S EARLY WARNING SIGNS

ADULTS

C Change in bowel or bladder habits.
A A lesion or sore that does not heal.
U Unusual bleeding or discharge.
T Thickening or difficulty swallowing.
I Indigestion or difficulty swallowing.
O Obvious changes in wart or mole.
N Nagging cough or persistent hoarseness.
(Note that the first letter of each sign spells "**CAUTION**").

CHILDREN

1. Marked changes in bowel and bladder; nausea and vomiting for no apparent cause.
2. Generally run-down condition; increased susceptibility to infection.
3. Spontaneous bleeding episode (epistaxis); failure to stop bleeding in normal time period.
4. Swellings, lumps or masses anywhere in the child's body.
5. Persistent crying or pain for which there is no apparent cause.
6. Any change in size of mole or birthmark.
7. Unexpected stumbling or lack of coordination in the child.

Source: American Cancer Society, *Cancer Facts and Figures*, (New York: American Cancer Society, 1992).

   a. Vascular system - cancer cells penetrate vessels and circulate until trapped. The cancer cells may penetrate the vessel wall and invade adjacent organs and tissues.
   b. Lymphatic system - cancer cells penetrate the lymphatic system and are distributed along lymphatic channels.
   c. Implantation - cancer cells implant into a body organ. Certain cells have an affinity for particular organs and body areas.
   d. Seeding - a primary tumor sloughs off tumor cells into a body cavity, such as the peritoneal cavity.

Early Detection

A. Identify client with increased risk factors.

1. Familial - the tendency of some lesions to follow familial characteristics.
2. Environmental - individuals working in asbestos and chemical plants.
3. Smoking - statistics indicate individuals who smoke have a significant increase in the development of cancer of the upper airway, mouth and lungs.
4. Radiation.
   a. Exposure to ultraviolet (sun) rays increases risk of skin cancer.
   b. Exposure to ionizing radiation .

c. Increased risk of a child developing cancer if exposed to x-ray during fetal life.

5. Hormones - use of estrogens during pregnancy and in postmenopausal syndrome.

B. Cancer's early warning signs (Table 2-4).

Treatment of Cancer

Diagnostics

A. Common cancer diagnostic studies.

1. X-ray.
2. Computerized axial tomography (CAT).
3. Magnetic resonance imaging (MRI).
4. Cytology (cell) studies.
5. Radioisotope scans.
6. Positron emission tomography (PET).

B. Biopsy.

1. Needle - tissues obtained by aspiration, or with a large bore needle; a sample is removed.
2. Incisional - tumor mass may be too large for removal; this may be done for staging the disease level.
3. Excisional - involves removal of the entire tumor.
4. Endoscope biopsy - direct biopsy through an endoscopy of the area (gastrointestinal, respiratory, genitourinary tracts).

Goals of Cancer Therapy

A. Cure - client will be disease-free and live to normal expectancy.

B. Control - client's cancer is not cured but controlled by therapy over long periods of time.

C. Palliative - maintain as high a quality of life for the client when cure and control are not possible.

D. Prophylaxis - provide treatment when no tumor is detectable but when client is known to be at risk for tumor development, spread, or recurrence.

Modalities of Cancer Treatment

A. Surgery — excision of the tumor, or extensive resection of tumor and surrounding tissue.

1. Evaluate any adverse effects of previous treatment and their implications for proposed surgery, (e.g., poor nutritional status or fibrosis from effects of radiation therapy which may lead to poor wound healing, leukopenia from chemo-therapeutic agents.)
2. Evaluate extent of disfigurement or debilitation caused by surgery and consider its impact on client (e.g., ostomy formation, amputation.)
3. Promote healthful self-image and return to normal lifestyle by recommending cancer support groups and other rehabilitation resources.

B. Chemotherapy - overall goal of chemotherapy is to attack the cancer cell during its most vulnerable stage.

1. Chemotherapy agents are administered in doses large enough to damage or kill cancer cells, but small enough to limit adverse effects to safe and tolerable levels.
2. Nursing implications in chemotherapy (Table 2-6).

a. Collect data on client for symptoms of bone marrow depression (increased bruising and bleeding, sore throat, fever).

b. Prevent exposure of client to people with communicable diseases.

c. Prior to therapy, establish a baseline regarding intake and output, bowel habits, oral hygiene, psychological status, and family relationships.

d. Monitor fluid intake and output; maintain adequate hydration to prevent urinary complications.

e. Client education.

(1) Client should avoid all OTC medications while on chemotherapy.

(2) If treated on an out-patient basis, client should not alternate dosages and should maintain schedule of administration.

NCLEX ALERT: *Follow procedures when handling biohazardous materials (sharps, radioactive materials, etc.).*

Table 2-5: RADIATION SAFETY PRECAUTIONS - Internal Source

- Private room and bath.
- Plan care so minimal time is spent in the room.
- When prolonged care is required, wear a lead shield or apron.
- Wear a monitoring device to measure exposure.
- Mark on the room and in the kardex that pregnant women, infants, and young children should not come in contact with the client during treatment.
- Check all linens and materials removed from the bed for presence of foreign bodies that could be a source of radioactivity.
- Keep long handled forceps and lead container in the room of a client with an implant in place.

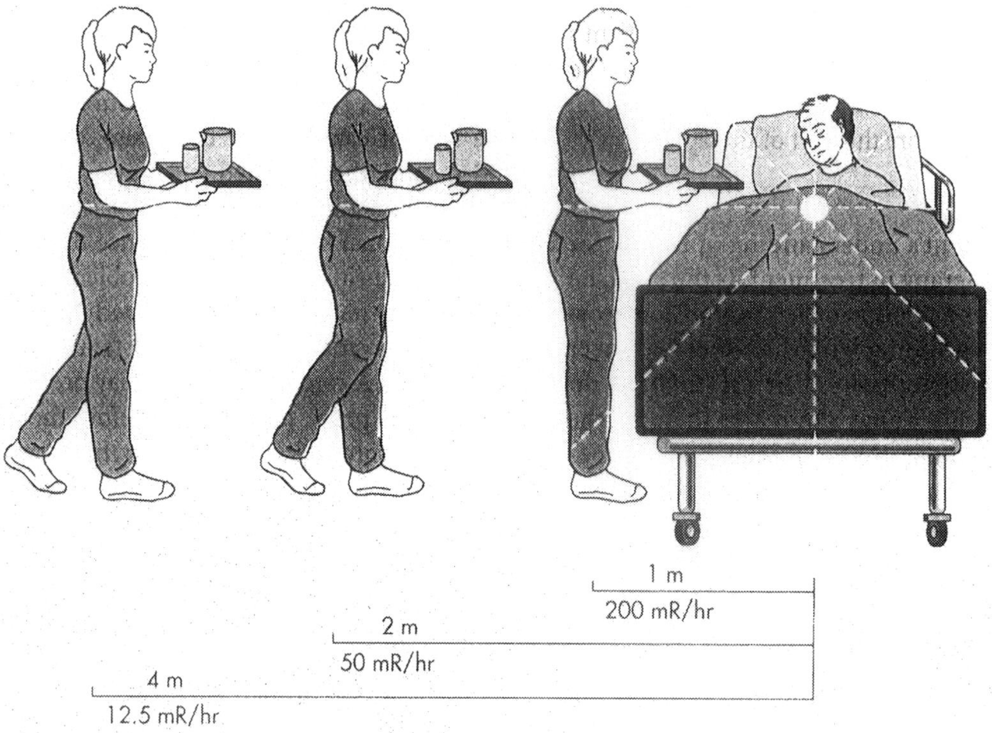

Figure 2-2: Radiation Safety
The nurse nearest the source of radioactivity (the client) is more exposed. at two feet, exposure is 15 times that at eight feet.
Reprinted with permission: Phipps, WJ, Sands, JK, & Marek, JF, (1999). *Medical Surgical Nursing: Concepts & Clinical Practice*, 6th ed. Philadelphia: Mosby, p. 291.

C. Radiation therapy.

1. The purpose of radiation therapy is to destroy the rapidly dividing cancer cells. Cells that are reproducing rapidly are more sensitive to the radiation.

***NURSING PRIORITY:** Adverse effects are related to radiation dose delivered within a specified time, method of delivery, and client's overall health status.*

2. Prevent excessive exposure (Figure 2-2).
   a. Time - client care should be coordinated to allow greatest amount of care to be given in shortest time framework possible.
   b. Distance - except when giving direct care, attempt to maintain distance of six feet from the source of radiation.
   c. Shield - some institutions provide lead shielding; generally not necessary if time and distance principles are observed.
3. Common side effects of radiation therapy.
   a. Gastrointestinal disturbances.
      (1) Nausea and vomiting.
      (2) Anorexia.
      (3) Diarrhea and constipation.
      (4) Stomatitis.
   b. Blood dyscrasias.
      (1) Anemia.
      (2) Leukemia.
      (3) Thrombocytopenia.

NCLEX ALERT: Observefor side effects of radiation therapy.

4. Nursing implications for a client with an internal radiation source (implant, or sealed source).
   a. Private room and bath.
   b. A lead container and tongs should be present in the client's room.
   c. If implant becomes dislodged, it should be picked up with the forceps and returned to the lead container. Notify radiation therapist or officer immediately.
   d. Observe time, distance, and shield precautions.
   e. Examples of this type of radiation therapy include uterine implants, testicular implants, implants used in head and neck tumors.
   f. Inform all people coming in contact with the client of the specific precautions necessary.

Table 2-6: Nursing Implications And Chemotherapy

PROBLEM	NURSING IMPLICATIONS
Bone marrow depression: Increased bleeding, anemia, decreased resistance to infection (leukopenia)	1. Observe for bleeding tendency (bruising, hematuria, bleeding gums, etc.). 2. Report any unexplained temperature elevation. 3. No active vaccinations while on medication. 4. Report any unusual fatigue. 5. Decrease invasive procedures, minimize injections.
Hyperuricemia (increased serum levels of uric acid)	1. Encourage fluid intake up to 3,000 cc daily if allowed. 2. Assess for flank and abdominal pain. 3. Assess for swelling of the lower extremities and joint pain. 4. May be treated with allopurinol.
Alopecia	1. Encourage client to obtain a wig after beginning of symptoms. 2. Ice packs to the scalp may reduce hair loss. 3. A scalp tourniquet during medication infusion may also reduce hair loss.
Stomatitis (mucositis)	1. Good oral hygiene. a. Frequent mouth rinse to keep mucous membranes moist. b. Brush teeth with a small, soft toothbrush. 2. Avoid alcohol, spicy or hot foods.
GI: anorexia, nausea, vomiting, diarrhea, and constipation	1. Assist client to maintain good nutrition. a. Discuss food preferences with client and dietician. b. Correlate meals with antiemetic medications. c. Treat stomatitis with anesthetic mouthwashes to decrease discomfort while eating. 2. Evaluate client for fluid and electrolyte imbalances. 3. Evaluate skin around anal area in the client with diarrhea; prevent excoriation. 4. Identify clients prone to constipation and maintain high fluid and high fiber intake. 5. Observe for occurrence of paralytic ileus. 6. May need to withhold food and fluid 4 to 6 hours before treatment. 7. Small feedings and high fluid intake.
Tissue irritation, necrosis, ulceration	1. The health care professional preparing the chemotherapy solution should avoid all skin contact with the solution. Gloves should be worn when mixing the preparation. 2. Extra precaution should be taken to prevent extravasation (infusion of chemotherapy medication into subcutaneous tissue). *If extravasation occurs notify RN, (a)anticipate stopping the infusion, (b) do not remove the needle.*

NCLEX ALERT: *Observe client for side effects of chemotherapy or radiation therapy.*

g. Utilize badges or radiation monitors for caregivers having direct client contact.

h. List on the chart.

(1) Type of radiation.

(2) Time inserted.

(3) Anticipated removal time.

(4) Specific precautions for the type radiation utilized.

NURSING PRIORITY: *Check linens, bedpans, and other items for signs of a dislodged implant. Move client away from implant and use tongs to place it in a protective safety lead container, which should be in the client's room. Notify radiation therapy department.*

5. Nursing implications for the client receiving systemic radiation therapy.

a. Systemically administered radionuclides (radioisotopes) may cause radioactive body secretions. Wear gloves when handling client's bodily secretions.

b. May be necessary to have the linens and trash checked for radioactivity prior to removing them from the room.

Nursing Intervention

✦ *Goal: to maintain client at optimum psychosocial level.*

1. Encourage verbalization.
2. Assist client to understand disease process and therapeutic regime.
3. Include family in the care.
4. Assist client to cope with changes in body image due to hair loss.

a. Encourage to select and wear a wig or turban.
b. Instruct client with regards to hair care.
(1) Use mild protein-based shampoo and cream conditioner to help prevent hair dryness.
(2) Advise client to shampoo only every 3 to 5 days.
(3) Teach client to pat, *not rub*, hair dry after shampooing to avoid excessive handling of brittle hair.
(4) Encourage client to avoid excessive brushing to prevent tearing or unnecessary manipulation of hair.
(5) Suggest client sleep on a satin pillowcase to decrease hair tangles and friction.
(6) Encourage client to discontinue use of electric hair dryers, hot rollers or crimpers, hair clips, sprays, dyes, or permanents to prevent further hair damage.
c. Prevent or minimize hair loss by applying cold packs to scalp.
5. Recognize client's emotional outbursts and anger as part of his coping process.
6. Encourage measures to maintain ego.
a. Allow him to participate in his own care and make decisions.
b. Maintain active listening.
c. Encourage personal lifestyle (clothing, makeup, hobbies, etc.).

NCLEX ALERT: *Implement measures to protect the immunocompormised client.*

✦ *Goal: to maintain nutrition.*
1. Diet - appropriate to age level.
a. Increase calories, increase protein.
b. Supplemental vitamins.
c. Small frequent feedings.
d. Increase fluid intake.
e. Between meal supplements.
2. Hyperalimentation (See Chapter 13).
3. Prevent and/or decrease complications associated with nutrition.
a. Anorexia.
b. Nausea and vomiting.
c. Stomatitis.
(1) Good oral hygiene after each meal and at bedtime.
(2) Observe oral mucosa daily.
(3) Provide nonirritating foods.
(4) Keep mucous membranes moist; encourage fluid intake to prevent dehydration.

✦ *Goal: to maintain normal elimination pattern.*
1. Provide adequate fluids and fiber in diet to prevent constipation.
2. Prevent and/or decrease complications of diarrhea.
a. Antidiarrheal medications.
b. Low residue, high protein, bland diet.
c. Evaluate fluid status.
d. Prevent anal irritation.
(1) Thorough cleansing of rectal area with mild soap and water.
(2) Avoid irritation of the rectal area.
(3) Use ointments and sprays to decrease discomfort and promote healing.
3. Prevent urinary tract infections, primarily cystitis.
a. Maintain adequate fluid intake—3000cc/day.
b. Frequent assessment for symptoms of cystitis (See Chapter 18).
c. Avoid bladder catheterization if possible.
4. Minimize embarrassment of incontinence and provide appropriate hygiene measures.

✦ *Goal: to prevent and/or decrease infectious process.*
1. Careful assessment of all temperature elevations.
2. Administer antibiotics.
3. Good personal hygiene.
4. Child should be isolated from communicable diseases, especially chicken pox.
5. Frequent assessment for potential infectious processes.
6. Do not clean bird cages or cat litter boxes.
7. Thoroughly wash fruit and vegetables or peel them.

✦ *Goal: to prevent and/or decrease hematological complications (See Chapter 9).*
1. Observe for bleeding problems associated with bone marrow depression.
a. Increased bruising.
b. Bleeding gums.
c. Hematuria.
d. Anemia (↓ hemoglobin).
e. Nosebleed (epistaxis).
f. Presence of blood in the stool.

NURSING PRIORITY: *Advise client to use electric razor and a soft-bristle toothbrush, and avoid dental flossing.*

2. Anemia.
   a. Maintain adequate rest, encourage client to pace activities to avoid fatigue.
   b. Assess respiratory and cardiac systems and report changes to RN.
   c. Encourage a diet high in protein, vitamins, and iron.

✦ *Goal: to maintain activity level.*

1. Encourage daily activities appropriate to developmental level.
2. Assist client to evaluate activity patterns and encourage periods of rest.
3. Avoid fatigue.

✦ *Goal: to relieve pain (See Chapter 3).*

1. Evaluate client's and family's response to pain.
2. Evaluate characteristics of pain.
3. Promote general comfort.
4. Administer medications for pain relief.

✦ *Goal: to recognize complications specific to radiation and chemotherapy. (Table 2-6)*

1. Alopecia.
2. Hemorrhagic problems.
3. Gastrointestinal distress.
4. Bone marrow depression (myelosuppression).
5. Skin reactions.
6. Decreased immune response.

Study Questions—Health Implications

1. The nurse finds the client's radiation implant in the bed. What is the best nursing action?

① using tongs, replace it in the lead container in the room.
② immediately evacuate the client and all others from the room.
③ wearing gloves, replace the implant into the body cavity.
④ call radiation control to come pick up the implant.

2. What immunizations will be given to the infant within the first 6 months?

① varicella, diphtheria, polio, and hepatitis-B
② diphtheria, pertussis, tetanus, hepatitis-B, polio.
③ polio, measles, mumps, rubella, diphtheria, tetanus.
④ varicella, measles, mumps, rubella, diphtheria.

3. The mother of a newborn asks when she can begin to give her infant some fruits. What is the best nursing care?

① Begin cereals at 3 months, then begin fruits at 6 months.
② start fruits as the first solids at 6 months, then vegetables.
③ fruits can be started at 3 months, followed by cereal.
④ cereals are started at 6 months, followed by fruit.

4. The mother brings her 9 month old infant in for a well baby check. What observation would cause the most concern?

① cannot sit alone without support.
② shows no interest in walking.
③ anterior fontanel remains open.
④ does not respond to name.

5. What is the treatment of a malignant disease process by a chemical medication called?

① chemotherapy.
② antibiotic therapy.
③ immunotherapy.
④ palliative therapy.

6. The nurse understands that the following is an example of palliative surgery for cancer?

① gastrostomy.
② colectomy.
③ nephrectomy.
④ craniotomy.

7. What are the major side effects of antineoplastic drugs?

① tachycardia and orthostatic hypotension.
② electrolyte and mineral imbalance.
③ nausea and bone marrow suppression.
④ constipation and stomach cramping.

8. What is important to teach a client regarding self-care during radiation therapy?

① remove the skin dye tattoos between treatments.
② avoid exposure to sun and do not remove the skin dye markings.
③ reduce carbohydrates and protein intake during treatments.
④ decrease fluids and increase carbohydrate intake after treatments.

9. A client on antineoplastic therapy is experiencing nausea and vomiting. What is the best nursing action?

① give antiemetics and check for dehydration.
② administer oral care and assess for mouth lesions.
③ decrease fluid intake and moisten dry food.
④ record daily weights and encourage small meals.

10. At what age does a child begin to discriminate between the mother's face and a stranger's face?

① one month.
② six weeks.
③ four months.
④ thirty weeks.

11. What is true regarding the beginning of physiological development that occurs during puberty ?

① two years earlier for girls.
② one year earlier for boys.
③ four years earlier in girls.
④ three years earlier in boys.

12. What is characteristic of the developmental socialization in an adolescent?

① is not attracted to peer groups, prefers time alone.
② spends more time with siblings than peers.
③ prefers to spend all their time with the members of their immediate family.
④ uses their peer group as a standard against which to compare themselves.

13. A client is receiving chemotherapy for lung cancer. The nurse understands that the medication can cause renal damage. What is an important nursing action?

① encourage fluids to increase acidity of urine.
② monitor daily weight, intake and output.
③ decrease fluids to reduce edema formation.
④ monitor the urinalysis for level of bacteria.

14. A client is on furosemide (Lasix) for treatment of his heart condition. What foods should he be encouraged to eat?

① breads and fortified cereals.
② dried fruits and juices.
③ leafy green vegetables.
④ lean red meat and whole grains.

15. The DPT immunization for infants should start at what age?

① four months.
② three months.
③ two months.
④ one month.

16. At what age is the MMR vaccination recommended to be started?

① at birth
② 1 month
③ 6 months
④ 12 months

17. Chickenpox (varicella) is characterized by which symptoms?

① vesicles that rupture with clear fluid.
② erythematous, fine macular rash on the trunk.
③ pustules that are filled with pus.
④ papules that are confined to the face and trunk.

18. A client comes to the emergency room with a penetrating wound he received while working in the forest clearing lumber. What is the best initial nursing response to this client?

① cleanse the wound with antibiotic solution.
② administer gamma globulin intramuscularly.
③ anticipate notifying poison control for plant toxicology.
④ determine when client received last tetanus injection.

19. Which foods would be limited on a low-cholesterol diet?

① eggs.
② skim milk.
③ apples.
④ carrots.

20. What food would be added to a diet to increase protein and not fat in the diet?

① eggs.
② nonfat milk.
③ cereal.
④ carrots.

Nursing Concepts

BASIC HUMAN NEEDS

A. Maslow's Hierarchy of Basic Human Needs.
  1. Human behavior is motivated by a system of needs.
  2. Client will focus or attempt to satisfy needs at the base of the pyramid before focusing on those higher up (Figure 3-1).

B. Characteristics of human needs.
  1. Human needs are *universal*, however, some may be modified by cultural influence.
  2. Human needs may be altered by individual priorities.
  3. Human needs may be deferred.
  4. Human needs may be met in different ways.
  5. Human needs are interrelated.
  6. Human needs are aroused by stimuli that are either external or internal to the body.
  7. When a human need is not satisfied, it results in the disruption of normal body activities and frequently leads to illness.

NCLEX ALERT: *Maslow's Hierarchy is very useful in answering test questions related to setting priorities. Always remember the physiological needs at the base of the pyramid must be satisfied in order to focus on other needs and that* ***oxygenation is always first priority.***

STEPS OF THE NURSING PROCESS

The categories of the nursing process and the activities in each category vary somewhat according to nursing authors. The nursing process as presented here correlates with the categories of the NCLEX-P.N.

Data Collection

A. Collecting data.
  1. Objective data are nursing observations.
    - Example: Client weighs 125 pounds; 50 cc. of green drainage via the nasogastric tube.
  2. Subjective data is information given by the client.
    - Example: "My side hurts; I am scared about surgery."
  3. Client data is collected utilizing three skills.
    a. **Observation** - what can be seen.
    - Example: Is the client awake or asleep; is the client obese or underweight; is the client smiling or frowning?

    b. **Auscultation** - what can be heard.
    - Example: Is the client laughing; are there breath sounds present; do you hear hyperactive bowel sounds?

    c. **Palpation** - what can be felt.
    - Example: Is the client's skin warm and dry; does the client have a pedal pulse; is the client's abdomen soft?

Planning

A. Assign priority to the nursing care activities.

B. Specify goals reflecting desired outcome of nursing care.
  1. Develop short-term and long-term goals.
  2. Identify nursing interventions for goal attainment.
  3. Establish outcome criteria.

C. Develop the written nursing care plan.
  1. Involve client and family in all aspects of planning.
  2. Keep care plan current and flexible.

Implementing

A. Initiate and carry out planned nursing activities.

B. Coordinate activities of client and family members along with health team members.

C. Record and document client's responses to nursing actions.

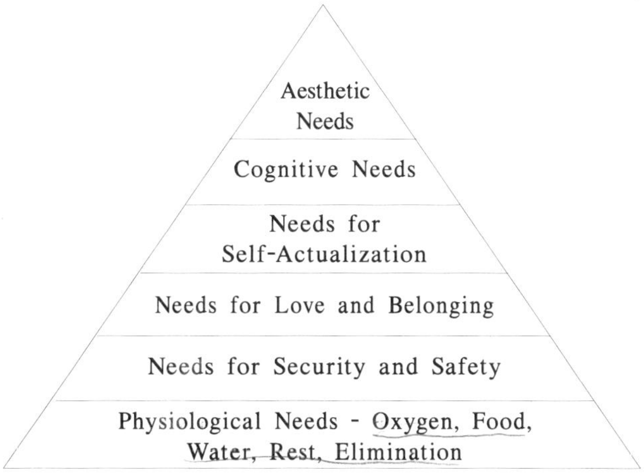

Figure 3-1: Maslow's Hierarchy of Needs

Evaluating

A. Collect objective data and determine if goals were achieved.

B. Identify and make revisions to the nursing care plan.

HEALTH ASSESSMENT

Subjective Health Assessment

Health History

The health history is a primary source of client information. The source of the information can be the client, relatives, friends, old records, or any combination of these. A predetermined format should be used as a guide for the interview.

NCLEX ALERT: *Collect a health history, or risk assessment (e.g., life style, family history, etc.)*

A. Demographic data.
 1. Name, address, phone, age, sex, marital status.
 2. Race, religion, usual source of medical care.

B. Chief Complaint/reason for visit.
 1. Chief complaint (CC) is main reason client sought health care.
 2. CC is recorded in client's own words.
 - *Example*: "I have been vomiting blood since this morning."

C. History of the present illness.
 1. Chronologic narrative story of the history of the present state of health.
 2. Includes relevant family history.

D. Past History.
 1. Childhood diseases.
 2. Immunizations.
 3. Allergies.
 4. Hospitalizations and serious illnesses.
 5. Accidents and injuries.
 6. Medications.
 7. Prenatal, labor and delivery, or neonatal history (recorded for all children under age of 5 and older children with a congenital or developmental problem).

E. Review of Systems (ROS).
 1. Is a verbal rundown from head to toe of the client's overall state of health.
 2. Contains subjective data given by the client; *does not* contain information from the physical examination.
 - Specific assessment data for each body system can be found at the beginning of each chapter.

NCLEX ALERT: *Collect baseline physical data (e.g., admission data, vital signs, etc.)*

HEALTH PROMOTION

Levels of prevention

❑ **Preventive health care is more dynamic than health maintenance. Focuses on health enhancement and health promotion, whereas health maintenance is concerned with maintaining the status quo.**

A. Primary—prevention of disease
 1. Goal is to achieve maximum functioning in each health potential area.
 - *Examples:* Stop smoking, practice safe sex, maintain body weight, limit alcohol intake, follow a regular exercise program, and healthy diet.

B. Secondary—early diagnosis and treatment.
 1. Emphasis is determining intervention priorities.
 - *Examples:* Screening for tuberculosis, yearly glaucoma, pap smear, self-breast examination and self- testicular examination.

C. Tertiary—prevention of complications.
 1. Focus is on the prevention and rehabilitation after the disease or condition has already occurred.
 - *Examples:* Have CBC drawn before chemotherapy, speech therapy after a CVA, cardiac rehabilitation.

NCLEX ALERT: *Determine client's understanding of lifestyle choices and disease prevention n (smoking, diet, etc.)*

Nursing Intervention

1. Providing health education programs.
2. Enhancing behavior change.
 a. Encourage motivation by identifying client's needs.
 b. Focus on factors which motivate client.
 c. Realize resistance is a healthy, normal response to threat and change.

3. Role modeling (the nurse) healthy lifestyle choices.

HEALTH TEACHING

Principles of Client Education

A. Common characteristics of the adult learner.

NURSING PRIORITY: *The first step in the education process is to determine what the client already knows.*

1. The adult client's background of experience, skills, and attitudes will form the base for any new information received. Frequently, the client has had no positive experiences in a hospital environment.
2. The level of adult development will greatly affect his readiness to learn. If a client is in a mid-life transition, it may be very difficult for him to learn new attitudes and skills which threaten his self image.
   - *Example:* a man in his early 40s may have difficulty accepting any education regarding his colostomy.

A. Factors contributing to the teaching-learning process.

1. Readiness to learn.
   a. The client must feel the material is relevant to his health, and he must be willing to put forth the effort to learn.
   b. The client must have the mental capacity to learn, as well as the physical ability to perform the skills.
   c. The client must have his physical and safety needs met before he can focus on learning. If a client exerts all of his energy to cope with the physical stress, then he has little energy for learning.
   d. Comfort.
      (1) Physical comfort-discomforts (such as pain, nausea, hunger, need to void) are distracters to the learning process.
      (2) Psychological comfort-anger, frustrations, fear, and guilt severely hamper the learning process.
   e. Before the teaching-learning process can begin, the client and the nurse need to discuss and agree on specific long-term and short-term goals. The nurse must carefully evaluate the client's knowledge of the problem.

B. Factors relating to the presentation.

1. State the specific objective of each teaching session: exactly what the client is to gain.
2. Use vocabulary and terminology appropriate to client's understanding and to his or her developmental level. Utilize correct terms for body parts.
3. Try to stimulate as many senses as possible. Utilize charts, handouts, and pieces of equipment when appropriate.
4. Repetition is an integral part of learning. Be ready to repeat the material, or to have the client repeat the skill until he does it correctly and becomes comfortable with the skill.
5. The more active the client is in the process; the better he/she will retain the information.
6. Plan short sessions; do not overwhelm the client with too much information at one time.
7. When appropriate, actively involve the family and significant others.
8. Be generous with positive reinforcement.

NCLEX ALERT*: Instruct client about healthy behaviors, health risks and health promotion (exercise, risky behaviors, breast/testicular exams, etc.)*

C. Pediatric factors influencing the learning process.

1. Intellectual development moves from the concrete to the abstract.
2. The nurse needs to assess the developmental level of the child before planning the educational approach.

NURSING PRIORITY: *A typical "No" response from a toddler when being taught a new activity (e.g., combing hair) is usually an assertion of their independence, not that they will not learn.*

   a. Preschooler.
      (1) Preschool children frequently experience fears of body injury. Explanations should be simple.
      (2) Separation anxiety is a problem at this age range; include parents in teaching session.
      (3) Preschool children are aware of the physical and mechanical causes of problems they can see; they are unaware of physical and mechanical forces they cannot see.

NURSING PRIORITY: *It is important to emphasize to the preschooler that treatment is not punishment.*

b. School age.
(1) Benefit from tours, drawings, anatomical dolls.
(2) Learn well from role playing and puppets.
(3) Need to include parents in teaching session for reinforcement and to maintain consistency.

c. Adolescent.
(1) Needs to be as independent as possible in management of health problem.
(2) Needs assistance in coping with loss of independence and self-direction.
(3) Educational programs need to help him or her deal with changes in body image and in maintaining ego.

D. Geriatric clients.

Geriatric Priority: *Elderly clients tend to be solitary learners and consideration of ill health and sensory deficits needs to occur (e.g., large type books for reading).*

1. Determine their functional losses (i.e., hearing or vision impairment, memory loss).
2. Identify social support to aid the older adult; this often increases compliance with information being taught.
3. Determine hearing and visual acuity and make adjustments to leaning process.
4. Determine if the client is experiencing any confusion or disorientation. Ask client to include family member in teaching activity.

BASIC NURSING SKILLS

Hygienic Nursing Measures

A. Beds and comfort measures.
1. Avoid shaking linens or tossing them into the hamper.
2. Hold all soiled linens away from your uniform.
3. Mattresses.
a. Alternating pressure mattress.
(1) Provides a continuous shift of pressure by alternating inflation and deflation of air or water every two to five minutes.
(2) Used to prevent development of or to treat pressure sores.
b. Eggcrate mattress.
(1) Foam rubber mattress with projections that look like an eggcrate.
(2) Placed on top of a regular mattress.
(3) Used to prevent pressure areas from developing in a bedfast client.

NCLEX ALERT: *Assist in performance of activities of daily living.*

B. Bathing.
1. Types of bath.
a. Bed bath.
b. Partial bath.
c. Shower.
d. Therapeutic bath — sitz bath or medicated bath.
2. Nursing implications.
a. Room should be kept warm.
b. To prevent dry skin, irritation, and infection, carefully rinse all surface areas and dry them.
c. Keep client warm by using a bath blanket and controlling room temperature.
d. Ensure quiet and privacy.
e. Moisturize skin with lotion.

NURSING PRIORITY: *Clients who receive radiation treatment should not be bathed with soap over the radiation site, which will be marked with ink. Lotions and powder should not be used.*

3. Levels of personal care.
a. Complete care — client requires total assistance from nurse because client is able to do little or nothing without assistance.
b. Partial care — client performs as much of his or her own care as possible, nurse usually completes remaining care.
c. PM care (HS care or hour of sleep care) — provided to prepare client for a relaxing, uninterrupted period of sleep; includes oral care, possible partial bathing, skin care, soothing back massage, straightening or changing the bed linen, and offering the bedpan or urinal.

C. Oral hygiene.
1. Includes care of the client's teeth or dentures, gums, tongue, and lips.
2. When providing oral care to unconscious client, turn the client's head to the side to prevent aspiration.

D. Hair care.
1. Newborn infants need scalp scrubbed daily to prevent cradle cap.

2. Adolescents usually require more frequent shampooing due to increase in oily secretions.
3. Geriatric clients will need to shampoo less often.

Body Alignment and Range of Motion

A. Characteristics of correct body alignment in bed.
  1. Head up with eyes looking straight forward.
  2. Neck and back straight.
  3. Arms relaxed and supported at sides.
  4. Legs parallel to hips with knees slightly flexed.
  5. Feet separated and parallel to the legs with the toes pointed upward and slightly outward.

B. Range of motion (ROM)
  1. Active ROM
    a. Client performs exercise without assistance.
    b. Used for client who independently performs activities of daily living (ADLs), but for some reason is immobilized or limited regarding activity.
    c. Muscle strengthening is the goal.
  2. Passive ROM
    a. Client can not actively move.
    b. Cannot contract muscles, therefore muscle strengthening *cannot* be accomplished.
    c. Goal is joint flexibility.

C. Principles of ROM exercises.
  1. Stretch muscles by moving the body part; avoid movement to the point of discomfort.
  2. Perform ROM at least twice daily on immobile clients, with a minimum of 4-5 repetitions of each exercise.
  3. Always support extremity above and below the joint when doing passive ROM on extremities.
  4. Involve the client in planning their exercise program.

NCLEX ALERT: *Implement prescribed measures to maintain a client's range of motion (ambulation, passive or active exercise, etc.)*

Asepsis

NCLEX ALERT: *Use aseptic/sterile technique when handling equipment or supplies.*

A. Medical asepsis.
  1. Designed to reduce the number of pathogens in an area and decrease the likelihood of their transfer (e.g., hand washing).
  2. Often referred to as *clean technique.*
  3. Administration of oral medications, enemas, tube feedings, daily hygiene practices are all carried out with clean technique.

***NURSING PRIORITY:** Proper hand washing is one of the most important procedures for preventing transfer of micro-organisms. Be aware it is frequently the first step in nursing procedures.*

B. Surgical asepsis.
  1. Designed to *not* just simply reduce the number of pathogens but to make the object free of all micro-organisms.
  2. Also known as *sterile technique.*
  3. Surgical asepsis is reserved primarily for sterile dressing changes, performing sterile catheterizations, and surgical procedures in the operating room (Table 3-1: Procedures Requiring Sterile Technique).

Wound Care

❑ **A wound is a disruption in normal tissue caused by traumatic injury; also may be surgically created.**

A. Major goals.
  1. Promote healing.
  2. Prevent further damage.
  3. Prevent infection.

B. Wound healing is affected by:

Table 3-1: STERILE TECHNIQUE: PROCEDURES AND GUIDELINES

Procedures Requiring Sterile Technique
- Surgical procedures in the operating room, (i.e., TURP, appendectomy).
- Biopsies in the operating room or client's room.
- Catheterizations of the heart, bladder, or other body cavities.
- Injections: IM, SQ, Intradermal.
- Infusions: IV, instillations or infusions of medication or radioactive isotopes into body cavities.
- Dressing changes:
  Usually first postoperative dressing change is done using sterile technique.
  Dressings over catheters inserted into body cavities, (i.e., Hickman catheter, subclavian lines, dialysis access sites).
  Dressings of clients with burns, immunologic disorders, and skin grafts.

Guidelines For Sterile Field
- Never turn your back on a sterile field.
- Avoid talking.
- Keep all sterile objects within view (i.e., below waist is not within sterile field).
- Moisture will carry bacteria across/through a cloth or paper barrier.

1. Nutritional status.
2. Circulation to the wound.
3. Characteristics of the wound.
4. Presence of existing disease, (i.e., diabetes).
5. Location and approximation of wound.

NCLEX ALERT: *Monitor wound drainage; Perform wound care; Promote progress of wound healing.*

C. Nursing intervention.
1. Cleansing of wound.
   a. Horizontal wound — cleansed from center of incision outward, then laterally.
   b. Vertical wound — cleansed from top to bottom, then laterally.
   c. Drain or a stab wound — cleansed in a circular motion.

***NURSING PRIORITY:** When cleansing an area, always start at the cleanest area and work away from that area. Never return to an area you have previously cleaned. Be sure to discard cleansing swab after each horizontal or vertical stroke.*

2. Drain — inserted into open wounds to prevent the accumulation of secretions and exudate.
   a. Safety pins are inserted into Penrose drains to prevent them from slipping back into the wound.
   b. Frequent dressing changes are preferable to reinforcing the same dressing.
3. Jackson-Pratt catheter or drainage system — bulb must be compressed to allow air to escape and then is re-capped to maintain suction.
   a. Hemovac - evacuator must be compressed at least every four hours to provide suction; be sure to empty drainage from pouring spout.
4. Wet-to-dry dressings.
   a. Purpose is to trap necrotic tissue in the dressing as it dries.
   b. Dressing should be moist when applied and allowed to dry for four to six hours.

***NURSING PRIORITY:** Wring out excessive moisture from dressings. The dressings should be thick and wet enough to dry between dressing changes. Protect the skin around the wound.*

5. Obtain a specimen of wound drainage.
   a. Gently roll a sterile swab in the purulent drainage.
   b. Obtain wound specimen before any medication or antimicrobial agent has been applied to wound area or administered to client.

Heat and Cold Applications

NCLEX ALERT: *Evaluate client's physiological response to prescribed therapy.*

A. Heat applications.
1. Purpose of heat application is to soften exudate, encourage formation of pus, and promote healing.
2. General principles.
   a. Take vital signs before, during, and after heat application, if it is applied to a large area.
   b. Moist heat penetrates deeper than dry heat.
   c. Unless a physician orders continuous heat applications, treatment time is usually 20 minutes.
3. Types of heat application.
   a. Moist heat pack.
   b. Aquamatic or Aqua K-pad — circulates warmed water through the pad to distribute dry heat to body parts.
   c. Heat lamp or heat cradle.
   d. Sitz bath.

B. Cold Applications
1. The purpose is to promote vasoconstriction, decrease edema or temperature, stop bleeding, or stop pain by numbing pain receptors.
2. Types of cold applications.
   a. Ice bag, ice collar, or ice glove.
   b. Cold compress or cold pack.
   c. Hypothermia blanket.
3. Reduces edema if applied immediately after an injury.

***NURSING PRIORITY:** Do not use cold applications with conditions of impaired circulation, (i.e., peripheral vascular disease or diabetes).*

Specimen Collection

NCLEX ALERT: *Collect specimens (urine, sputum, etc.)*

A. General principles.

Table 3-2: NORMAL VITAL SIGNS

Neonate:	
Respiration	30 to 60
Pulse	110 to 160
Child 2 to 4 years:	
Respiration	24 to 32
Pulse	90 to 130
Child 6 to 10 years:	
Respiration	20 to 26
Pulse	100
Blood Pressure	80/40 to 110/80
Adult:	
Respiration	12 to 18
Pulse	60 to 100
Blood Pressure	90/60 to 140/90

NCLEX ALERT: Monitor vital signs.

1. Use sterile equipment to obtain specimen and prevent contamination from outside sources.
2. Use the correct container for each specimen - preservatives, anticoagulants, or chemicals may be required.
3. Always observe universal precautions when obtaining specimens.
4. Properly label the specimen. Collect the correct amount at the correct time.

B. Types of specimen.

1. Urine (Appendix 18-3).
2. Stool (Appendix 13-13).
3. Sputum, throat or nasopharyngeal (Appendix 10-8).
4. Blood.
5. Wound specimen.

Vital Signs

***NURSING PRIORITY:** Know the range of normal for vital signs at different age levels. This is critical in identifying changes in a client's status as well as being specific criteria for medication administration.*

A. Normal values (see Table 3-2: Normal Vital Signs).

B. Assessment.

1. Respirations.
   a. Evaluate an infant's respiratory pattern prior to stimulation.
   b. Check thoracic cavity for symmetrical excursion.
   c. Breath sounds are best evaluated with client in sitting position.
2. Pulse.
   a. Irregular radial pulse, weak volume, or low rate should be assessed by taking an apical pulse for a full minute.
   b. Apical pulse is auscultated at the fifth intercostal space at the mid-clavicular line (point of maximal intensity—PMI).
   c. Apical-radial pulse is determined by two people counting both the apical and the radial at the same time. This provides information about *pulse deficit*, which is the difference in the two values.
   d. A weak peripheral pulse may be evaluated by Doppler ultrasound.
3. Temperature.
   a. Temperature affected by mouth breathing and temperature of oral intake.
   b. Oral temperature is taken unless otherwise indicated.

Table 3-3: BLOOD PRESSURE ASSESSMENT

Procedure:
The inflatable cuff is wrapped tightly around the upper ⅔ of the arm.
The cuff is inflated 20-30 mm Hg above the point at which radial pulsation disappears.
As the cuff is deflated, a sound is produced within the brachial artery just below the cuff and is audible with the stethoscope. This sound (*Korotkoff sound*) coincides with each pulse beat. Usually when the cuff pressure is below diastolic, the sound will cease or become muffled.
It is important to ascertain and record when the sound becomes muffled. If there is any doubt, the BP may be recorded as a tripartite pressure (120/70/50) implying that the sound became muffled at 70 mm Hg and disappeared at 50 mmHg.

Nursing Implications:
Size of cuff should be 20% wider than the diameter of the limb.
If the cuff is too large (i.e., child's arm), the BP obtained will be substantially lower than the true BP. Hence, the importance of obtaining a pediatric BP cuff for measuring a child's BP.
If the cuff is too small (i.e., obese person's arm), the BP obtained will be higher than the true BP.
The difference of BP in right and left arms should be no more than 5 mm Hg.

***NURSING PRIORITY:** The BP of a hypertensive person should be measured lying down, sitting, and then standing. It is measured in both right and left arms.*

4. Blood pressure assessment (See Table 3-3).

NCLEX ALERT: *Determine if vital signs are abnormal (e.g., hypotension, hypertension, bradycardia, etc.*

Change of Shift Report

A. Purpose is to inform the oncoming nurse of the immediate needs and progress of the client. The oncoming nurse is responsible for the nursing care required on their shift.

1. Do not read everything on the care plan.
2. Plan ahead what information is important to report.
   a. Status of IV's and amount of fluid to count.
   b. Any abnormal conditions (e.g., vital signs, pain, special treatment).
   c. Status of client with regard to their diagnosis.
   - *Example:* cardiac client — presence or absence of chest pain and dysrhythmias
     surgical client — voiding, incision status
     orthopedic client —circulation distal to cast or traction.

B. Report any information that is important for the oncoming nurse to know in order to meet the client's needs.

NCLEX ALERT: *Give report to other health care team members (end of shift, telephone, etc.)*

Disaster Planning

A. A. Fire

1. Immediately return to your unit if a fire code is called.
2. If clients on your unit are not in immediate danger, close all of the doors to the client rooms and to the unit.
3. If your unit is evacuated because of immediate danger, evacuate clients in this order
   a. First - ambulatory clients first because they can move the quickest and you can remove more client's quickly.
   b. Second - clients in wheel chairs or walkers, or client's that need assistance are next to be evacuated.
   c. Third - clients that require the most assistance-ventilator clients, those who are totally bedridden.
   d. Know the types of fire extinguishers:
      (1) Class A - water or solution for paper or linens.
      (2) Class B - foam extinguisher for grease, chemicals, or electric fires.
      (3) Class C - multipurpose for paper, linens, electrical fires.

B. Response acronym - RACE
R-Rescue
A-Alert
C-Confine
E-Evacuate

NCLEX ALERT*: Participate in activities to prepare for internal/external disasters.*

IMMOBILITY

❑ ***Immobility* is the therapeutic or unavoidable restriction of a client's physical activity.**

A. Causes of restricted movement.

1. Spinal cord or neuro injury.
2. Presence of severe pain-arthritis, surgery, or injury.

B. Therapeutic reasons for restricted movement.

1. To decrease pain.
2. To immobilize a wound.
3. To limit exercise and activity (e.g., clients with cardiac problems).
4. To reduce effects of gravity on edema, varicosities.

Adverse Physical Effects of Immobility

The primary nursing goal in the care of the immobilized client is the *prevention* of complications. This is achieved by initiating nursing activities to prevent complications and by careful assessment of major organ systems for specific data indicating the effects of immobility.

NCLEX ALERT: *Provide measures to prevent the complications of immobility.*

A. Cardiovascular System.

1. Physical effects.
   a. Orthostatic hypotension (↓ BP when standing).
   b. Decrease in ability of the heart to maintain output.
   c. Venous stasis.
   d. Increase in cardiac workload.
2. Nursing implications.

a. Position body to enhance circulation.
b. Change position frequently.
c. Passive and active range of motion.
d. Begin activity gradually; allow client to sit before standing.

B. Respiratory System.
1. Physical effects.
a. Decrease in thoracic excursion.
b. Decrease in O_2/CO_2 exchange.
c. Increase in pulmonary infections.
d. Increase in collection of fluids in the lung.
2. Nursing implications.
a. Elevate head of bed.
b. Maintain adequate hydration.
c. Have client turn, cough, and deep breathe every 2 hours.
d. Promote increase in activity as soon as possible - have client sit up in chair at bedside.
e. Assess pulmonary secretions for infection.

C. Urinary System.
1. Physical effects.
a. Urinary stasis.
b. Increased calcium in urine, precipitating stone formation.
c. Urinary tract infections.
2. Nursing implications.
a. Have client sit up to void, if possible.
b. Increase fluid intake.
c. Decrease calcium intake.
d. Assess for urinary retention and urinary tract infection.

D. Musculoskeletal System.
1. Physical effects.
a. Demineralization of bones - decrease in bone strength.
b. Muscle weakness and atrophy, paralytic ileus.
c. Loss of motion in joints leads to fibrosis and contractures.
2. Nursing implications.
a. Perform range of motion exercises.
b. Active contraction and relaxation of large muscles.
c. Position body to maintain proper alignment.
d. Encourage daily weight bearing (standing at bedside) when possible.

E. Gastrointestinal System.
1. Physical effects.
a. Anorexia.
b. Ineffective movement of feces through colon that leads to constipation.
c. Diarrhea secondary to impaction.
2. Nursing implications.
a. Establish bowel program - every other day, or three times a week.
b. Encourage diet with adequate protein, bulk, and liquids.
c. Check for impaction.

F. Integumentary System.
1. Physical effects.
a. Decrease in tissue perfusion leading to decubitus ulcer.
b. Decrease in sensation in an area of increased pressure.
2. Nursing implications.
a. Maintain cleanliness.
b. Promote circulation through frequent positioning.
c. Protect bony prominences when turning.
d. Prevent pressure areas from tight clothing, cast, braces.
e. Frequent visual inspection of pressure areas.

NCLEX ALERT: *Identify potential for skin breakdown.*

LONG-TERM CARE

❑ **Long-term care includes those services provided in institutional settings, such as a nursing home, rehabilitation center, or adult day care program *after the acute phase of the illness* has passed. Often involves restorative care for clients with chronic health care problems.**

A. Types of long-term care facilities.
1. Nursing home—provides services ranging from maintenance to restorative care with skilled nursing, use of certified nursing assistants (CNAs), LPNs, and RNs.
2. Adult day care home—client lives at home during the evening and night and spends the day in a facility that provides a range of care from skilled nursing to restorative care.
3. Hospice care—care provided in both the home and in-patient care settings; funded by Medicare for the terminally ill older adult, with other programs available for other age groups.

a. Does not institute life support by extraordinary means.

b. Emphasis on pain control for client and support of family members through dying process.

4. Respite care—a type of short-term care for the primary care giver (often a family member) to give him/her a rest from the daily responsibilities of taking care of the long-term client.
5. Rehabilitation center—facility that provides multiple services for the client and family to make adjustments to daily living.
6. Home care—nursing care is provided in the home to clients who do not need hospitalization, but do need additional assistance with medical problems.
7. Adult housing or assisted living centers—places where clients can live under minimal supervision; meals and other services are offered to the residents.

Rehabilitation

NCLEX ALERT: *Refer client/significant others to appropriate resources.*

❑ ***Rehabilitation* means the restoration of an individual to his optimum level of functioning. This includes physical, mental, social, vocational, and economic parameters.**

A. Rehabilitation: term used when an individual has lost functional ability due to illness or injury.

B. Habilitation: term used to refer to congenital problems or deficiencies.

Goals of Rehabilitation

NURSING PRIORITY: *Rehabilitation is an area that affects all levels of nursing care. A primary goal in planning any client's care is to prevent complications.*

In order for the rehabilitation client to achieve the highest level of productivity, the rehabilitation process must begin when the condition becomes evident, or when the disease is diagnosed.

A. Prevention of deformities and complications.

1. Maintain function and prevent deterioration of unaffected organs or areas.
2. Prevent further injury to affected area or organ.
3. Prevent or reduce complications of immobility.

B. Assist client to perform his activities of daily living (ADL) with minimum or no assistance, depending on his or her level of disability.

- *Examples* of ADLs: eating, dressing, bathing.

C. Assist client with independent activities of daily living (IADL).

- Examples of IADLs: shopping for groceries, paying bills, lawn care.

D. Promote continuity of care when the client is discharged or transferred.

Psychological Responses to Disability

Not every client will progress through all stages of grief in an orderly fashion. Clients will fluctuate between emotional crises.

A. Initial responses of confusion, disorganization, and denial represent a state of internal conflict. Conflict is precipitated by:

1. Forced dependency.
2. Loss of self-esteem.
3. Threat to personal and family integrity.

B. A period of depression may occur as the client mourns for the lost body function or activity.

C. An anger stage may occur as client projects blame and hostility on family and health care providers.

D. Adaptation and adjustment will come as the client begins to redirect his or her energy toward coping with the disability.

E. New situations (going home, new job, etc.) may precipitate emotional outbursts and trauma.

F. Some clients will refuse to accept their disability and will not put forth any effort to adapt to everyday living.

CHRONIC HEALTH CARE

A chronic illness may be defined as an illness or condition that is present for more than three months in a year and interferes with daily function and lifestyle.

NURSING PRIORITY: *As the geriatric population increases, there is an increase in the practical nurse's role to provide initial health care and to assist in planning, as well as providing long-term care. Situations may involve a specific illness, but questions may focus on the conceptual care of the chronically ill client.*

Nursing Considerations

A. Client may remain free from symptoms, but must remain in contact with health care provider in order to maintain optimum level of wellness.

B. The condition of the client and the level of the disease will have a variable impact on the client's life style and coping strategies.

C. The majority of clients with extended health care needs are suffering from at least two chronic health conditions. These conditions may or may not be interrelated.

D. The focus of care for the chronically ill client is on assisting the client to control their disease and manage their lifestyle.

1. Prevention and management of medical crises.
2. The control of disease symptoms, which may focus on pain control and comfort measures.
3. The implementation of the prescribed therapeutic regimens.
4. Psychosocial implications and adjustment of lifestyle, frequently requires dealing with social isolation.
5. Adjustments of lifestyle as disease and/or condition changes.
6. Financial strain to pay for medical care and supplies.
7. Coping with strain on marriage and on family structure.

E. The majority of clients with chronic health care needs are over 65 years old. The feeling of powerlessness is not uncommon in the elderly.

NURSING PRIORITY: In planning the nursing or health care for a client with a chronic disease, it is very important to assist the client to maintain control over his condition and his lifestyle. Frequently, health care providers and family tend to take control of the situation and further the feeling of powerlessness in the individual.

Nursing Considerations in the Chronically Ill Pediatric Client

The diagnosis of a child's chronic illness is a major situational crisis in the family. Support systems, perception of the problem, and coping mechanisms will ultimately determine the resolution of the crisis.

A. Focus care on the child's developmental age rather then the chronological age. Emphasis should be made on the child's strengths rather the on the child's disabilities.

B. Promote the child's maximum level of growth and development. Current trend is to return the child to the academic environment with his peer group. A variety of supplemental programs are being developed in the school systems to meet the needs of these children.

C. Assess the family response to the child's illness and evaluate for parental overprotection. Overprotection by the parents prevents the child from developing self esteem, independence, and self-control over disease and activities of daily living. The practical nurse should observe for the following parental characteristics.

1. Inconsistency with discipline; discipline often differs from that of the other children in the family.
2. Attempts to protect the child from every discomfort, both physical and psychosocial, frequently restricts play with peers for fear of injury and/or rejection by peers.
3. Makes decisions for the child without involving the child.
4. Does not allow the child the opportunity to learn self care; frequently afraid the child cannot handle the requirements for self-care. For example, encouraging and assisting the diabetic child to become responsible for administration of his own insulin.
5. Continues to do things for the child, even when the child is capable of doing for himself.
6. Self-sacrifice and isolation of family from social interactions.

NURSING PRIORITY: Questions involving pediatrics often encompass the concepts of care of the chronically ill child. The question may involve a specific disease or condition, but the answer is frequently based on concepts of a chronic illness in the pediatric client.

PAIN

❑ **Pain is a complex, universal experience. Most definitions include the following points: (1) Pain is a sensory perceptual experience; (2) Pain is a totally subjective personal experience; (3) Pain is an early warning system, its presence triggers an awareness that something is wrong in our body (Figure 3-2).**

NCLEX ALERT: *Plan measures to care for clients with anticipated or actual alteration in comfort; provide alternative measures for pain relief (e.g., imagery, massage, repositioning).*

Types of Pain

- Acute pain—short, predictable duration (6 months), immediate onset, reversible or controllable with treatment.
  Example: postoperative pain that will disappear after the wound heals.
  Example: postoperative pain which disappears as wound heals.

- Chronic pain—lasts 6 months; continual or persistent and recurrent.
  Example: malignant (cancer) or arthritis.
- Cutaneous pain—client can identify specific area of pain which may sting or burn; may occur along a dorsal sensory nerve root.
  Example: abrasions on skin, herpes zoster.
- Visceral pain—affects any of the large body cavities (abdominal viscera); characterized as diffuse, poorly localized, vague, and dull.
  Example: acute pancreatitis, peptic ulcer disease, cholecystitis.
- Somatic pain—pain affecting skeletal muscle, joints, and ligaments; generally diffuse and less localized than cutaneous pain.
  Example: rheumatoid arthritis, osteomyelitis.
- Referred pain—does not occur at the point of injury.
  Example: myocardial ischemia felt in the left arm or shoulder; shoulder pain with cholecystitis.

Pathologic pain syndromes

- Vascular pain—associated with blood vessels; may be induced by cold.
  Example: migraine headaches, peripheral vascular disease.
- Pain due to inflammation—redness, swelling, heat are common findings.
  Example: peritonitis
- Phantom pain—follows an amputation of a body part; described as throbbing, burning, stabbing, boring, vice-like, or in a cramped, twisted position.
  Example: client feels "phantom sensations" in the area of the amputation, as if the part were still present.
- Malignant pain—pressure on nerve endings or interference of blood supply to area due to cancer.
- Pretended pain (malingering)—client expresses that there is pain when he actually has no pain.

Box 3-1: Pediatric Pain Assessment

*Use a variety of pain assessment strategies to question pediatric clients such as **QUEST**.*
***Q**uestion the child.*
***U**se pain rating scales*
***E**valuate behavior*
***S**ecure parent's involvement*
***T**ake into account pathology.*

- Psychogenic pain—due to emotional factors rather than physiologic dysfunction.

Pain Assessment

NURSING PRIORITY: *In addition to the pain and discomfort associated with a surgical procedure, it is important to assess other possible sources of discomfort, such as full bladder, occluded catheter or tube, gas accumulation, IV infiltration, or compromised circulation due to position/pressure.*

A. Subjective data collection.
1. Discussion of pain location, onset, precipitating and alleviating factors.
2. Assessment of duration, intensity, and severity of pain.
3. Characteristics of pain (e.g., stabbing, throbbing, knife-like, crushing, cramping, suffocating, etc.)
4. Meaning of the pain experience to the client.

NCLEX ALERT: *Assess client's discomfort or pain (severity, specific type, associate symptoms, etc.)*

B. Objective data collection.
1. Appearance, motor behavior, facial expression.
2. Affective behavior (e.g., crying, irritability, withdrawal, etc.).
3. Verbal behavior (e.g., expressions of anger, fear, frustration).
4. Increased blood pressure, pulse, and respirations.
5. Dilated pupils, decreased urinary output, increased muscle tension, nausea, vomiting.
6. Inspection and palpation of painful area and range of motion of involved part.
7. See Table 3-4: Mnemonic to Evaluate Pain, Table 3-5: Assessing the Harmful Effects of Pain, and Box 3-1: Pediatric Pain Assessment.
8. Move these tables to the text content or follow it.

NURSING PRIORITY: *The most significant aspect of pain relief is the relationship that exists between the nurse and the client. The client is aware that the nurse has the power to relieve pain or withhold pain relief. Anticipatory anxiety is created by this situation.*

Noninvasive Pain Relief Measures

Behavioral Techniques

A. Relaxation Techniques.

Table 3-4: MNEMONIC TO EVALUATE PAIN

P:	Provoking or palliative factors
Q:	Quality
R:	Region
S:	Severity
T:	Timing

NURSING PRIORITY: *Low levels of anxiety or pain are easier to reduce or control than are higher levels. Consequently, pain relief measures should be utilized before pain becomes severe.*

1. Relaxed muscles result in decreased pain level.
2. Typical relaxation exercises focus on deep breathing and alternate tensing and relaxing of various body parts in a systematic manner.
3. Meditation—focuses attention away from pain.
4. Rhythmic breathing—method of relaxation and distraction by focusing on the breath.
5. Music may assist in relaxation.

Table 3-5: ASSESSING THE HARMFUL EFFECTS OF PAIN

ACUTE PAIN	CHRONIC PAIN
Disturbs sleep	Fatigue
Appetite decreases	Weight gain
Fluid intake decreases	Poor concentration
Nausea and vomiting	Job loss
	Divorce
	Depression

NCLEX ALERT*:* *Provide nonpharmacological measures for pain relief (e.g. imagery, massage, repositioning, etc.)*

B. Guided imagery.

1. Creative visualization is the therapeutic use of images from one's imagination to focus away from pain sensation by emphasizing pleasant memories and experiences.
2. Often combined with relaxation and biofeedback.

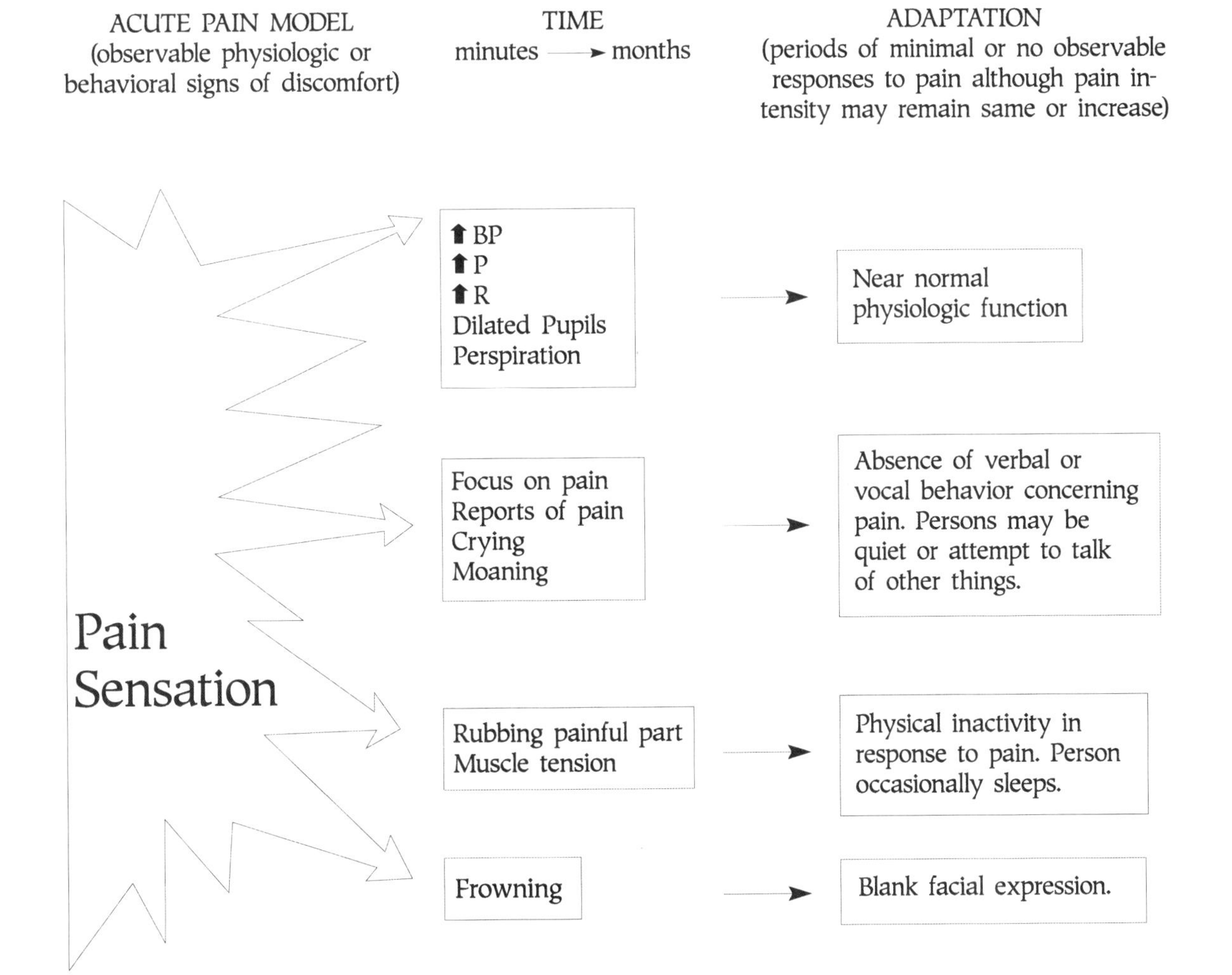

Figure 3-2: Pain

C. Hypnosis is also used to produce a state of altered consciousness which is characterized by extreme responsiveness to suggestion.

D. Biofeedback—provides client with information about changes in bodily functions of which he is usually unaware, (i.e., blood pressure, pulse).

E. Cutaneous stimulation—alleviates pain through stimulation of skin.

1. Provide cutaneous stimulation through pressure, massage, bathing, and heat or cold therapy to promote relaxation.
2. Change positions frequently and support body parts.
3. Encourage early ambulation after surgery.
4. Elevate swollen body parts.
5. Check drainage tubes to ensure that they are not stretched, kinked, or pulled.

F. Transcutaneous electric nerve stimulation (TENS).

1. Delivers an electrical current through electrodes applied to the skin surface of the painful region or a peripheral nerve.
2. TENS unit procedure.
   a. Identify trigger points (areas which are extremely sensitive when stimulated) and place electrode.
   b. Determine whether the electrodes are water conductive (moisten with water) or are gel conductive (moisten with gel).
   c. Instruct client to adjust TENS unit intensity until it creates a pleasant sensation and relieves the pain.

NCLEX ALERT: *Provide holistic complementary therapy to promote comfort.*

G. Therapeutic touch—holistic approach using touch to realign energy fields (laying on of hands); involves 3 steps.

1. Nurse is centered or focused in a meditative state.
2. Nurse assesses energy fields (vibrations around client) by passing the hands over the client's body at a distance of 2-6 inches above body.
3. Last step is treatment where nurse helps clean up client's energy field and return it to normal.

H. Acupressure—pressure or massage is applied over acupuncture points to decrease pain.

Medications for Pain Relief

A. Administer PRN analgesic medications (Appendix 3-2: Analgesics).

NURSING PRIORITY: *Utilize a preventive approach in alleviating pain by giving narcotics before the pain occurs (if it can be predicted), or at least before it reaches severe intensity. This is particularly important in regards to care of the new postoperative client.*

1. Steps in administering PRN medications.
   a. Assess client to determine source and quality of pain.
   b. Check client's chart.
      (1) Last medication received and how administered.
      (2) The time administered.
      (3) Current physician's order.
   c. Analyze nursing assessment data and determine most appropriate nursing intervention.
   d. Implement and document pain intervention.
   e. Decrease stimuli in room and determine other factors influencing discomfort.
   f. At 15 and 30 minute intervals, assess client's response to pain intervention and document nursing actions.

NCLEX ALERT: *Determine client's need for administration of a PRN medication.*

2. Types of medications.
   a. Narcotic analgesics are used for relieving severe pain.
   - *Example:* Morphine, codeine, hydromorphone (Dilaudid), meperidine (Demerol), oxycodone (Percodan).

   b. Non-narcotic analgesics act at peripheral sites to reduce pain.
   - *Example:* Propoxyphene (Darvon), pentazocine (Talwin).

   c. Potentiating drugs used to intensify the action of the narcotic agent—promethazine (Phenergan), hydroxyzine (Vistaril, Atarax), diazepam (Valium).
   d. Nonsteroidal anti-inflammatory drugs have analgesic, anti-inflammatory, and anti-pyretic properties.
   - *Example:* Acetylsalicylic acid (ASA) or aspirin, acetaminophen (Tylenol), ibuprofen (Motrin, Advil), naproxen (Naprosyn).

NCLEX ALERT: *Monitor functioning of an infusion pump (e.g. IV, feeding, PCA, etc.)*

B. Patient-controlled analgesia (PCA).
1. Client controls delivery of pain medication via a PCA pump.
2. PCA pump procedure.
a. A common order is to give 1-4 mg of Morphine q10min until pain is relieved.
3. Advantages of PCA.
a. More effective pain control.
b. Decreased client anxiety (doesn't have to wait for medication).
c. Increased client independence.
d. Decreased level of sedation.
e. Clients tend to use less narcotics.

NURSING PRIORITY: *Fear of addiction is often a major concern of clients (and their families) who are receiving pain medication at home. The client should be assured that pain medication when taken as directed will relieve the pain and will not lead to addiction. The nurse should administer PRN pain medication to clients experiencing acute pain without fear of addicting the client to the medication.*

Evaluation of Pain Control

NCLEX ALERT: *Observe for effects of medications. Determine client's need for PRN medications.*

A. Identify client behavior response prior to the intervention and compare with response following intervention.
B. Use ongoing assessment and modify nursing interventions in accordance with results and client's status.

Geriatric Priority: *Analgesics tend to last longer; there is increase risk for side effects and toxic effects.*

PERIOPERATIVE CARE

Surgical procedures, whether planned or emergency, represent a crisis in a client's life. However minor, surgical procedures always carry some degree of risk, physical discomfort, and financial stress.

A. Perioperative refers to the entire operative experience (preoperative, intraoperative, and postoperative care).
B. Preoperative phase - the period of time prior to the surgical procedure.
1. Assessment and correction of physiological and psychological problems that may increase the client's risk factors.
2. Client teaching regarding the surgery.
3. Client teaching regarding postoperative care and activities.
4. Client planning for any anticipated changes in lifestyle at time of discharge.
C. Intraoperative phase - The period of time the client is in the operating room.
D. Postoperative phase - The period begins with the admission of the client to the post anesthesia recovery (PAR) area, and includes the rest of the client's hospitalization and recovery period.

Preoperative care

A. Client Profile.
1. Age - The elderly and the infant have more difficulty maintaining homeostasis than do the adult and child. The elderly are more likely to have chronic health problems complicating surgery.

Geriatric Priority: *The older client has less physiologic reserve (the ability of an organ to return to normal after a disturbance in its equilibrium) than younger clients.*

2. Weight - Obesity predisposes the client to postoperative complications of infection and wound dehiscence. Fatty tissue is more susceptible to the infectious process.
3. Preoperative interview.
a. Chronic health problems and previous surgical procedures.
b. Past and current drug therapy, including over-the-counter medications.

NCLEX ALERT: *Evaluate client's use of medications (prescriptive, over the counter).*

c. History of drug allergies and dietary restrictions.
d. Client's perception of his or her illness and impending surgery.
e. Determine client's level of orientation and any visual or auditory problems that would hinder communication.

f. Discomfort or symptoms he/she is currently experiencing.
g. Religious affiliation.
h. Family or significant others.

4. Psychosocial needs - Fear of the unknown is the primary cause of preoperative anxiety in the mentally stable client. The surgical experience is unique to each client and represents a time of crisis.

Geriatric Priority: *Assess for use of medications over prolonged period and report medications to RN.*

5. Check routine laboratory studies.
   a. Complete blood count.
   b. Urinalysis.
   c. VDRL or FTA-ABS.
   d. Chest x-ray.
   e. Electrocardiogram (EKG).

NCLEX ALERT: *Determine if client is prepared for a procedure/surgery.*

B. Preoperative Teaching - The goal is to decrease the client's anxiety and to prevent postoperative complications.
1. Evaluate the client's current understanding of his/her illness and of the anticipated surgical intervention.
2. Use terminology the client will understand.
3. Do not overwhelm the client with too much information at one time; allow adequate time for client questions.
4. Involve the client's significant others in the preoperative teaching.
5. Preoperative teaching content.
   a. Deep breathing and coughing exercises.
   b. Turning and extremity exercises.
   c. Pain medication policy - PRN, PCA.
   d. Adjunct equipment used for breathing - incentive spirometry, nebulizer, O_2 mask.
   e. Explanation of NPO policy.

NCLEX ALERT: *Explain/teach about scheduled treatments or procedures.*

C. Physical Preparation.
1. Skin preparation - the operative site and the surrounding area should be clean either by the client bathing or specific cleansing of the site.
   a. Food and fluid restriction for approximately 6 hours preoperatively.
   b. Enemas or some type of gastrointestinal cleansing is usually administered the evening prior to surgery involving the GI tract, pelvic area, retroperitoneal area. This assists to prevent fecal contamination in the peritoneal cavity.
2. Promote sleep and rest - After the preoperative procedures are completed the client generally receives a sleeping medication to promote rest. Common medications used are the barbiturates.

D. Legal Implications.
1. The physician should give the client a full explanation of the procedure, including complications and alternatives.
2. The client's informed consent record (permit) must be signed by the physician, the client, and a witness; the witness is frequently the staff nurse.

***NURSING PRIORITY:** The informed consent record (permit) must be signed prior to the client receiving the preoperative medication.*

3. The signed consent record (permit) is part of the permanent chart record and must accompany the client to the operating room.

NCLEX ALERT: *Inform client of his or her rights. The signed informed consent form provides evidence the consent process has occurred. The nurse should verify with the client that the physician has discussed the risks and benefits of the surgery and the client understands their rights.*

Day of Surgery

A. Nursing Responsibilities.
1. Have client follow routine hygiene care.
2. Record vital signs within four hours of client going to surgery.
3. Secure and/or remove valuables according to hospital policy; wedding bands may be taped on finger.
4. Remove fingernail polish or acrylic nails from at least 2 fingers.
5. Dress client in appropriate clothing.
6. Inform client that dentures and removable bridge work must be removed before surgery. Check young children for the presence of loose teeth.

7. Make sure the NPO policy has been initiated according to orders and the client has adhered to it.
8. Check the client's identification band; validate the information and see it is secure.
9. Identify family and significant others who will be waiting for information regarding client's progress.
10. Check the chart for completeness regarding laboratory reports, consent form, significant client observations, history and physical records.

B. Preoperative Medications (Appendix 3-3).

NCLEX ALERT: *Administer medications, observe for effects of medications.*

1. Purpose.
   a. Decrease anxiety and provide sedation.
2. Nursing Responsibilities.
   a. Ask client to void prior to administration of medication.
   b. Obtain baseline vital signs.
   c. Administer medication on call to OR usually 45 minutes to 1 hour prior to surgery.
   d. Raise the siderails and instruct the client not to get out of bed.
   e. Remove dentures, partial plates (if removable type).
   f. Observe for desired effects as well as side effects of medication.
   g. Maintain quiet environment prior to being transported to the operating room.
   h. Allow parent to accompany child as far as possible.

Geriatric Priority: *Spinal anesthesia may be used for clients undergoing TURP, inguinal herniorrhaphy, orthopedic procedures, and for poor-risk clients who would not tolerate inhalation anesthesia very well.*

C. Nursing Considerations for Spinal Anesthesia.

1. Requires anesthesiologist for administration.
2. Client will not be able to feel any sensation below level of anesthesia.
3. Vasodilation below level of anesthesia may precipitate hypotension.
4. Client may experience post-anesthesia headache.
5. Client may remain awake throughout procedure.
6. May be used in major surgical procedures below the level of the diaphragm.

Box 3-2: Elderly Care Focus

Preoperative and Postoperative Considerations

Elderly clients are at increased risk due to decreased response of the immune system which delays healing and the increased incidence of chronic disease.

Cardiovascular—decreased cardiac output and peripheral circulation along with arrhythmias and increased incidence of arteriosclerosis and atherosclerosis can lead to hypotension or hypertension, hypothermia, and cardiac problems.

Respiratory—decreased vital capacity, reduced oxygenation, and decreased cough reflex can lead to an increased risk of atelectasis, pneumonia, and aspiration.

Renal—decreased renal excretion of wastes and renal blood flow along with increased incidence of nocturia can lead to fluid overload, dehydration, and electrolyte imbalance.

Musculoskeletal—increase incidence of arthritis and osteoporosis can lead to trauma on bones and joints with positioning in the operating room, if pressure points and limbs are not padded.

Sensory—decreased visual acuity and reaction time can lead to safety problems associated with falls and injuries.

The older client may require repeated explanation, clarification, and positive reassurance.

Elderly clients often have a poor nutritional status which can directly influence healing and postoperative recovery.

NCLEX ALERT: *Provide care that meets special needs of older adult clients.*

D. Conscious sedation — the administration of an IV medication to produce sedation, analgesia, and amnesia.

1. Characteristics
   a. Client can respond to commands, maintains his protective reflexes, and does not need assistance to maintain his airway.
   b. Amnesia most often occurs after the procedure.
2. Nursing Implications.
   a. Client is assessed continuously, vital signs are recorded every 5-15 minutes.
   b. Monitor level of consciousness, client should not be unconscious, but relaxed and comfortable.
   c. Client should respond to physical and verbal stimuli, protective airway reflexes remain intact.

d. Potential complications include loss of gag reflex, aspiration, hypoxia, hypercapnia, and cardiopulmonary depression.

e. Does not require extensive post recovery time.

Immediate Postoperative Recovery

NURSING PRIORITY: *The client's respiratory status is a priority concern on admission to and throughout the recovery room period.*

A. Admission of client to recovery area.

1. Obtain baseline assessment.
   a. Vital signs.
   b. Status of respirations.
   c. General color.
   d. Type and amount of fluid infusing.
   e. Special equipment.
   f. Dressings.

Nursing Intervention

✦ *Goal: to maintain respiratory function.*

1. Leave airway in place until pharyngeal reflex (gag reflex) has returned.
2. Position client to maintain ventilation and prevent aspiration.
3. Encourage coughing and deep breathing.
4. Administer humidified oxygen as necessary.
5. *Notify RN of significant changes in respiratory status.*
6. Listen to the chest for a decrease in breath sounds. Notify RN as necessary.

✦ *Goal: to maintain cardiovascular stability.*

1. Check vital signs every 15 minutes until stable; compare with preoperative vital signs.
2. *Notify RN of blood pressure that is continually dropping 5 to 10 mm Hg with each reading.*
3. *Notify RN of consistently increasing bradycardia or tachycardia.*
4. Evaluate quality of pulse and presence of irregular pulse.

✦ *Goal: to maintain adequate fluid status.*

1. Monitor rate of IV infusion.
2. Measure urine output if bladder catheter is present (minimum of 30 cc per hour for an adult).
3. Evaluate for bladder distention if there is no catheter.
4. Observe amount and character of drainage on dressings or drainage in collecting containers.
5. Assess amount and character of gastric drainage if nasogastric tube is in place.
6. Nausea and vomiting frequently occur as client is recovering from anesthesia. Evaluate the amount and characteristics of the vomitus.

NCLEX ALERT: *Use measures to prevent aspiration, prevent aspiration by positioning on the left side and suctioning if appropriate.*

✦ *Goal: to maintain incisional areas.*

1. Evaluate amount and character of drainage from incision and drains.
2. Check and record status of Hemovac, Jackson-Pratt, or any other wound drains.

✦ *Goal: to maintain psychological equilibrium.*

1. Speak to client frequently in calm, unhurried manner.
2. Continually orient client.
3. Maintain quiet, restful atmosphere.
4. Promote comfort by maintaining proper body alignment.
5. Explain all procedures, even if client is not fully awake.
6. Remember that in the anesthetized client, the sense of hearing is the last to be lost and the first to return.

✦ *Goal: client meets criteria to return to room.*

1. Vital signs stable and within normal limits.
2. Client awake and reflexes have returned.
3. Dressings intact with no evidence of excessive drainage.
4. Client can maintain a patent airway without assistance.

GENERAL POSTOPERATIVE CARE

NCLEX ALERT: *Monitor client during or after a procedure/surgery. Anticipate questions regarding basic postoperative nursing care, as well as questions that apply to a specific surgical condition or procedure. Nursing implications for specific surgical procedures may be found under the major systems in the care of the medical-surgical client.*

✦ *Goal: to maintain cardiovascular function and tissue perfusion.*

1. Monitor vital signs, usually every four hours, after full recovery.

2. Evaluate skin color and nail beds for paleness and cyanosis.
3. Assess client's tolerance to increasing activity.
4. Encourage early activity and ambulation.
5. Monitor for circulatory complications of immobility.

✦ *Goal: to maintain respiratory function.*

1. Have client turn, cough, and deep breathe every 2 hours.
2. Use blow bottles, incentive spirometry to promote deep breathing.
3. Maintain adequate hydration to keep mucus secretions thinned and easily mobilized.
4. Encourage early ambulation.
5. Evaluate sputum for presence of infection.

✦ *Goal: to maintain adequate nutrition and elimination.*

1. Assess for return of bowel sounds and normal peristalsis.
2. Assess the client with a nasogastric tube for return of peristalsis.
3. Encourage fluids after client demonstrates tolerance to fluids.
4. Assess client's tolerance of PO fluids; usually begin with clear liquids.
5. Diet is usually progressive as client's condition and appetite indicate.
6. Record bowel movements; normal bowel function should return as evidenced by normal bowel movement on the second or third postoperative day (provided the client is eating).
7. Assess urinary output.
   a. Client should void 8 to 10 hours after surgery.
   b. If bladder catheter is present, client should average at least 30 cc per hour.
   c. Promote voiding by allowing client to stand or use bedside commode, if not contraindicated.
   d. Avoid catheterization if possible.

✦ *Goal: to maintain fluid balance.*

1. Monitor IV infusions for correct fluid and rate of infusion.
2. Assess for adequate hydration.
   a. Moist mucous membranes.
   b. Adequate urine output.
   c. Good skin turgor.
   d. Vital signs stable.
   e. Alert and oriented.
3. Assess character and amount of gastric drainage through the nasogastric tube.

✦ *Goal: to promote comfort.*

1. Anticipate pain, assess and administer appropriate analgesics.
2. Administer antiemetic as ordered for nausea and vomiting.
3. Maintain hygiene (dressings, gown, etc.).
4. Change client's position every 2 hours.
5. Allow for periods of rest after analgesics.

POSTOPERATIVE COMPLICATIONS

Respiratory Complications

Atelectasis

❑ **Atelectasis is a collapse of a portion of the lung, producing an airless state in the alveoli (Chapter 10).**

Data Collection

1. Dyspnea.
2. Decreased or absent breath sounds over affected area.
3. Asymmetrical chest expansion.
4. Tachycardia.
5. Increased anxiety and restlessness.

Nursing Intervention

1. Prevention.
   a. Have client turn, cough and deep breathe every 2 hours., incentive spirometry every 2 hours.
   b. Maintain adequate hydration (3,000 cc per day, unless contraindicated).
   c. Avoid large doses of analgesics in clients with increased susceptibility.
   d. Prevent abdominal distention.
   e. Encourage ambulation as soon as possible.
2. Stimulate coughing.
3. Maintain humidification of inspired air.

Pneumonia

❑ **An acute inflammatory process of the alveolar spaces; the alveoli fill with fluid, thereby interfering with normal pulmonary function (Chapter 10).**

Data Collection

1. Rapid, shallow respirations.
2. Fever.
3. Wet breath sounds (rales, rhonchi) or absent breath sounds over affected area.

4. One side of the chest may expand more on inspiration.
5. Productive cough — thick yellow or green sputum.
6. Client with advanced hypoxia may demonstrate circumoral and nail bed cyanosis.
7. Tachycardia.

Nursing Intervention

1. Position in semi- to high-Fowler's.
2. Maintain adequate hydration (3,000 cc per day).
3. Administer antibiotics and antipyretics.
4. Have client turn, cough, and deep breathe every 2 hours.
5. Maintain humidification of air and oxygen.
6. Take measures to decrease fever and promote comfort.

Hemothorax, Pneumothorax

- see Chapter 10

CIRCULATORY COMPLICATIONS

Shock (Hypovolemic)

A decrease in cardiac output due to loss of circulating blood volume (Chapter 11).

> ***Geriatric Priority:*** *The incidence of shock is greater in older client's due to impairment of the cardiovascular, pulmonary, or renal system. They cannot tolerate a reduction of blood volume or hypotension, since the heart and blood vessels do not constrict as readily.*

Data Collection

1. Decreased/falling blood pressure (systolic <70 mm Hg).
2. Weak, thready pulse.
3. Shallow respirations.
4. Cool, clammy skin.
5. Oliguria (urine output ↓ 30 cc per hour).
6. Changes in sensorium (restlessness, anxiety, confusion, eventually coma).
7. Excessive thirst.
8. Incisional area, surgical drains or tubes may show excessive amount of bright red blood.

Nursing Intervention

1. Anticipate the RN will initiate an IV access for IV fluids.
2. Place client in supine position unless contraindicated.
3. Maintain airway and promote ventilation.
4. Monitor vital signs every 15 minutes, or as necessary.
5. Do not administer medications PO, IM or subq; with decreased peripheral circulation, the meds will not be absorbed.

Pulmonary Embolism

❑ **The movement of a thrombus from its venous origin into the pulmonary artery (Chapter 10). Thrombus formation is often precipitated by venous pooling due to immobility and by thrombophlebitis of the lower extremities.**

Data Collection

1. Chest pain - ranging from pleuritic in nature to severe stabbing pain.
2. Mild transient dyspnea to severe dyspnea.
3. Tachycardia.
4. Anxiety, apprehension.
5. Diaphoresis.
6. Changes in sensorium.
7. Hypotension.

Nursing Intervention

1. Position client in semi-Fowler's.
2. *Notify RN immediately of chest pain or difficulty in breathing.*
3. Administer oxygen as indicated.
4. Maintain bed rest.
5. Anticipate administration of anticoagulants.
6. Remain with client in acute distress.

WOUND COMPLICATIONS

Wound Infection

❑ **An infection of the surgical incision area.**

Data Collection

1. Redness, tenderness, heat in area of incision.
2. Presence of purulent wound drainage.
3. Fever.
4. Tachycardia.
5. Pain.

Nursing Intervention

1. Prevention.
   a. Identify clients susceptible to wound infections.
   b. Use sterile technique in dressing change.
2. Culture incisional area before starting antibiotic.

3. Evaluate progress of infection.
4. Prevent skin excoriation around wound.

Wound Dehiscence and Evisceration

❑ ***Dehiscence*** **is the unintentional opening of the surgical wound; may be sudden or gradual.** ***Evisceration*** **is the protrusion of body contents through the wound (characteristically protrusion of a loop of bowel).**

Data Collection

1. Separation of incision.
2. Visual evidence of bowel protruding through incision.
3. Client may complain of increase in pain.

Nursing Intervention

1. Evaluate client's vital signs.
2. *Notify RN.*
3. If bowel protruding, cover with sterile dressing soaked with sterile normal saline.
4. Decrease abdominal tension.

> **NCLEX ALERT:** *Respond to life threatening situations (wound evisceration)*

URINARY COMPLICATIONS

Urinary Retention

❑ **Client is unable to void normally due to depression of urinary reflexes by general anesthesia, preoperative medications, or type of procedure (Chapter 18).**

> **NCLEX ALERT:** *Use alternative methods to promote voiding (pour water over perineum, etc.)*

Data Collection

1. Unable to void 8 to 10 hours postoperative.
2. Palpable bladder.
3. Frequent voiding of small amounts.
4. Discomfort in suprapubic area.

Nursing Intervention

1. Maintain adequate hydration.
2. Position client in normal voiding position if not contraindicated.
3. Have client practice using bedpan or urinal preoperatively.
4. Provide privacy.
5. Run tap water.
6. Pour tap water over client's perineal area.

> ***NURSING PRIORITY:*** *Catheterize only if client is unable to void after trying preceding nursing measures.*

GASTROINTESTINAL COMPLICATIONS

Gastric Dilatation

❑ **Gastric dilatation is caused by decreased peristalsis leading to gastric distention.**

Data Collection

1. Nausea, vomiting.
2. Decreased bowel sounds.
3. Distended abdomen.
4. Abdominal discomfort.

Nursing Intervention

1. Anticipate insertion of nasogastric tube and connection to added suction.
2. Evaluate nasogastric drainage.
3. Evaluate serum electrolytes.
4. Position in semi-Fowler's to prevent aspiration of vomitus and to facilitate respirations.
5. Instruct client not to take anything by mouth.
6. Maintain adequate hydration by IV.

Paralytic Ileus

❑ **A decrease of neuromuscular innervation leading to decreased peristalsis in intestinal area.**

Etiology

Same as gastric dilatation although not as common.

Data Collection

1. Decreased or absent bowel sounds.
2. Failure to pass normal stool or flatus.
3. Nausea, vomiting.
4. Abdominal distention.
5. Abdominal tenderness and discomfort.

Nursing Intervention

1. Anticipate insertion of nasogastric tube with added suction.
2. Evaluate gastric drainage.
3. Maintain adequate hydration by IV.
4. Instruct client not to take anything by mouth.

Intestinal Obstruction - See Chapter 13

LEGAL IMPLICATIONS

Responsibility for Practice

A. Individual Liability.

1. Every person is liable for his or her own conduct.
2. Liability may be shared by another person or group, (i.e., the doctor, another nurse, or the hospital), but it cannot be removed by the statements or actions of another.
3. If an RN is not available, the practical nurse may not carry out functions that are recognized to be an exclusive area of registered professional nursing.
4. If a practical/vocational nurse assumes the responsibilities of a registered nurse, then he or she is held to the standards of performance of a professional registered nurse.

NCLEX ALERT: *Identify ones professional practice limitations (refuse to perform tasks outside the scope of practice.)*

B. Unethical Nursing Care:

1. Medication errors that are made and not reported/corrected
2. Physical and verbal client abuse.
3. Providing care while under the influence of alcohol or drugs.
4. Breech of client confidentiality.
5. Jeopardizing a client's well being by withholding care or treatment.
6. Providing care outside the protocol for safe, ethical nursing practice according to the individual state nurse practice act.
7. The practical/vocational nurse should follow the line of authority within the institution for reporting the incident.

NCLEX ALERT: *Report a health care provider's unsafe practice.*

C. Standard of Care - the legal concept of a fictional, reasonable, prudent individual of the same education and profession against which another professional's performance is judged.

1. Established by considering:
   a. Curriculum in schools of nursing.
   b. Actual practice of practical nurses using "expert witnesses".
   c. Statement of nursing standards.
      (1) Practice Acts, and rules and regulations.
      (2) Joint commissions.
      (3) Professional organizations.
   d. Policy and procedures manuals.
   e. Prior court decisions.
2. Need not meet maximum level of performance.
3. Used to determine when a breach of duty has occurred.

D. Good Samaritan Act.

   a. Purpose: to encourage health care providers to assist at accidents and emergencies.
   b. Elements.
      (1) Services given without payment.
      (2) Protection from ordinary negligence when performing nursing type activities at accident or emergency.
      (3) No protection for serious misconduct or for care considered to be outside the health care provider's realm of knowledge.

Legal Implications

A. Negligence - unintentional harm to another which occurs through failure to act in a reasonable and prudent manner.

B. Malpractice - nursing practice which injures someone through failure to meet the proper standard of care.

1. Elements of malpractice suit.
   a. Nurse-client relationship is established.
      (1) Assignment to specific nursing team or client.
      (2) Nursing care given to client regardless of formal assignment.
      (3) Emergency or need for immediate care by any client.
   b. The practical nurse must breach the duty by doing something wrong or not doing something needed.
   c. Harm must occur to client.
   d. Direct cause-and-effect relationship between the breach and the harm.
   e. Foreseeability: a practical nurse of equal education and preparation could reasonably expect injury to occur as a result of the breach of duty.

C. Invasion of Privacy - Protection of constitutional right to be free from undesired publicity and exposure to public view.

NCLEX ALERT: *Provide for client privacy.*

a. Proper covering of physical body.

b. Medical records.

(1) Release with client consent.

(2) Release for medical "need to know" limited to care-givers only.

c. Belongings must be protected and may not be searched without specific authorization. A client's list of belongings should be explained to and signed by the client.

d. Conversations confidential; in some states protected by specific statute.

e. Photographs and viewing of procedures require consent of client.

f. Control of visitor access to client and client information.

g. Reporting laws are an exception.

(1) Communicable diseases.

(2) Gunshot and knife wounds.

(3) Child abuse.

(4) Others defined by state statute.

h. Rights may be waived by the client but never by medical personnel.

D. Valid consent (informed consent).

1. Timely - some states or institutions have specific time restrictions on when consents are signed.
2. Written - for all invasive procedures.
3. Witnessed signature - do not witness unless you know client has all information needed to make informed decision.
4. Procedure specified in terms the client can understand.
5. Client understanding of significant risks of procedure.
6. Client understanding of alternatives to procedure.
7. Signed while client is free from mind-altering drugs or conditions.
8. Withdrawal of consent can be written or verbal and may occur at any time prior to the procedure.

E. Orders - Doctors/primary health care provider

1. Question any order that is not clearly written and understood.
2. Each medication order should contain the medication name, the route of administration, the dosage amount, time of administration and frequency.
3. Single dose orders are most often for a medication to be given one time.
4. "Stat" orders - procedure or medication should be given/carried out immediately; orders should be scanned initially to determine if any are present.
5. The nurse is responsible for questioning any medication order if the order is not clear, or the nurse feels there may be an error in the order.

NCLEX ALERT: *Review the accuracy of client orders.*

Important Protective Procedures

A. Documentation - written record of events surrounding client's hospital stay.

1. Protects client by promoting good communication among health care providers.
2. Provides evidence in court of care given.

a. Courts will not assume care is given unless it is recorded.

b. Demonstrates meeting of standard of care.

c. Demonstrates decision-making of practical nurse.

B. How to document (Table 3-6: Guidelines for Defensive Charting).

1. Be sure notes conform to the format required by the agency or institution.
2. Use the format correctly.

a. Complete all portions of format (i.e., SOAP or SOAPIE notes).

b. Use opinions only in assessment portion of charting, never in areas requiring factual data.

c. Complete an honest record of events.

(1) Exclude reference to "incident report" filed.

(2) Do not alter record at any time.

(3) Record all events, even unusual events, factually.

(4) Give all appropriate information about each note (i.e., status of incision -presence of and type of drainage, inflammation of area, foul odor, and type of dressing if any).

(5) Explain omissions in care.

d. Time, date, and sign all entries.

e. Do not skip lines, do not leave any blank spaces for other people to chart.

f. Correct errors properly.

(1) Draw a straight line through error; date, initial, and write word *error.*

(a) No white-out on error.

Table 3-6: GUIDELINES FOR DEFENSIVE CHARTING

✦ All entries should be accurate.

✦ Make corrections appropriately and according to agency or hospital policies. Do not obliterate any information that is in the chart.

✦ If there is information that should have been charted and was not, then the nurse should make a "late entry" noting the time the charting actually occurred and the specific time the charting reflects. Example: 10/13/03. 10:00am late entry, charting to reflect 10/12/03.

✦ All identified client problems, nursing actions taken, and the client responses should be noted. Do not describe a client problem and leave it without including nursing actions taken and the client response.

✦ Be as objective as possible in charting. Rather then charting the client tolerated the procedure well, chart the specific parameters checked to determine that conclusion. Example: "ambulated, tolerated well" would be more effective if charted "ambulated complete length of hall, no shortness of breath noted, pulse rate at 98, respirations at 22."

✦ Each page of the chart should contain the current date and time. Frequently, chart forms are stamped ahead of time. Each time you enter information on a new page, make sure it reflects the current time of charting.

✦ Follow through with who saw the client and what measures were initiated. Particularly note when the doctors visited; if you had to call a doctor for a problem, record the doctor's response. If orders were received, be sure they are signed according to policy. This is especially important, if you had to make several calls to the doctor.

✦ Make sure your notes are legible and clearly reflect the information you intended. It is a good idea to read over your nurse's notes from the previous day to see if they still make sense and accurately portray the status of the client. If the notes do not make sense to you the next day, imagine how difficult it would be to decipher the information at a later date.

(b) No obliteration or erasure of error.

(c) No recopying of page to omit note.

(2) Add omitted information by an "addendum", or "late entry" - give date and time of original note as well as date and time of addendum.

g. Use meaningful, specific language. Do not use words you do not understand or unaccepted abbreviations.

NCLEX ALERT: *Document client care.*

C. Client Identification.

1. Clients and situations at increased risk:

a. . Confused/unconscious client - unable to verbalize or acknowledge treatments or procedures.

b. Surgical procedures - always check the chart against the client's arm band prior to taking them to the operating room.

c. Labor and delivery - when it is necessary to separate mother and infant, identification should be placed on infant before he is ever taken from the delivery area.

d. Newborn infant - in newborn nurseries all infants should have identification that correlates to mothers identification.

2. Always have objective, verifiable evidence of client's identification - client's ID band, medication administration record, client's chart, etc.

NCLEX ALERT: *Verify the identify a client.*

D. Know Your Limits.

1. Physical-Emotional - be aware of fatigue and confusion, and compensate for them.

2. Practice competency - do not perform procedures without adequate preparation, knowledge and experience. Request supervision if unsure of your skills.

3. Never allow anyone to talk you into doing something you are not sure of by letting them agree to take the liability or telling you it is simple.

E. Continuing Education.

1. Mandatory in some states.

2. Important to keep knowledge and skills current.

Specific Situations of Risk

A. Physical Injury to Client.

1. Inappropriate siderail usage.

2. Inadequate attention during ambulation.

3. Obstacles or dangers on floor or in path.

4. Improper transportation.

a. Inadequate locks.

b. Inadequate restraints.

c. Inadequate supervision

5. Improper use of restraints.

B. Medication Errors.

1. Use five rights to protect client.

2. Basic knowledge of all medications administered.
   a. Reason the client is receiving the medication.
   b. Major side effects.
   c. Anticipated client response to medication.
3. Never give drugs without complete order with name, route, dose, frequency.
4. *When medication orders are not complete or there is an obvious contraindication to the administration of the medication, the practical nurse must notify the RN.*

C. Administration of narcotics.
1. Never sign out for a narcotic you do not personally administer.
2. Do not sign as a witness for narcotic wasting unless you actually observed the procedure.
3. Have another licensed person (RN or LPN/VN) co-sign whenever it is necessary to waste a narcotic.

D. Telephone and Other Verbal Orders.
1. Practical nurses must be aware of policies and procedures of the institution regarding telephone and verbal doctor's orders. Some institutions do not allow the PN to take doctor's orders. The practical nurse is legally obligated to follow the policy of the employing institution.
2. Verify all orders at the time they are received, and again, should any questions arise.
3. Obtain needed signature promptly.

E. Consents.
1. Do not witness client signature unless client understands procedure or refuses to receive information.
2. Carefully document events around signature of consent.
3. Take withdrawal of consent seriously.

F. Changes in client's condition.

NCLEX ALERT: *Notify other health care team members about change in client's status.*

1. Notify appropriate individuals.
2. Challenge failure to provide appropriate care.

G. Restraints - Any device that the client cannot remove and restricts freedom of movement or access to one's body.
1. Restraints are used only when ono other option is available.
2. A physician's order is required to utilize a restraint on a client.
3. The client's family should be involved in the plan of care and consulted if the health care team determines restraints are necessary.
4. In an emergency, a physical restraint should be applied only after assessing the client. An order for the restraint should be obtained within an hour.
5. Safe nursing practice includes:
   a. Check restrained client every 30 minutes.
   b. Every 2 hours restraints should be removed and range of motion performed on extremities.
   c. Documentation should include time of each check and status of client's extremities with regard to circulatory status of the restrained extremity.
   d. Restraints should be removed as soon as possible.
   e. Orders for restraints should be renewed every 24 hours.

Management of Client Care

Supervision of Unlicensed Health Care Workers

A. Delegation, according to the NCSBN is "entrusting the performance of selected nursing tasks to competent persons in selected situations. The nurse retains the accountability for the total nursing care of the individuals." (NCSBN, 1990.) Most often delegation is considered to be the role of the r*egistered nurse.*

B. Supervision, according to the NCSBN is "provision of guidance by a qualified nurse for the accomplishment of nursing task or activity with initial direction of the task or activity and periodic inspection of the actual act of accomplishing the task or activity (NCSBN, 1990.).

NCLEX ALERT: *Assign client care to assistive personnel (e.g. CNAS's, etc.)*

C. Role of the practical nurse in supervision.
1. To make sure the unlicensed person understands the directions of what they are supposed to do. They should acknowledge to the nurse they understand the direction.
2. The practical nurse should make periodic checks to determine that the unlicensed person is performing the tasks as directed.

3. If the unlicensed person does not carry out the tasks correctly, the practical/vocational nurse should correct the action in a professional manner and if the problem is nor resolved, the registered nurse should be notified.
4. The practical/vocational nurse should assign tasks to the CNAS that are clearly defined and have very specific guidelines - bathing, ambulating, obtaining equipment, client hygiene, etc.

D. Prioritizing client care assignments.

1. Identify the most ill or unstable client on your assignment - evaluate and care for that client first.
2. Physiological needs are a priority - education and communication are needs that can wait until physiological needs are met. Of the physiological needs airway, breathing and circulation (ABC's) are priority.
3. Initially review the assigned client list, considering the report received on each client, determine which client needs immediate physical assistance in order to maintain their safety.

NCLEX ALERT: *Organize and prioritize care for an assigned group of clients.*

Study Questions—Nursing Concepts

1. Under what category would data relating to a client's problems be placed?

① planning.
② assessment.
③ evaluation
④ nursing diagnosis.

2. In the nursing process, what is the role of the practical nurse in the assessment phase?

① is involved in preventive and therapeutic nursing delivery.
② through observations and evaluations makes appropriate changes in the plan of care.
③ assists in the development of the database by the collection of client-based information.
④ functions only in the implementation of the nursing care plan.

3. Information reported by the client or family is considered what type of information?

① assessment information.
② objective data.
③ evaluative information.
④ subjective data.

4. What is the best position for a client who is on bed rest?

① semi-Fowler's.
② supine.
③ left lateral Sims.
④ prone.

5. At 5pm the nurse begins to chart, after entering the initial information, she realizes that she is charting on the wrong chart. What is the best way to correct the error?

① white out the error and initial it.
② erase the information.
③ recopy the information on another page.
④ draw a line through the error and initial it.

6. What is the rationale for an NPO order?

① to reduce the possibility of abdominal ascites.
② to increase the production of digestive enzymes.
③ to assist in the stimulation of peristalsis.
④ to reduce the possibility of vomiting and aspiration.

7. What are the common preoperative medications?

① antiemetics, sedative, and drugs to increase secretions.
② anticonvulsant, diuretic, and cardiac stimulant.
③ antiemetics, narcotic, and drugs to decrease secretions.
④ antibiotic, antidepressant, and diuretic.

8. Why should surgical clients void before receiving a preoperative medication?

① give an accurate account of their I & O for that day.
② reduce the risk of bladder pain during surgery.
③ promote the physiological safety of the client during surgery.
④ decrease the possibility of infection.

9. What is the most probable cause of shock in the postoperative client?

① increased blood pressure.
② decreased blood volume.
③ decreased body temperature.
④ increased metabolism.

10. What potential problem should the practical nurse anticipate when too much strain is placed on the suture line?

① thrombosis.
② infection.
③ evisceration.
④ dehiscence.

11. What condition occurs when peristalsis is absent?

① gas pain.
② paralytic ileus.
③ diarrhea.
④ abdominal cramps.

12. A wound is left open after surgery and allowed to heal from the inside to the outside. This describes what type of healing?

① first intention.
② second intention.
③ primary healing.
④ superficial healing.

13. A client with a dehiscence is placed on bed rest. What is the purpose of bed rest for this client?

① to decrease oxygen consumption.
② to increase the healing of the site.
③ to prevent development of pneumonia.
④ to prevent the occurrence of evisceration.

14. What nursing measure is used to prevent the complication of atelectasis and pneumonia in the hospitalized client?

① turn, cough, and deep breathe.
② range of motion exercise.
③ clear liquid diet with frequent suctioning.
④ bed rest with frequent vital signs.

15. Prior to a surgical procedure, the nurse asks a client to sign an informed consent form. What is important for the nurse to validate prior to the client signing this form?

① the physician has discussed the surgery with the client.
② the client understands the postoperative nursing care.
③ the physician has discussed the possible complications.
④ the client understands the surgery and the risks involved.

16. Postoperative pain and cancer pain may be considered predictable. How can the effectiveness of the analgesics be increased?

① give them PRN.
② administer once a day.
③ plan around the clock dosing.
④ administer twice a day.

17. Geriatric clients are considered high risk for respiratory problems based on problems of immobility and aging changes. What are these changes related to?

① decreased lung expansion and reduced breathing capacity.
② increased breathing and lung capacity.
③ deceased posture and size of chest cavity.
④ increased lung size and decreased tidal volume.

18. With the client in a prone position, the bony prominence most susceptible to skin breakdown include the anterior superior iliac spines and what other area?

① sacrum.
② scapulae.
③ patellae.
④ trochanter.

Appendix 3-1:
NURSING PROCEDURE ■ POSITIONING ■

POSITIONS	PLACEMENT	USE
Fowler's	Head of bed 60-90 degree angle; hips flexed	Thoracic surgery, severe respiratory conditions
Semi-Fowler's	Head of bed 30- 60 degree angle; hips flexed.	Cardiac, respiratory, neurosurgical conditions
Low Fowler's	Head of bed 15-30 degree angle; hips may or may not be flexed	Postoperative, gastrointestinal conditions
Knee-gatch	Slightly elevate section of bed under knees	For client comfort; contraindicated for vascular disorders
Trendelenburg	Head of bed lowered and foot raised	Thoracic percussion, vibration, and drainage procedure
Lateral (side-lying or Sim's)	Head of bed lowered; pillows under arm and legs	For client comfort; increases uterine perfusion in pregnancy and prevents supine vena caval syndrome
Lithotomy	On back with thigh flexed against abdomen and legs supported by stirrups	Examination of female reproductive tract and rectum, cystoscopy, and surgical procedures
Prone	Head of bed flat, client on abdomen, head turned to side	To promote drainage postoperative tonsillectomy, to prevent contractures in AKA clients, imperforate anus, spinal bifida

✓ Key Points: Turning to a Prone Position
- Lower the head of the bed to a position that client can tolerate.
- Move the client to the side of the bed away from the side where the client will finally be positioned.
- Position pillows on the side of the bed for the client's head, thorax, chest and feet.

✓ Key Points: Moving the Client Up in Bed
- Lower the head of the bed so that it is flat or as low as the client can tolerate.
- Place one arm under the client's shoulders and the other arm under the client's thighs.
- Face the direction of the move, flex your knees and feet should be placed to provide wide base for support.
- Instruct the client to bend legs, put feet flat on bed, and push.

✓ Key Points: Moving the Client with Assistance
- Remove pillow; place it at the head of the bed.
- Hold drawsheet firmly with one hand at client's shoulders and one hand at client's thighs.
- Move close to client for proper support

✓ Key Points: Dangling at the Bedside
- Raise the head of the bed until the client is sitting upright.
- Place one arm around shoulders and grasp knees with the other arm.
- In one motion, swing client's legs over bedside to sitting position.

✓ Key Points: Moving from Bed to Chair
- Move client to the side of the bed closest to the edge where the client will be getting up.
- Raise head of bed to assist client in pivoting to the side of the bed.
- Move client to edge of bed and place feet flat on floor.
- Have client reach across chair and grasp arm.
- Stabilize client by positioning your foot at the outside edge of client's foot.
- Pivot client into chair using leg muscles instead of back muscles.
- Pull client back and up in wheelchair for better posture.

✓ Key Points: Logrolling the Client
- Used for neck and back injury or surgical client.
- Maintain proper alignment of client's head and back areas while turning.
- Before moving patient, place a pillow between knees.
- Move client in one coordinated movement.

Clinical Tips for Problem Solving

If client is unable to assist with movement, then —

- ❏ Use a turn sheet to provide more support for client.
- ❏ Obtain additional assistance to help in moving the client.

If client is unable to maintain any type of position without assistance, then —

- ❏ Use trochanter roll made from bath blankets to align the client's hips to prevent external rotation.
- ❏ Use foam bolsters to maintain side-lying positions.
- ❏ Use folded towels, blankets, or small pillows, position client's hands and arms to prevent dependent edema.

If skin begins to break down, then —

- ❏ Keep client off affected area until healed.
- ❏ Change client's position every two hours.
- ❏ Check with physician for therapeutic mattress or medications for pressure sores.

Appendix 3-2: ANALGESICS

MEDICATIONS	SIDE EFFECTS	NURSING IMPLICATIONS

❖ GENERAL NURSING IMPLICATIONS ❖

— Tell client to take oral doses with food to minimize GI irritation.
— Discuss with client anticipated relief of pain.

1. Assess pain parameters, blood pressure, pulse, and respiratory status before and periodically after administration.
2. Administer before pain is severe for better analgesic effect.
3. Regular administration may be more effective than doses as needed.
4. Caution should be used in clients with increased intracranial pressure.
5. Elderly or debilitated patients may require decreased dosages.
6. Instruct patient to change position slowly to minimize orthostatic hypotension.
7. Warn patient to avoid activities requiring alertness until effects of drug are known.
8. Discuss ways to minimize dry mouth and constipation.

NARCOTIC ANALGESICS: Alter the perception of and emotional response to pain. Controlled substances (Schedule II).

Strong Opiod Analgesics

MEDICATIONS	SIDE EFFECTS	NURSING IMPLICATIONS
Morphine sulfate (MS):PO, SQ, IM, IV Meperidine (**Demerol**): PO, SQ, IM Fentanyl Citrate (**Fentanyl, Sublimzae**) IM, IC, PO, transdermal	Respiratory depression Orthostatic hypotension Sedation, dizziness, lightheadedness, dysphoria Constipation Tolerance, physical and psychological dependence	1. Morphine and meperidine are commonly used for PCA. 2. Demerol has an increased toxicity and seizures in children and geriatrics, 3. Use with caution in clients with respiratory compromise. 4. Requires documentation as required by law.

Moderate to Strong Opiod Analgesics

MEDICATIONS	SIDE EFFECTS	NURSING IMPLICATIONS
Hydromorphone (**Dilaudid**): PO, SQ, IM, IV, rectal suppository Codeine: PO, SQ Oxycodone (**Percodan, Percocet, Tylox**): PO Propoxyphene (**Darvon, Darvocet**): PO	Sedation, euphoria, Respiratory depression, Constipation, Urinary retention Cough suppression.	Usually administered by mouth Codeine is extremely effective cough suppressant Warn client to avoid activities requiring mental alertness until effects of drug are known.

Moderate Opiods

MEDICATIONS	SIDE EFFECTS	NURSING IMPLICATIONS
Butorphanol (**Stadol**): IM, IV, nasal spray Nalbuphine (**Nubain**) SQ, IV, IM Pentazocine (**Talwin, Talwin Nx**): PO, SQ, IM, IV		

***NURSING PRIORITY:** Concurrent administration with non-narcotic analgesics may enhance pain relief because they act at different sites. CNS depression occurs with alcohol, antihistamines, and sedative/hypnotics.*

Appendix 3-2: ANALGESICS

MEDICATIONS	SIDE EFFECTS	NURSING IMPLICATIONS
NON-NARCOTIC ANALGESICS: Act peripherally to prevent the formation of prostaglandins in inflamed tissue, inhibiting the stimulation of pain receptors. Also, inhibit prostaglandin synthesis in the CNS and stimulate peripheral vasodilation to cause antipyresis.		
Acetaminophen (**Tylenol, Datril, Tempra**): PO Aspirin (**ASA**, Acetylsalicylic acid): PO Ibuprofen (**Motrin, Nuprin, Advil**): PO Naproxen (**Naprosyn**); PO Naproxen sodium (**Anaprox**): PO Piroxicam (**Feldene**): PO Sulindac (**Clinoril**): PO	GI pain and upset, nausea, vomiting, diarrhea, heartburn Dizziness, headache, tinnitus (aspirin)	1. Nonsteroidal anti-inflammatory agents may prolong bleeding time and increase the effects of oral anticoagulant, use is contraindicated in pregnancy and preoperatively. 2. Chronic use of acetaminophen may cause renal and liver damage. 3. ***Uses:*** **Mild to moderate pain**: acetaminophen, aspirin, ibuprofen, naproxen. **Fever:** acetaminophen, aspirin, ibuprofen **Inflammation:** aspirin, naproxen **Arthritis:** aspirin, ibuprofen, naproxen, piroxicam, sulindac **Dysmenorrhea:** ibuprofen, naproxen

NURSING PRIORITY: *Advise patient that CDC warns against giving aspirin to children or adolescents with influenza.*

MEDICATIONS	SIDE EFFECTS	NURSING IMPLICATIONS
NARCOTIC ANTAGONISTS: Competitively block the effects of narcotics, without producing analgesic effects.		
Naloxone (**Narcan**)	Hypotension, hypertension, dysrhythmias	1. Assess respiratory status, blood pressure, pulse, and level of consciousness until narcotic wears off. Repeat doses may be necessary if effect of narcotic outlasts the effect of the narcotic antagonist. 2. Remember that narcotic antagonists reverse analgesia along with respiratory depression. Titrate dose accordingly and monitor pain level. 3. ***Uses***: Used to reverse CNS and respiratory depression in narcotic overdose. 4. ***Contraindications and precautions:*** Use with caution in narcotic-dependent patients; may cause severe withdrawal symptoms.

Appendix 3-3: PREOPERATIVE MEDICATIONS

CLASSIFICATION	SIDE EFFECTS	NURSING IMPLICATIONS
SEDATIVES: Decrease anxiety the evening prior to surgery.		
Amobarbital (**Amytal**): PO Pentobarbital (**Nembutal**): PO, rectal Secobarbital (**Seconal**): PO, IV, IM, rectal Lorazepam **(Ativan)**: PO, IM, IV	May produce paradoxical effects in elderly Confusion and dizziness	1. Decreased stimuli in room after administration. 3. Offer emotional support to anxious client. 4. **Ativan** has decreased incidence of paradoxical response. 5. Versed commonly used for conscious sedation.
Midazolam hydrochloride (**Versed**) IM, IV	Decreased respirations, pain at IM or IV site, Nausea, vomiting	
ANTIHISTAMINES: Potentiates effect of preoperative narcotic, decreases postoperative nausea, and has sedative effects.		
Promethazine hydrochloride (**Phenergan**): PO, IM Hydroxyzine hydrochloride (**Vistaril, Atarax**): PO, IM	Blurred vision, hypotension, flushed skin	1. Frequently administered with **Demerol** as preoperative medication. 2. **Vistaril** must be given deep IM (preferably Z track) to prevent tissue irritation.
ANTICHOLINERGIC: Reduces oral, bronchial, gastrointestinal secretions, decreases gastrointestinal motility, bronchodilates, decreases incidence of laryngospasm.		
Atropine: PO, IM, IV Scopolamine: PO, IM	Flushed face Dilated pupils Increased cardiac rate Urinary retention Children more susceptible to side effects.	1. Elderly and children are at higher risk for side effects. 2. Advise clients regarding atropine flush. 3. Administer with caution to the glaucoma, MI, and CHF client. 4. Postural hypotension may result if client ambulates after parenteral administration. 5. Monitor for urinary retention and decreased bowel sounds.
TRANQUILIZERS: Decrease anxiety prior to surgery.		
Diazepam (**Valium**): PO Droperidol (**Inapsine**): PO Lorazepam **(Ativan)**: PO	Hypotension. May cause dizziness, clumsiness, or confusion.	1. Decrease stimuli in room after administration. 2. Offer emotional support to anxious client.

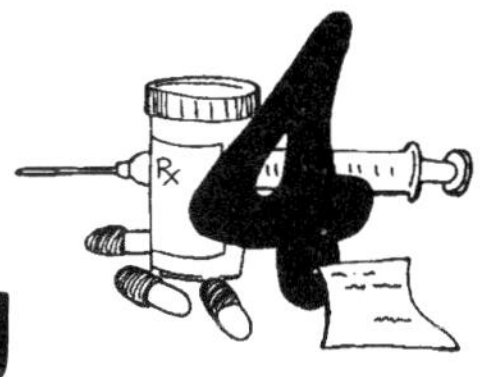

Pharmacology

GENERAL CONCEPTS OF PHARMACOLOGY

❑ **No medication has a single action; all medications have the potential to alter more than one body function.**

NURSING PRIORITY: *Many medications have several actions that are desirable. Carefully evaluate the questions as to what is the desired response of the medication for the specific client situation. Example: Aspirin—prophylactic for stroke or MI; relieve inflammation in the arthritic client.*

1. Desired action—the desired, predictable response for which the medication is administered.
2. Side effects (drug reaction)—the undesirable, or unwanted response; frequently predictable.
3. Unpredictable response—the unusual response to a medication.
   a. Idiosyncratic reaction—an individual, unexpected response to a medication.
   b. Allergic reaction—does not occur with the initial dose of medication; occurs with subsequent doses because it requires that the immune system respond with the production of antibodies in order to trigger the allergic reaction.

A. The Drug Amendments of 1962 made it mandatory that each medication have one official name.
   1. Generic name (nonproprietary)—the official designated name which the medication is listed under in official publications.
   2. Chemical name—designates the specific chemical composition of the medication.
   3. Trade (proprietary name, brand)—the name designated and registered by a specific manufacturer.

NCLEX ALERT: *Typically, the medications on the exam will be identified with both the generic and trade name, i.e., diazepam **(Valium)**.*

B. Factors influencing dosage—response relationships.
   1. Age—the young infant and the elderly are generally more sensitive to medications.
   2. Medication history—the prior administration of medications may greatly affect the client's response.
      a. Tolerance—medications administered repeatedly begin to produce progressively decreased effects.
      b. Cumulative effects—more medication is being administered than is being removed.
      c. Medication interactions—the effects of one medication may be increased, decreased, or eliminated by the prior administration of another medication.
   3. Presence of disease process, specifically kidney and liver problems.
   4. Method of administration.
   5. Adequate cardiac output.
   6. Emotional factors—clients are more likely to respond to a medication in a positive manner if they have confidence in their physician and anticipate the therapeutic effects.

Drug Interactions

A. Pharmacokinetic Interaction

❑ **Drug interaction can be defined as an altered or modified action or effect of a drug as a result of interaction with one or more drugs. It is not to be confused with adverse drug reaction or drug incompatibility.**

1. Drug interaction can change the absorption, distribution, metabolism, or excretion of one or both drugs. Letters **ADME** are often used to represent these processes .
   a. **A**bsorption—drugs can block, decrease, or increase absorption. Does this by an ↑ or ↓ in gastric emptying time, changing gastric pH, or by forming drug complexes.
   b. **D**istribution—altered distribution occurs when two drugs that bind to the same plasma proteins are taken.
   c. **M**etabolism—a drug may affect the metabolism of another drug by stimulating or inhibiting enzymes secreted from the liver.
   d. **E**xcretion—a change in urine pH or cardiac output can effect the excretion of a drug.
2. Adverse drug reaction—undesirable drug effect ranging from mild untoward effects to severe responses, including hypersensitivity reaction and anaphylaxis.

3. Drug incompatibility—a chemical or physical reaction that occurs among two or more drugs *in vitro* (outside the body).

B. Pharmacodynamic Interactions

1. Additive effect—get twice the effect.
   - *Example:* Desirable additive effect occurs when giving a diuretic and a beta blocker for hypertension or giving two analgesics (e.g., aspirin and codeine) for increased pain relief. Undesirable additive effect can occur from two vasodilators (**Apresoline** and nitroglycerin) for angina can lead to severe decreased BP.
2. Synergistic or potentiation effect—greater than twice the effect.
   - *Example:* Desirable synergistic effect is when **Demerol** and **Phenergan** are combined causing **Phenergan** to potentiate the effect of **Demerol**.

C. Drug—food interactions.

1. Food can bind with drugs and delay drug absorption.
   - *Example:* Tetracyclines bind with dairy products → decrease in plasma tetracycline.
2. Food increases the absorption of nitrofurantoin (**Macrodantin**)—anti-infective, metoprolol (**Lopressor**)—beta blocker, and lovastatin (**Mevacor**)—anti-lipemic.
3. MAO inhibitors (**Marplan**)—antidepressants when taken with tyramine-rich foods (i.e., cheese, wine, organ meats, beer, yogurt) may lead to a hypertensive crisis.

D. Drug-laboratory interactions.

1. Abnormal plasma or serum electrolytes can affect drugs.
   - *Example:* Digitalis toxicity can occur when a client's serum potassium and magnesium are decreased or serum calcium increased.

Geriatric Pharmacology Considerations

1. See Table 4-1.

MEDICATION ADMINISTRATION

> ***NURSING PRIORITY:*** *The nurse's responsibility in administering medication is influenced by three primary factors: nursing guidelines for safe medication administration, pharmacological implications of the medication, and the legal aspects of medication administration.*

Nursing Responsibilities in Medication Administration

A. Administer according to the "5 Rights."

1. Right medication.
2. Right dosage.
3. Right route of administration.
4. Right time.
5. Right client.
6. Sixth right—right charting (documentation).

B. A nurse should administer only those medications which she has prepared.

C. Be familiar with medication.

1. General purpose the client is receiving the medication.
2. Common side effects.
3. Average dose or range of safe dosage.
4. Any specific safety precautions prior to administration (digitalis—check apical pulse, heparin—check clotting times).

D. Document medication against physician's orders according to institution policy.

E. Evaluate client's overall condition and assess for changes which may indicate the medication is contraindicated. (e.g., morphine would be contraindicated in a client developing increased intracranial pressure).

> **NCLEX ALERT:** *Observe for effects of medications (e.g., therapeutic effects, adverse effects, side effects.)*

F. Evaluate compatibility with other medications the client is receiving.

G. Use appropriate aseptic technique in preparing and administering medication.

H. Do not leave medications at the client's bedside without a doctor's order to do so.

I. If client is to administer his own medication, review with him correct administration (i.e., eye drops).

> **NCLEX ALERT:** *Evaluate clients use of medications (prescription, over-the-counter, home remedies.)*

LEGAL IMPLICATIONS

Nurse's Legal Responsibilities in Administration of Medication

A. The nurse administers a medication only by order of a licensed physician and according to provisions of the specific institution.

Table 4-1: GERIATRIC PHARMACOLOGY AND NURSING IMPLICATIONS

PHYSIOLOGIC CONSIDERATIONS	BODY EFFECTS & POSSIBLE DRUG RESPONSES
ABSORPTION	
GI: ↑ pH (alkaline) gastric secretions ↓ Peristalsis with delayed intestinal emptying time	↓ Gastric acidity alters absorption of weak acid drugs, such as aspirin. ↓ In gastrointestinal motility rate (peristalsis) may delay onset of action.
Cardiac: ↓ Cardiac output ↓ Blood flow	↓ Blood flow to the gastrointestinal tract (40-50% less) is due to a ↓ in cardiac output. Because of the reduction of blood flow, absorption is slowed but not decreased.
DISTRIBUTION	
↓ Body water and fluids ↑ Fat to water ratio ↓ Serum protein and albumin	Water-soluble drugs are more concentrated. Fat-soluble drugs are likely to accumulate. There are fewer protein-binding sites, resulting in more free drug. Drugs with a high affinity for protein compete with other drugs for protein-binding sites. Drug interactions result due to a lack of protein sites and an increase in free drugs.
METABOLISM	
Liver: ↓ Enzyme function ↓ Blood flow ↓ Total liver function	↓ Liver function causes a reduction in drug metabolism. With a reduction in metabolic rate, the half-life of drugs increases, and drug accumulation can result. Metabolism of a drug inactivates the drug and prepares it for elimination via the kidneys. Drug toxicity might occur when the half-life is prolonged.
EXCRETION	
Renal: ↓ Blood flow by 40-50% ↓ Functioning nephrons (kidney cells) ↓ Glomerular filtration rate by 40-50%	With a decrease in renal function, there is a decrease in drug excretion and drug accumulation results. Drug toxicity should be assessed continually while the client is on the drug.

B. The nurse should not automatically carry out an order if the dosage is outside the normal range or if the route of administration is not appropriate; he/she should consult the physician.

NCLEX ALERT: *Pay particular attention to medications that have specific nursing implications. Questions may be based on when you would contact the physician regarding the appropriateness of a medication order.*

C. The nurse is legally responsible for the medication he/she administers, even when the medication is administered according to a physician's order.

D. The nurse is responsible for evaluating the client prior to and after the administration of a prn medication.

E. The nurse must administer the medication according to the nursing responsibilities previously discussed.

F. The medication should be charted as soon as possible after administration.

G. When taking verbal orders on the phone, carefully repeat all the orders to verify they are correct.

H. Medication errors:

1. If an error is found in a physician's drug order, it is the nurse's responsibility to question the order.

2. Always report medication errors to the physician immediately.
3. It is the nurse's responsibility to carefully assess the client for effects of the erroneous medication.
4. Medication errors should be documented in an incident report and on the client's chart.

Methods of Medication Administration

(Note: This section on medications should not be used as a procedure guideline. The purpose is to note specific characteristics of each method. All medications are administered according to previously discussed nursing responsibilities in medication administration.)

NCLEX ALERT: *Administer medications via oral, topical, subcutaneous, or IM routes*

A. Oral medication.
  1. Assess level of consciousness and ability to follow directions.
  2. Evaluate swallow reflex.

B. Topical medications.
  1. Skin application—evaluate condition of skin in area medication is to be applied; if appropriate, rotate sites to prevent irritation.
  2. Sublingual—allow medication to dissolve under the tongue; client should not chew or swallow.
  3. Nasal—position client to allow nose drops or spray to enter nares directly without contaminating the eyes.
  4. Eyes—medication must be specifically indicated for ophthalmic use.
    a. Instill one or two drops in the middle of the lower conjunctival sac.
    b. Do not allow tip of applicator to come in contact with the eye.
    c. Do not drop medication directly on the cornea.
    d. Direct client to close their eyes gently to distribute the medication.
    e. Make sure you administer the correct medication in the correct eye.
  5. Ears—medication is instilled into the auditory canal.
    a. Position client with affected ear upward.
    b. Children under three—pull pinna down and backward.
    c. Older children, adults—pull pinna up and backward.
    d. Administer solution at room temperature.
    e. Keep client in the same position for appropriate time to prevent medication from coming out.
  6. Suppositories
    a. Rectal—absorption from rectal mucosa is slower and less predictable than in systemic medications.
      (1) Frequently given for nausea and vomiting.
      (2) May be preferred route for infant.
      (3) Insert with blunt end advanced first through the rectal sphincter, especially if client is having difficulty retaining when the suppository is inserted with the tapered end first.
    b. Vaginal—absorption across vaginal mucous membranes.
      (1) Should maintain supine position after insertion.
      (2) Should not douche unless advised by physician.

C. Transdermal medication—medication is stored in a patch or is measured on a dose-determined applicator that is placed on the skin; absorption occurs through the skin.
  1. Provides more consistent blood levels and avoids GI problems.
  2. Patch sites should be rotated and areas cleansed after use.
  3. Patch should not be applied over inflamed areas.
  4. Do not allow transdermal medications to come in contact with your skin, since absorption of medication can then occur in the nurse.
  5. Patch needs to come in contact with skin (excessive body hair may need to be removed).

D. Inhalation medication—medication is in an aerosol form and is inhaled and absorbed throughout the respiratory tract.
  1. Position in semi-Fowler's.
  2. Check instructions for inhaler use and make sure client understands.

E. Parenteral medications—the administration of medications by some method of injection.
  1. Intradermal injection—administered just below the skin surface.
    a. Use syringe with appropriate calibrations since amount is very small in volume (.01 to .10 cc).
    b. Use small gauge (26) needle; $\frac{3}{8}$ to $\frac{3}{8}$ inch long.
    c. Select area where skin is thin (inner surface of forearm, middle of back).

d. Insert needle bevel edge up at 15° angle.

e. Frequently used for tuberculin testing, local anesthetic, allergy testing.

2. Subcutaneous injection—medication injected into fatty tissue, just below the dermis.
   a. Medication should be small in volume (0.5 to 1.5 cc) and nonirritating.
   b. Area on outer surface of upper arm, anterior surface of the thigh, or the abdomen are frequent sites.
   c. Use 25 or 26 gauge needle, $\frac{1}{2}$ to 1 inch long, and insert at 45° angle or 90° depending on body size and location.

3. Intramuscular injection—injection of medication into the muscle.
   a. The amount of medication is usually 0.5 to 3.0 cc.
   b. Appropriate sites (Figure 4-1).
      (1) Deltoid and dorsal gluteal.
      (2) Ventrogluteal and vastus lateralis.
   c. Use 1 to $1\frac{1}{2}$ inch needle; gauge of needle depends on viscosity of medication; insert needle at 90° angle.
   d. Aspirate when needle is in place; if no blood returns, administer medication.

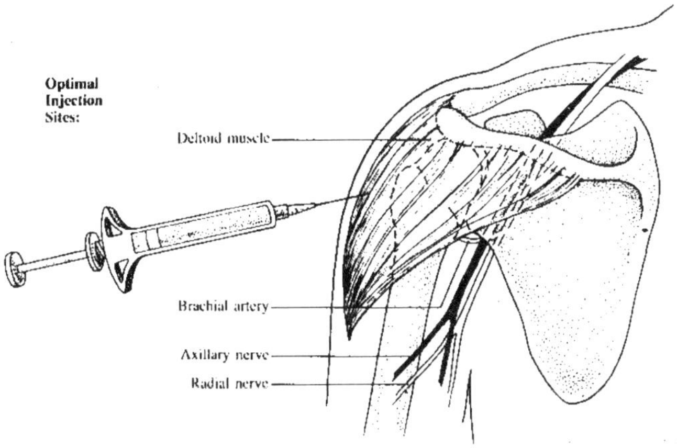

Deltoid

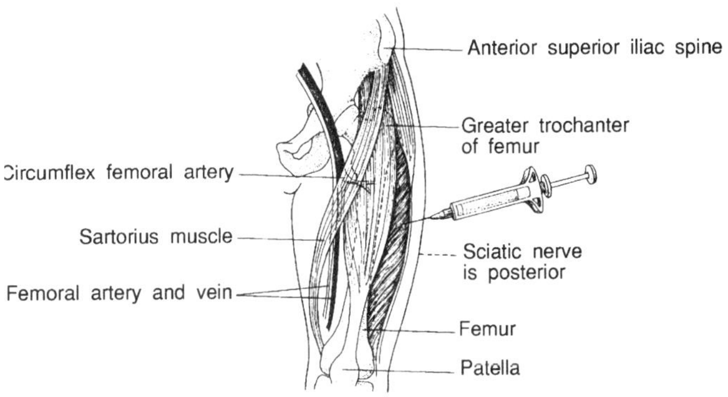

Vastus lateralis

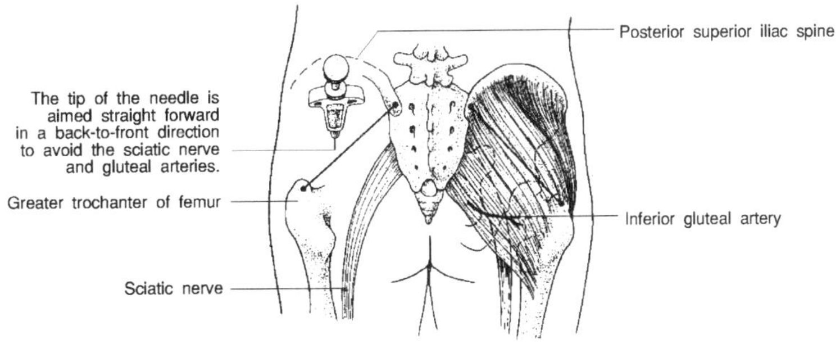

Dorsogluteal

Figure 4-1: Intramuscular Injection Sites

e. Z-track technique is utilized to prevent medication from leaking back through the needle track and irritating or staining subcutaneous tissue.
(1) After medication is drawn up, change the needle.
(2) Pull skin over to one side at the injection site.
(3) Inject medication through taut skin into the muscle at site selected.
(4) Remove the needle and release the skin. As the stretched tissue returns to its original position, the needle track is sealed.
(5) The most preferable site is the dorsogluteal area.

f. Intramuscular injections in children.
(1) Vastus lateralis is common site in infants.
(2) Dorsogluteal area is generally not used unless child is walking.
(3) Needle is inserted about 1 inch.

Forms of Medication Preparations

A. Solids.
1. Capsule—medication is placed in cylindrical gelatin container.
2. Pills, tablets—medication is pressed into solid form of various shapes and colors.
   a. Enteric coated—prevents medication from being released in stomach; dissolves in intestine (do not crush enteric coated tablets.)
   b. Lozenge—flavored tablet that is held in the mouth for slow release of medication.
3. Suppositories—generally kept in cool area; will melt at body temperature; may produce local or systemic effect.
   a. Rectal.
   b. Vaginal.
   c. Urethral.
4. Ointments—used for external application.
5. Powders—finely ground medications which are stable only in dry form; frequently mixed with solution prior to administration.

B. Solutions.
1. Spirits—alcohol solutions of volatile substances (camphor spirits).
2. Syrups—medication prepared in an aqueous sugar solution.
3. Elixirs—solutions containing alcohol, sugar and water; may or may not have medicine ingredients.
4. Suspensions—finely ground particles of medication dispersed in a liquid; shake all suspensions well before preparing dose (antacids).
5. Emulsions—medication is dispersed in an oil or fat solution; shake all emulsions well before preparing dose.
6. Liniments, lotions—medication is dispersed in a mixture of oil, soap, alcohol, water; used for external application.

Calculation of Medication Dosages

Frequently, medications are not ordered by the physician in the amounts supplied by the pharmacy. In these situations, it is necessary for the nurse to calculate the correct dosage. Another important area of calculation is in the administration of intravenous solutions. It is essential that the nurse have a good working knowledge of the fundamental principles of mathematics in order to calculate medications correctly.

- **Equivalent Conversions—medication dosages used in a mathematical formula must be in the same system of measurement**

Convert grains to milligrams: multiply by 60 (60 mg = 1 gr).

$$\frac{1}{2} gr = ?\ mg$$

$$\frac{1}{2} gr \ x \ \frac{60}{1} = 30\ mg$$

Convert milligrams to grains: divide number of milligrams by 60.

$$30\ mg = ?\ gr$$

$$30\ div\ by\ 60 = \frac{1}{2}\ gr$$

Convert grams to milligrams: multiply by 1,000.

$$5\ gm = 5{,}000\ mg$$

Convert milligrams to grams: divide by 1,000.

$$500\ mg = .5\ gm$$

- **Oral medication calculations**

$$\frac{Dose\ desired}{Dose\ on\ hand} = amount\ \ to\ \ give$$

- **Example:** Order reads to give **Keflex** 500 mg. Dose on hand is 250 mg capsules.

$$\frac{500}{250} = 2\ capsules$$

$$\frac{Dose\ desired}{Dose\ on\ hand}\ x\ quantity = amount\ to\ give$$

- **Example:** Order reads to give ampicillin 350 mg. Dose on hand is 250 mg. in 5 cc.

$$\frac{350}{250} x\ 5 = X$$

$$350\ div\ by\ 250 = 1.4$$

$$1.4\ x\ 5cc = 7cc$$

The problem can also be set up in algebraic proportion:

$$\frac{350mg}{X} = \frac{250mg}{5cc}$$

$$250X = 1{,}750$$

$$X = 7cc$$

▪ Parenteral medication calculations

$$\frac{Dose\ desired}{Dose\ on\ hand} x\ quantity\ of\ solution = amount\ to\ give$$

- **Example:** Order reads 75 mg of **Demerol**. On hand is 100 mg in 1 cc.

$$\frac{75mg}{100mg} x\ 1cc = X$$

$$75\ div\ by\ 100 = .75$$

$$.75\ x\ 1cc = .75cc\ or \frac{3}{4}\ cc$$

Set up in algebraic proportion, the equation reads:

$$\frac{75mg}{x} = \frac{100mg}{1cc}$$

$$100X = 75$$

$$X = .75cc\ or \frac{3}{4}\ cc$$

- **Example:** Order reads to give ⅙ gr Morphine sulfate. On hand is 15 mg in 2 cc.

$$\frac{1}{6} gr = ?\ mg$$

$$\frac{1}{6} x \frac{60}{1} = 10mg$$

$$\frac{10mg}{15mg} x\ 2cc = amount\ to\ give$$

$$10\ div\ by\ 15 = .67cc$$

$$.67\ x\ 2cc = 1.3cc$$

▪ Intravenous medication calculation

To determine how long an infusion will run, divide the total number of cc's to infuse by the hourly infusion rate.

$$\frac{Amount\ to\ infuse}{Hourly\ rate} = Number\ of\ hours$$

- **Example:** Order reads 1,000 cc at 125 cc per hour. How long will it take the 1,000 cc to infuse?

$$\frac{1000}{125} = X$$

$$1000\ div\ by\ 125 = 8\ hours$$

To determine how many cc per hour an infusion will run, divide the total number of cc to infuse by the infusion time.

$$\frac{Amount\ to\ infuse}{Total\ infusion\ time} = cc\ per\ hour$$

- **Example:** Order reads 1,000 cc to run every 8 hours. How many cc's per hour?

$$1000cc\ div\ by\ 8\ hours = 125cc\ per\ hour$$

Calculating drop factors—check the intravenous equipment to determine how many drops are delivered in 1 cc. For example purposes, a drop factor of 10 gtt per 1 cc is used. The following are two formulas to calculate this factor.

$$\frac{Total\ cc}{Times\ in\ minutes} = cc\ per\ \min\ x\ drop\ factor\ = gtt\ per\ \min$$

- **Example:** 1,000 cc is ordered to infuse in 8 hours. Set drop factor is 10 gtt per cc.

$$\frac{1000cc}{480min} = 2.08\ cc\ per\ minute$$

$$2.08\ x\ 10 = 20.8\ or\ 21\ gtt / \min$$

- **Example:** 500 cc is ordered to infuse in 2 hours. Set calibration is 10 gtt per cc.

$$\frac{500cc}{120min} = 4.16\ x\ 10 = 41.6\ or\ 42\ gtt / \min$$

Determine the number of cc per hour and divide by 60 (60 minutes in 1 hour). This equals the number of cc (ml) per minute. Multiply by set calibration of number of gtts per cc.

$$\frac{Number\ of\ cc\ per\ hour}{60} = cc\ per\ \min$$

$$cc\ per\ minute\ x\ set\ calibrations = gtt / \min$$

- **Example:** 500 cc is ordered to infuse in 2 hours. Set calibration is 10 gtt per cc. (250 cc/hr to infuse).

$$\frac{250cc}{60} = 4.16cc\ per\ \min$$

$$4.16cc\ x\ 10 = 41.6\ or\ 42\ gtt / \min$$

- **Note:** There may be a 2 to 4 gtt difference when using different formulas.

Study Questions—Pharmacology

1. What should the nurse take into consideration when giving medication to an elderly client?

① multiple simultaneous drugs can be dangerous.
② the elderly client metabolizes and excretes the drugs differently from younger and more active clients.
③ medication affects the elderly client during the early hours of the morning.
④ medication has an effect on the respiratory system of the elderly.

2. A client has an order for Prozac 20mg in the AM and at noon; 10mg tablets are available. How many will the client receive each day?

① 8
② 6
③ 4
④ 3

3. A client has ordered Mellaril elixir 300mg qd at HS. You have Mellaril elixir on the floor at 500 mg/ml. How many ml will the client receive?

① 0.3
② 1.3
③ 0.6
④ 0.5

4. Gentamcin 60 mg IM is ordered for a client. Available is a multi-dose vial with 40mg/cc. What is the correct amount to give?

① 1.5cc
② 1.25cc
③ 2cc
④ 1.75cc

5. To ensure that the right medication was being given, the first step for the nurse would be:

① check the client's ID band.
② read the information insert for directions as to correct administration.
③ check the order with the medication administration sheet.
④ check the expiration date on the medication.

6. The nurse pours a dose of medication then finds that the client no longer needs the dose. What action should the nurse take?

① record the dose as taken to keep the count correct.
② charge for the dose because the dose must be paid for.
③ record the medication as "not taken" and waste the poured dose.
④ pour the medication back into the container.

7. Different medication preparations of drugs are absorbed in the body at different rates of time. Which preparation of a drug absorbs more rapidly?

① ointment applied to the skin.
② liquid medicine given orally.
③ oral gelatin capsules.
④ enteric-coated tablets.

8. Medications taken orally must undergo a change after contact with body fluids in order to be used by the body. This process is know as:

① concentration.
② elimination.
③ transference.
④ absorption.

9. The nurse is verifying whether or not to give a medication to a client. It would be important to first check the :

① client's name.
② expiration date of the drug.
③ route of delivery.
④ chart to see if the drug was ordered.

10. A client is to get Demerol 75 mg IM for pain. While drawing up the medication, the nurse draws up an extra 0.3cc of air in the syringe in order to:

① seal the injection site with an air bubble.
② give the site enough space in case the client is a bleeder.
③ clear the drug from the needle and seal the site.
④ decrease the possibility of infection at the site.

11. What is a characteristic of effective intradermal injection?

① they form a bleb in the dermal are a of the skin.
② the injection is given at a 40 degree angle.
③ the injection site is pressed and rubbed in a circular motion.
④ a small 16 gauge needle is used.

12. What is the correct method for administering eye drops to a geriatric client?

① drop the medication directly on the cornea.
② instruct the client to rapidly open and close their eye to distribute the medication.
③ place the applicator tip on the lower conjunctival sac and instill the drops.
④ instill the drops in the lower conjunctival sac.

13. The nurse is giving an IM injection a 10-month-old infant. Where is the best site to administer the IM injection?

① left upper deltoid area.
② the outer left quadrant of the gluteus.
③ the upper forearm.
④ vastus lateralis muscle of the thigh.

14. There is an order for chlorphreniramine (Chlor-trimeton) 2.5 mg qid. Chlor-trimetron comes in a concentrate of 5mg/ml. What is a single measured dose in milliliters?

① 0.5
② 0.25
③ 2.5
④ 0.15

15. What is important for the nurse to understand about the administration of transdermal medications?

① the medication should be thoroughly rubbed into the skin.
② it should be applied topically PRN throughout the day.
③ the nurse should use the same site every day.
④ avoid touching the medication with hands.

16. Which physiologic changes in the elderly should be given the greatest consideration when administering medications?

① increased cardiac output.
② increased peristalsis.
③ reduced fat to water ratio.
④ reduced liver function.

17. What is the correct method for administering a medication by Z track?

① use a 25 gauge, 5/8 inch needle and infuse the medication slowly and avoid rubbing after the injection to prevent staining and bruising.
② gently pinch a fold of skin up and inject deep IM into the muscle mass, making sure that the injection is into the thick part of the muscle.
③ pull the skin laterally approximately 1/2 inch and insert medication, followed by removing the needle and then releasing the skin.
④ insert the needle halfway into the muscle, retract the skin laterally, and slowly infuse the remaining part.

Appendix 4-1:
CONVERSIONS

▪ Celsius to Fahrenheit

$$\textit{Fahrenheit reading} = \frac{9}{5} \times \textit{Celsius reading} + 32$$

Example: Celsius is 50°.

$$\textit{Fahrenheit} = \frac{9}{5} \times 50 + 32$$

$$90 + 32 = 122 \backslash \textit{ Fahrenheit}$$

▪ Kilograms and pounds

1 kilogram = 2.2 lbs.

To convert kilograms to pounds, multiply the number of kilograms by 2.2.

10 kg x 2.2 lb. = 22 lb.

To convert pounds to kilograms divide the number of pounds by 2.2.

$$\frac{44}{2.2} = 20\ kg.$$

▪ Pounds and grams

1 lb = 454 grams

To convert pounds to grams, multiply the number of pounds by 454.

7.5 x 454 = 3,405 gm.

To convert grams to pounds, divide the number of grams by 454.

Example: An infant weighs 3,405 gm.

$$\frac{3{,}405}{454} = 7.5\ lb.\ or\ 7\ lb.\ 8\ oz.$$

▪ Grains and milligrams

1 grain = 60 milligrams

To convert grains to milligrams, multiply the number of grains by 60.

$$\tfrac{1}{8}\ gr = ?\ mg$$

$$\tfrac{1}{8} \times 60 = 7.5\ mg$$

To convert milligrams to grains, divide the number of milligrams by 60.

$$7.5\ \text{mg} = ?\ \text{gr}$$

$$7.5 \div 60 = .125$$

$$\frac{125}{1000} = \frac{1}{8}$$

Appendix 4-2:
ABBREVIATIONS AND SYMBOLS

aa	of each
ac	before meals
ad lib	as desired
bid	twice daily
$\bar{c}$	with
Ca	calcium
CBC	complete blood count
Cl	chlorine
dr	dram
et	and
ext	extract
fl or fld	fluid
GI	gastrointestinal
gm	gram
gr	grain
gt/gtt	drop/drops
H_20	water
H_20_2	hydrogen peroxide
HS	bedtime (hour of sleep)
in	inch
K	potassium
L	liter
lb or #	pound
liq	liquid
lytes	electrolytes
m	minim
ml	milliliter
Mg	magnesium
N	nitrogen
Na	sodium
NPO	nothing by mouth
od	once daily
OD	right eye
OOB	out of bed
OS	left eye
os	mouth
OU	both eyes
oz	ounce
pc	after meals
po	by mouth
prn	as needed
q	every
qd	every day
qid	four times a day
qod	every other day
qs	as much as required
qt	quart
q2h	every 2 hours
q3h	every 3 hours
$\bar{s}$	without
ss	one half
stat	immediately
tab	tablet
tbs	tablespoon
tid	three times a day
tsp	teaspoon
WBC	white blood count

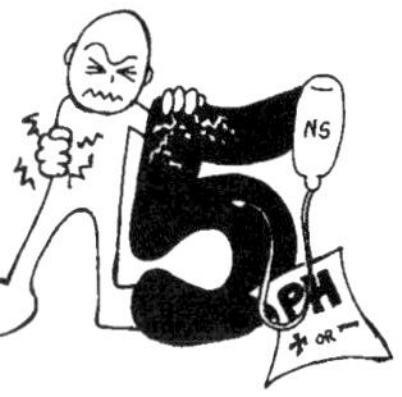

5 Homeostasis

❑ ***Homeostasis*, for the purposes of this chapter, is defined as the mechanism for maintaining a steady state in the body.**

STRESS AND ADAPTATION

❑ ***Stress* is a state produced by a change in the environment that is perceived as challenging, threatening, or damaging to the individual's equilibrium.**

❑ ***Adaptation* is a constant, ongoing process that occurs along the time continuum, beginning with birth and ending with death.**

Stressors

1. Physiologic stressors - change or stimulus which evokes stress.
   a. Chemical agents - drugs, poisons, alcohol.
   b. Physical agents - heat, cold, radiation, electrical shock, trauma.
   c. Infectious agents - viruses, bacteria, fungi.
   d. Faulty immune mechanisms.
   e. Genetic disorders.
   f. Nutritional imbalance.
   g. Hypoxia.
2. Psychosocial stressors.
   a. Accidents and the survivors.
      - *Example:* Airplane crash survivors, prisoners of war, hurricane and earthquake survivors.
   b. Experiences of others in our social network.
      - *Example:* Death of a close friend, neighbor being robbed and beaten.
   c. Horrors of history: Auschwitz, Hiroshima, Chernobyl.
   d. Fear of aggression, mutilation, and destruction.
   e. Events of history brought into our living room.
      - Example: Wars, starvation, robbery.
   f. Changes of the narrower world in which we live and the rapidity in which it occurs.
      - *Example:* Alvin Toffler's *Future Shock* which includes demographic, technologic, economic, and scientific changes.
   g. Life crises - situational, developmental, role, etc.
   h. Inherent conflicts in all social relations.

Stress Response

> ***NURSING PRIORITY:** Understanding of the stress response is basic to many nursing interventions. Identify effects of environmental stressors. Teach stress reduction techniques.*

1. Sympathetic-Adrenal-Medullary Response: **"Fight or Flight."**
   - *Example:* Increased heart rate, blood glucose, and coagulability of blood; pupils dilated; mental activity enhanced; cold, clammy skin; respirations rapid and shallow.
2. What is ***hardiness***? Ability to resist the effects of stress.
   a. Three characteristics.
      (1) Hardy people have a sense of *commitment* to life and work—provides them with a sense of satisfaction and motivation.
      (2) Hardy people look at life's occurrences as *challenges*, not threats—curious about life, not afraid of change.
      (3) Hardy people have a sense of *control* over their lives—don't feel helpless.
   b. Techniques to increase hardiness.
      (1) Decrease time spent watching TV, join volunteer organizations, develop hobbies and interests.
      (2) Take controlled risks (trying a new sport), vary daily activities.
      (3) Set aside time daily and weekly for doing exactly what you want.

Stress Reduction Methods

1. Proper nutrition.
2. Regular exercise, physical activity, and recreation.
3. Meditation, breathing exercises, creative imagery.
4. Communication, time management.
   - *Example:* Expression of feelings, talking it out, organizing time and space to be less hectic.
5. Biofeedback, rolfing (massage of deep connective tissue to achieve realignment of body structure), therapeutic touch, bioenergetics (decrease muscle tension by releasing feelings through physical exertion and verbal techniques).
6. Relaxation response.
   a. Quiet environment.
   b. Passive attitude.

c. Comfortable position.

d. A mental device or object, such as a word, sound, or phrase to occupy the mind and keep out thoughts.

7. Group process and social support.

- *Example:* Groups—Reach for Recovery, Alcoholics Anonymous, etc.

8. Thought stopping - refocusing on more positive thought.

9. Self-hypnosis.

FLUID AND ELECTROLYTES

Physiology

A. Basic concepts of body fluid.

1. Water is a primary body fluid. It is used to transport nutrients as well as to remove waste products.

a. Infant — 70 to 80 percent of body weight is water.

b. Adult —50 to 60 percent of body weight is water.

c. Elderly adult—45 to 55 percent of body weight is water.

2. Electrolytes - electrically charged particles: electrolytes found in intracellular fluid and in extracellular fluid are essentially the same; however, the concentrations differ.

3. Intracellular fluid - fluid located within the cell wall.

a. Approximately 40 to 50 percent of total body fluid.

b. Potassium is the primary electrolyte.

4. Extracellular fluids (ECF) - fluid located outside the cell wall.

a. Approximately 30 to 40 percent of total body water.

b. An infant maintains a larger percentage of extracellular fluids than does an older child or adult.

c. Vascular - circulating plasma volume.

d. Interstitial - fluid surrounding tissue cells.

e. Sodium is the primary electrolyte.

B. Dynamic transport of fluid and electrolytes.

1. Diffusion - movement of molecules from an area of high concentration to an area of low concentration.

2. Osmosis - movement of water through a semipermeable membrane from an area of low electrolyte concentration to an area of high concentration; *osmotic pressure* is term used to describe osmosis (water goes where the salt is.)

3. Filtration - the movement of water and electrolytes through a semipermeable membrane from an area of high pressure to an area of low pressure; *hydrostatic pressure* is term used to describe the force of filtration.

C. Plasma to interstitial fluid shift.

1. Edema - accumulation of fluid in interstitial spaces.

2. Hypovolemia may occur as a result of excessive fluid shift into the interstitial spaces, resulting in circulatory collapse.

Fluid Imbalances (ECF)

NCLEX ALERT: *Monitor client's hydration status (I&O, edema, signs & symptoms of dehydration).*

A. Fluid deficit - dehydration.

1. Sensible fluid loss—fluid loss of which an individual is aware, such as urine.

2. Insensible fluid loss— fluid loss of which an individual is not aware (approximately 1,000 cc of fluid is lost every 24 hours through the skin and lungs in a normal adult.)

3. Causes of fluid deficit (result from loss of both water and sodium).

a. Decrease in or absence of fluid intake.

b. Failure to absorb or reabsorb water, as in diarrhea and intestinal disorders.

c. Loss of fluid through the gastrointestinal tract, as in vomiting, nasogastric suctioning.

d. Excessive fluid loss through skin and lungs due to febrile state.

e. Impaired integrity of the skin as in burns, wounds, and hemorrhage.

4. Clinical manifestations.

a. Thirst.

b. Dry skin and dry mucous membranes.

c. Poor skin turgor (collect data on skin on the abdomen or the inner thigh in children.)

d. Weight loss.

e. Urine.

(1) Under 30 cc/hr—oliguria.

(2) Concentrated, dark, foul-smelling.

(3) Increased specific gravity.

f. Depressed fontanelles in the infant.

g. Postural hypotension.

5. Laboratory findings

a. Increeased specific gravity of urine.

b. Incresed blood urea nitrogen (BUN>25mg without increase in creatinine.

c. Increased hematocrit-normal ratio of hematocrit to hemoglobin is three to one, for example if there are 12 grams of hemoglobin, there should be a 36% hematocrit.

d. Hyperglycemia (>120mg/dl)

B. Fluid excess (over hydration) - retention of both water and sodium.

1. Causes of fluid excess.
   a. Excessive oral fluid intake.
   b. Failure to excrete fluids, as in renal disease and congestive heart failure.
2. Clinical manifestations.
   a. Generalized edema.
   b. Pulmonary edema.
   c. Bradycardia.
   d. Weight gain.
   e. Lethargy.
   f. Variable urine volume.
   g. Cerebral edema resulting in seizures.
3. Laboratory findings
   a. Decreased urine specific gravity (<1.010)
   b. Decreased hematocrit - loss of hemoglobin/hematocrit 1:3 ratio.
   c. Decresed serum sodium.

C. Nursing management of client with fluid imbalances.

NCLEX ALERT: *Monitor output (e.g., NG drainage, emesis, stools, urine, etc.) Adjust intake to improve fluid and electrolyte balance.*

1. Data Collection
   a. Evaluate client's history and predisposing factors contributing to the problem.
   b. Collect data for direction of fluid problem: fluid excess or deficit.
   c. Evaluate client's ability to tolerate and correct the problem.
2. Nursing intervention.
   a. Maintain accurate intake and output records.
   b. Obtain accurate daily weight.

***NURSING PRIORITY:** Daily weight is the most reliable indicator of fluid loss or gain in all clients, regardless of age.*

   c. Evaluate for presence of peripheral edema.
   d. Monitor all intake as indicated.
   e. Monitor vital signs; blood pressure is not a reliable indicator of problems of fluid balance in young children.
   f. Maintain good skin care to prevent breakdown.
3. See Appendices on Electrolyte Imbalances and Replacement (Appendices 5-1 through 5-6).

NCLEX ALERT: *Modify client's care based on results of diagnostic/lab tests.*

INTRAVENOUS FLUID REPLACEMENT THERAPY

Goals of Fluid Therapy

✦ *Goal: Maintain adequate fluid balance.*

1. Client NPO.
2. Unable to take fluids by mouth due to disease process.

✦ *Goal: Correct a fluid deficiency.*

1. Electrolyte imbalance.
2. Fluid deficits.

✦ *Goal: Maintain nutritional requirements (caloric replacement)*

1. Nutritional requirements are in excess of the intake, as in burns.
2. Malabsorption syndromes.

Intravenous Infusions

NCLEX ALERT: *Monitor client receiving peripheral IV fluids.*

1. Factors influencing rate of fluid administration.
   a. Type of fluid.
   b. Age of client.
   c. Cardiac and renal status.
   d. Size of the vein and gauge of catheter/needle.
   e. Client's response to fluids.
2. Maintain accurate intake and output records.
3. Average maintenance fluid rate is 3,000 cc over 24 hours.
4. Heparin lock.
   a. Utilized for intermittent administration of medication or fluid.

b. May be flushed with a heparin flush solution or saline solution at regular intervals to maintain patency.

c. Site may be converted to fluid infusion if necessary.

5. IV infusion sites are changed on a regular basis, preferably prior to inflammation, irritation, or fluid extravasation occurring at the site.

6. Pediatric Considerations.

a. Children are very conducive to rapid fluid shifts resulting in cerebral edema. IV solutions of normal saline or percentages of normal saline are frequently used to decrease the possibility of an untoward fluid shift.

b. Children should be restrained appropriately in order to protect the infusion site. Restraints should be checked on a regular basis and observations charted.

c. Volume chambers holding no more that a 2 hour supply of fluid, or controlled infusion devices, should be used on children, to prevent the inadvertent rapid infusion of too much fluid.

Geriatric Priority: *(1) Fluids are generally administered at a slower rate due to decreased ability of the heart and kidney to handle fluids.(2) Elderly clients are prone to circulatory overload. (3) Poor skin turgor is not a reliable indicator of fluid status in elderly.*

Indications for Use of Infusion Control Devices

1. To deliver a medication that requires a precise rate of administration (dopamine, pitressin, aminophylline).
2. To deliver fluids that would precipitate adverse effects if administered too rapidly - (total parenteral nutrition -TPN.)
3. To deliver fluids in controlled amounts to a client very sensitive to volume administered (infants, children under 10 years old, clients with pulmonary edema).

Complications of Intravenous Therapy Infiltration

NCLEX ALERT: *Monitor client receiving peripheral IV fluids. Inspect intravenous site for infiltration and/or extravasation and report to RN.*

1. ***Common causes*** - dislodging of the needle by client movement or obstruction of fluid flow, bevel of needle pushed through posterior aspect of vein during insertion, placement of catheter in area of flexion, not taped or anchored properly.
2. ***Signs and symptoms*** - edema, blanching of skin, discomfort at site, fluid which is flowing slowly or has stopped; cooler skin temperature, IV solution is much cooler than client's body temperature.
3. ***Preventive nursing management*** - use an arm board to stabilize catheter especially in restless, confused clients, or those with catheters placed in the antecubital fossa area; check frequently for coolness of skin around site; avoid looping tubing below bed level; check IV flow rate at least every 2 hours.
4. ***Nursing interventions*** - *Advise RN if IV site is over 72 hours old;* apply cold compress if within first 30 minutes of infiltration, then apply warm moist heat to increase fluid absorption if not contraindicated; *if infiltrated solution has irritating medication, advise RN of increasing irritation in the area.*

Phlebitis

1. ***Common causes*** - overuse of a vein, irritating infusion solutions or medications, catheter in vein for too long of period of time, or use of large gauge catheters.
2. ***Signs and symptoms*** - tenderness, pain along the course of the vein, edema, redness at insertion site, red streak along course of vein, arm with IV feels warmer than other arm.
3. ***Preventive nursing management*** - *Advise RN and anticipate the solution will be discontinued and the catheter removed.* Stabilize cannula, infuse at prescribed rates.
4. ***Nursing interventions*** - apply warm compresses to stimulate circulation and promote absorption.

Circulatory Overload

1. ***Common causes*** - IV infuses too rapidly, positional IV, pre-existing medical conditions that make client more prone to develop pulmonary edema (more frequent in elderly clients and infants).
2. ***Signs and symptoms*** - rise in blood pressure and CVP, neck vein engorgement with client's head elevated, shortness of breath, increased respirations, coughing, syncope, shock.
3. ***Preventive nursing management*** - maintain infusion at prescribed rate; monitor flow of solution

frequently; place client in semi-sitting position during infusion; be especially attentive to elderly clients, infants, or clients with existing heart conditions.

4. ***Nursing interventions*** - reduce infusion rate to a "keep open" rate; *notify RN and/or physician*; position client in semi-Fowler's.

ACID-BASE BALANCE

NCLEX ALERT: *Modify care based on diagnostic or lab results.*

Basic Concepts of Acid-Base Balance

A. Terms used to describe acid-base balance.

1. pH - the chemical abbreviation for negative logarithm of hydrogen ion concentration.
2. CO_2: carbon dioxide.
3. PCO_2: pressure of dissolved carbon dioxide gas in the blood.
4. O_2: oxygen.
5. PO_2: pressure of dissolved oxygen gas in the blood.
6. HCO_3^-: bicarbonate.
7. mmHg: millimeters-mercury.
8. H^+: hydrogen ion concentration.

B. Normal blood gas values.

1. pH 7.4 (7.35-7.45).
2. PO_2: 80-100 mmHg.
3. PCO_2: 35-45 mmHg.
4. HCO_3^-: 22-26 mEq/L.

C. The hydrogen ion (H^+) concentration determines the acidity or alkalinity of a solution. The higher the H^+ concentration, the more acid the solution. The increased H^+ concentration is reflected by a decrease in the pH.

D. Acid-base ratio is determined by sampling arterial blood. This provides a reliable index of overall body function.

E. The body maintains a normal or neutral state of acid-base balance. The stable concentration of H^+ balance is reflected in arterial blood with a relatively constant pH of 7.35-7.45.

Regulation of Acid-Base Balance

A. Buffer system - the most rapid-acting of the regulatory systems. The buffer system is activated where there is an excess acid or base present.

1. A buffer is a chemical that helps maintain a normal pH.
2. The buffer system chemicals are paired. The primary buffer chemicals are sodium bicarbonate and carbonic acid. The buffers are capable of absorbing or releasing hydrogen ions as necessary.
3. An effective buffer system depends on normal-functioning respiratory and renal systems.

B. Respiratory system - the second most rapid response in the regulation of acid-base balance. Carbonic acid is transported to the lungs via the veins, where it is converted to carbon dioxide and water, then excreted.

1. Carbon dioxide is considered an acid substance because it combines with water to form carbonic acid.
2. Increased respirations will decrease carbon dioxide levels, thus decreasing the carbonic acid concentration and resulting in decreased H^+ and an increase in the pH.
3. Decreased respirations will cause a retention of carbon dioxide, increasing the carbonic acid concentrations and resulting in increased H^+ concentration and a decrease in the pH.
4. With excessive acid formation the respiratory center in the medulla is stimulated, which results in an increase in the depth and rate of respirations. This causes a decrease in the carbon dioxide levels and attempts to return the pH to a more normal point.
5. With excessive base formation, the respiratory rate slows in order to promote retention of carbon dioxide and decrease the alkalotic state. The PCO_2 levels are influenced only by respiratory causes.

C. Renal system - the slower but most effective mechanism of acid-base regulation.

1. The kidneys reabsorb sodium (Na), and produce and conserve sodium bicarbonate ($NaHCO_3$).
2. In acidosis the kidney will attempt to excrete more H^+

Alterations in Acid-Base Balance

A. **Respiratory acidosis** - characterized by an excessive retention of carbon dioxide due to hypoventilation.

1. Primary causes - conditions which cause decreased respiratory function.
   a. Head injuries.
   b. Over sedation with sedatives and/or narcotics.
   c. Infection of CNS.
   d. Postoperative anesthesia.

e. Conditions affecting pulmonary function.
  (1) Obstructive pulmonary diseases.
  (2) Pneumonia.
  (3) Cystic fibrosis.
  (4) Atelectasis.
  (5) Occlusion of respiratory passages (asthma).

2. Clinical manifestations.
  a. Dyspnea on exertion.
  b. Rapid, shallow respirations.
  c. Disorientation, decreased level of consciousness.
  d. Tachycardia, arrhythmias.
  e. Muscle weakness.

3. Blood gas values.
  a. pH decreases below 7.35.
  b. PCO_2 increases above 45.
  c. HCO_3^- may remain within normal limits.

4. Nursing management.
  a. Use preventive management.
    (1) Have client turn, cough, and deep breathe every two hours postoperative.
    (2) Use narcotics sparingly in the immediate post-op period.
    (3) Maintain adequate hydration.
  b. Use semi-Fowler's position to facilitate breathing.
  c. Thoroughly assess client's pulmonary function.
  d. Try postural drainage and percussion followed by suction to remove excessive pulmonary secretions.
  e. Anticipate use of bronchodilator either systemically or aerosol.
  f. *Report to the RN any changes in the client's respiratory status.*

NCLEX ALERT: *Implement measures to prevent respiratory complications. The concept of respiratory acidosis may be tested in a variety of situations, particularly in situations that involve an alteration or decrease in respiratory function).*

B. **Respiratory alkalosis**-characterized by a low PCO_2 most often due to hyperventilation.

1. Primary cause of respiratory alkalosis.
  a. Emotional origin (hysteria, fear, apprehension).
  b. Hyperventilation due to disease entity.
  c. Salicylate poisoning.
  d. CNS infection (encephalitis).

2. Clinical manifestations.
  a. Deep, rapid breathing.
  b. Seizures.
  c. Confusion.
  d. Muscle twitching.
  e. Hyperreflexia.
  f. Tingling of extremities.

3. Blood gas values.
  a. pH increases above 7.45.
  b. PCO_2 decreases below 35.
  c. HCO_3^- may remain within normal limits.

4. Nursing Management.
  a. Identify and eliminate (if possible) causative factor.
  b. Evaluate need for sedation.
  c. Use re-breathing devices to increase CO_2 levels.
  d. Remain with client to decrease anxiety levels.

C. **Metabolic alkalosis** - characterized by an increase in the bicarbonate levels in the serum.

1. Primary causes.
  a. Diuretic therapy - loss of H^+, Cl^-, K^+ precipitates an increase in the bicarbonate level in the serum.
  b. Excessive loss of H^+ ions.
    (1) Prolonged nasogastric suctioning without adequate electrolyte replacement.
    (2) Excessive vomiting resulting in loss of hydrochloric acid and K^+.

2. Clinical manifestations.
  a. Nausea, vomiting, diarrhea.
  b. Increased irritability, disorientation.
  c. Restlessness.
  d. Muscle twitching.
  e. Shallow, slow respirations.
  f. Arrhythmias.

3. Blood gas values.
  a. pH increases above 7.45.
  b. PCO_2 normal.
  c. HCO_3^- increases above 26.

4. Nursing management.
  a. Preventive.
    (1) Provide foods high in potassium and chloride for client on diuretics.
    (2) Administer potassium supplement to clients on long-term diuretics.
    (3) Administer IV solution with replacement electrolytes.
  b. Maintain accurate intake and output records.

D. **Metabolic Acidosis** - characterized by a decrease in bicarbonate level in the serum.

1. Primary causes (deficit of a base or an increase in acid).
   a. Diabetic acidosis.
   b. Abnormal loss of alkaline substances.
      (1) Deep, prolonged vomiting may precipitate acidosis due to a loss of base products.
      (2) Severe diarrhea and loss of pancreatic secretions may precipitate an acidotic state.
   c. Renal insufficiency - kidney loses ability to retain HCO_3^- and to excrete H^+.
   d. Salicylate poisoning due to accumulation of ketone bodies produced as a result of the increased metabolic rate.
2. Clinical manifestations.
   a. Disorientation.
   b. Deep, rapid respirations (Kussmaul's).
   c. Changes in level of consciousness (drowsiness, stupor, coma).
   d. Muscle twitching.
   e. Arrhythmias.
3. Blood gas values.
   a. pH decreases below 7.35.
   b. PCO_2 remains normal.
   c. HCO_3- decreases below 22.
4. Nursing management.
   a. Assist in identification of underlying problem.
   b. Maintain accurate intake and output records.
   c. Evaluate client for hydration due to excessive fluid loss.
   d. Support respiratory system.

INFLAMMATION

❑ ***Inflammation*** **is the tissue response to localized injury or trauma.**

Basic Concepts of Inflammation

A. Three major categories.

1. Simple acute.
   a. Occurs most quickly and may leave with no residual damage.
   b. Neutrophils (WBC) are usually the predominant cell.
   - *Example:* Skin infection, tonsillitis.
2. Delayed hypersensitivity.
   a. Typical inflammatory response.
   b. Directly caused by an antigen-sensitized lymphocyte reaction.

Table 5-2: CARDINAL SIGNS OF INFLAMMATION

CLINICAL SYMPTOM	PATHOPHYSIOLOGY
Redness	Hyperemia from vasodilation.
Heat	Increased metabolism at site and local vasodilation.
Pain	Pressure from fluid exudate on adjacent nerve endings which leads to nerve stimulation; change in local pH.
Edema/swelling	Fluid shift and accumulation in interstitial spaces.
Loss of function	Decreased movement due to swelling and pain.

   c. Involves a longer time to develop.
   - *Example:* tuberculin skin testing, subacute bacterial endocarditis (SBE), and organ transplant rejection.
3. Chronic.
   a. Characterized by pain, redness, and swelling.
   b. Does not subside in two weeks, but has a damaging course that lasts for weeks, months, or even years.
   c. Predominant cell types are lymphocytes, plasma cells, and macrophages.
   - *Example:* rheumatoid arthritis, tuberculosis, chronic glomerulonephritis.

B. Concepts of the inflammatory response.

1. The movement of blood and fluid into an injured area is necessary to promote healing of the damaged tissue. This is particularly true of a surgical client.
2. Problems occur when the area of edema impedes tissue perfusion. This is particularly true of edema and swelling with orthopedic injuries (fractured extremities in a cast or traction).
3. Anti-inflammatory meds (corticosteroids) may be administered to the client when the swelling is impeding tissue perfusion.
4. Anti-inflammatory meds are not routinely administered to the surgical client. Anti-inflammatory meds administered to this client may hamper the healing process and mask the symptoms of an infection.

C. Cardinal signs of inflammation .

1. Local response (see Table 5-1).
2. Systemic response.
   a. Fever.
   b. Leukocytosis (shift to the left with increased numbers of neutrophils in circulation).

c. Malaise.
d. Nausea and anorexia.
e. Weight loss.
f. Increased pulse and respiration.

D. Healing process.
1. Primary intention healing.
a. Healing takes place with wound margins neatly approximated.
b. *Example:* a surgical incision.
2. Secondary intention healing.
a. Wound edges are wide and irregular and may not be approximated; large amounts of exudate may be present.
b. Increased amount of granulation tissue; healing takes place upward and from the edges inward.
c. Example: a wound that is left open and allowed to heal from the inside out.

E. Factors delaying the healing process.
1. Nutritional deficiency, specifically protein and vitamin C.
2. Decreased blood supply (edema or peripheral vascular disease, etc.).
3. Infection.
4. Advanced age.
5. Obesity.
6. Long-term intake of steroids.

INFECTION

❑ **Infection is the process by which an organism (pathogen, pathogenic agent) invades the host and establishes a parasitic relationship.**

NCLEX ALERT: *Identify signs and symptoms of an infection. Be able to apply this concept to all ages and categories of client care.*

Chain of Transmission

A. Pathogens.
1. Incubation period—the period of time from exposure to the pathogen until symptoms of infection occur in the host.
2. A person can be asymptomatic and still transmit a pathogen that will produce an infection in someone else (carrier).
3. Pathogens vary in how they interact with the host.
4. Toxigenicity refers to the destructive potential of the toxin that is released by the pathogen.
5. Types of pathogens.
a. Viruses.
b. Bacteria—gram negative and gram positive.
c. Fungus.
d. Chlamydia.
e. Protozoa.
f. Mycoplasm.

B. Reservoir.
1. Environment within which the organism can live and multiply; is provided by some organic substance, human or animal.
2. Provides essential needs for organism survival.
3. A carrier provides an environment for the pathogen to grow and multiply, but shows no symptoms of the infection.

C. Exit port.
1. How the infection leaves the host.
2. Common ports of exit include feces, secretions, and body fluids.
3. Understanding port of exit is necessary to prevent transmission of pathogen.

D. Route of transmission.
1. Method by which the pathogen moves to another host.
2. Direct transmission is immediate transfer from one host to another, as in sexually transmitted diseases; inhalation or contaminated droplets from respiratory infections.
3. Indirect transmission occurs via an intermediate carrier, mosquitos, contaminated water, contaminated food.

E. Port of entry into susceptible host.
1. May enter the host via inhalation, ingestion, through the mucous membranes, or percutaneously.
2. Whether an infectious disease will occur depends on the defense system of the invaded host. Biological and personal characteristics of the new host will determine the lines of defense the host will have against the invading pathogen.

F. Control of transmission.
1. Transmission of a contagious disease can be broken by interfering with any link of the transmission chain.
2. Treatment is aimed at breaking the transmission chain at the most vulnerable and cost effective point.
a. Barrier precautions—gloves, gowns, condoms.
b. Proper handling of food and water supplies.

c. Avoidance of high risk behavior—unsafe sex, IV drug use.

d. Good hand washing technique and good personal hygiene.

3. Important to consider chain of transmission in order to protect health care workers .
4. Host susceptibility can be greatly reduced through immunizations (see Table 2-1).

Nursing Intervention

✦ *Goal: to provide adequate nutrition.*

1. Increase fluid intake.
2. Diet high in protein, carbohydrates and vitamins, specifically vitamins A, B complex and C.

✦ *Goal: to promote healing by decreasing the inflammatory process when the inflammatory response impedes circulation or causes pain and discomfort.*

1. Administer anti-inflammatory medications.
2. Immobilize the inflamed area with a cast, splint, or bandage.
3. Provide adequate rest.
4. Administer antipyretic medications (See Appendix 5-7).

✦ *Goal: to diminish pain.*

1. Heat and cold applications are controversial.
   a. Apply cold after initial trauma to decrease swelling and pain.
   b. Heat is used later to promote healing and to localize the inflammatory agents.
2. Elevate the injured area to decrease edema and promote venous return.

✦ *Goal: to prevent infection.*

1. Monitor vital signs - increase in pulse, respiration, and temperature occurring four to five days postoperatively may indicate infectious process.
2. Evaluate wounds for purulent drainage, may be staphylococcus and/or *Pseudomonas.*
3. Maintain meticulous aseptic technique in dressing changes and in wound irrigations.
4. Initiate infection control procedures as necessary (See Appendix 5-9).
5. Administer antibiotic medications (See Appendix 5-10).

NCLEX ALERT: *Apply principles of infection control (e.g., isolation, standard precautions, communicable disease reporting.)*

✦ *Goal: to prevent complications.*

1. Report any indications of spreading infection, or poor response to treatment.
2. Determine whether client has impaired circulation.
3. Protect healing wounds from injury such as pulling or stretching.

✦ *Goal: to decrease fever.*

1. Sponge bath with tepid water.
2. Administer antipyretics.

Methicillin Resistant Staphylococcus Aureus (MRSA)

❑ **A strain of bacteria that has developed a resistance to common antibiotics.**

A. Bacteria is commonly carried in nasal passages. It is not harmful to healthy person, but will cause infection in susceptible host.

B. Clients who have received multiple antibiotics and who have had multiple hospitalizations are at increased risk.

Treatment

Cultures then antibiotics sensitive to bacteria.

Nursing Intervention

✦ *Goal: Decrease spread of infection*

1. Routine cultures of health care workers.
2. Identification of clients at increased risk.
3. Add contact isolation barrier to the standard precautions:
   - Private room.
   - Gown and gloves.
   - Masks are not necessary unless the client has lower respiratory infection.
   - Teach family importance of gloves and gowns.
4. Notify nurse epidemiologist when client is diagnosed with MRSA.
5. Hand washing is critical, even after removal of gloves.

IMMUNE SYSTEM

Physiology of the Immune System

❑ **The immune system cannot be divided into specific compartments. Immunity includes all physiologic mechanisms that enable the body to protect itself against invasion of foreign substances or protein. An *immunological reaction* is the homeostatic protective response through which the body reorganizes and destroys foreign agents (antigens).**

Table 5-3: ACQUIRED IMMUNITY

TYPE	CHARACTERISTICS	EXAMPLES
Active: antibodies synthesized by body in response to antigen stimulation.	***Natural***: contact with an antigen through exposure; develops slowly, often lifetime protection.	Recovery from childhood diseases (e.g., chicken pox, measles, mumps).
	Artificial: immunization with an antigen develops slowly; may provide protection for several years but "boosters" may be required.	Immunization with live or attenuated vaccines (polio, measles). Toxoid immunization (tetanus toxoid, diphtheria toxoid).
Passive: antibodies produced in one individual and transferred to another.	***Natural:*** immunity from placenta and colostrum transferred from mother to child; provides immediate temporary protection.	Maternal immunoglobin in the neonate.
	Artificial: injection of serum from immune human or animal; short-lived but immediate immunity.	Gammaglobulin; injection of animal hyperimmune serum (diphtheria antitoxin, tetanus antitoxin).

A. The immune system serves three primary functions.
   1. Defense against infection, protection of the body against invading microorganisms.
   2. Maintain homeostasis by removing old cells; the primary organ involved is the spleen.
   3. Surveillance of circulating cells with identification and destruction of the abnormal cells.

B. The body recognizes foreign proteins that are not part of the normal body. These foreign proteins, antigens, elicit a response from the immune system. The immune system produces antibodies which attack and destroy the invading antigens.

Immunological Responses

A. Properties of the immunologic response.
   1. Specificity - the formation of a specific antibody for each antigen. Antibodies produced against one bacteria will not protect the body from other type of bacteria.
      - *Example:* Antibodies against chicken pox will not protect body against measles.
   2. Memory - the ability to remember the specific antigen and make the appropriate antibody. Once the body responds to a particular antigen, memory cells are produced. This produces a stronger immune response the next time the body comes in contact with the same antigen.
      - *Example:* The body remembers how to make the antibody against the chicken pox virus.
   3. Self-recognition - the ability of the body to recognize its own proteins and differentiate them from foreign protein. This allows foreign protein to be attacked without injury to the body's own cells.
      - *Example:* When the body does not recognize its own cells, the condition is called autoimmune, an autoimmune disease, or disorder.

B. Types of specific immunity.
   1. Natural immunity - no prior contact with an antigen; may be related to genetic tendency or species specific.
   2. Acquired immunity - develops either actively or passively (See Table 5-2).

Factors Affecting the Immune Response

1. **Age** - The infant's immune system is not fully developed, and in the elderly the immune response is hypoactive.
2. **Metabolism** - Thyroid and adrenal hormone deficiencies decrease the immune response, steroids inhibit the inflammatory response.
3. **Emotional stress** - May precipitate a decrease in a normal production of cells for the immune response.
4. **Hormonal influences** - Females have a greater incidence of autoimmune diseases then do males.
5. **Environment and lifestyle** - Unsanitary living conditions and exposure to pathogens may increase susceptibility to infections.
6. **Nutrition** - Poor nutrition can decrease the overall immune response.

> ***NURSING PRIORITY:*** *Clients that have a compromised immune system should not participate in any immunization program until they have checked with their doctor.*

DISORDERS OF THE IMMUNE SYSTEM

Autoimmune

A. When the immune system can no longer recognize normal tissue and begins to destroy healthy tissue, an autoimmune response has occurred. Antibodies (autoantibodies) are then formed against the body's own antigens.

B. Some autoimmune responses are very tissue specific and only invade that tissue, while another response may cause body wide affects.

C. Autoimmune response may be systemic or organ specific.

1. Systemic diseases.
   a. Systemic lupus erythematosus (SLE).
   b. Rheumatoid arthritis.
2. Organ specific diseases.
   a. Myasthenia gravis.
   b. Hyperthyroidism (Graves' Disease).
   c. Addison's Disease.
   d. Insulin dependent diabetes (Type I).

Anaphylactic Reaction

❑ **An antigen-antibody response that precipitates the release of histamine, causing profound vasodilatation and increased capillary permeability.**

Data Collection

1. Clinical Manifestations
   a. Hypotension to vascular collapse.
   b. Urticaria, diffuse erythema, periorbital edema.
   c. Hoarseness, wheezing.
   d. Bronchospasm, progressing to respiratory failure.
   e. Vomiting.
   f. Generalized burning and/or itching.
   g. Sense of impending doom.

> **NCLEX ALERT:** *Initiate measures to manage life-threatening emergencies. Progression of symptoms is very rapid. Death from an anaphylactic reaction is most often due to bronchoconstriction.*

Diagnostics

(According to symptoms and exposure to allergen)

Treatment

1. Maintain patent airway.
2. Epinephrine (dosage and route of administration depend on the client's condition).
3. Benadryl, IM or IV.
4. Oxygen.
5. IV fluids (Ringer's lactate or 5% Dextrose).
6. Continuous cardiac monitoring.
7. Corticosteriods to reduce inflammatory response.

Nursing Intervention

✦ *Goal: to collect data for client's predisposition to hypersensitivity reactions.*

1. Obtain client history, specifically with regard to antibiotics (penicillin) and insect bites.
2. If hypersensitivity is suspected, a localized skin test may be done prior to the administration of substance.

✦ *Goal: to maintain adequate ventilation.*

1. Comfortable position, preferably in bed.
2. High oxygen concentrations.
3. Anticipate utilization of airway adjuncts (oral airways, endotracheal intubation).
4. Anticipate administration of medications to reverse bronchospasm. (bronchodilators, corticosteriods, epinephrine).

✦ *Goal: to restore adequate circulation.*

1. Anticipate IV fluids to correct loss of fluid.
2. *Carefully titrate fluid replacement with vital signs and advise RN of significant changes.*

> ***NURSING PRIORITY:*** *Monitor the client carefully. As fluid begins to shift back into the vascular compartment, it is very easy to fluid overload the client.*

3. Client may be placed in supine position with the feet and legs elevated, provided this does not compromise ventilation.

✦ *Goal: client teaching to prevent recurrence.*

1. Once causative agent is identified, instruct client accordingly.
2. Depending on causative agent, client may be candidate for desensitization.
3. Advise client to wear identification tag or bracelet.

Systemic Lupus Erythematosus (SLE)

❑ **An autoimmune disorder that affects multiple organs. Tissue injury in SLE results from the attack of the autoantibodies and the deposition of the immune complex throughout the body. The course of the disease varies greatly in the severity of symptoms. There are exacerbations and remissions.**

Data Collection

1. Primary clinical manifestations for diagnosis.
   a. Skin rash - erythematous rash on areas of the body exposed to sunlight, maybe a characteristic "butterfly" rash over face.
   b. Arthritis - does not cause bone erosion or joint deformity; generally affects 2 or more peripheral joints.
   c. Renal system involvement - proteinuria, hypertension.
   d. Neurologic disorders - seizures and or psychoses.
   e. Hematologic disorders - anemia, decreased white cells (leukopenia).
   f. Respiratory system - pleuritis.
   g. Pericarditis.

Treatment

(There is no known cure.)

1. Corticosteroids.
2. Immunosuppressants (Appendix 5-11).

Nursing Intervention

✦ *Goal: to prevent exacerbations.*

1. Maintain good nutritional status.
2. Avoid exposure to infections.
3. Teach client regarding skin problems and observation for complications.
4. Teach client personal hygiene to prevent urinary tract infections.
5. Take medications; it is important the client does not skip or discontinue any of their medications.
6. Review with client signs and symptoms of infection; call doctor for fever, chills, anorexia, or worsening of symptoms.
7. Avoid exposure to sunlight; use a heavy sun screen when exposure is unavoidable.
8. Teach client to contact physician before participating in any immunization procedures.

✦ *Goal: to maintain good renal function.*

1. Monitor for edema, hypertension, hematuria, decreased output.
2. Maintain on bed rest if renal involvement is severe.
3. Monitor BUN and creatinine levels.
4. Careful evaluation for urinary tract infections.

Acquired Immunodeficiency Syndrome (AIDS)

❑ **A condition resulting from severe impairment of the immune system's ability to respond to invading pathogens. AIDS ultimately affects all body systems.**

A. Occurs as a result of being infected with the human immunodeficiency virus (HIV).

B. After exposure to the virus, the immune system is compromised. Initially, the client may experience flu-like symptoms - fever, chills, fatigue, and lymphadenopathy.

C. For the most optimum effect of treatment, medications should begin early.

D. After exposure to the virus, the client may develop symptoms within 6-12 weeks, however symptoms may not develop for 6 months.

E. The infections that occur in the AIDS clients are called *opportunistic* because they take advantage of the suppressed immune system. These infections tend to resist treatment. The type of infection and its extent varies with each client, depending on the extent of immunosuppression.

1. Pneumocystis carinii pneumonia (PCP) is the most common opportunistic infection associated with AIDS.
2. Fungal infections.
   a. Candidiasis - may involve the oral cavity (thrush), GI tract, or respiratory tract or cause vaginal and urinary tract problems in women.
   b. Extrapulmonary cryptococcoses - may involve the brain.
   c. Histoplasmosis - may disseminate throughout the body.
3. Viral infection - cytomegalovirus (CMV) in the spleen, liver or lymph nodes; both herpes simplex and zoster may occur.
4. Bacterial infections: *Salmonella*, and *Mycobacterium tuberculosis*.

F. Malignancies - Kaposi's sarcoma most common.

Transmission of HIV

A. Blood transmission.

1. Transfusion of contaminated blood or blood products. Screening of transfused blood began in 1985.

2. Sharing of contaminated needles, or accidental needle sticks from an infected person.
   a. Infected IV drug users are the main bridge to other adults through their heterosexual contacts.
   b. Female IV drug users are a source of transmission of HIV to their children through perinatal transmission.
3. Exposure to an infected client's blood via open wounds or mucous membranes.

B. Sexual transmission.
1. Homosexual males.
2. Heterosexual; either partner can infect the other.
3. Anal sex is considered to be a high risk sexual activity.
4. Any sexual activity that involves direct contact with vaginal secretions and semen may transmit HIV.

C. Perinatal transmission.
1. Intrauterine exposure via maternal circulation.
2. HIV is present in breast milk.

D. HIV dies quickly outside the body because it needs living tissue to survive. It is easily killed by soaps, cleansers, hot water, and general household disinfectants, especially household bleach (1:10 dilution).

E. HIV *may not* be transmitted by:
1. Hugging, kissing, holding hands, or other nonsexual contact.
2. Inanimate objects (money, doorknobs, bathtubs, toilet seats, etc.).
3. Dishes, silverware, or food handled by an infected person.
4. Animals or insects.

Prevention of Transmission in Health Care Setting

NCLEX ALERT: *Use standard precautions (Appendix 5-9).*

A. Consider all blood and body fluids from all clients to be contaminated.

B. Avoid contaminating outside of container when collecting specimens.

C. Do not recap needles and syringes.

D. Cleanse work surface areas with appropriate germicide (household bleach in concentrations of 1:100 to 1:10 is effective).

E. Clean up spills of blood and body fluid immediately. Wash the area with a germicide solution.

***NURSING PRIORITY:** It is essential that you know the modes of transmission of HIV, activities that do not transmit the virus, and the nursing care to protect yourself, your AIDS client and other clients you are caring for.*

Clinical Manifestations

1. HIV positive - client has tested positive for the human immunodeficiency virus. No symptoms are observed at this time.
2. Early non-specific changes (AIDS- related complex - ARC).
   a. Chronic fatigue.
   b. Progressive weight loss.
   c. Persistent fever.
   d. Diarrhea.
   e. Night sweats.
   f. Decreased energy.
   g. Generalized lymphadenopathy.
   h. For definite diagnosis of ARC, the client must test positive for HIV antibody.
3. Lymphadenopathy syndrome - lymph glands in at least two extra inguinal sites stay swollen for at least 3 months.
4. HIV wasting syndrome.
   a. Involuntary loss of weight that exceeds 10% of the client's baseline weight.
   b. Chronic diarrhea (2 stools per day for 30 days).
   c. Intermittent weakness and fever lasting more than 30 days.
5. HIV encephalopathy (AIDS dementia, subacute encephalitis).
   a. May be reversed if treatment is started early.
   b. Confusion, disorientation, impaired concentration, loss of coordination.
   c. Hallucinations, impaired judgment, delusions, restlessness, withdrawal.
   d. Dysarthria, ataxia, hyperreflexia, tremor, impaired fine motor function, leg weakness.
   e. Anorexia.
   f. Enuresis, incontinence.
6. Kaposi's sarcoma.
   a. Cherry red or purple slightly raised lesions may occur anywhere over the body.
   b. May obstruct the lymphatic system causing head, neck, and leg edema.

c. May invade deeper body organs, especially the GI tract.

7. Pneumocystis carinii pneumonia (PCP).

a. The most common of the opportunistic infections.

b. Dyspnea and tachycardia on exertion.

c. Chest X-ray showing diffuse bilateral infiltrates.

d. Fever.

e. PaO_2 of 70mm Hg. or less.

Diagnostics

1. CD4+ cell count - (receptor cell on the T4 helper cell) - dramatic decrease in cell count after primary infection (T4, T4 helper, CD4+ are synonymous).

2. Enzyme immunoassay (EIA) testing - after the primary invasion there is an increase in the viral load and decrease in CD4+ count, at this time the client begins to develop antibodies to the HIV. The EIA detects these antibodies.

3. If the EIA test is positive, then the Western blot test is done to confirm the HIV positive results.

4. Testing is done is two stages: first with the HIV antibody test - (ELISA -enzyme-linked immunosorbent assay) indicates that the client has been exposed to the virus and has produced antibodies against it. Does not mean the person has AIDS. The confirming test is the Western blot. If a client tests negative, he should be retested if it has been 12 weeks or less since a possible exposure. (Usually, these tests become positive within 1 month of infection; almost all infected persons have an HIV+ test within 3-6 months of exposure and remain HIV+ indefinitely.)

5. Antigen test - (HIVAGEN) can detect antigens as early as 2 weeks after infection. When the antigen appears along with the antibody, then the virus is active.

Treatment

1. Medications - antivirals (Appendix 5-12).

2. Other medications are utilized to treat the opportunistic infections, according to area of involvement.

3. Chemotherapeutic drugs may be used to treat Kaposi's sarcoma.

***NURSING PRIORITY:** Frequently, the treatment for the AIDS client causes problems in other areas. The high dose antibiotics may increase the level of leukopenia. The chemotherapy medications will further decrease the bone marrow functions. The AIDS client on chemotherapy is going to be even further immunosuppressed.*

Nursing Intervention

✦ *Goal: client and public education regarding transmission of disease.*

***NURSING PRIORITY:** Public and client teaching regarding the transmission of HIV is vital in the control of this disease.*

1. Safe sex.

a. Maintain monogamous relationships.

b. Do not have sex with female or male prostitutes.

c. Avoid all sexual activities that cause cuts or tears in the vagina, on the penis, or in the rectum.

d. Affected client should wear a condom for all sexual activity.

e. If the HIV status of either sexual partner (male or female) is not known, a condom should always be used during intercourse.

f. Anyone who has been involved in any high-risk sexual activities, or has injected IV recreational drugs, should have a blood test to determine presence of the HIV.

Self-Care

1. Maintain personal hygiene; wash hands frequently.

2. Do not share personal items such as toothbrushes, razors, and enema equipment.

3. Do not get pregnant.

4. In a health care setting, always advise of HIV positive status.

5. Do not receive a live-virus vaccine.

6. Kitchen and bathroom facilities may be shared, provided normal sanitary practices are observed.

7. Clean up spills of body fluids or waste immediately with a solution of 1 part bleach to 10 parts water. A bleach solution should be used to disinfect kitchen and bathroom floors, showers, sinks, and toilet bowls.

8. Towels and washcloths should not be shared without laundering.

9. Sanitary napkins, tampons, and any bloody dressing should be wrapped in a plastic bag and placed in a trash container.

10. Needles should not be recapped. Dispose of them in an impenetrable sealed container.
11. Clients with AIDS do not have to remove pets. Have someone else change litter boxes and birdcages, when possible; if this is not feasible, use gloves.
12. Do not donate blood or plasma, body organs, or semen.
13. HIV positive women should not breast feed.

✦ *Goal: to maintain ventilation.*

1. Client frequently on limited activities or bed rest.
2. Supplemental oxygen.
3. Avoid contact with upper respiratory infections.
4. Adequate fluid intake, humidifier.
5. Frequent data collection for pulmonary changes and hypoxemia.
6. Coughing and deep breathing exercises.
7. Carefully evaluate respiratory function if narcotic analgesics are used.
8. Carefully collect data for activity tolerance.

✦ *Goal: to assist client to minimize the effects of neurologic changes.*

1. Frequent data collection pertaining to neurologic status.
2. Collect data pertaining to visual changes.
3. If client is confused, provide care directed to reorientation.
4. Provide a safe and supportive environment, according to the neurological deficits.

✦ *Goal: to assist client to maintain psychosocial equilibrium.*

1. Encourage client to express his feelings and concerns.
2. Do not be judgmental regarding client's lifestyle.
3. Maintain frequent contact with the client.
4. Encourage client to maintain as much independence as possible.
5. Assist client to take advantage of services available - social worker, financial aid, support groups.

Pediatric AIDS

❑ **Majority of children with AIDS are infected in the perinatal period.**

Data Collection

1. Infants who become symptomatic prior to their first birthday have a poor long term prognosis.
2. Failure to thrive is a primary symptom in infants.
3. Failure to meet developmental milestones.
4. Diagnostics - same as adult.

Treatment

Essentially same as for adult.

Nursing Intervention

✦ *Goal: to maintain homeostasis .*

1. Children should receive only killed vaccines.

> ***Pediatric Priority:*** *Oral polio vaccine should not be used in children with AIDS or in families with children who are either infected or suspected of being infected with the HIV virus.*

2. High caloric, high protein diet.
3. Clean the umbilical stump carefully until completely healed.
4. Generally, HIV positive infants are not circumcised.
5. See "Care of Immunosuppressed Client."

Self-Care

1. Teach the parents how to care for the child.
2. Teach parents how to prevent transmission of disease.
3. Teach parent to identify measures to control opportunistic infections.

Nursing Interventions for the Immunologically Suppressed Client

A. Regardless of the disease process or immunosuppressive state, clients on immunosuppressive medications have common nursing concerns.

Nursing Intervention

✦ *Goal: to monitor for and/or prevent opportunistic infections.*

1. The type, location, and severity of the infection depend on the disease progress and the client's immunosuppressive state.
2. Observe and/or teach client signs of opportunistic infections.
   a. Carefully evaluate temperature elevations; may be low grade (100° F.) or significantly elevated (103° F.).
   b. Assess for presence of common infections.
      (1) Urinary tract infection.
      (2) Respiratory infections, especially PCP.
      (3) Poor healing and infection of abrasions and ulcerations.
      (4) Persistent weight loss and diarrhea.

(5) White spots in the mouth (thrush).

(6) Herpes simplex abscesses in the mouth.

(7) Stomatitis.

(8) Vaginal yeast infections in women.

3. Severely immunocompromised client may require reverse isolation for protection.
4. Decrease invasive nursing procedures (IMs, bladder catheterizations).
5. Monitor for chronic diarrhea.
6. Do not clean pet litter boxes or bird cages, if necessary to do so, wear gloves.

✦ *Goal: Decrease side effects from medications and not immunosupressive state.*

1. Maintain regular checks on CBC and hemoglobin.
2. Good oral hygiene.
3. No active vaccines while immunosupressed.
4. Close observation for signs and symptoms of common infections.
5. Frequent hand washing (nurse and client) to protect client as well as prevent transmission of infection from the client.

✦ *Goal: to prevent excessive fatigue.*

1. Evaluate respiratory status and tolerance to activity.
2. Evaluate hemoglobin levels and tolerance of activity.
3. Encourage activity within tolerance level.
4. May require oxygen if anemia is severe.

✦ *Goal: to identify early indications of renal problems.*

1. Nephrotoxicity related to immunosuppressive medications is frequently dose and duration related.
2. Carefully monitor intake and output.
3. Evaluate BUN and creatinine for indications of renal problems.
4. Evaluate weight gain and loss.

✦ *Goal: to maintain adequate nutritional intake.*

1. Teach client regarding nutrition and caloric intake.
2. Encourage high calorie snacks through out the day.
3. Encourage client to eat several small meals throughout the day.
4. May need to include liquid dietary supplements.
5. Antiemetics prior to meals may increase appetite.
6. Avoid foods or beverages that may cause oral, esophageal, or gastric irritation.
7. Tube feedings or parenteral nutrition may be necessary.

✦ *Goal: to prevent decubiti formation and excoriation of the skin.*

1. Wash perineal and anal area; allow to dry thoroughly.
2. Observe bony prominences for adequacy of circulation and development of decubiti.
3. Do not put any lotions on reddened areas or open lesions.
4. Teach client importance of frequent change in position.

✦ *Goal: to assist client to maintain psychological equilibrium.*

1. Encourage client to express feelings and concerns.
2. Encourage client to maintain as much independence as possible.
3. Assist client to take advantage of community services available.
4. Advise client of patient rights and consent for treatment.

Study Questions — Homeostasis

1. A client is on steroid therapy, what is important to teach him regarding his medication?

① increase fluid intake.

② increase dose as needed.

③ do not discontinue medication abruptly.

④ do not take medication with food.

2. What type of reaction quickly deteriorates into severe respiratory difficulty and shock?

① anaphylaxis.

② allergic reaction.

③ serum sickness.

④ hay fever.

3. What is the process when a person's immune system reacts against itself?

① anaphylaxis.
② macrocytosis.
③ phagocytosis.
④ autoimmunity.

4.Which category of medications significantly decreases the body response to infection?

① beta blockers.
② corticosteroids.
③ anticoagulants.
④ calcium channel blockers.

5. What is the condition that occurs when a client's body is unable to defend itself from an invading microorganism?

① immunodeficiency.
② anaphylaxis.
③ phagocytosis.
④ autoimmunity.

6. When a client's body is exposed to foreign antigens by a vaccination, what type of immunity does this provide?

① autoimmune.
② natural active immunity.
③ acquired passive immunity.
④ acquired active immunity.

7. A client is exposed to an antigen through an illness. What is developed in the client's body due to this exposure?

① macrophage.
② eosinophil.
③ erythrocytes.
④ antibodies.

8. A client is dehydrated, what condition can develop secondary to this problem?

① edema.
② hypovolemia.
③ congestive failure.
④ hypothermia.

9. What is the most accurate measurement to determine changes in a client's fluid balance, either fluid loss or retention?

① adequacy of skin turgor.
② daily body weight.
③ measure intake and output.
④ measure circumference of the legs.

10. The nurse is checking a client's foot for edema and finds barely detectable pitting. What is this level of edema?

① 4+.
② 3+.
③ 2+.
④ 1+.

11. What organ system regulates the fluid and electrolyte balance in the body?

① kidneys.
② heart.
③ parathyroid.
④ liver.

12. Which problem can occur as the result of a fever?

① fluid loss.
② hyponatremia.
③ hypokalemia.
④ fluid overload.

13. The nurse observes flushed, dry skin on a client. The nurse should further evaluate this client for the development of what condition?

① edema.
② shock.
③ dehydration.
④ hypervolemia.

14. The nurse is assessing an elderly client and determines the presence of dry mucous membranes and confusion. The nurse should continue to assess the client for what complication?

① hypertension.
② hypervolemia.
③ dehydration.
④ hypocalcemia.

15. Which of these clients would be at the greatest risk for having a significant fluid imbalance if their fluid intake was significantly reduced?

① 46 year old diabetic.
② 3 week old infant.
③ 12 year old underweight teenager.
④ 25 year old obese adult.

16. When should the nurse utilize protective eye wear?

① emptying urinals and bedpans.
② administering an IM injection.
③ performing direct client care on a client in respiratory isolation.
④ whenever there is a chance of splashing blood or body fluids.

17. A postoperative client is experiencing a problem with respiratory acidosis. What nursing care is important for this client?

① increase fluid intake.
② provide oxygen via face mask.
③ observe for confusion.
④ turn, cough and deep breath.

18. What is the primary method of transmission of the human immunodeficiency virus?

① via sexual contact with an infected individual.
② through contact with contaminated blood.
③ from the mother via the placenta at birth.
④ sharing a bathroom with an infected individual.

19. In caring for the client who is immunosuppressed, what is a priority nursing concern?

① maintaining therapeutic communication.
② preventing opportunistic infections.
③ promoting good skin care and wound healing.
④ maintaining adequate elimination.

20. Ototoxicity is a serious side effect of what medication?

① penicillin (Omnipen)
② gentamicin (Garamycin)
③ tetracycline (Achromycin V)
④ erythromycin (E-Mycin)

Appendix 5-1:
ELECTROLYTE IMBALANCES: POTASSIUM

CAUSES	SYMPTOMS	NURSING IMPLICATIONS
NORMAL SERUM LEVELS (POTASSIUM): 3.5 - 5.0 mEq/L		
HYPOKALEMIA: Serum K below 3.5 mEq/L		
Decreased intake of K GI loss: vomiting, diarrhea, fistulas, nasogastric suction, without replacement Excessive renal excretion: diuretics, aldosterone Alkalosis Steroid therapy	Muscle weakness and cramps Hyporeflexia Confusion, drowsiness, fatigue Tachycardia Postural hypotension GI: anorexia, vomiting, diarrhea	1. Identify source of depletion. 2. Monitor K levels. 3. Encourage foods high in K. 4. Replace K (oral and IV). 5. Maintain accurate intake and output records. 6. Evaluate for digitalis toxicity (lowered K potentiates digitalis) and for alkalosis. 7. Provide client education regarding diuretics. 8. Administer potassium supplements.
HYPERKALEMIA: Serum K above 5.0 mEq/L		
Decreased urinary excretion: renal failure, ↓ aldosterone Massive tissue injury: burns, trauma Excessive administration of IV K Acidosis	Drowsiness Muscle weakness to flaccid paralysis Hyperreflexia EKG changes Tachycardia, bradycardia Cardiac arrest Oliguria, anuria	1. Identify origin of increase. 2. Monitor K levels. 3. Administer diuretics, if renal function adequate. 4. Administer hypertonic glucose and insulin to initiate K transfer into cell. 5. Utilize exchange resins: (**Kayexalate**). 6. Administer sodium bicarbonate if client is acidotic; be prepared for a cardiac emergency. 7. Maintain accurate intake and output records.

Appendix 5-2:
MEDICATIONS TO CORRECT POTASSIUM IMBALANCE

MEDICATIONS	ACTION	NURSING IMPLICATIONS
POTASSIUM SUPPLEMENTS		
ORAL: Potassium chloride (KCl) Potassium triplex Potassium citrate Potassium gluconate **(Kaon)** **IV:** Potassium chloride Potassium acetate	Principle intracellular action and essential for many physiological processes. Used in treatment and prevention of hypokalemia.	1. Oral preparations generally have unpleasant taste; administer with full glass of water or juice. 2. Potassium is irritating to gastric mucosa. 3. Pediatric implications: make sure child/infant is urinating adequately before beginning supplement. **Do not give K by IM or subcutaneously**. 5. IV potassium solutions are irritating to the vein. If pain occurs notify the RN. 6. Administer with caution to cardiac clients and those on digitalis preparations.
EXCHANGE RESIN		
Sodium polystyreal sulfonate **(Kayexalate)**: PO or rectal retention enema	In the intestine the hydrogen ion is exchanged for the potassium; this binds excess potassium and removes it from the serum. Medication is not absorbed systemically.	1. Laxatives are given to facilitate excretion of the resin. 2. Cleansing enema must precede the **Kayexalate** retention enema. 3. Carefully evaluate the client with CHF and/or hypertension. 4. Monitor serum electrolytes. 5. Use with caution in clients requiring sodium restriction.

Appendix 5-3:
ELECTROLYTE IMBALANCES: SODIUM

CAUSES	SYMPTOMS	NURSING IMPLICATIONS
NORMAL SERUM LEVELS (SODIUM) 135 - 145 mEq/L		
HYPOVOLEMIC HYPONATREMIA: Serum Na below 135 mEq/L		
Inadequate Na intake Decreased renal excretion: diuretics, adrenal insufficiency, increased ADH Edema Excessive administration of D_5W Fresh water near drowning Cystic fibrosis Excessive sweating Gastrointestinal losses Diabetic acidosis Massive tissue injury: burns, trauma	*Solution deficit (sodium loss):* CNS problems: decreased level of consciousness, seizures, weakness, restlessness, oliguria, abdominal cramps, postural hypotension, increased hematocrit, flushed skin *Dilutional hyponatremia (water excess):* CNS problems: confusion, headache, seizures, muscle twitching, increased urine	1. Decreased hematocrit. Identify source of depletion. 2. Maintain accurate intake and output records and daily weight (best measurement of fluid status). 3. Irrigate nasogastric tubes with normal saline. 4. Restrict fluid intake if client has fluid excess. 5. Elderly and infants at higher risk because of variations in total body water. 6. Occurs in clients who are NPO, on diuretics, or have excessive perspiration, vomiting, diarrhea, burns, or excessive administration of D5W. 7. Occurs in renal disease, Addison's disease, and diabetic acidosis. 8. Carefully monitor clients receiving only D5W.
HYPERNATREMIA: Serum Na above 145 mEq/L (sodium retention or water loss)		
Decreased fluid intake Excessive salt intake Increased renal retention: renal disease Cushing's syndrome (adrenal hyperfunction) decreased ADH Salt water near-drowning	*Fluid excess (sodium retention):* Pitting edema Weight gain Lethargic Decreased CVP Decreased hematocrit *Fluid deficit: (hemoconcentration of Na, water loss)* Concentrated urine Dry mucous membranes Flushed skin Tachycardia Increased temperature	1. Identify origin of increase. 2. Maintain accurate intake and output records and daily weight. 3. Administer diuretics to remove excess Na. 4. Restrict fluid intake if client has fluid excess. 5. Assess skin condition. 6. Assess for pitting edema. 7. Assess for CHF.

Appendix 5-4:
MEDICATIONS TO CORRECT SODIUM IMBALANCE

MEDICATION	ACTION	NURSING IMPLICATIONS
SODIUM SUPPLEMENTS		
Sodium chloride (NaCl, table salt) Saline solutions: 0.9% and 0.45% saline solution for infusion	Necessary ion in maintaining osmotic pressure in intravascular and extracellular fluids. Necessary component for acid-base buffer system.	1. Caution clients with CHF, renal problems, edema, or hypertension to use salt sparingly. 2. Maintain daily weights, I & O to evaluate fluid retention. 3. Evaluate serum Na levels.

Appendix 5-5: ELECTROLYTE IMBALANCES: CALCIUM

CAUSES	SYMPTOMS	NURSING IMPLICATIONS
NORMAL SERUM LEVELS (CALCIUM): 8 - 10.5 mg % or 4.5 - 5.5 mEq/L		
HYPOCALCEMIA: Serum Ca below 8.6 mg % or below 4 mEq/L, or 3.5 mEq/L - infants		
Acute pancreatitis Steatorrhea Dietary lack of Ca and vitamin D Renal failure Hypoparathyroid Excessive transfusion of citrated blood Metabolic alkalosis Overuse of antacids and laxatives **Infants:** ***Early onset*** - decreased activity of parathyroid; infants of diabetic mothers; premature infants; exchange transfusion ***Late onset*** - decreased dietary intake	Tetany: + Chvostek's sign + Trousseau's sign Neuromuscular irritability Numbness and tingling in extremities Seizures Abdominal cramping and distention Hyperreflexia Arrhythmias ***Early onset in infant***: edema, apnea, intermittent cyanosis, vomiting, abdominal distention ***Late onset in infant:*** Increasing CNS excitability	1. Identify origin of deficiency. 2. Keep Ca replacement medications easily accessible for postoperative thyroid and parathyroid clients. 3. Assess for tetany. 4. Evaluate adequacy of Ca intake in infants. 5. Reduce environmental stimuli in both adults and infants. 6. Institute seizure precautions. 7. Provide client education regarding Ca intake.
HYPERCALCEMIA: Serum Ca above 10.5 mg% or above 5.5 mEq/L		
Metastatic malignancy Hyperparathyroidism Thiazide diuretics Prolonged immobilization	Anorexia Nausea, constipation CNS depression Decreasing muscle tone Renal calculi Pathological fractures Arrhythmias	1. Identify origin of increase. 2. Administer diuretics to facilitate removal of serum Ca. 3. Increase client's fluid intake to 3,000 to 4,000 cc daily to decrease calculi formation. 4. Decrease Ca intake. 5. Encourage client mobility. 6. Handle client carefully to prevent pathological fractures. 7. Assess client on digitalis for symptoms of toxicity.

Appendix 5-6: MEDICATIONS TO CORRECT CALCIUM IMBALANCE

MEDICATION	ACTION	NURSING IMPLICATIONS
CALCIUM SUPPLEMENTS		
Calcium lactate, PO Calcium gluconate (**Kalcinated**) IV, PO Calcium carbonate, PO (Loop diuretics are used to enhance excretion of calcium.)	Primary component of bones and teeth Activator for coagulation enzyme factors Necessary for cardiac muscle function IV infusion for treatment of hypocalcemic tetany Adjunctive therapy to prevent hypocalcemia during exchange transfusion.	1. May be given in conjunction with vitamin D to enhance absorption. 2. PO supplements utilized best if given 1½ hours before meals. 3. Do not add Ca preparations to solutions containing carbonates or phosphates. 4. Use with caution for client receiving digitalis.

Appendix 5-7: ANTI-INFLAMMATORY MEDICATIONS

❖GENERAL NURSING IMPLICATIONS❖
— Give oral medications with or after meals.
— IV injection should be over at least 1minute.
— Withdrawal from steroids should be gradual.
— Increased amounts of adrenocorticosteroids may be required during stress periods such as surgery.
— Assess for complications associated with prolonged usage (infections, psychological changes, fluid retention).

MEDICATION	SIDE EFFECTS	NURSING IMPLICATIONS
ADRENOCORTICAL STEROIDS: ***Anti-inflammatory action:*** Inhibit release of proteolytic enzymes during inflammation, decreases the number of lymphocytes, used as an immunosuppressant for delaying organ rejection ***Cardiovascular:*** Potentiate vasoconstriction effects of norepinephrine; elevated blood pressure. ***Carbohydrate, fat protein metabolism***: produce hyperglycemia, glycosuria; facilitate breakdown of protein in muscle, and promote mobilization of fatty acids from adipose tissue. ***Stress effect:*** During stress (sympathoadrenal response) a release of corticosteroids occurs.		
Cortisone acetate (**Cortisone**): PO, IM, topical ophthalmic ointment Hydrocortisone: IM, PO Dexamethasone (**Decadron**): PO, topical, IM or ophthalmic Prednisone (**Deltasone, Meticorten**): PO Methylprednisolone sodium succinate (**Solumedrol**): PO, IM, IV	Increased susceptibility to infections GI upset Osteoporosis Psychological disturbances (depression, euphoria) Hypocalcemia Hyperglycemia Hypertension (caused by sodium and water retention) Cushing's syndrome: moon face, buffalo hump, distended abdomen, thin arms and legs, excessive hair growth	1. Administer medication before 9 a.m. to decrease adrenal cortical suppression. 2. Encourage daily dose with breakfast. 3. Monitor for psychological changes. 4. Decrease salt intake in diet; encourage high protein and potassium. 5. Weigh daily. 6. Topical steroids usually do not provoke physical evidence of absorption unless applied to large areas or over prolonged periods. ***Teaching:*** Take medication with food. Diet should include adequate K intake and decreased Na intake. Do not stop taking the medication without a doctor's order. Avoid immunizations if on long-term therapy. Report to health care provider: stress situations, sore throat, fever, or other signs of infection, or a weight gain of 5 lb or more in a week.

Appendix 5-8: NON-STEROID ANTI-INFLAMMATORY (NSAID) MEDICATIONS

MEDICATIONS	SIDE EFFECTS	NURSING IMPLICATIONS
❖ GENERAL NURSING IMPLICATIONS ❖ — Give with a full glass of water, either with food or just after eating. — Drink increased water during the day (2-3 quarts). — Store in child-proof containers and out of reach of small children. — Do not exceed recommended doses.		
NSAIDs: Inhibit prostaglandin synthesis.		
Acetaminophen: (**Tylenol, Datril, Tempra**): PO, rectal	Very little gastric irritation; does not affect prothrombin time. Hepatotoxic in large doses: vomiting, anorexia, diaphoresis, weakness, RUQ tenderness, jaundice, fever, ↑liver function studies.	1. Assess for toxicity by observing symptoms of CNS stimulation. 2. If used concomitantly with anticoagulants, dosage may need to be reduced to avoid hemorrhage. 3. Available in flavored liquid and tablets for children. 4. ***Uses***: analgesic for relief of headache, joint pain; reduces fever.
Acetylsalicylic Acid: (**Aspirin, ASA**): PO	***Salicylism:*** skin reactions, redness, rashes, ringing in the ears, GI upset, hyperventilation, sweating and thirst. ***Severe salicylate poisoning:*** stimulation of CNS followed by depression, incoherent speech, stupor, respiratory failure. ***Long-term usage:*** erosive gastritis with bleeding. Associated with Reye's syndrome in children.	1. Interacts with oral anticoagulants and may significantly increase the prothrombin time. 2. If available, administer as enteric-coated or buffered tablets. 3. Be aware that aspirin is the most common agent responsible for accidental poisoning in small children. 4. Do not give aspirin to children unless under the specific direction and supervision of a physician. 5. Observe clients who are on anticoagulant therapy and also diabetic patients who may have symptoms of hypoglycemia, because salicylate potentiates antidiabetic oral drugs. 6. ***Uses:*** pain, fever, inflammatory conditions such as arthritis, gout.
Ibuprofen (**Advil, Motrin**): PO	Dyspepsia (heartburn, nausea, epigastric distress) Dizziness Rash, dermatitis	1. May increase effects of anticoagulants. 2. Do not crush enteric-coated form. 3. Avoid taking it concurrently with aspirin. 4. ***Uses:*** arthritis, fever, pain, muscle cramps.
Naproxen (**Naprosyn**): PO	Headache Dyspepsia Dizziness, drowsiness Peripheral fluid retention.	1. May increase effects of anticoagulants. 2. Avoid tasks requiring alertness until response to drug is established. 3. ***Uses:*** arthritis, primary dysmenorrhea, pain.
Indomethacin: (**Indocin**): PO	GI upset Nephrotoxicity Lightheadedness Fatigue	1. Caution client against performing hazardous task requiring mental alertness or physical coordination. 2. Assess renal function in clients on long-term therapy. 3. ***Uses***: rheumatoid arthritis, osteoarthritis; relieves pain and swelling in acute gouty arthritis.
Celecoxib (**Celebrex**): PO	GI upset Headache	1. Should not be used in clients with history of asthma. 2. Should not be used by clients who have a history of allergy to apsirin. 3. *Uses:* osteo and rheumatoid arthritis, dysmenorrhea.

Appendix 5-9:
INFECTION CONTROL PROCEDURES

GENERAL INFORMATION:

- ✓ Many patients with disease-specific isolation precautions now require only standard precautions.
- ✓ The specific substances covered by standard precautions include blood and all other body fluids, body secretions, and body excretions, except sweat, even if blood is not visible.
- ✓ Transmission-based precautions are followed, in addition to standard precautions, whenever a patient is known or suspected to be infected with contagious pathogens.

STANDARD PRECAUTIONS:

1. Wash your hands immediately if they become contaminated with blood or body fluids; also wash your hands before and after patient care and after removing gloves.
2. Wear gloves if you will or could come in contact with any body fluid, or contaminated surfaces or objects.
3. Change your gloves between tasks and procedures on the same patient.
4. Wear a gown, eye protection (goggles, glasses), or face shield, and a mask during procedures likely to generate droplets of blood or body fluids.
5. Carefully handle used patient care equipment soiled with body fluids.
6. Ensure that hospital procedures for routine care, cleaning and disinfection of environmental surfaces, beds, bed rails, and bedside equipment are followed.
7. Handle contaminated linens in a manner that prevents contamination and transfer of microorganisms.
8. Handle used needles or other sharp implements carefully. Do not bend, break, reinsert them into their original sheaths, or handle them unnecessarily. Discard them intact immediately after use into an impervious disposal box.
9. Place patients who cannot maintain appropriate hygiene or who contaminate the environment in a private room.
10. If the care giver has an exudative lesion, they should avoid all direct patient contact until the condition has resolved.

AIRBORNE TRANSMISSION-BASED PRECAUTIONS:

1. Place the patient in a private room that has monitored negative air pressure in relation to surrounding areas.
2. Wear respiratory protection (masks or face shields) when entering the room.
3. Limit patient transport and patient movement out of the room.
4. Utilized in clients with measles, varicella, tuberculosis.

DROPLET TRANSMISSION-BASED PRECAUTIONS:

1. Place the patient in a private room.
2. Wear a mask when working within 3 feet of the patient.
3. Keep visitors 3 feet from the infected patient.
4. Limit movement of the patient from the room. If the patient must leave the room, have him wear a surgical mask, if possible.

CONTACT TRANSMISSION-BASED PRECAUTIONS:

1. Place the patient in a private room.
2. Wear gloves whenever entering the room. Always change gloves after contact with infected material. Remove gloves before leaving the patient's room and wash hands.
3. Wear a gown when entering the patient's room if clothing will have extensive contact with the patient, environmental surfaces, or if the patient has diarrhea or is incontinent. Remove the gown before leaving the patient's room.
4. Limit movement of the patient from the room.
5. Avoid sharing any patient care equipment.
6. Gastrointestinal, respiratory, skin, and wound infections are easily transmitted by direct contact.

NCLEX ALERT: *Apply principals of infection control.*

Appendix 5-10:
ANTIBIOTIC MEDICATIONS

MEDICATIONS	SIDE EFFECTS	NURSING IMPLICATIONS

❖ GENERAL NURSING IMPLICATIONS ❖

— Cultures should always be taken prior to the administration of the first dose.
— Teach the client to finish the entire prescribed course of medication even though he may feel well.
— Schedule at evenly spaced intervals around the clock.
— Give most oral antibiotic drugs on an empty stomach (1 hour before or 2 hours after meals).
— Take drugs with a full glass of water.
— Observe for hypersensitivity:
  anaphylaxis—hypotension, respiratory distress, urticaria, angioedema, vomiting, diarrhea.
  serum sickness—fever, vasculitis, generalized lymphadenopathy, edema of joints, bronchospasm.
— Observe for superinfection:
  stomatitis—sore mouth, white patches on oral mucosa, black furry tongue
  diarrhea
  monilial vaginitis—rash in perineal area, itching, vaginal discharge
  new localized signs and symptoms—redness, heat, edema, pain, drainage, cough
  recurrence of systemic signs and symptoms—fever, malaise

PENICILLIN: Bactericidal; interferes with the formation of the bacterial cell wall.

MEDICATIONS	SIDE EFFECTS	NURSING IMPLICATIONS
Penicillin G (**Bicillin**): PO, IM Penicillin V (**PenVee K, V-Cillin K**): PO Amoxicillin (**Amoxil**): PO with clavulanate — (**Augmentin**): PO Ampicillin (**Omnipen, Polycillin**): PO, IM, IV Cloxacillin (**Tegopen**): PO Ticarcillin (**Ticar**): IM, IV	Parenteral injection is more hazardous than oral administration. Diarrhea ***Allergic reactions:*** skin rashes, joint pain, dermatitis, kidney damage. ***Anaphylactic reaction*** (hypersensitivity): decreased B/P, increased pulse, respiratory distress, diaphoresis.	1. Observe for allergic reactions and have emergency equipment available. 2. Amoxicillin can be scheduled without regard to meals. 3. Observe client for 30 minutes after IM or IV administration for symptoms of allergic reactions. 4. Clients with beta hemolytic strep infections should be on penicillin for a minimum of 10 days to prevent development of rheumatic fever or glomerulonephritis. 5. May reduce the effectiveness of oral contraceptives. 6. Discard liquid forms of penicillin after 7 days at room temperature and 14 days when refrigerated. 7. ***Uses:*** pneumonia, meningitis, gonorrhea, otitis media, urinary tract infections, syphilis, and as prophylaxis for clients with rheumatic fever.

AMINOGLYCOSIDE: ***Bactericidal:*** interferes with formation of bacterial cell wall.

MEDICATIONS	SIDE EFFECTS	NURSING IMPLICATIONS
Gentamycin (**Garamycin**): IM, IV Amikacin (**Amikin**): IM, IV Kanamycin sulfate (**Kantrex**): PO, IM, IV Neomycin sulfate (**Mycifradin** sulfate): PO, IM, topical, ophthalmic	***Toxicity:*** Ototoxicity—hearing loss is irreversible, Nephrotoxicity—albuminuria, cast, oliguria Skin rash, headache, hypotension, pain, and tenderness at injection site.	1. Neurotoxicity may be increased if given soon after surgery. 2. Assess for ototoxicity (change in hearing, ringing in the ears, dizziness, or unsteady gait) and nephrotoxicity (monitor BUN and creatinine). 3. Are generally not used for long-term therapy. 4. Drink 2000-3000 ml. of fluid daily. 5. ***Uses:*** broad spectrum; primarily used for gram- negative sepsis and serious gram-negative infections including, *E. coli*, *Klebsiella*, *proteus*, and staphylococcus; infections of the urinary tract, and neonatal meningitis.

Bet J 4/1 1800 200 0160

Appendix 5-10:
ANTIBIOTIC MEDICATIONS

MEDICATIONS	SIDE EFFECTS	NURSING IMPLICATIONS
CEPHALOSPORINS: ***Bacteriostatic:*** broad spectrum, interferes with the formation of the bacterial cell wall.		
1st generation—Cefadroxil **(Duricef, Ultracef)**:PO Cephalexin **(Keflex)**: PO Cephalothin sodium (**Keflin**): IM, IV Cefazolin (**Kefzol, Ancef**): IM, IV 2nd generation—Cefuroxime **(Ceftin)**: PO, IM, IV Loracarbef (**Lorabid**): PO Cefoxitin (**Mefoxin**): IM, IV 3rd generation—Cefixime **(Suprax)**: PO Ceftriaxone (**Rocephin**): IM, IV	Hypersensitivity Superinfection GI upset, neutropenia (decreased WBC), pain at injection site, renal damage seizures	1. Give oral cephalosporins with food or milk. 2. Administer IM medications deep into the muscle. 3. Use with caution in clients known to be allergic to penicillin. 4. Ceftriaxone (**Rocephin**) is only drug approved for once-daily dosing.
TETRACYCLINES: ***Bacteriostatic:*** broad spectrum; interferes with protein synthesis of infectious organisms and thus diminishes its growth and reproduction.		
Tetracycline (**Achromycin**): PO, IV, IM Doxycycline (**Vibramycin**): PO, IV Demeclocyline (**Declomycin**): PO Minocycline (**Minocin**): PO, IV	Loose stools, diarrhea, sore throat, photosensitivity, deformity in teeth in children up to eight years old and in newborns whose mothers have received the drug.	1. Administer on empty stomach; withhold antacids, dairy foods, and foods high in calcium at least 2 hours after PO administration. Do not administer with milk. 2. Can give doxycycline and minocycline with food. 3. Do not give at the same time with iron preparations. Give them as far apart as possible (i.e., 2-3 hours). 4. Advise client to avoid direct or artificial sunlight. 5. Prevent or treat pruritus ani which occurs as a side effect by cleansing the anal region several times each day and after each BM. 6. ***Uses***: severe respiratory tract and urinary tract infections, septicemia, osteomyelitis. 7. Observe for suprainfections
SULFONAMIDES: ***Bacteriostatic:*** interferes with the utilization of para-aminobenzoic acid (PABA, required by bacteria for growth); halt multiplications of bacteria but do not kill fully formed microorganisms.		
Sulfamethoxazole **(Gantanol)**: PO Sulfisoxazole (**Gantrisin**): PO Sulfamethoxazole-trimethoprim **(SMZ-TMP, Bactrim, Septra)**: PO, IV	Blood dyscrasia, renal dysfunction (crystalluria, hematuria, oliguria); skin and mucous membrane lesions, dizziness, headache, fatigue. Rash (Stevens-Johnson syndrome) May reduce the synthesis of vitamin K, leading to hemorrhage.	1. Encourage adequate fluid intake to prevent crystalluria. 2. Assess for side effects. 3. **Sulfamylon**: use for treatment of burns; causes pain on application; give pain medication 30 - 45 minutes prior to applying. 4. **Azulifidine**: urine may turn orange yellow. 5. ***Uses:*** treatment of acute and chronic cystitis, ulcerative colitis, lymphogranuloma venereum, toxoplasmosis, and chancroid.
MACROLIDES: ***Bacteriostatic and bactericidal:*** inhibit microbial protein synthesis.		
Erythromycin base **(Ilosone, E-mycin)**: PO, IV, Azithromycin ***(Zithromax)***: PO Clarithromycin (**Biaxin**): PO	Nausea, vomiting, abdominal distress, diarrhea Hepatotoxic: abnormal liver function studies, jaundice, fever	1. Do not administer with or immediately prior to fruit juice or other acid drinks. 2. **Ilosone**: observe for jaundice, usually after 10 - 14 days of therapy. Also, do not store **Ilosone** suspension longer than two weeks at room temperature. 3. ***Uses:*** suppression of intestinal bacteria before colonscopy or bowel surgery, Legionnaire's disease, and as a substitute for penicillin.

Appendix 5-10:
ANTIBIOTIC MEDICATIONS

MEDICATIONS	SIDE EFFECTS	NURSING IMPLICATIONS
QUINOLONES: ***Bacteriostatic and bactericidal:*** broad-spectrum; inhibit microbial protein synthesis.		
Ciprofloxacin (**Cipro**): PO Ofloxacin (**Floxin**): PO, IV	Nausea, vomiting, abdominal distress, diarrhea Crystalluria Hepatotoxic: abnormal liver function studies, jaundice, fever	1. Not used in pediatric clients due to potential damage to cartilage and joints. 2. Increase fluid intake and avoid calcium-containing antacids to prevent crystalluria. 3. ***Uses:*** suppression of intestinal bacteria before colonscopy or bowel surgery, Legionnaire's disease, and as a substitute for penicillin.
OTHER ANTIBIOTICS:		
Chloramphenicol sodium: (**Chloromycetin**): PO, IV	Blood dyscrasia (aplastic anemia), irreversible bone marrow depression, GI upset; in neonates, may cause the gray syndrome: ashen gray color, vomiting, loose green stools, vasomotor collapse.	1. Not to be used for minor infections. 2. Observe for bone marrow depression, e.g. weakness, sore throat, bruising. 3. Monitor CBC, platelets, serum iron, reticulocyte counts (q3days). 4. Assess for optic and peripheral neuritis which is an indication for immediate discontinuance of the drug. 5. Observe for GI side effects, neurotoxic reactions, and jaundice.
Astreonam (**Azactam**): IM, IV	Diarrhea, rash, blood dyscrasias, elevated liver enzymes	1. Effective against gram-negative bacterial infections. 2. Used for UTIs, lower respiratory tract infections, and gynecologic/abdominal infections.
Vancomycin (**Vancocin**): PO, IV	Ototoxicity, nephrotoxicity	1. Used in severe penicillin-resistant staphylococcal infection. 2. Peak and trough levels are monitored.
Metronidazole (**Flagyl**): PO, IV, Intravaginally	Anorexia, nausea, vomiting, dry mouth with a metallic taste Abdominal cramps, and uterine pain (if given intravaginally) Superinfection	1. Used to treat anaerobic infections (e.g., intra-abdominal, gynecologic, bone, and joint). 2. Urine may turn dark red-brown. 3. Avoid alcohol and alcohol containing elixirs.

Appendix 5-11: IMMUNOSUPPRESSIVE MEDICATIONS

MEDICATIONS	SIDE EFFECTS	NURSING IMPLICATIONS

IMMUNOPSUPPRESIVE MEDICATIONS: Inhibits the immunological response.

❖ GENERAL NURSING IMPLICATIONS ❖

— Avoid exposure to infection; wash hands frequently.
— Wear protective clothing; use sunscreen.
— Report any sore throat, fever, or other signs of infection to health care provider.
— Take medication at the same time each day to maintain consistent blood levels.
— No vaccines or immunity-conferring agents while client is immunosuppressed.
— Depending on level of immunosuppression, client may need protective isolation.

MEDICATIONS	SIDE EFFECTS	NURSING IMPLICATIONS
Azathioprine (**Imuran**): PO or IV	Dose-and duration-dependent. Bone marrow suppression: leukopenia, thrombocytopenia, anemia. Nausea, vomiting, anorexia. Alopecia, rash.	1. Interacts with allopurinol. 2. Avoid use in pregnancy. 3. Take with food or milk to decrease GI upset. 4. Should not be given to client with active infection. 5. Follow up CBCs at least monthly while on medication. 6. Closely monitor client for development of infections.
Cyclosporine (**Sandimmune**): PO, IV Methotrexate **(Mexate)** Cyclophosphamide **(Cytoxan)**	Dose-and-duration dependent. Infections, nephrotoxicity, hypertension, hirsutism, gum hyperplasia, tremors.	1. Monitor renal function as nephrotoxicity occurs frequently. 2. Avoid use in pregnancy. 3. Use the pipette supplied by manufacturer to measure dose, mix with 4-8oz. of water, milk, or juice. 4. Evaluate blood pressure and report elevations 5. Monitor liver and renal function studies. 6. Good oral hygiene to reduce gum problems. 7. Teach client that he should not stop taking the medication or change dosage without physician's order. 8. Serum blood levels are monitored at regular intervals. 9. Hirsutism that occurs is reversible.
Anti-lymphocyte globulin **(ALG)** Murine monoclonal anti-lymphocyte therapy **(OKT3)**	Fever, chills, hypotension, bronchospasm, Aseptic meningitis—**(OKT3)**	1. Over 50% of clients experience a fever. 2. Have epinephrine and supportive emergency care available, as allergic reaction can occur at any time during therapy.
Methylprednisolone sodium **(SoluMedrol)**	See Appendix 5-7	

Appendix 5-12: ANTIVIRALS MEDICATIONS

MEDICATIONS	SIDE EFFECTS	NURSING IMPLICATIONS

ANTIVIRAL MEDICATIONS: Inhibit viral DNA or RNA replication in the virus, preventing replication and leading to viral death.

❖ GENERAL NURSING IMPLICATIONS ❖

— Medications may be used in combination to obtained better therapeutic results.
— Avoid exposure to infection; wash hands frequently.
— Advise client to report any sore throat, fever, or other signs of infection to health care provider.
— No vaccines or immunity-conferring agents while client is immunosuppressed.
— Depending on level of immunosuppression, client may need protective isolation.
— Most of the medications are to be avoided during pregnancy.
— Medications do not cure AIDS or reduce the risk of transmission of HIV.

MEDICATIONS	SIDE EFFECTS	NURSING IMPLICATIONS
Nucleoside Reverse Transcriptase Inhibitors (NRTIs)		
Zidovudine (**AZT, Retovir**): PO Stavudine (**d4T, Zerit**): PO Didanosine (**ddl, Videx**): PO Zalcitabine (**ddC, Hivid**): PO	Anemia, severe headache, nausea, insomnia	1. Monitor CBC. 2. Schedule/take medications around the clock. 3. Take Didanosine on an empty stomach. Chew tablets thoroughly or crush and disperse in 3 oz of water. Do not mix with fruit juice. 4. Closely monitor client for development of infections.
Protease Inhibitors (PIs)		
Indinavir (**Crixivan**): PO	Nephrolithiasis, GI upset, abdominal pain, headache	1. Monitor renal function. 2. Take one hour before or after low-fat meals.
Nelfinavir (**Viracept**): PO	Diarrhea, nausea, flatulence	
Non-Nucleoside Reverse Transcriptase Inhibitors (NNRTIs)		
Nevirapine (**Viramune**): PO	Possible severe rash (Steven-Johnson syndrome), hepatotoxic, fever, nausea	1. Monitor liver function studies.
Delavirdine (**Rescriptor**): PO	Rash, GI upset	
Nucleoside Analogs		
Acyclovir (**Zovirax**): PO, IV, topical Famciclovir (**Famvir**): PO Valacyclovir (**Valtrex**): PO	Nausea, vomiting, headache, CNS disturbance (especially in elderly)	1. Needs to be administered within 24 hours of herpes zoster outbreaks.

Notes

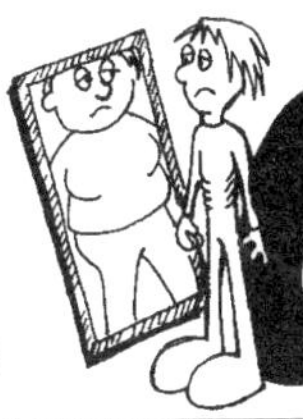

6 Psychiatric Nursing Concepts And Care

SELF-CONCEPT

A. Definitions.

1. Self-concept - all beliefs, convictions and ideas that constitute an individual's knowledge of himself and influence his relationships with others.
2. Self-esteem - an individual's personal judgement of his own worth obtained by analyzing how well his behavior conforms to his self-ideal.

B. Components of a Healthy Personality.

1. Positive and accurate body image.
2. Positive self-concept and high self-esteem.
3. Satisfying role performance.
4. Clear sense of identity.

> ***NURSING PRIORITY:*** *A healthy self-concept, (i.e., a positive self-esteem), is essential to psychologic well being; it is universal,(i.e., something everyone wants and needs).*

Data Collection

A. Factors affecting self-esteem.

1. Parental rejection in early childhood experiences.
2. Lack of recognition and appreciation by parents as child grows older.
3. Over-possessiveness, over-permissiveness, and control by one or both parents.
4. Unrealistic self-ideals or goals (tyranny of the shoulds).

> ***Geriatric Priority:*** *The use of wheelchairs, canes, walkers, hearing aids, or any combination of these will impact the self-esteem of the elderly client.*

B. Behaviors associated with low self-esteem.

1. Self-criticism - describes himself as stupid, no good, a born loser.
2. Minimizes one's ability.
3. Guilt and worrying.
4. Postponing decisions and denying oneself pleasure.
5. Disturbed interpersonal relationships.
6. Self-destructiveness and boredom.
7. Polarizing view of life.

Nursing Intervention

> ***NURSING PRIORITY:*** *Promoting a positive self-concept is basic to all psychotherapeutic interventions. Look for options that focus on this concept; acknowledging the client as a person is an example.*

1. Promote an open, trusting relationship.
2. Work and expand on whatever ego strength the client possesses.
3. Maximize the client's participation in the therapeutic relationship.
4. Encourage the client to accept his own feelings and thoughts.
5. Assist the client to clarify his concept of self and relationship with others through appropriate self-disclosure.
6. Explore with client maladaptive thinking patterns such as:
   a. Catastrophizing - thinking that the worst will happen.
   b. Minimizing and maximizing - tendency to minimize the positive and maximize the negative.
   c. Black-and-white thinking - tendency to look at situations in extremes, no middle ground.
   d. Over-generalization - if something happens once, it will happen again.
   e. Self-reference - tendency to believe that people are particularly aware of their mistakes.
   f. Filtering - selectively pulling out certain details out of context while neglecting to look at more positive facts.
7. Communicate empathically, not sympathetically, and encourage client that he has the power to change himself.
8. Encourage client to define and identify problem.
9. Identify irrational beliefs such as:
   a. "I must be loved by everyone."
   b. "I must be competent and not make mistakes."
   c. "My whole life is a disaster, if it doesn't turn out exactly as planned."
10. Identify areas of strength by exploring areas such as hobbies, skills, work, school, character traits, personal abilities, etc.

Pediatric Priority: *If parents assist children to accomplish goals that are important to them, children begin to develop a sense of personal competence and independence.*

11. Explore client's adaptive and maladaptive coping responses.
    a. Determine "pay-offs" for maintaining self-defeating behaviors such as:
       (1) Procrastination.
       (2) Avoiding risks and commitments.
       (3) Retreating from the present situation.
       (4) Not having to accept responsibility for one's action.
    b. Identify the disadvantages of the maladaptive coping responses.

A. Realistic planning.
1. Assist client to identify alternative solutions.
2. Encourage creative visualization to enhance self-esteem through goal setting.
3. Assist client to set realistic goals by encouraging him to participate in new experiences.

B. Commitment to action.
1. Providing opportunity for client to experience success is essential.
2. Reinforce strengths, abilities, and skills.

NURSING PRIORITY: *An individual's functional level of overall self-esteem may change markedly from day to day and moment to moment.*

NCLEX ALERT: *Identify dynamics of family interactions. strengths of client and family/significant others. Promote positive self-esteem in client with a psychosocial disorder.*

CULTURAL COMPETENCE

A. Definitions.
1. Culture - the individual, group, or community's beliefs, values, and norms that are used in everyday life.
2. Cultural competence - process whereby the nurse develops cultural awareness, knowledge, and skills to promote effective health care.
3. Cultural diversity - unique differences in areas such as age, gender, socioeconomic status, religion, race, and ethnicity.

B. Barriers to culturally competent care.
1. Miscommunication.
2. Failure to assess for cultural perspective.
3. Differences in understanding the way in which people function, interact, and behave everyday.
4. Patients use culturally specific language to describe medical symptoms or problems.
5. *Example:* Native Americans may express depression symptoms as "having heart pain or heartbroken." Hispanics may say that their soul is lost because of another's ability to put an "evil eye" on them.

NURSING PRIORITY: *Recognize cultural issues that could impact client and family understanding/acceptance of diagnosis and respect personal choices/lifestyle of client (e.g., sexual orientation, health care decisions, and cultural considerations.*

BODY IMAGE

Evaluation of Body Image Alteration

A. Types of body image disturbances.
1. Changes in body size, shape, and appearance (rapid weight gain or loss, plastic surgery, pregnancy).
2. Pathological processes causing changes in structure or function of one's body (arthritis, Parkinson's disease, cancer, heart disease).
3. Failure of a body part to function properly (paraplegic or stroke).
4. Physical changes associated with normal growth and development (puberty, aging process).
5. Threatening medical or nursing procedures (catheterization, radiation therapy, organ transplants).

B. Principles.
1. Body characteristics that have been present from birth or acquired early in life seem to have less emotional significance than those arising later.
2. Body-image changes, handicaps, or changes in body function that occur abruptly are far more traumatic than ones that develop gradually.
3. The location of a disease or injury greatly affects the emotional response to it; internal diseases are generally less threatening than external diseases (trauma, disfigurement).
4. Changes in genitals or breasts are perceived as a great threat and reawaken fears about sexuality and virility.

Specific Situations of Altered Body Image and Nursing Intervention

NCLEX ALERT: *Provide support to client with changes in body image (e.g., mastectomy, amputation, alopecia, etc.).*

Obesity

Data Collection

A. Body weight exceeds 20% above the normal range for age, sex, and height.
B. Feeding behavior is gauged according to external environmental cues (i.e., availability of food, odors, stress) rather than hunger (increased G.I. motility).
C. Increased incidence of diabetes, cardiovascular disease, and poor healing.
D. Often has symptoms of depression, fatigue, dyspnea, tachycardia, and hypertension.

Nursing Intervention

A. Encourage behavior modification programs.
B. Promote activities and interests not related to food or eating.
C. Identify client's need to eat and relate the need to preceding events or situations.
D. Decrease guilt and anxiety related to being obese.
E. Encourage an exercise program.

Stroke (CVA)

Data Collection

A. Change of body function due to loss of bowel and bladder control, speech, and cognitive skills.
B. Disordered orientations in relationship to body and position sense in space; body image boundaries disrupted.

Intervention

A. Decrease frustration related to speech problems by encouraging speech effort, speaking slowly, and clarifying statements.
B. Promote reintegration of altered body image due to paralyzed body part by tactile stimulation and verbal reminders of the existing body part.

Amputation

Data Collection

A. Feelings of loss; lowered self-esteem; guilt; helplessness.
B. Depression, passivity, and increased emotional vulnerability.
C. Phantom limb pain in most clients - increased experience if amputation occurs after four years of age, and almost universal experience after age eight.
D. Phantom limb pain stronger in upper limbs and lasts longer than in lower limbs.

Intervention

A. Discussion of phantom limb phenomenon and exploration of client's fears regarding amputation.
B. Acknowledge phantom limb pain; administer analgesics; reassure client that this is a normal process.

Pregnancy

Data Collection

A. Produces marked changes in a woman's body, resulting in major alterations in body configuration within a short period of time.
B. Second trimester - becomes aware that her body is widening and requires more body space.
C. Third trimester - very much aware of increased size; may feel ambivalent about the changes in her body.
D. Perceives her body as vulnerable, yet as a protective container for the unborn.
E. Mate experiences changed body image and sympathetic symptoms during woman's pregnancy.

Intervention

A. Explanation and reassurance of the normal physiologic changes that are occurring.
B. Provide discussions of alterations in body image for both mates.
C. Encourage verbalization of feelings relating to changed body image.

Cancer

Data Collection

A. Cancer clients may suffer many changes in body image.
B. Removal of sex organs (breasts, uterus) has a significant impact on client's sexuality.
C. Disfiguring head and neck surgery has devastating impact to body image, since the face is one of the primary means by which people communicate.
D. Symptoms of depersonalization, loss of self-esteem, and depression may occur.

Intervention

A. Provide anticipatory guidance to help client cope with crisis of changed body image.

B. Set long-term goals to help cancer client adjust to physiological and psychological changes occurring.

Enterostomal surgery

Data Collection

A. Client often shocked at initial sight of ostomy.

B. May experience lowered self-esteem, fear of fecal spillage, alteration in sexual functioning, feelings of disfigurement and rejection.

Intervention

A. Preoperative explanation by use of drawings, models, or pictures of how stoma will appear.

B. Reassurance that reddish appearance of stoma and large size will diminish in time.

C. Encourage discussion and recognize importance of client taking with a "successful ostomate."

HUMAN SEXUALITY

A. Effect of illness and injury on sexuality.

1. Depression episodes often precipitate a decrease in libido.
2. Sexual preoccupations and overtones may be experienced in the psychotic client.
3. Certain medications contribute to sexual dysfunction (e.g., antihypertensives, SSRI's, antipsychotics, phenothiazines).
4. Clients with spinal cord injuries may lose sexual functioning because of full or partial paralysis.
5. Trauma and disfigurement can lead to dysfunction.

B. Effect of the aging process on sexuality.

1. Physiological changes in the woman relate to decreasing estrogen supply: decrease in vaginal lubrication, shrinkage in size and elasticity of vaginal canal, and decrease in breast size.
2. Physiological changes in the man include a decrease in testosterone, decrease in spermatogenesis, a longer length of time to achieve erection along with a decrease in the firmness of erection.

CONCEPT OF LOSS, DEATH, DYING

NCLEX ALERT: *Assist client with expected life transitions (e.g., losses, impending death) and provide emotional support to client/family/significant others.*

Definition

1. Includes both biological and physiological aspects; loss of function.
2. Components of loss include death, dying, grief, and mourning.
    a. Death: represents finality, the end of one's biological being.
    b. Dying: the social process of organizing activities that prepare for death; provides others, as well as the client, a way to prepare for the future.
    c. Grief: the sequence of subjective states that follow loss and accompany mourning.
    d. Mourning: the psychological processes that are aroused by the loss of a loved object or person.

Data Collection

A. Characteristic stages.

1. Death and dying (Kübler-Ross, 1969).
    a. Denial and isolation.
    b. Anger.
    c. Bargaining.
    d. Depression.
    e. Acceptance.
2. Grief.
    a. Shock and disbelief.
    b. Developing awareness.
    c. Restitution or resolution of the loss.

B. Clinical Signs.

1. Impending death.
    a. Loss of muscle tone.
        (1) Bowel/bladder incontinence.
        (2) Difficulty speaking, swallowing, loss of gag reflex.
        (3) Decreased GI motility (e.g., flatus, abdominal distention, retention of feces).
    b. Slowing of the circulation.
        (1) Mottling and cyanosis of extremities.
        (2) Cool skin: first in feet, later the hands, ears and nose.
    c. Changes in vital signs.
        (1) Decreased pulse (weaker) and blood pressure.
        (2) Rapid, shallow, irregular, or abnormally slow respirations; mouth breathing.
    d. Sensory impairment.
        (1) Blurred vision.
        (2) Impaired senses of taste and smell.

Box 6-1:
Understanding Defense Mechanisms

NAME OF DEFENSE MECHANISM	DEFINITION
Compensation	Attempting to make up for or offset deficiencies, either real or imagined by, concentrating on or developing other abilities
Denial	Blocking out or disowning painful thoughts or feelings
Displacement	Feelings are transferred, redirected, or discharged from the appropriate person or object to a less threatening person or object
Introjection	Acceptance of another's values and opinions as one's own
Projection	Attributing one's own unacceptable feelings and thoughts to others
Rationalization	Attempting to justify or modify unacceptable needs and feelings to the ego, in an effort to maintain self-respect and prevent guilt feelings
Regression	Retreating to an earlier, more comfortable level of adjustment
Repression	An involuntary, automatic submerging of painful, unpleasant thoughts and feelings into the *unconscious*
Sublimation	Diversion of unacceptable instinctual drives into personally and socially acceptable areas to help channel forbidden impulses into constructive activities
Suppression	Intentional exclusion of forbidden ideas and anxiety producing situations from the *conscious* level; a voluntary forgetting and postponing mechanism

***NURSING PRIORITY:** Hearing is thought to be the last sense lost.*

2. Imminent death.
   a. Dilated, fixed pupils.
   b. Inability to move; loss of reflexes.
   c. Faster, weaker pulse, lowered blood pressure.
   d. Cheyne-Stokes respirations.
   e. Noisy breathing, often referred to as the death rattle, due to collection of mucus in the pharynx.
3. *Clinical* death.
   a. Total lack of response to external stimuli.
   b. No muscular movement, especially breathing.
   c. No reflexes.
   d. Flat encephalogram.
4. The *biological* signs of death are traditionally considered to be cessation of apical pulse, respirations, and blood pressure.

Nursing Intervention

✦ *To acknowledge the pain of the loss.*
1. Assist the griever to recognize that they must yield to the painful process of grief.
2. Explain how grief affects all areas of one's life.
3. Try and view the loss from the griever's perspective.

✦ *To assist the grieving and/or dying client to accept the reality of loss and/or death.*
1. Encourage expression and verbalization of feelings with interruption,(i.e., crying, talking).
2. Listen nonjudgementally with acceptance.
3. Reach out and make contact with client and family—let genuine concern and caring show.

✦ *To provide for spiritual needs of the grieving and/or dying client.*
1. Ask clergy to visit.
2. Pray with client and family (if requested to do so), read inspirational literature, play music.
3. Encourage the griever to give self-respite times from the grieving process.

✦ *To promote adjustment to life and living after the experience of loss.*
1. Encourage re-investing energies into new undertakings and relationships.
2. Promote letting go and moving on.

PSYCHOSOCIAL DATA ASSESSMENT

❑ **Complete data collection includes descriptions of the intellectual functions, behavioral reactions, emotional reactions, and dynamic issues of the client.**

***Geriatric Priority:** Allow ample time to gather psychosocial data from elderly clients, as they are often starved for someone to listen to them.*

A. Purpose: to obtain data from multiple sources, (e.g. client, family, friends, police, mental health personnel), in order to identify patterns of functioning that are healthy as well as patterns that create problems in the client's everyday life.

B. Psychosocial data to obtain.

1. Chief Complaint (CC) - main reason client is seeking psychiatric help.
2. History of the Presenting Illness (HPI) - onset and development of symptoms or problems.
3. Past Medical History (PMH) - Previous mental health hospitalizations or treatment; information concerning client's birth, growth and development, illnesses, occupation, marital history, religious practices, use of tobacco, alcohol, or drugs, etc.
4. Family history - have any immediate family members sought psychiatric treatment or counseling?
5. Personality profile - client's interests, feelings, mood, and usual leisure or hobby activities.

***NURSING PRIORITY:** Assess level of consciousness, vision, and hearing first (alert, lethargic, stuporous, comatose) and ability of the client to comprehend the interview (mental status exam).*

COPING OR DEFENSE MECHANISMS

A. Specific defense processes used by individuals to relieve or decrease anxieties caused by uncomfortable situations that threaten self-esteem.

B. Related principles.

1. The primary functions are to decrease emotional conflicts, provide relief from stress, protect from feelings of inadequacy and worthlessness, prevent awareness of anxiety, and maintain an individual's self-esteem.
2. Everyone uses defense mechanisms to a certain extent. If used to an extreme degree they distort reality, interfere with interpersonal relationships, limit one's ability to work productively, and may lead to pathological symptomatology.

C. Common defense mechanisms (Box 6-1).

NCLEX ALERT: *Identify coping mechanisms.*

D. Nursing management.

1. Accept coping mechanisms.

Box 6-2:
Ineffective Responses and Behaviors

- Not listening; talking too much
- Looking too busy
- Seeming uncomfortable with silence
- Avoiding sensitive topics
- Changing the subject
- Laughing nervously; smiling inappropriately
- Showing a closed body posture
- Focusing on personal issues of the nurse
- Making flippant comments

2. Discuss alternative coping mechanisms and problem-solving situations.
3. Assist the client in learning new or alternative coping patterns for a healthier adaptation.
4. Utilize techniques to decrease anxiety.

THERAPEUTIC NURSING PROCESS

❑ **Therapeutic Interpersonal Relationship is the interaction between two persons: the *nurse* promotes goal-directed activities that help to alleviate the discomfort of the *client* by promoting growth and satisfying interpersonal relationships.**

Characteristics

- Goal- directed.
- Empathetic understanding.
- Honest, open communication.
- Concreteness; avoid vagueness and ambiguity.
- Acceptance; non-judgmental attitude.
- Involves nurse's understanding of self, and personal motives and needs.

Phases

1. Initial phase - goal is *to build trust.*
   a. Explore the client's perceptions, thoughts, feelings and actions.
   b. Identify problem.
   c. Assess levels of anxiety of self and client.
   d. Mutually define specific goals to pursue.
2. Working phase - goal is *to establish objectives* or working agreement (a contract).
   a. Encourage client participation.
   b. Focus on problem-solving techniques; choose between alternate courses of action and practice skills.
   c. Explore thoughts, feelings, and emotions.

Table 6-1:
THERAPEUTIC COMMUNICATION

RESPONSE	EXAMPLE
1. Exploring	"What seems to be the problem?" "Tell me more about..."
2. Reflecting	"I am really mad at my mother for grounding me." "You sound angry."
3. Focusing	"Give an example of what you mean." "Let's look at this more closely."
4. Clarifying	"I'm not sure that I understand what you're saying." "Do you mean...?"
5. Using general leads	"Go on..." "Talk more about..."
6. Broad opening leads	"Where would you like to begin?" "Talk more about..."
7. Validating	"Did I understand you to say...?
8. Informing	"The time is..." "My name is..."
9. Accepting	"Yes." "Okay." Nodding "Uh hmm."
10. Sharing observations	"You appear anxious. I noticed that you haven't been coming to lunch with the group."
11. Presenting reality	"I do not hear a noise or see the lights blinking." "I am not Cleopatra; I am your nurse."
12. Summarizing	"During the past hour..."
13. Using silence	Nurse remains silent.
NONTHERAPEUTIC COMMUNICATION	
1. False reassurance	"Don't worry, you will be better in a few weeks." "Don't worry, I had an operation just like it; it was a snap."
2. Giving advise	"What you should do is..." "If I were you, I would do..."
3. Rejecting	"I don't like it when you..." "Please, don't ever talk about..."
4. Belittling	"Everybody feels that way." "Why, you shouldn't feel that way."
5. Probing	"Tell me more about your relationship with other men."
6. Overloading	"Hi, I am JoAnn, your student nurse. How old are you? What brought you to the hospital? How many children do you have? Do you want to fill out your menu right now?"
7. Underloading	Not giving enough information so that the meaning is clear; withholding information.
8. Cliches	"Gee, the weather is beautiful outside."

d. Develop constructive coping mechanisms.
e. Increase independence and self-responsibility.

3. Termination phase - goal is *to evaluate goals* set forth and terminate relationship.
   a. Plan for termination early in formation of relationship (in initial phase).
   b. Discuss client's feelings about termination.
   c. Evaluate client's progress and goal attainment.

Levels of Communication

❑ **Verbal communication—occurs through the medium of words, spoken or written.**

❑ **Nonverbal communication — includes everything that does not involve the spoken or written word; involves the five senses.**

1. Vocal cues — tone of voice, quality of voice, nervous coughing and sounds of hesitation.
2. Action cues — body movement, posture, facial expressions, gestures and mannerisms.
3. Object cues — dress, appearance to convey a certain "look" or message.
4. Space — distance between two people; intimate, personal, public space.
5. Touch — universal and basic to all nurse-client relationships; response to it is influenced by the setting, cultural background, type of relationship, sex of communicators, and expectations.

Therapeutic Nurse-Client Communication Techniques

NCLEX ALERT: *Listen to client's/family's concerns; acknowledge differences between client's views/feelings and the health care provider's views/feelings; establish rapport with client or family.*

1. Demonstrate active listening-face-to-face contact.
2. Demonstrate unconditional positive regard, interest, congruence, respect.
3. Develop trusting relationship; accept client's behavior, and display non-judgmental objective attitude.
4. Be supportive, honest, and authentic.
5. Focus on emotional needs and emotionally charged area.
6. Focus on here and now behavior and expression of feelings.
7. Attempt to understand another point of view.
8. Develop an awareness of the client's likes and dislikes.
9. Encourage expression of both positive and negative feelings.
10. Use broad openings and ask open-ended questions; avoid questions that can be answered by yes or no.
11. Use reflections of feelings, attitudes and words.
12. Explore alternatives rather than answers or solutions.
13. Focus feedback on *what* is said rather than *why* it is said.
14. Paraphrase to assist in clarifying client statement.
15. Promote sharing of feelings, information, and ideas rather than giving advice.

INTERVENTION MODALITIES

Crisis Intervention

❑ **A crisis is a self-limiting situation in which usual problem-solving or decision-making methods are not adequate.**

1. A crisis offers opportunities for growth and renewal.
2. Crisis intervention strategy views people as capable of personal growth and able to control their own lives.
3. Types of crisis intervention strategies:
   a. Individual crisis counseling.
   b. Crisis groups.
   c. Telephone counseling.
4. Crisis intervention requires support, protection, and enhancement of the client's self-image.

Group Therapy

❑ **A structured or semi-structured process in which individuals (7 - 12 members ideal size) are interrelated and interdependent and who may share common purposes and norms.**

1. Emphasis on clear communication to promote effective interaction.
2. Disturbed perceptions can be corrected through consensual validation.
3. Socially ineffective behaviors can be modified through peer pressure.

Geriatric Priority: *Reality-testing ability in the client is an important consideration in the selection of group members. An elderly psychotic client would not be good selection as a group member.*

NCLEX ALERT: *Participate in a group session for clients with psychosocial disorders.*

Family therapy

NCLEX ALERT: *Help client/significant other adjust to roles changes; assess family's emotional reaction to client's illness (e.g., chronic disorder, terminal illness); assess dynamics of family interactions.*

❑ **A treatment modality designed to bring about a change in communication and interactive patterns between and among family members.**

1. A family can be viewed as a system that is dynamic. A change or movement in any part of the family system affects all other parts of the system.
2. Family seeks to maintain a balance or "homeostasis" among various forces that operate within and upon it.
3. Emotional symptoms or problems of an individual are an expression of the emotional symptoms or problems in the family.
4. Therapeutic approaches involve helping the family members look at themselves in the here-and-now and recognize the influence of past models on their behavior and expectations.

Milieu

NCLEX ALERT: *Maintain a therapeutic milieu/environment (e.g., structured environment if needed, etc.).*

❑ **A scientifically planned, purposeful manipulation in the environment aimed at causing changes in the behavior and personality of the client.**

1. Nurse is viewed as a facilitator and a helper to clients rather than a therapist.
2. The *therapeutic community* is a very special kind of milieu therapy in which the total social structure of the treatment unit is involved as part of the helping process.
3. Emphasis is placed on open communication both within and between staff and client groups.

Somatic Therapies

1. Restraints (Box 6-2).
   a. Mechanical restraints include camisoles, wrist and ankle restraints, sheet restraints, and cold wet sheet packs.

Box 6-3:
Use Of Restraints

- Obtain a consent to apply restraints.
- Selecting a restraint — should restrict movement as little as possible, least obvious to others, does not interfere with client's treatment, is readily changeable, and is safe for age of client (active child would have a jacket restraint versus a wrist restraint to keep in bed).
- Secure restraint—check for adequate blood circulation to extremities.
- Pad bony prominences (wrists & ankles) before applying restraint.
- Always tie limb restraint with a knot (e.g., clove hitch) that will not tighten will pulled.
- Never tie ends of restraint to a side rail or to part of fixed bed frame if the bed position is going to be changed.
- *Assess restraint q30 min and document.*
- *Release all restraints q2-4h, provide ROM, and skin care — stay with client when restraint is removed and document.*
- Keep in mind the *principle of least restriction* — restrain the client to the extent necessary to accomplish restraint's purpose.

NCLEX ALERT: *Apply restraints or other safety devices per protocol (e.g., vests, etc.)*

   b. Chemical restraints include the use of medications — antianxiety or antipsychotics.
2. Seclusion.
   a. Confinement to a room that may be locked. Often, the room is without a mattress or linens and the client is in a hospital nightgown.
   b. There is limited opportunity for communication.
   c. Legal requirements for the care of the secluded client vary from state to state.

Psychosurgery

❑ **Surgical interruption of selected neural pathways that govern transmission of emotion between the frontal lobes of the cerebral cortex and the thalamus.**

1. Recent resurgence of interest in psychosurgery as knowledge of neuroanatomy; "mapping" the cerebral cortex has become more sophisticated.
2. Area of moral and ethical debate, especially since nerve tissue once damaged can not regenerate.

Electroconvulsive Therapy (ECT)

Table 6-2:
ASSESSMENT OF ANXIETY

PHYSIOLOGICAL	PSYCHOLOGICAL
SYMPATHETIC RESPONSES	BEHAVIORAL RESPONSES
Tachycardia	Restlessness
Elevated blood pressure	Agitation
Increased perspiration	Tremors (fine to gross shaking of the body)
Dilated pupils	Startle reaction
Hyperventilation with difficulty breathing	Rapid speech
Cold, clammy skin	Lack of coordination
Dry mouth	Withdrawal
Constipation	
PARASYMPATHETIC RESPONSES	COGNITIVE RESPONSES
Urinary frequency	Impaired attention
Diarrhea	Poor concentration
	Forgetfulness
	Blocking of thought
	Decreased perceptual field
	Decreased productivity
	Confusion

Table 6-3:
NURSING MANAGEMENT OF ANXIETY

LEVEL OF ANXIETY	ASSESSMENT	GOAL	NURSING MANAGEMENT
MILD	Increased alertness, motivation, and attentiveness.	To assist client to tolerate some anxiety.	1. Help client identify and describe feelings. 2. Help client develop the capacity to tolerate mild anxiety and use it consciously and constructively.
MODERATE	Perception narrowed, selective inattention, physical discomforts.	To reduce anxiety; Long term goal directed toward helping client understand cause of anxiety and new ways of controlling.	1. Provide outlet for tension such as walking, crying, working at simple, concrete tasks.
SEVERE	Behavior becomes automatic; connections between details are not seen; senses are drastically reduced.	To assist in channeling anxiety.	1. Recognize own level of anxiety. 2. Link client's behavior with feelings. 3. Protect defenses and coping mechanisms. 4. Identify and modify anxiety-provoking situations.
PANIC	Overwhelmed; inability to function or communicate; possible bodily harm to self and others; loss of rational thought.	To be supportive and protective.	1. Provide nonstimulating, structured environment. 2. Avoid touching. 3. Stay with client. 4. Medicate client with tranquilizers if necessary.

❑ **ECT is an electric shock delivered to the brain through electrodes that are placed on the head. The shock artificially induces a seizure.**

1. Indications
   a. Severe depression, when other treatment modalities are ineffective.
   b. Acute schizophrenia (catatonic type).
   c. Number of treatments: usually given in a series which vary according to the client's presenting problem and response to therapy; 2 - 3 treatments per week for a total of 6-12 treatments. May also see maintenance or continuation of ECT (once per month for 6-12 months).
2. Nursing Intervention
   a. Assess client's record for routine preoperative type checklist for information (informed consent).
   b. NPO for 6-8 hours prior to treatment.
   c. Remove dentures, hairpins, contact lens, and hearing aids.
   d. Administer preoperative medication (atropine sulfate) after electrodes are applied and before convulsion occurs.
   e. Care immediately following treatment.
      (1) Provide orientation to time.
      (2) Temporary memory loss is usually confusing; explain that this is a common occurrence.
      (3) Assess vital signs for 30 minutes to 1 hour after treatment.
      (4) De-emphasize preoccupation with ECT; promote involvement in regularly scheduled activities.

Other Therapies

1. Psychodrama—the use of structured and directed dramatization of client's emotional problems and experiences.
2. Activities therapy—a number of vital programs come under this, such as, music therapy, occupational therapy, art therapy, recreational therapy, dance or movement therapy, etc.

ANXIETY

NCLEX ALERT: *Identify a client's potential for a physical/emotional reaction to a crisis event; determine ability of family/support system to provide care for client; use crisis intervention techniques to assist client to cope with anxiety.*

A. Definition.
   1. An emotion, a subjective experience.
   2. A feeling state that is experienced as vague uneasiness, tension, or apprehension.
   3. Occurs when the ego is threatened.
   4. Provoked by the unknown; precedes all new experiences.

B. Data Collection (Table 6-2).

C. Nursing management (Table 6-3).

D. Specific disorders of anxiety (Table 6-4).

Problems Associated with Anxiety

❑ **This group of problems has anxiety as the primary disturbance. In the past, these were grouped together as neuroses. Anxiety can be a predominant disturbance (panic and generalized anxiety), or anxiety is experienced as a person attempts to confront a dreaded situation (phobic disorder) or resist the obsessions and compulsions of an obsessive-compulsive disorder. In general, these are common responses to emotional problems that are very seldom treated in a psychiatric setting, as the person has no great defect in reality testing nor demonstrates severe antisocial behavior.**

Interpersonal Withdrawal

❑ ***Interpersonal Withdrawal* is characterized by avoidance of interpersonal contact and a sense of unreality.**

1. Physical Withdrawal - client sits or stands apart from others; may hide, assume a catatonic posture, or in extreme form attempt suicide.
2. Verbal withdrawal - avoidance through silence or, extreme form, mutism; silence may indicate resistance, a pensive moment, or the indication that nothing more is to be said.

Nursing Intervention

1. Avoid punishment of client.
2. Decrease isolation.
3. Invite the client to speak.
4. State the amount of time you are willing to stay with the client whether he/she chooses to speak or not.
5. Change the context of the contact (for example, go for a walk together).
6. Encourage the client to share responsibility for the continuance of the relationship.

Regression

❑ ***Regression* is retreating to earlier, childish, or less complex patterns of behavior which once brought the client attention or pleasure.**

Nursing Intervention

1. Avoid fostering dependency and childlike attitudes.
2. Be patient and understanding.
3. Confront client directly about his/her plan.
4. Compliment client when he/she does something unusually well or assumes more responsibility.
5. Promote problem solving, reality orientation, and involvement in social activities.
6. Avoid punishment following periods of regression; instead, explore the meaning of the regressive behavior.

Anger

❑ ***Anger*** **is the unconscious process used in order to obtain relief from anxiety that is produced by a sense of danger; it involves a sense of powerlessness.**

> ***NURSING PRIORITY:*** *Fear of expressing anger is related to fear of rejection.*

Nursing Intervention

1. Have client acknowledge or name feelings.
2. Explore source of personal fear or perceived threat, (e.g., illness, disability, disfigurement or emotional crisis).
3. Encourage verbalization of anxiety.
4. Explore appropriate external expression of feelings.
5. Avoid arguing with client.
6. Acting out behavior is often an indirect expression of anger; it attracts attention and often represents the feelings the person is experiencing.

> ***NURSING PRIORITY:*** *Non-therapeutic responses to a client's anger are defensiveness, retaliation, condescension, and avoidance.*

Hostility/Aggressiveness

❑ ***Hostility or aggressiveness*** **is an antagonistic feeling; the client wishes to hurt or humiliate others; the result may be a feeling of inadequacy or self-rejection due to a loss of self-esteem.**

Nursing Intervention

> **NCLEX ALERT:** *Use interventions to assit client to control behavior (e.g., contract, behavior modification, set limits, etc.).*

1. Prevent aggressive contact by early recognition of increased anxiety.
2. Maintain client contact rather than avoid it.
3. Encourage verbalization of feelings associated with a threat of frustration (helplessness, inadequacy, anger).
4. Reduce environmental stimuli.
5. Avoid reinforcement behavior, (i.e., joking, laughing, teasing, competitive games).
6. Encourage an alternative expression of aggression such as use of Bataccas (cylindrical clubs of a soft, padded material so that injury is avoided), pillows, or foam balls.
7. Use distraction, or remove the client from the immediate environment to reestablish self-control.
8. Set limits on unacceptable behavior.
9. Protect other clients.

> ***NURSING PRIORITY:*** *When two clients are arguing, engage the dominant client first by using distraction or removing the client from the setting to allow time for de-escalation and processing of the situation.*

Violence

❑ ***Violence*** **is behavior that is physically assaultive and risks injury to the self, others, and environment.**

Nursing Intervention

> ***NURSING PRIORITY:*** *Immediate intervention should focus on control and safety, followed by discussion to alleviate guilt and identify alternative behaviors to help prevent future episodes of violence.*

1. Establish eye contact.
   a. Conveys attention and concern.
   b. Elicits more information.
   c. Ask the person to look at you.

> ***Geriatric Priority:*** *Expect some elderly clients to have vision problems; they may not know who you are.*

2. Avoid asking, "Why?"; instead ask, "What's bothering you?"
   a. *Why* questions are threatening and decrease self-esteem.
   b. Open-ended questions identify the problem, convey concern, and produce more information.

Table 6-4:
SPECIFIC DISORDERS OF ANXIETY

Problem	Description	Nursing Intervention
Phobia: an intense,irrational fear of a specific object, activity, or situation.	Fear of being alone or in public places. Claustrophobia (fear of close places) and acrophobia (fear of heights).	**Goal: to reduce phobic behavior.** 1. Do not force client to come in contact with the feared object or source of anxiety. 2. Have client focus on awareness of self. 3. Distract client's attention from phobia.
Obsessive-Compulsive Disorder: unconscious control of anxiety by the use of rituals, thoughts, obsession, or compulsions.	**Obsessions:** recurrent, persistent ideas, thoughts, or impulses that are not voluntarily produced. *Most common obsessions include thoughts of violence, contamination, and doubt.* **Compulsions:** repetitive, ritualistic behaviors that are performed in a certain fashion that relieve an unbearable amount of tension. *Most common compulsions include handwashing, counting, checking.*	**Goal: to assist in coping with the compulsive behavior.** 1. Accept rituals and avoid punishment or criticism; do not interrupt ritual, as this will increase anxiety. 2. Plan for extra time, due to slowness and client's need for perfection. 3. Prevent physical deterioration or harm, and set limits only to prevent harmful acts (such as handwashing excessively) that removes the skin from the hand surface. **Goal: to encourage client to develop different ways of handling anxiety.** 1. Reduce demands on the individual. 2. Convey acceptance of client regardless of behavior. 3. Encourage alternative activity.
Post-Traumatic Stress Disorder: involves the development of characteristic symptoms following a traumatic psychological event in which the individual is unable to adapt or adjust (e.g., rape, military combat, airplane crashes, death camps, torture or abuse).	Client re-experiences the traumatic event. Client withdraws, becomes isolated or herself and restricts emotional response. Experienes hyperalertness, insomnia, nightmares, depression and anxiety.	**Goal: to determine precipitating stress factor in client's reaction.** 1. Reduce and prevent chronic disability. 2. Encourage verbalization of the traumatic event. **Goal: to maintain personal integrity.** 1. Provide physical, social, or occupational rehabilitation. 2. Somatic therapies are used to decrease anxiety (e.g., anti-anxiety agents, etc.)
Conversion Disorder: a loss of or alteration in physical functioning that suggests a physical disorder, but is related to expression of a psychological conflict or need.	Physical symptoms associated with disorder are *not* under voluntary control.	**Goal: to identify primary or secondary gain.** 1. Primary gain: symptom has symbolic meaning to client; keeps client unaware of internal conflict and anxiety. 2. Secondary gain: a gain of attention and sympathy along with reinforcement of maladjusted behavior. **Goal: to avoid reinforcing the client's symptoms.** 1. Focus on feelings and not on symptoms. 2. Reduce pressure and anxiety-provoking situations around client. 3. Divert attention from symptoms. 4. Provide recreational activity. 5. Avoid pity and sympathetic approach to client's "illnesses" or "symptoms."

> ***Geriatric Priority:** Hearing problems occur with the elderly; don't shout or talk rapidly.*

3. Speak to client softly, slowly, and with assurance.
4. Give directions clearly and concisely. Tell the patient what you want him or her to do.
5. Encourage client to verbalize feelings.
   a. Give the person an outlet for the physical tension, "Walk with me — tell me what happened."
   b. Keep the conversation slow. Pace yourself. "Wait, I can't follow that. Tell me what you said."
   c. Listen more than talk.
   d. Let the person walk, move, or pound, and vent the tension before you talk.
6. Position yourself near the door.
   a. Don't block the door.
   b. Don't box the patient into a corner.
7. Self-protection and protection of other clients is a primary concern.

a. Never see a potentially violent client alone, call security or other personnel.

b. Keep a comfortable distance from client, don't intrude on his or her personal space.

(1) With mild or moderate anxiety in the patient — sit near, about 2 feet away.

(2) With severe or panic anxiety — stay 4 to 6 feet back (or farther).

c. Be prepared to move quickly; violent clients act fast and unpredictably.

d. Ascertain that client has no weapons before approaching.

e. Be supportive and intervene to increase client's self-esteem.

f. Be honest — tell the person you are concerned that he or she is out of control, but you are not going to let anyone get hurt.

g. Stay with the person, but don't touch until you've asked permission and it has been given to you.

8. When client is in control, review and process the situation in order to alleviate client's guilt and to discuss alternatives should client become anxious or angry in the future.

NCLEX ALERT: *Identify disruptive or destructive behavior of client and intervene to increase client understanding of his/her behavior.*

Manipulation/Acting Out

❑ ***Manipulation/Acting Out* is a type of controlling behavior in which an individual uses others to meet his/her own needs or to achieve specific goals; often disguises underlying feelings of inadequacy, inferiority, and unworthiness; an attempt to protect against failure or frustration and to gain power over another.**

Nursing Intervention

1. Be consistent and firm in the expectations of behavior.
2. Allow some freedom within set limits.
3. Consistent enforcement of set limits.
4. Be alert to client's attempt to intimidate; allow verbal anger.
5. Avoid involvement and intellectualization.
6. Watch carefully for client's use of manipulative patterns; be alert to the many guises in which it may be manifested.
7. Keep staff united, firm, and consistent.
8. Encourage open communication about real needs and feelings.
9. Maintain a sense of authority.
10. Do not accept gifts, favors, flattery or other guises of manipulation.

Dependence

❑ ***Dependence* is a behavior pattern characterized by adopting a helpless, powerless stance; a reliance on other people to meet a basic need.**

Nursing Intervention

1. Assess client's abilities and capacities.
2. Set firm and consistent limits on behavior.
3. Provide only help needed.
4. Encourage problem-solving and decision-making skills; emphasize accountability
5. Avoid making decisions or assuming responsibility for client's ability to make decisions.
6. Maintain an attitude of firmness and confidence in client's ability to make decisions.
7. Discourage reliance beyond actual needs.
8. Give positive reinforcements for development of independent growth-facilitating behavior.
9. Encourage successful participation in social relationships.

Shame

❑ ***Shame* is the inner sense of being completely diminished or insufficient as a person, (e.g., feeling less than).**

Nursing Intervention

1. Assist client to begin to *externalize* rather than internalize feelings of shame.
2. Encourage client to share feelings honestly with individuals they feel "safe" with.
3. Involve clients in "debriefing," which is writing and talking about past shame experiences.
4. Encourage client to make positive self-affirmations, involve themselves in creative visualization activities to improve self-concept.

Detachment

❑ **Detachment is characterized by aloofness, superficiality, denial, and intellectualization in interpersonal contact.**

Nursing Intervention

1. Establish awareness of the process of detachment.
2. Explore fears and fantasies inhibiting emotional expression.

3. Encourage verbalization from global generalities to specific personal comments.
4. Provide clarification of client's unclear responses.
5. Emphasize awareness and exploration of feelings.

ABUSE

***NURSING PRIORITY:** Report client abuse to authorities and act as a client advocate.*

Types of Abuse

A. ***Physical abuse***—non-accidental, intentional injury inflicted on another person, often seen as elder abuse or child abuse.

B. ***Physical neglect***—willing deprivation of essential care needed to sustain basic human needs and to promote growth and development.

C. ***Emotional abuse***—use of threats, verbal insults, or other acts of degradation that are intended to be injurious or damaging to another's self-esteem.

D. ***Emotional neglect***—absence of a warm, interpersonal atmosphere that is necessary for psychosocial growth, development, and the promotion of positive feelings of self-worth and self-esteem.

E. ***Sexual abuse***—lack of comprehension and consent on the part of the individual involved in sexual activities that are either exploitative or physically intimate in nature, (e.g., fondling, oral or genital contact, masturbation, unclothing, etc).

F. ***Incest***—sexual activity performed between members of a family group.

Intrafamily Abuse and Violence

❑ **Patterns of dysfunctional, violent families can frequently be traced back for several generations. Adult behavior and role models for parenting are influenced by the childhood experiences within the family system.**

A. The incorporation of violence within the family teaches the children that the use of violence is appropriate. When the children grow up and form their own families, they tend to recreate the same parent-child, husband-wife relationships experienced in their original family.

B. Frequently the abuser has inappropriate expectations of family members; they may expect perfection and may be obsessed with discipline and control.

C. Family members are confused regarding their role in the family; parents may be unable to assume an adult role in the family. Adult family members who feel inadequate in their role may use violence in an attempt to prove themselves and to maintain superiority.

D. Family is usually isolated, both physically and emotionally. The family tends to have few friends, and frequently is isolated from the extended family. Family members are ashamed of what is occurring and tend to withdraw from social contacts in fear that the family activities might become known to others.

Characteristics of Abuse

A. The person who abuses.
   1. Inability to control impulses; explosive temper; low tolerance for frustration.
   2. Possesses greater physical strength than the victim.
   3. Low self-esteem.
   4. Tends to project shortcomings and inadequacies onto others.
   5. Emotional immaturity; decreased capacity to delay satisfaction.
   6. Suspicious of everyone; fear of being exposed; tend to isolate themselves from their families.
   7. High incidence of drug and alcohol abuse.

B. Victim.
   1. Low self-esteem and depression.
   2. Experiences feelings of dependency, helplessness, or powerlessness.
   3. If he has experienced abuse as a child, there is a greater tendency to demonstrate violence in his adult relationships.
   4. Feels responsible for abuse or neglect that is inflicted upon him; may feel guilty that he is at fault.

C. Common similarities between person who abuses and victim.
   1. Poor self-concept and feelings of insecurity.
   2. Feelings of helplessness, powerlessness, and dependence.
   3. Difficulty or inability to handle anger.

D. Physical abuse symptoms in elders and children (Box 6-3: Elderly Care Focus: Elder Abuse).
   1. Symptoms.
      a. Bruises and welts from being beaten with a belt, strap, stick, coat hanger or from being slapped repeatedly in the face.
      b. Rope burns from being tied up or beaten with a rope.
      c. Human bite marks.
      d. Burns.

Table 6-5:
DOCUMENTATION FOR SUSPECTED ABUSE

Procedure:
1. Obtain the client's or parent's permission before photographing the victim.
2. Do not make assumptions as to whom the assailant or abuser was; chart the exact client/child's words used to describe the abuser.
3. Record information very objectively; do not record your feelings, assumptions, or opinions of the incident or how it occurred.

History:
1. Specific time, date, and location the client says the incident occurred.
2. Reported sequence of events prior to the abuse/attack.
3. Period of time between the abuse/attack and initiation of medical attention.
4. Presence of other people/children in the immediate vicinity of the abuse/attack.
5. Include verbal quotations from the client.
6. Be very specific and objective in recording observations of the client and the person who brought the client to the emergency room; observe and record the interaction of the child and the parents.

Physical Examination:
1. Be very specific in describing the location, size, shape of bruises and lacerations. If possible, photograph the client to demonstrate the extent of the injury.
2. If possible, describe the location and extent of injuries on an anatomical diagram.
3. Identify presence of other injuries.
4. Describe the victim's reaction to pain, level of pain and location of pain.

(1) Burns on the buttocks from being immersed in hot water.

(2) Pattern of burns—round, small burns from cigarettes; patterns that suggest an object was used.

(3) Burns frequently are on the buttocks, in genital area, or on the soles of the feet.

e. Evidence of various fractures in different stages of healing.

f. Internal injuries from being hit repeatedly in the stomach.

g. Head injuries—skull, facial fractures.

h. Severe dehyration, poor hygiene, and malnutrition in elders.

2. Behavior symptoms.

a. Withdrawal from physical contact with adults or caretakers.

Box 6-4: Elderly Care Focus
Elder Abuse

- Types of elder abuse—physical, psychological, sexual, financial, and neglect.
- Neglect indicators—poor hygiene, poor nutrition, poor skin integrity, contractures, urine burns/excoriation, pressure ulcers, dehydration, bruising on inner surfaces of extremities.

b. Inappropriate response to pain or injury, failure to cry or seek comfort from parents or residential caretakers.

c. Infant may stiffen when held; child may stiffen when approached by adult or parent.

d. Children—very little eye contact with adults.

e. Child may try to protect abusing parent for fear of punishment if abuse is discovered.

3. Parent or caretakers.

a. Conflicting stories regarding accident or injury.

b. Explanation of accident is inconsistent with injuries sustained (fractured skull and broken leg from falling out of bed).

c. Initial complaint is not associated with child's injury (child is brought to the ER with complaints of the "flu,"and there is evidence of a skull fracture).

d. Exaggerated concern or lack of concern related to level of child's injury.

e. Refusal to allow further tests or additional medical care and long delay in treatment of an injury.

f. Lack of nurturing response to injured or ill child; no cuddling, touching, or comforting child in distress.

g. Repeated visits to various medical emergency facilities.

h. Do not have realistic expectations of the child; do not understand stages of growth and development (severe spanking or beating a 1-year-old for lack of response to toilet training).

Nursing Intervention

✦ *Goal: to establish a safe environment.*

1. It is important for the nurse to be knowledgeable of the legal responsibilities in regard to state practice acts and child abuse laws, and assault and battery with regards to the elder adult (See Table 6-5: Documentation for Suspected Abuse).
2. All fifty states have a designated agency that is available on a 24-hour basis for reporting and assistance with child abuse.

3. All states have mechanism for removing the child from the immediate abusive environment.
4. Report elder abuse suspicions to licensing bodies associated with the agency in question.

✦ *Goal: to educate families and help them identify assistance for long term supportive care.*

1. Educate parents in regard to normal growth and development of children, the role of discipline, and the necessity for having realistic expectations.
2. Educate caretakers to the normal process of aging, (i.e., forgetfulness, need for assistance, etc).
3. Become familiar with available community resources such as crisis centers, crisis hotlines, parent effectiveness training groups, Parents Anonymous groups, etc.

Rape

A. The legal definition of rape varies from state to state. The most general definition is that of forced, violent, sexual attack on an individual without their consent. Some states include sex acts other than forced intercourse as rape, some states do not recognize rape by the husband.

B. Sexual assault is not a means of sexual gratification; it is a violent physical and emotional attack. Men attack women in an attempt to demonstrate their power and dominance. They attempt to control, terrify, and degrade the woman.

C. Victims are in all age ranges; highest risk age group is between 12 and 20 years old.

D. The majority of rapes are not sudden and impulsive; they are well-planned.

E. Studies reveal that most women know the rapist; most rape assaults occur between people of the same race.

Physical Assessment

1. Woman may experience a wide range of emotional responses—rape trauma syndrome symptoms include sleep disturbances, nightmares, loss of appetite, fears, anxiety, phobias, suspicion, disruptpion in realtionships with partner, family, and friends, along with low self-esteem, feelings of worthlessness, self-blame, guilt, and shame.
2. Complete physical assessment—important for as much evidence as possible to be obtained.
3. If possible, advise the woman to not "clean up," the physical evidence may be destroyed. She should come immediately to the emergency room.

Nursing Intervention

✦ *Goal: to assist the client through the initial phase after the rape experience.*

1. Encourage the client to verbalize her feelings regarding the attack.
2. Assist her to set priorities and immediate needs.
3. Warm, respectful, accepting response from the nurse; protect the client from becoming overwhelmed and distressed from the initial physical examination and questioning.
4. Discuss need for follow-up care and physical examination regarding possible pregnancy and venereal disease.
5. Provide information regarding physical and emotional responses to rape.
6. Provide referral information and plan for follow -up contact within the next week.

✦ *Goal: to assist the client to work through the emotional phases that commonly occur after the initial trauma.*

1. Encourage mental health counseling the first few days after the assault.
2. Assist the client to understand and recognize the period of reorganization which frequently follows the sexual attack.
   a. Victim may experience sexual problems.
   b. May experience a strong urge to discuss the incident and feelings related to the attack.
   c. During the reorganization phase, client should have professional counseling to assist her to cope positively with the situation.

PSYCHIATRIC DISORDERS

***NURSING PRIORITY:** It is important to note that emotional disturbances must be evaluated within the context and framework of normal growth and development since behavior that is part of normal growth and development at one age may be a symptom of a pathology at another age.*

Mental Retardation

❑ ***Mental retardation* is associated with developmental disabilities, intellectual deficits, and lack of adaptive behaviors.**

Data Collection

A. Causes.

1. Down's syndrome (trisomy of the 21st chromosome).
   a. Incidence with maternal age.

b. Head: small in size; face has flat profile, sparse hair.
c. Eyes: inner epicanthal folds.
d. Nose: small and depressed nasal bridge (saddle nose).
e. Ears: small and sometimes low- set.
f. Mouth: protruding, thick tongue.
g. Neck: short and broad.
h. Abdomen: protruding.
i. Genitalia: small penis, undescended testes.
j. Hands: short, stubby fingers; simian crease (transverse palmar crease).
k. Muscles: hypotonic.

2. Phenylketonuria (PKU) — metabolic deficiency.
   a. Needs to be treated early.
   b. Newborn screening in nursery.
3. Fetal Alcohol Syndrome (See Alcoholism).
4. Rubella.
5. Kernicterus (elevated bilirubin).
6. Anoxia.

B. Additional characteristics.
1. Irritability, temper tantrums, stereotyped movements.
2. Dysfunction with vision, hearing, or seizure activity.
3. IQ below 70.

Nursing Intervention

✦ *Goal: to promote optimum development within a family and community setting.*
1. Promote feelings of self-esteem, worth, and security.
2. Educate the parent regarding dealing with child's developmental, not chronological; age.
3. Involve child and parent in early stimulation program.
4. Promote self-care skills.
5. Encourage parents to enroll child in special daycare programs and education classes.
6. Emphasize to parent that child has same needs of play, discipline, and social interaction as other children.

✦ *Goal: to promote independence by setting realistic goals.*
1. Teach skills in simple terms with steps outlined.
2. Utilize behavior modification as a method for behavior control.
3. Utilize the principles of *repetition, reinforcement* and *routine* when providing information for understanding and learning.

✦ *Goal: to prevent physical problems associated with Down's syndrome.*
1. Prevent respiratory infections by teaching parents about postural drainage and percussion.
2. Encourage use of cool mist vaporizer.
3. Stress importance of changing infant's position frequently.
4. Explain to parents about feeding difficulties; encourage small, frequent feedings; feed solid food by pushing food back inside of mouth; provide foods that will form bulk to prevent constipation.

✦ *Goal: to prevent Down's syndrome.*
1. Encourage pregnant women at risk (over thirty-five years, family history of Down's, or a previous birth of a child with Down's syndrome) to consider amniocentesis prior to the sixteenth week to rule out Down's syndrome.

Eating Disorders

❑ **This group of disorders is characterized by gross disturbances in eating behavior; it includes anorexia nervosa, bulimia, and pica.**

Data Collection

A. Anorexia nervosa.
1. Intense fear of becoming obese.
2. Disturbance of body image.
3. Weight loss of at least 15 - 25 percent or original body weight.
4. No known physical illness.

B. Bulimia.
1. Recurrent episodes of binge eating (consuming high carbohydrate food — 5,000 to 10,000 calories in a single sitting).
2. Awareness that eating pattern is abnormal.
3. Fear of not being able to stop eating voluntarily.
4. Depressed mood following the eating binges.
5. Purging — induced vomiting, use of diuretics or laxatives.

C. Pica.
1. Persistent eating of non-nutritive substances.
2. Infants: eat paint, plaster, cloth.
3. Older children: eat sand, bugs, rocks.
4. Adults: eat chalk, starch, paper.

Nursing Intervention

✦ *Goal: to exhibit no signs or symptoms of malnutrition.*

1. If client is unable or unwilling to maintain adequate oral intake, a liquid diet may be administered via nasogastric tube. Nursing care of the individual receiving tube feedings should be administered according to established hospital procedures.
2. Client may need to be accompanied to bathroom if self-induced vomiting is suspected.
3. Strict documentation of intake and output.
4. Do not discuss food or eating with client, once protocol has been established. Do, however, offer support and positive reinforcement for obvious improvements in eating behaviors.

✦ *Goal: to increase self-esteem.*

1. Assist client to re-examine negative perceptions of self and to recognize positive attributes.
2. Offer positive reinforcement for independently made decisions influencing client's life.

✦ *Goal: to identify eating disorder and rule out physiological etiology.*

✦ *Goal: to recognize anorexia nervosa as a life-threatening emergency - up to 15% of cases die of malnutrition and many are prone to suicide.*

J	Judgement
A	Affect
M	Memory
C	Confusion
O	Orientation

Psychiatric Considerations of Geriatric Client

❑ ***Delirium* is a syndrome which usually develops over a short period of time. The symptom picture typically fluctuates and is often reversible and temporary.**

❑ ***Dementia* is a syndrome characterized by loss of intellectual abilities (See Table 6-6: Key Points of Dementia).**

Data Collection

A. Causes of dementia.
   1. Alzheimer's disease.
   2. Stroke.
   3. Parkinson's disease.
   4. Injury.
   5. Medication therapy.

B. Alzheimer's Disease.
   1. More commonly seen in elderly geriatric clients.
   2. Irreversible.
   3. FAST — Functional Assessment Staging of Alzheimer's Disease (See Table 6-7).
   4. Special concerns.
      a. Recent memory loss. Client can recall events and activities of 10 years ago, but not 10 minutes ago.
      b. Sundowner's syndrome — confused, disoriented behavior that becomes noticeable after the sun goes down and during the night.
      c. Wandering behavior.
         (1) Restlessness and activity-seeking behavior.
         (2) The "stalking of old haunts."
         (3) Disorientation and inability to sustain intentions; the person forgets what she or he set out to do.
      d. Catastrophic reactions - heightened anxiety occurring during interviewing or questioning when a person cannot answer or perform.
      e. Combative behavior.

Geriatric Priority: *The cardinal rule is: do not push too fast in getting information, assisting with activities of daily living, or insisting that the person socialize. Continued pressure and insistence on a task may result in combative behavior. Potential situations that can lead to combative behavior are threats to self-image, new things or people in environment, illusions, pressure to remember, and direct confrontation.*

Nursing Intervention

NCLEX ALERT: *Plan interventions to manage confusion and intervene to maintain independence in client with dementia.*

✦ *Goal: to provide a quiet, structured environment in order to increase consistency and promote feelings of security.*

1. Avoid dependency.
2. Establish routine for activities of daily living.
3. Meet client's physical needs.
4. Do not isolate client from others in the unit.
5. Provide handrails, walkers, and wheelchairs.
6. Do not change schedules suddenly - *routine, reinforcement*, and *repetition* are the key aspects of care.
7. Check for hazards in the environment (rugs on floor); make sure environment is well-lighted; do not move client suddenly into darkness.
8. Provide quiet, non-stimulating environment to prevent hallucinations.

✦ *Goal: to promote contact with reality.*

Table 6-6:
KEY POINTS — ORGANIC MENTAL SYNDROMES

✦ Clients have varying degrees of awareness of the changes that are occurring which is emotionally painful to them.

✦ Often depression is mistaken for the early onset of dementia.

✦ Dementia disrupts the elderly couple's final stage of family development (generativity, retirement, etc.).

✦ Dementia interferes with family intergenerational development where adult offspring are unable to rectify past injustices, conflicts, and disappointments with parent.

✦ Caregiver coping is highly stressful and can be handled in a more positive approach when there is a focus on problem solving and education.

✦ Alzheimer's Disease (AD) clients have loss of memory, intellectual functioning, orientation, affective regulation, motor coordination, personality, with eventual loss of bowel and bladder control to the point of total incapacitation.

1. Make brief and frequent contact.
2. Give feedback and praise whenever possible.
3. Supply stimulation to motivate client to engage in activities.
4. Use concrete ideas in communication.
5. Maintain reality orientation by encouraging reminiscing.

Geriatric Priority: *Reminiscence and life review help the client resume progression through the grief process associated with disappointing life events and increase self-esteem as successes are reviewed.*

6. Frequently orient client to reality and surroundings. Allow client to have familiar objects around him or her. Use other items, such as clock, calendar, and daily schedules, to assist in maintaining reality orientation.
7. Use simple explanations and face-to-face interaction when communicating with client. Do not shout message into client's ear.
8. Allow sufficient time for client to complete projects.
9. Reinforce reality-oriented comments and continually orient clients to time, place, and date.
10. Use memory joggers — frequent notes, messages on calendars to decrease forgetful incidents.

Table 6-7:
FUNCTIONAL ASSESSMENT STAGING OF ALZHEIMER'S DISEASE—FAST

Stage	Characteristics
Stage 1	—Capable of self-care.
Stage 2	—Complaint of forgetting locating of objects. —Subjective work difficulties. —Capable of self-care.
Stage 3	—Decreased ability in a demanding work setting is evident to peers. —May have difficulty in traveling to new areas. —Capable of self-care regarding activities of daily living.
Stage 4	—Decreased ability to perform complex tasks, cooking, shopping, and management of finances. —Partial self-care; needs supervision and assistance.
Stage 5	—Requires assistance selecting attire. —May need to be coaxed to bathe; fear ofbathing may develop. (Elders often complain of being cold when they are exposed on the way to and from the bathing or shower area. A shower could frighten a person accustomed to tub baths and vice versa.)
Stage 6	—Decreased ability to put on clothing properly and perform personal hygiene measures. —Urinary incontinence. —Fecal incontinence. —Possible seizures. —Sundowner's syndrome.
Stage 7	—Vocabulary reduced to few words, then to just one word. —Loss of ambulatory ability, ability to sit, smile, and eventually to hold up head.

Geriatric Priority: *Speaking slowly and in a face-to-face position is most effective when communicating with an elderly individual experiencing a hearing loss. Visual cues facilitate understanding. Shouting causes distortion of high-pitched sounds and in some instances creates a feeling of discomfort for the client.*

✦ *Goal: to manage and minimize wandering behavior.*

1. A protective environment is needed for the wanderers as well as room to move about.

2. Bed rails should be avoided (place mattress on floor if necessary).
3. Limit cash in wallet to a few dollars and coins to minimize danger of financial loss.
4. Have patient wear a Medic-Alert bracelet or necklace which cannot be removed (give name, address, telephone number).
5. Place name, address, and phone number on items of clothing where the person cannot remove them.
6. Install complex door locks opened by actions demanding thought rather than sheer strength.
7. Implement a buddy system in an institution.
8. Spend extra time with newly admitted persons; provide frequent reassurance, and attend to orientation carefully.

✦ *Goal: to promote self-esteem.*

1. Client should wear own clothing; no night clothes during daytime hours.
2. Makeup should be available for women.
3. Client should carry purse or wallet; and have a monthly allowance to spend or a few coins to carry.
4. Use praise whenever possible.
5. Use affection.
6. Let client make choices whenever possible, but offer only two.

✦ *Goal: to provide diversion activities that enhance self-esteem.*

1. Provide occupational therapy, physical therapy, and recreational therapy that client enjoys.
2. Maintain a flexible schedule and keep client from becoming bored and easily distracted.
3. Recognize specific accomplishments.
4. Encourage family involvement and provide emotional support.
5. Devise methods for assisting client with memory deficit. Examples:
   a. Name sign on door identifying client's room.
   b. Identifying sign on outside of dining room door.
   c. Large clock, with oversized numbers and hands, appropriately placed.
   d. Large calendar, indicating one day at a time, with month, day, and year identified in bold print.

NURSING PRIORITY: *Do not try to force the client to eat, take medication, or participate in any activity. Leave him alone, return in a few minutes and try again. Take advantage of recent memory loss.*

Psychophysiologic Disorders

❑ ***A psychophysiologic disorder* is a physical illness that is strongly influenced by psychological factors. In previous terminology it was entitled psychosomatic disorder. It is thought that stress and anxiety arouse specific conflicts in an individual, which result in damaging effects on particular organs or organ systems pathophysiologically under the autonomic nervous system control.**

NCLEX ALERT: *Assess for mental status changes associated with physiological conditions.*

Data Collection

A. Respiratory — hyperventilation syndrome, bronchial asthma.
B. Cardiovascular — essential hypertension, angina, migraine headaches, tachycardia.
C. Gastrointestinal— peptic ulcer disease, ulcerative colitis, colic.
D. Integumentary — dermatitis, pruritus, excessive sweating, atopic dermatitis.
E. Musculoskeletal — cramps, rheumatoid arthritis.
F. Endocrine — diabetes mellitus, sexual dysfunctions, hyperemesis gravidarum, hyperthyroidism.
G. Genital/Urinary — amenorrhea, impotence, secondary outbreaks of herpes genitalis Type II (HVH II).

Nursing Intervention

Pathophysiology and nursing intervention of the above disorders will be thoroughly discussed in the chapters under the appropriate body system affected.

PERSONALITY DISORDERS

❑ **Personality disorders are characterized by inflexible and maladapted behaviors. Those with personality disorders clash with society and cultural norms, and are often placed in correctional systems, mental hospitals, and child placement facilities.**

Data Collection

1. Problems expressed through behavior rather than as a physical symptom of stress.

2. Disruptive lifestyle is deeply ingrained and quite difficult to change.
3. Often comes in conflict with others.
4. Unable to develop meaningful relationships with others and communicate effectively.
5. Rarely acknowledges that there is a problem.
6. Types.
   a. Paranoid personality.
   b. Schizoid personality.
   c. Schizotypic personality.
   d. Antisocial personality.
   e. Borderline personality.
   f. Narcissistic personality.
   g. Avoidance personality.
   h. Dependent personality.
   i. Passive-aggressive personality.

Nursing Intervention

✦ *Goal: to promote communication and socialization in the suspicious client.*

1. Decrease social isolation.
2. Verbal and nonverbal messages should be clear and consistent.
3. To decrease anxiety, plan several brief contacts rather than one prolonged contact.
4. Promote trust by following through on commitments.
5. Be open and honest to avoid misinterpretation.

✦ *Goal: to promote a positive therapeutic, interpersonal relationship.*

1. Set realistic expectations.
2. Provide a model of mature behavior.
3. Use problem-solving technique to encourage client to make change.
4. Anticipate and deal with depression in clients who gradually develop enough insight to realize and accept responsibility for their behavior.
5. Common sources of frustration to practical nurses.
   a. Client's immature behavior.
   b. Poor communication skills.

✦ *Goal: to minimize manipulation and "acting out" behaviors and encourage verbal communication.*

1. Set firm, consistent limits without being punitive.
2. Be aware of how client may manipulate other staff members (e.g., playing one against the other).
3. Promote expression of feelings versus acting out.
4. Promote client's acceptance of responsibility of his/her own actions and a social responsibility to others.

✦ *Goal: to assist client to manage anxiety.*

1. Anticipate client needs before he/she demands attention.
2. Teach client to express his/her ideas and feelings assertively.

✦ *Goal: to set realistic limits.*

1. Support clients who are gradually making more decisions on their own.
2. Offer assistance *only* when needed.

NCLEX ALERT: *Identify signs and symptoms of substance abuse/chemical dependency.*

Alcohol Dependence

❑ ***Alcoholism* is chronic pattern of pathological alcohol use. It is characterized by impairment in social or occupational functioning along with tolerance or withdrawal symptoms.**

Data Collection

A. Risk factors.
   1. History of alcoholism in family.
   2. History of total abstinence.
   3. Broken or disrupted home.
   4. Last or near-last child in a large family.
   5. Heavy smoking.
   6. Cultural groups: Irish, Eskimo, Scandinavian, Native American.

B. General personality characteristics of alcoholics.
   1. Dependent behavior,along with resentment of authority.
   2. Demanding, domineering, and a low tolerance for frustration.
   3. Dissatisfied with life; tendency toward self-destructive acts, including suicide.
   4. Low self-esteem and self-concept.

C. Signs and symptoms of possible alcohol abuse.
   1. Sprains, bruises, and injuries of questionable origin.
   2. Diarrhea and early morning vomiting.
   3. Chronic cough, palpitations, and infections.
   4. Frequent Monday morning illnesses; blackouts (inability to recall events or actions while intoxicated).

D. Alcohol withdrawal syndrome.

1. ***Alcohol withdrawal.***
   a. Anorexia, nausea, and tremulousness.
   b. Insomnia, nightmares, irritability, hyperalertness.
   c. Tachycardia, increased blood pressure, and diaphoresis.
   d. Clears up within five to seven days.
2. ***Alcohol withdrawal delirium.***
   a. Autonomic hyperactivity — tachycardia, sweating, increased blood pressure.
   b. Vivid hallucinations, delusions, confusion.
   c. Coarse, irregular tremor is almost always seen; fever may occur.
   d. Onset within twenty-four to seventy-two hours after the last ingestion of alcohol; delirium tremens usually last two to three days.
   e. Convulsions/seizures may occur ("rum fits").
   f. First episode occurs after five to fifteen years of heavy drinking.
3. ***Alcohol hallucinosis***.
   a. Auditory hallucinations.
   b. Occurs within forty-eight hours after heavy drinking episode.
   c. Often persecutory delusions.
   d. May be potentially suicidal or homicidal.
   e. Spontaneous recovery within one week.
   f. Wernicke's encephalopathy.
      (1) An acute, *reversible* neurologic disorder.
      (2) Triad of symptoms: confusion, ataxia, and eye movement abnormality (nystagmus).
      (3) Occurs primarily in chronic alcoholics; may develop in illnesses that interfere with thiamine (B_1) absorption, (e.g., gastric cancer, malabsorption syndrome, regional enteritis).
      (4) Treatment: high doses of thiamine usually reverses eye signs within 2-3 hours of treatment.

E. ***Korsakoff's syndrome (alcohol amnesiac disorder)***.
   1. A chronic, *irreversible* disorder, often following Wernicke's encephalopathy.
   2. Triad of symptoms: memory loss, learning deficit, confabulation (filling in of memory gaps with plausible stories).

F. Other disorders associated with chronic alcoholism; esophageal varices, cirrhosis, pancreatitis, diabetes (These will be discussed in Unit 4 under the appropriate system.).

Nursing Intervention

✦ *Goal: to assess for alcoholism in client through careful questioning.*

1. *Identify the alcoholic client in the preoperative period and report to RN.*
   a. Often alcoholics are undiagnosed at the time of surgery and may go into withdrawal or DTs after the NPO period.
   b. Postoperative period usually takes longer for client to be fully responsive; susceptible to severe respiratory complications; has more difficulty with healing due to poor nutritional state.

✦ *Goal: to assist in the medical treatment of alcohol withdrawal.*

1. **Librium** or **Valium** for agitation.
2. Tranquilizers (**Thorazine**) for nausea and vomiting.
3. Anticonvulsants (**Dilantin**) or magnesium sulfate given.
4. Encourage multivitamins, especially B complex and vitamin C.
5. Encourage fluids but do not force.

✦ *Goal: to provide for the basic needs of rest, comfort, safety, and nutrition.*

1. Safety measures such as bed rest and bed rails may be necessary.
2. *If client is in DTs, stay with him or her and call for RN.*
3. Have room adequately lit to help reduce confusion, and avoid shadows and unclear objects.
4. Monitor vital signs q 1-4 hours and PRN.
5. Encourage a high carbohydrate, soft diet.

✦ *Goal: to recognize complications of alcohol use.*

1. Obstetric implications.
   a. Use of alcohol during pregnancy can lead to fetal alcohol syndrome.
   b. Alcohol withdrawal syndrome may occur in the intrapartal period as early as twelve to forty-eight hours after the last drink.
   c. Delirium tremens may occur in the postpartum period.
2. Neonatal implications (Fetal Alcohol Syndrome - FAS).
   a. Teratogenic effects may be seen along with growth and developmental retardation.
   b. Increased risk for anomalies of the heart, head, face and extremities.

c. Withdrawal symptoms can occur shortly after birth; characterized by tremors, agitation, sweating, and seizure activity.

d. *Maintain seizure precautions and report any seizure activity to RN.*

3. Medical complications of alcohol abuse.

a. Trauma — related to falls, burns, hematomas.

b. Liver disease — cirrhosis, esophageal varices, hepatic coma.

c. Gastrointestinal disease — gastritis, bleeding ulcers, pancreatitis.

d. Nutritional disease — malnutrition, anemia due to iron or B_{12} deficiency, thiamine deficiency.

e. Infections, especially pneumonia.

f. Neurologic disease — polyneuropathy and dementia.

✦ *Goal: to assist in the long-term rehabilitation of client.*

1. Avoid sympathy as clients tend to rationalize and use dependent, manipulative behavior to seek privileges.
2. Maintain a nonjudgmental attitude.
3. Set behavior limits in a firm but kind manner.
4. Place responsibility of sobriety on client; do not give advice, punish or reprimand client for failures.
5. Provide opportunities to decrease social isolation and encourage social groups and activities.
6. Encourage client to develop alternative coping mechanisms other than alcohol to deal with stress.
7. Refer clients to available community resources.

a. Alcoholics Anonymous (AA) - a self-help group focusing on education, guidance, and the sharing of problems and experiences unique to the individual.

b. Alanon - a self-help support group for the spouses and significant others of the alcoholic.

c. Alateen - the support group for teenagers with an alcohol parent.

8. Promote adherence to prescribed therapeutic regimes.

a. Disulfiram (**Antabuse**) — a drug therapy that produces intense side effects after ingestion of alcohol (severe nausea, vomiting, flushed face, hypotension, and blurred vision).

b. Aversion therapy — a form of deterrent therapy attempting to induce alcohol rejection behavior by administering alcohol with an emetic.

Drug Abuse and Dependence

❑ **The chronic or occasional use of drugs other than alcohol or tobacco can be categorized as either *substance abuse* or *dependence*.**

NCLEX ALERT: *Identify signs and symptoms of substance abuse/chemical dependency, withodrawal or toxicity.*

General Concepts

A. Incidence.

1. A social, widespread problem which costs an estimated fifty billion dollars a year in health and medical expenses.
2. Often, the person who abuses one drug abuses others (alcohol included).

B. Effects of use.

1. Relieves anxiety.
2. Overdose can occur.

C. General personality characteristics.

1. Inability to cope with stress, frustration, or anxiety.
2. Rebellious, immature; desire for immediate gratification.
3. Low self-esteem and passivity.
4. Difficulty forming warm, personal relationships.
5. Uses defense mechanisms related to escaping - denial, rationalization, intellectualization.

Data Collection

A. General Assessment.

1. Determine the pattern of drug use.

a. What drugs are the client using?

b. How much does client use and how often?

c. How long has client been using drugs?

d. What combination of drugs is being used?

2. Determine if there are any physical changes present, (e.g., needle track marks, swollen nasal mucous membranes, reddened conjunctiva).

B. Narcotic dependence.

1. Common drugs: opium, heroin, morphine, meperidine (**Demerol**), codeine, methadone.
2. Administration.

a. Heroin: sniffed, smoked, injected IV (mainlining), injected SQ (skin popping).

b. Other narcotics usually taken orally or injected.

3. Symptoms of use.

a. Drowsiness, decreased blood pressure, pulse and respiratory rate.

b. Pinpoint pupils, needle tracks, scarring.

4. Withdrawal symptoms.
   a. Onset of symptoms approximately eight to twelve hours following the last dose.
   b. Lacrimation, sweating, sneezing, yawning.
   c. Gooseflesh (piloerection), tremor, irritability, anorexia.
   d. Dilated pupils, abdominal cramps, vomiting, involuntary muscle spasms.
   e. Symptoms generally subside within seven to ten days.

C. Sedative-hypnotic dependence.
1. Common drugs: barbiturates (**Quaalude**, **Equanil**) and the benzodiazepines (**Librium**, **Valium**).
2. Administration: oral or injected.
3. Symptoms of use.
   a. Alterations of mood, thought, behavior.
   b. Impairment in coordination, judgment.
   c. Signs of intoxication: slurred speech, unsteady gait, decreased attention span or memory.
   d. Barbiturate use: often violent, disruptive, irresponsible behavior.
4. Withdrawal symptoms.
   a. Insomnia, anxiety, profuse sweating, weakness.
   b. Severe reactions of delirium, grand mal seizures, cardiovascular collapse.

D. *Cocaine abuse.*
1. Administration: intranasal ("snorting") or by IV or SQ injection, smoked in pipe (free-basing).
2. Symptoms of use.
   a. Euphoria and a sense of well-being.
   b. Amphetamine-stimulant-like effects such as increased blood pressure, racing of the heart, paranoia, anxiety.
   c. Taken regularly, may disrupt eating and sleeping habits leading to irritability and decreased concentration.

NURSING PRIORITY: *Crack (rock) has been labelled the most addictive drug known to man. It is a potent form of cocaine hydrochloride mixed with baking soda and water, heated, allowed to harden, and then is broken or "cracked" into little pieces and smoked in cigarettes or glass water pipes. Cardiac arrhythmias, respiratory paralysis, and seizures are some of the dangers associated with crack use.*

3. Withdrawal symptoms.
   a. Severe craving.
   b. Coming down from a "high" often leads to a severe "letdown," depressed feeling.
   c. Psychological dependence often leads to cocaine becoming a total obsession.

E. Amphetamine dependence - **Benzedrine**.
1. Administration: oral or injected.
2. Symptoms of use.
   a. Elation, agitation, hyperactivity, irritability.
   b. Increased pulse, respiration and blood pressure.
   c. Fine tremor, muscle twitching, and mydriasis (pupillary dilatation).
   d. Large doses: convulsions, cardiovascular collapse, respiratory depression, coma, death.
3. Withdrawal symptoms.
   a. Appear within two to four days after the last dose.
   b. Depression, overwhelming fatigue, suicide attempts.

F. PCP - phencyclidine abuse.
1. Administration: snorted, smoked, or orally ingested; usually smoked along with marijuana.
2. Symptoms of use.
   a. Euphoria, feeling of numbness, mood changes.
   b. Diaphoresis, eye movement changes (nystagmus), hypertension, catatonic-like stupor with eyes open.
   c. Seizures, shivering, decerebrate posturing, possible death.
   d. Synesthesia (seeing colors when a loud sound occurs).
3. Overdose symptoms ("bad trip").
   a. User may become violent, destructive, and confused.
   b. Users have been known to go berserk; may harm self and others.
   c. Intoxicating symptoms lighten and worsen over a period of forty-eight hours.

G. Hallucinogen abuse.
1. Common drugs: LSD, psilocybin ("magic mushroom"), mescaline (peyote), DMT, MDA.
2. Administration: usually oral, but LSD and mescaline can be injected.
3. Symptoms of use.
   a. Pupillary dilation, tachycardia, sweating.
   b. Visual hallucinations, depersonalization, impaired judgment and mood.
   c. "Flashbacks" and "bad trips."
   d. Usually no signs of withdrawal symptoms after discontinuing use.

H. Marijuana dependence.
1. Administration: oral, sniffed, and smoked.
2. Symptoms of use.
a. Euphoria, relaxation, tachycardia, and conjunctival congestion.
b. Paranoid ideation; impaired judgment.
c. Rarely, panic reactions and psychoses.
d. Heavy use leads to apathy and general deterioration in all aspects of living.
3. Withdrawal symptoms.
a. Anxiety, sleeplessness, sweating.
b. Lack of appetite, nausea, general malaise.

Nursing Intervention

✦ *Goal: to assess the drug use pattern.*

✦ *Goal: to assist in the medical treatment during detoxification or withdrawal.*

1. Narcotics.
a. Narcotic antagonists are administered intravenously for narcotic overdose.
b. Withdrawal is managed with rest and nutritional therapy.
c. Substitution therapy may be instituted to decrease withdrawal symptoms using propoxyphene (**Darvon**), for longer effects.
2. Depressants.
a. Substitution therapy may be instituted to decrease withdrawal symptoms using a long-acting barbiturate, such as phenobarbital (**Luminal**).
b. Some physicians prescribe oxazepam (**Serax**) as needed for objective symptoms, gradually decreasing the dosage until the drug is discontinued.
3. Stimulants.
a. Treatment of overdose is geared toward stabilization of vital signs.
b. IV antihypertensives may be used, along with IV diazepam (**Valium**) to control seizures.
c. Chlordiazepoxide (**Librium**) PO. may be administered for the first few days while client is "crashing."
4. Hallucinogens and cannabinols.
a. Medications are normally not prescribed for withdrawal from the substances.
b. In the event of overdose, diazepam (**Valium**) or chlordiazepoxide (**Librium**) may be given as needed to decrease agitation.
5. Awareness that gradual withdrawal, detoxification, or dechemicalization is necessary for clients addicted to barbiturates, narcotics, and tranquilizers.
6. Abrupt withdrawal, "cold turkey," is often dangerous and can prove fatal.
7. Maintain a patent airway have oxygen available.
8. Provide a safe, quiet environment, (i.e., remove harmful objects, use side rails).

✦ *Goal: to decrease problem behaviors of manipulation and "acting out" and promote alternative coping methods.*

1. Set firm, consistent limits.
2. Confront client with manipulative behaviors.
3. Encourage responsibility for own behavior.
4. Encourage the use of hobbies, exercise, or alternative therapies as a means to deal with frustration and anxiety.

✦ *Goal: to recognize complications of substance abuse.*

1. Obstetric implications.
a. Narcotic addiction.
(1) Increased risk of pregnancy-induced hypertension, malpresentation, and third trimester bleeding.

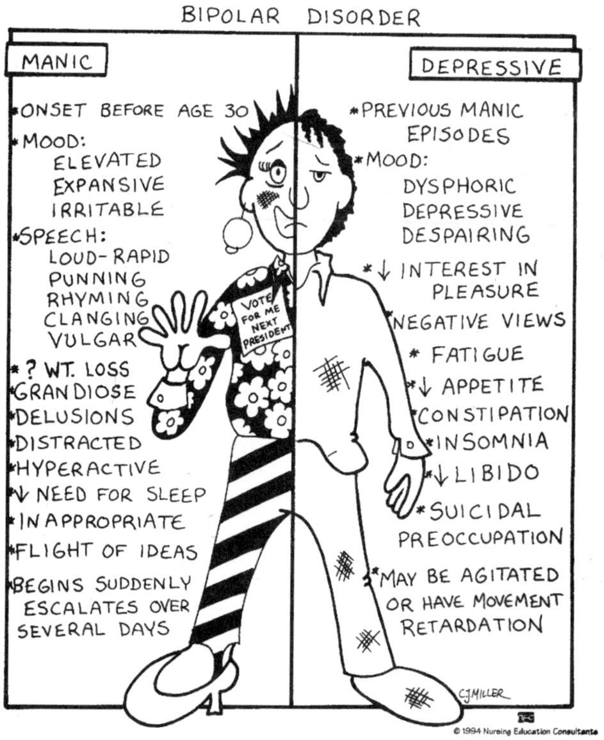

Figure 6-1: Bipolar Affective Disorder
Zerwekh, J. & Claborn, J. (2002). *Memory Notebook of Nursing*, Vol. 1, Dallas, TX: Nursing Education Consultants, Inc.

(2) Maintain on methadone for the duration of the pregnancy as withdrawal is not advisable due to risk to the fetus.

b. Other use of drugs provides increased risk to mother and fetus.

2. Neonatal complications.

a. Withdrawal symptoms depend on type of drug mother used.

b. Restlessness, jitteriness, hyperactive reflexes, high-pitched shrill cry, feeds poorly.

c. Maintain seizure precautions.

d. Administer phenobarbital or paregoric to treat withdrawal and prevent seizures.

e. Swaddle infant in snug-fitting blanket.

f. Increased risk for congenital malformations and prematurity.

3. Medical implications.

a. Increased risk of hepatitis, malnutrition, and infections in general.

✦ *Goal: to assist in the long-term process of client drug rehabilitation.*

1. Refer to drug rehabilitation programs.

2. Promote self-help residential programs which foster self-support systems and use ex-addicts as rehabilitation counselors.

3. Methadone maintenance programs.

a. Must be over the age of eighteen and addicted for more than two years, with a history of detoxification treatments.

b. Methadone is a synthetic narcotic which appeases desire for opiates.

(1) Controlled substance given only under urinary surveillance.

(2) Administered po; prevents opiate withdrawal symptoms.

Affective Disorders

❑ **The major *affective disorders* are characterized by disturbances of mood.**

Data Collection

A. *Bipolar disorder.*

1. Manic.

a. Onset before age thirty.

b. Mood: elevated, expansive, or irritable.

c. Speech: loud, rapid, difficult to interpret, punning, rhyming, clanging (using words that sound like the meaning rather than the actual word).

d. Cognitive skills: flight of ideas, grandiose delusions, easily distracted.

e. Psychomotor activity: hyperactive, decreased need for sleep, exhibitionalistic, vulgar, profane, may make inappropriate sexual advances and be obscene.

f. Course of manic episode: begins suddenly, rapidly escalates over a few days, and ends more abruptly than major depressive episodes.

2. Depressive.

a. Has had one or more manic episodes.

b. Mood: dysphoric, depressive, despairing, loss of interest or pleasure in most usual activities.

c. Cognitive process: negative view of self, world, and of the future; poverty of ideas; crying, and suicidal preoccupation.

d. Psychomotor: may see either agitation or retardation in movements, feelings of fatigue, lack of appetite, constipation, sleeping disturbances (insomnia or early morning wakefulness), decrease in libido.

3. Mixed.

a. Involves both manic and depressive episodes.

B. *Major depression.*

1. May occur at any age.

2. Differentiated as either a single episode or a recurring type.

3. Symptoms the same as those listed under "Bipolar disorder-depressed".

4. Severity and type of depression vary with the ability to test reality.

a. Psychotic: feels worse in the morning, better as the day goes on.

b. Neurotic: wakes up feeling optimistic, mood worsens as the day passes.

Nursing Intervention (manic episode)

✦ *Goal: to provide for basic human needs of safety and rest/activity.*

1. Reduce outside stimuli and provide a nonstimulating environment.

2. Monitor food intake - provide a high-calorie, high-vitamin diet with finger foods to be eaten as the client moves about.

> ***NURSING PRIORITY:** Physiological needs (food, hygiene, rest) are first priority in providing client care.*

3. Encourage noncompetitive solitary activities - walking, swimming, and painting.

4. Assist with personal hygiene.

✦ *Goal: to establish a therapeutic nurse-client relationship.*

1. Use firm, consistent, honest approach.
2. Assess client's abilities and involve in his/her own care planning.
3. Promote problem-solving abilities; recognize that false sense of independence is often demonstrated by loud, boisterous behavior.
4. Do not focus or discuss grandiose ideas.

✦ *Goal: to set limits on behavior.*

1. Instructions should be clear and concise.
2. Initiate regularly scheduled contacts to demonstrate acceptance.
3. Maintain some distance between self and client to allow freedom of movement and to prevent feelings of being overpowered.
4. Maintain neutrality and objectivity — realize that client can be easily provoked by harmless remarks and may demonstrate a furious reaction but calm down very quickly.
5. Employ measures to prevent overt aggression, (e.g., distraction, recognition of behaviors of increased excitement).

✦ *Goal: to promote adaptive coping with constructive use of energy.*

1. Do not hurry client, as this leads to anxiety and hostile behavior.

> ***NURSING PRIORITY:*** *In a hyperactive state, client is extremely distractible, and responses to even the slightest stimuli are exaggerated.*

2. Provide activities and constructive tasks that channel the agitated behavior, (e.g., cleaning game room, going for a walk, gardening, playing catch).

✦ *Goal: to assist in the medical treatment.*

1. Administer Lithium.
2. Teach client about Lithium medication instructions (Appendix 6-2).

Nursing Intervention (depressive episode)

> ***NURSING PRIORITY:*** *Depression and suicidal behaviors may be viewed as anger turned inward on the self. If this anger can be verbalized in a non-threatening environment, the client may be able to resolve these feelings, regardless of the discomfort involved.*

✦ *Goal: to assess for suicide potential.*

1. Recognition of suicide intent.
   a. *Self-destructive behaviors are viewed as attempts to escape unbearable life situations. Report any self-destructive behavior immediately to RN.*
   b. Anxiety and hostility are overwhelmingly present.
   c. There is the presence of ambivalence; life versus self-destructive impulses.
   d. Depression, low self-esteem, and a feeling of hopelessness are critical to evaluate, as suicide attempts are often made when the client feels like giving up.
   e. Assess for *indirect* self-destructive behavior - any activity that is detrimental to the physical well-being of the client where the potential outcome is death.
      (1) Eating disorders: anorexia nervosa, bulimia, obesity, and overeating.
      (2) Noncompliance with medical treatment, (e.g., diabetic who does not take insulin).
      (3) Cigarette smoking, gambling, criminal and socially deviant activities.
      (4) Alcohol and drug abuse.
      (5) Participation in high-risk sports, (e.g., automobile racing and sky diving).
2. Suicide danger signs.
   a. The presence of a suicide plan: specifics relating to method, its lethality, and a likelihood for rescue.
   b. Change in established patterns in routines, (e.g., giving away of personal items, making a will, and saying good-bye).
   c. Anticipation of failure: loss of a job, preoccupation with physical disease, actual or anticipated loss of a significant other.
   d. Change in behavior, presence of panic, agitation, or calmness; usually, as depression lifts, client has enough energy to act on suicidal feelings.
   e. Hopelessness: feelings of impending doom, futility, and entrapment.
   f. Withdrawal and rejection of help.
3. Clients at risk.
   a. Adolescents and the elderly; males usually complete the suicide act.
   b. Recent stress of a maturational or situational crisis.
   c. Clients with chronic or painful illnesses.
   d. Previous suicidal attempts or behavior.
   e. Withdrawn, depressed, or hallucinating clients.
   f. Clients with sexual identity conflicts and those who abuse alcohol and drugs.

✦ *Goal: to provide for basic human needs of safety and protection from self-destruction.*

1. Remove all potentially harmful objects, (e.g., belts, sharp objects, matches, lighters, strings, etc).
2. Maintain a one-to-one relationship and close observation.

***NURSING PRIORITY:** Be aware of special times when client might be suicidal, (e.g., when suddenly cheerful, when there is less staff available, upon arriving in the morning, or during a busy routine day).*

✦ *Goal: to provide for physical needs of nutrition and rest/activity.*

1. *Assess for changes in weight (weight loss may indicate deepening depression) and report to RN.*
2. Encourage increased bulk and roughage in diet along with sufficient fluids if constipated.

***NURSING PRIORITY:** Depressed clients are particularly vulnerable to constipation due to psychomotor retardation.*

3. Provide for adequate amount of exercise and rest; encourage client not to sleep during the day.
4. Assist with hygiene and personal appearance.

✦ *Goal: to promote expression of feelings.*

1. Encourage expression of angry, guilty, or depressed feelings.
2. Convey a kind, pleasant, interested approach to promote a sense of dignity and self-worth in the client.
3. Support the client in the expression of his/her feelings by allowing him/her to respond in his/her own time.
4. Seek out client; initiate frequent contacts.
5. Assist with decision making when depression is severe.

✦ *Goal: to provide for meaningful socialization activities.*

***NURSING PRIORITY:** The depressed client must have lots of structure in his or her life due to the impairment in decision-making/problem-solving ability.*

1. Encourage participation in activities, (e.g., plan a work assignment with client to do simple tasks: straightening game room, picking up magazines, etc.).
2. Assess hobbies, sports, or activities client enjoys and encourage participation.

Box 6-5:
Disturbances In Perception

- Hallucinations - false sensory perception with no basis in reality; auditory, olfactory, tactile, visual gustatory; auditory most common..
- Delusions - fixed, false beliefs, not corrected by logic; develop as a defense against intolerable feelings or ideas that cause anxiety.
- *Delusions of grandeur* - related to feelings of power, fame, splendor, magnificence.
  Delusions of persecution - people are out to harm, injure or destroy.
- Illusions - misinterpretation of reality, (e.g., seeing a mirror image turn into a monster).

3. Encourage client to participate in small group conversation or activity; practice social skills through role playing and psychodrama.
4. Encourage activities that promote a sense of accomplishment and enhance self-esteem.

✦ *Goal: to assist in the medical treatment.*

1. Administer antidepressant medication (See Appendix 6-3).
2. Assist in electroconvulsive therapy.

Schizophrenia

❑ ***Schizophrenia* is a maladaptive disturbance characterized by a number of common behaviors involving disorders of thought content, mood, feeling, perception, communication, and interpersonal relationships.**

Prepsychotic Personality Characteristics

A. Aloof, rejecting, and indifferent.
B. Social withdrawal, peculiar behavior.
C. Relatives and friends note a change in personality.
D. Unusual perceptual experiences, along with disturbed communication.
E. Lack of personal grooming.

Psychodynamics of Maladaptive Disturbances

A. Disturbance in thought processes.
   1. Thoughts are confused, chaotic and disorganized.
   2. Communication in symbolic language; all symbols have special meaning.
   3. Feeling that thoughts or wishes can control other people, (i.e., magical thinking).
   4. Retreat to a fantasy world, rejecting the real world of painful experience while responding to reality in a bizarre or autistic manner.

B. Disturbance of affect.

1. Difficulty expressing emotions.
2. Affect is either absent, flat, blunted, or inappropriate.
3. Inappropriate affect makes it difficult to form close relationships.

C. Disturbance in psychomotor behavior.

1. Display of disorganized, purposeless activity.
2. Behavior may be uninhibited and bizarre; abnormal posturing (agitated or retardative catatonia), waxy flexibility.
3. Often appears aloof, disinterested, apathetic, and lacking motivation.

D. Disturbance in perception (Box 6-3).

E. Disturbance in interpersonal relationships.

1. Establishment of interpersonal relationships is difficult due to inability to communicate clearly and react appropriately.
2. Difficulty relating to others.
   a. Unable to form close relationships.
   b. Has difficulty trusting others and experiences ambivalence, fear, and dependency.
   c. "Need-fear dilemma" - withdraws to protect self from further hurt and consequently experiences lack of warmth, trust, and intimacy.
   d. "As if" phenomenon - feels rejected by others which leads to increased isolation, perpetuating further feelings of rejection.

Data Collection

A. Classic four "A" symptoms — Eugene Bleuler's classic symptoms.

1. Associative looseness - lack of logical thought progression resulting in disorganized and chaotic thinking.
2. Affect - emotion or feeling tone is one of indifference, flat, blunted, exaggerated, or socially inappropriate.
3. Ambivalence - conflicting, strong feelings (e.g., love and hate) that neutralize each other, leading to psychic immobilization and difficulty expressing other emotions.
4. Autism - extreme retreat from reality characterized by fantasies, preoccupation with daydreams, and psychotic thought processes of delusion and hallucination.

B. Other symptoms.

1. Regression - extreme withdrawal and social isolation.
2. Negativism - doing the opposite of what is asked; typical behavior is to neither speak to no one nor answer no one; used to cover feelings of unworthiness and inadequacy.
3. Religiosity - excessive religious preoccupation.
4. Lack of social awareness - crudeness and social insensitivity; neglectful of personal grooming and hygiene.

Nursing Intervention

✦ *Goal: to build trust.*

> ***NURSING PRIORITY:** Building trust is the primary goal for the schizophrenic client.*

1. Encourage free expression of feelings, either negative or positive, without fear of rejection, ridicule, or retaliation.
2. Use nonverbal level of communication to demonstrate warmth, concern, and empathy as client often distrusts words.
3. Consistency, reliability, acceptance, and persistence build trust.
4. Allow client to set pace; proceed slowly in planning social contacts.

✦ *Goal: to provide a safe and secure environment.*

1. Maintain familiar routines. Make sure persons who come in contact with client are recognizable to client.
2. Avoid stressful situations or increasing anxiety.

> ***NURSING PRIORITY:** Stay with client to reduce fear and reduce sources of discomfort in the environment.*

✦ *Goal: to clarify and reinforce reality.*

1. Involve client in reality-oriented activities.
2. Help client find satisfaction in the external environment, and ways of relating to others.
3. Focus on clear communication and the immediate situation.

✦ *Goal: to promote and build self-esteem.*

1. Encourage simple activities with limited concentration and *no* competition.
2. Provide successful experiences with short-range goals realistic for client's levels of functioning.
3. Relieve client of decision making until he/she is ready.
4. Avoid making demands.

✦ *Goal: to encourage independent behavior.*

1. Anticipate and accept negativism.
2. Avoid fostering dependency.
3. Encourage client to make his/her own decisions using positive reinforcement.

✦ *Goal: to provide care to meet basic human needs.*

1. Determine client's ability to meet responsibilities of daily living.
2. Attend to nutrition, elimination, exercise, hygiene, and signs of physical illness.

✦ *Goal: to assist in the medical treatment.*

1. Administer antipsychotic medications (Appendix 6-4).
2. Assist with ECT; may be useful in some instances to modify behavior.

✦ *Goal: to deal effectively with withdrawn behavior.*

1. Establish a therapeutic one-to-one relationship.
   a. Initiate interaction by seeking out client at every opportunity.
   b. Maintain a nonjudgmental, accepting manner in what is said and done.
   c. Attempt to draw client into a response without demanding a response.
2. Promote social skills by helping client feel more secure with other people.
   a. Accept one-sided conversations.
   b. Accept staff reaction toward client's negativism without remarks.
3. Attend to physical needs of client as necessary.
4. Have client focus on reality.
5. Protect and restrain client from potential destructiveness to self and others.

✦ *Goal: to deal effectively with hallucinations.*

1. Clarify and reinforce reality.
   a. Help client recognize hallucination as a manifestation of anxiety.
   b. Provide a safe, secure environment.
   c. Avoid denying or arguing with client when he/she is experiencing hallucinations.
   d. Acknowledge client's experience, but point out that *you* do not share the same experience.
   e. Do not give attention to content of hallucinations.
   f. Direct client's attention to real situations.
   g. Protect client from injury to self or others when prompted by "voices" or "visions."
2. *Report any type of hallucinating behavior to RN.*

NCLEX ALERT: *Identify changes associated with psychsocial disoreders (e.g., hallucination, delusions, etc.).*

Paranoid Disorder

❑ ***Paranoid* behavior is characterized by delusions, usually persecutory, and extreme suspiciousness.**

Data Collection

A. Extreme suspiciousness and withdrawal from emotional contact with others.
B. Aloof, distant, hypercritical of others.
C. Frequent complaining by letter-writing or instigating legal action.
D. Resentment, anger, possible violence.
E. Delusions of grandeur, persecution, and hypochondriases.
F. Misinterpretation or distortion of reality; may refuse food and medications; insist they are poisoned despite evidence of proof.

Nursing Intervention

✦ *Goal: to establish a trusting relationship.*

1. Maintain calm, matter-of-fact attitude.
2. Keep promises made; be honest.
3. Avoid whispering or acting secretive.
4. *If client refuses medications, report to RN.*

✦ *Goal: to increase self-esteem by providing successful experiences.*

1. Allow client to set pace in closeness with others.
2. Avoid involvement in competitive, aggressive activities requiring physical contact (e.g., football, basketball).
3. Involve in solitary activities (e.g., drawing, photography, typing) and progress to intellectual activities with others using games (e.g., chess, bridge, word scrabble).
4. Reward completion of meaningful tasks.

✦ *Goal: to deal effectively with delusions.*

1. Clarify and focus on reality; use reality-testing.
2. Avoid confirming or approving false beliefs.
3. Point out that client's beliefs are not shared.
4. Divert attention from delusions to reality; focus on here and now.

Study Questions—Psychiatric Concepts

1. What are signs and symptoms of elder abuse?

① confusion and disorientation.
② recent hip fracture.
③ poor nutrition and hygiene.
④ unkempt house.

2. What is a priority of care for a confused client?

① neurological care.
② nutritional needs.
③ safety and comfort.
④ spiritual needs.

3. A nurse finds a client with dementia wandering around the unit. In considering this problem which nursing intervention would be appropriate?

① place new locks on doors in new areas to which the client might wander.
② keep the client confined to two rooms only during the day.
③ keep the client involved in activities during the day.
④ conduct reality orientation checks every hour.

4. A nurse whose family has a history of drug abuse makes derogatory comments while caring for a substance abuse client. What might be an explanation for the nurse's behavior? She has:

① an issue with denial and repression.
② feelings she is unaware of when working with this type of client.
③ a need to act out her feelings.
④ feelings that this type of client is insensitive and should be dealt with honestly.

5. A client is suspicious about her surroundings and paranoid with staff. What therapeutic approach should be avoided?

① silence.
② direct eye contact.
③ acceptance.
④ therapeutic touch.

6. A client is observed by the nurse opening and closing his fist while walking back and forth in his room. The nurse should:

① try to understand the meaning of the behavior.
② give PRN **Ativan** for anxiety.
③ call for help to restrain the client.
④ leave the client alone.

7. The nurse would recognize which of the following symptoms as indicative of depression?

① insomnia, loss of libido, and restlessness.
② anorexia, psychomotor retardation, poor grooming.
③ hypervigilance, overeating, poor grooming,
④ flight of ideas, weight loss, lack of interest.

8. An elderly client is diagnosed with bipolar disorder, manic type. What are common signs of this problem?

① frequent crying.
② poor grooming.
③ guilty feelings.
④ euphoria.

9. The nursing assessment of a client with schizophrenia would including which findings?

① delusions and hallucinations.
② ambivalence and delusions.
③ self-care deficits and delusions.
④ self-care deficits and flat affect.

10. A client is on antipsychotic drug therapy. What do Parkinson-like symptoms indicate?

① an allergic response to the drug.
② a therapeutic reaction to the drug.
③ extrapyramidal side effects.
④ cholingeric side effects.

11. A client is experiencing auditory hallucinations. What would the nurse be most concerned about?

① feelings of depression when the voices stop.
② how the voices were telling him to hurt someone.
③ feelings of happiness to hear the voices.
④ how the voices sound like a woman's.

12. What symptoms would the nurse recognize in a client that is hallucinating?

① sitting in the corner of a room facing the wall.
② movement of the head, as if trying to hear better and mumbling.
③ unable to sit still and poor concentration.
④ the client thinks she is a general in the Army.

13. The family of a client with Alzheimer's disease asks the nurse about caring for the client. What would the nurse advise the family to do?

① limit behaviors.
② identify stimuli which cause recurring episodes.
③ prioritize care and needs.
④ place locks on all rooms.

14. Familiar environment and routine to an elderly client fulfills which of Maslow's Hierarchy of Needs?

① self-actualization.
② biological integrity.
③ spiritual.
④ safety and security.

15. A child is brought into the emergency room with bruises and raised welts on the child's back. The nurse suspects child abuse. What would be the appropriate action?

① demand an explanation from the parents.
② observe the child's response to family members.
③ call the police.
④ call Child Protective Services.

16. A important nursing consideration when caring for an abused elderly client is that the abused elderly:

① are humiliated and defensive about abusive experiences.
② are usually unable to remember the event.
③ are confused about details regarding the event.
④ think that everyone is abusing them.

17. A client with a cocaine abuse problem is on a detoxification protocol. What is an important nursing action?

① increase fluid intake.
② check the vital signs.
③ encourage a high sodium diet.
④ check intake and output.

18. The family of an alcoholic asks the nurse where they can go for support in their community. Which of the following would be appropriate for the nurse to direct the family members to?

① an appropriate social worker.
② Alcoholics Anonymous.
③ Al-Anon.
④ the staff psychologist.

19. While interviewing a new admit on the substance abuse unit, the nurse is repeatedly told by the client that he is not a drug abuser, although his drug screen was positive for a variety of controlled substances. The nurse understands the client is using which defense mechanism?

① intellectualization.
② rationalization.
③ denial.
④ projection

20. What is the most important goal in planning the care for a client with a diagnosis of schizophrenia?

① to set limits.
② to build trust.
③ to encourage group participation in activites.
④ to promote expression of feelings.

21. Lithium at a toxic level would present which of the following signs and symptoms?

① tachycardia, hypertension, convulsions.
② urinary frequency, vomiting, febrile.
③ hypotension, bradycardia, increased thirst.
④ diarrhea, ataxia, seizures, lethargy.

Appendix 6-1: ANTI-ANXIETY AGENTS

❖GENERAL NURSING IMPLICATIONS❖

—Withhold or omit one or more doses if excessive drowiness occurs.
—Assess for symptoms associated with a withdrawal syndrome in hospitalized clients—anxiety, insomnia, (influenza-like symptoms) - vomiting, tremors, palpitations, confusion, and hallucinations.
—When discontinuing, the drug dosage should be gradually decreased over a period of days depending upon the dose and length of time on the medication.
—Schedule IV drug requires documentation.
—Promote safety with the use of siderails and assisting with ambulation as necessary.
—Teach client and family not to drink alcohol while taking an antianxiety agent not to abruptly stop taking the medication.

MEDICATIONS	SIDE EFFECTS	NURSING IMPLICATIONS
BENZODIAZEPINES: Reduce anxiety by enhancing the action of the inhibitory neurotransmitter GABA on its receptor. Also has anticonvulsant activity and skeletal muscle relaxation.		
Chlordiazepoxide (**Librium**): PO, IM, IV Diazepam (**Valium**): PO, IM, IV Clonazepam (**Klonopin**):PO Chlorazepate dipotassium (**Tranzene**): PO Midazolam (**Versed**): IM, IV	Central nervous system depression, drowsiness (decreases with usage), ataxia, dizziness, headaches, dry mouth. ***Adverse effects:*** Leukopenia, tolerance commonly develops, physical dependency.	1. Alters liver function tests. 2. Assess for symptoms of leukopenia, such as sore throat, fever, and weakness. 3. Encourage client to rise slowly from a supine position and to dangle feet before standing. 4. **Versed** is commonly used for induction of anesthesia and sedation prior to diagnostic tests and endoscopic exams. 5. Flumazenil (**Rocmazicon**) is approved for the treatment of benzodiazepine overdose; has an adverse effect of precipitating convulsions, especially with clients who have a history of epilepsy. 6. ***Uses:*** anxiety and tension, muscle spasm, preoperative medication, acute alcohol withdrawal, and to induce sleep.
NONBENZODIAZEPINE AGENTS: Interacts with serotonin and dopamine receptors in the brain to decrease anxiety. Lacks muscle relaxant and anticonvulsant effects, does not cause sedation or physical or psychological dependence, does not increase CNS depression of alcohol or other drugs.		
Buspirone (**Buspar**): PO	Dizziness, drowsiness, headache, nausea, fatigue, insomnia.	1. Not a controlled substance. 2. Some improvement can be noted in 7-10 days, however usually takes 3-4 weeks to achieve effectiveness. 3. ***Uses:*** short-term relief of anxiety and anxiety disorders.

Appendix 6-2:
ANTIMANIC MEDICATIONS

MEDICATION	SIDE EFFECTS	NURSING IMPLICATIONS
LITHIUM CARBONATE: Acts to lower concentrations of norepinephrine and serotonin by inhibiting their release; believed to alter sodium transport in both nerve and muscle cells. ***Uses:*** bipolar affective disorder—manic episode.		
(**Lithane, Lithobid**): PO	***High incidence:*** Increased thirst, increased urination (polyuria). ***Frequent:*** 1.5 mEq/L levels or less Dry mouth, lethargy, fatigue, muscle weakness, headache, GI disturbances, fine hand tremors. ***Adverse effects:*** 1.5—2.0 mEq/L may produce vomiting, diarrhea, drowsiness, incoordination, coarse hand tremors, muscle twitching. 2.0—2.5 mEq/L may result in ataxia, slurred speech, confusion, clonic movements, high output of dilute urine, blurred vision, hypotension. ***Acute toxicity:*** Seizures, oliguria, coma, peripheral vascular collapse, death.	1. Monitor lithium blood levels: blood samples taken 12 hours after dosage. 2. Teach client the following: a. symptoms of lithium toxicity. b. the importance of frequent blood tests (every 2-3 days) to check lithium levels at the beginning of treatment (maintenance blood levels done every 1-3 months). c. the importance of dietary intake and taking dose at same time each day, preferably with meals or milk. 3. Encourage a diet containing normal amounts of salt and a fluid intake of 3 liters per day; avoid caffeine due to its diuretic effect. 4. Report polyuria, prolonged vomiting, diarrhea, or fever to physician (may need to temporarily reduce or discontinue dosage). 5. Do not crush, chew, or break the extended-release or film-coated tablets. 6. Assess clients at high risk of developing toxicity: postoperative, dehydrated, hyperthyroid, those with renal disease, or those clients on diuretics. 7. Blood levels: a. extremely narrow therapeutic range; 0.5—1.5 mEq/liter. b. toxic serum lithium level is greater than 2 mEq/liter. 8. Management of lithium toxicity: administration of osmotic diuretics (e.g., urea or mannitol); aminophylline and **Diamox**. 9. Long-term use may cause goiter; may be associated with hypothyroidism. 10. No antidote available for lithium poisoning.
OTHER AGENTS: Both medications listed below were originally developed and used for seizure disorders. Both have mood-stabilizing abilities.		
Carbamazepine (**Tegretol**): PO	Drowiness, dizziness, visual problems (spots before eyes, difficulty focusing, blurred vision), dry mouth. ***Toxic reactions***: blood dyscrasias	1. Used primarily for clients who have failed to respond to lithium or who cannot tolerate the side effects. 2. Avoid tasks that require alertness, motor skills until response to drug is established. 3. **Tegretol** — monitor CBC frequently during initiation of therapy and at monthly intervals thereafter. 4. **Depakene** — monitor liver function studies.
Valproic acid (**Depakene**) : PO	Nausea, GI upsets, transient hair loss, weight gain, tremors, heptatotoxicity, and dose-realated thrombocytopenia.	

Appendix 6-3: ANTIDEPRESSANT MEDICATIONS

MEDICATIONS	SIDE EFFECTS	NURSING IMPLICATIONS
❖GENERAL NURSING IMPLICATIONS❖ — SSRIs are first line of drug of choice for depression followed by TCA and MAO. — MAOs have potential interactions with other drugs and certain foods. — Therapeutic effect has a delayed onset of 7-21 days. — Can potentially produce cardiotoxicity, sedation, seizures, and anticholingeric effects, as well as induce mania in bipolar clients (SSRIs less likely to cause these problems). — Drugs are usually discontinued prior to surgery (10 days for MAOs; 2-3 days for TCAs) because of adverse interaction with anesthetic agents.		
SELECTIVE SEROTONIN REUPTAKE INHIBITORS (SSRI): Causes selective inhibition of serotonin uptake and produces CNS excitation rather than sedation; has no effect on dopamine or norepinephrine.		
Fluoxetine (**Prosac**): PO Sertraline (**Zoloft**):PO Paroxetine (**Paxil**): PO	Nausea, headache, anxiety, nervousness, insomnia, weight loss, skin rash.	1. Give medication in the morning. 2. ***Uses:*** depression, obsessive-compulsive disorder, bulimia, suppress appetite in obese clients.
TRICYCLIC ANTIDEPRESSANTS (TCA): Prevent the reuptake of norepinephrine or serotonin, which results in increased concentrations of these neurotransmitters.		
Imipramine hydrochloride (**Tofranil**): PO, IM Nortriptyline hydrochloride (**Aventyl**): PO Doxepin hydrochloride (**Sinequan**): PO Amitriptyline hydrochloride (**Elavil**): PO, IM	Drowsiness, dry mouth, blurred vision, constipation, and hypotension. ***Adverse reactions:*** Cardiac dysrhythmias, nystagmus, tremor, hypotension, restlessness.	1. Should not be given at the same time with an MAO inhibitor; a lag time of 14 days is necessary when changing from one drug group to the other. 2. Because of marked sedation, client should avoid activities requiring mental alertness (driving or operating machinery). 3. Instruct client to move gradually from lying to sitting and standing positions to prevent postural hypotension. 4. **Sinequan** is tolerated better by the elderly; has less effect on cardiac status; dilute the concentrate with orange juice. 5. Contraindicated in clients with epilepsy, glaucoma, and cardiovascular disease. 6. Usually given once daily at bedtime. 7. Too high of dose of these drugs can be fatal due to the narrow therapeutic index. Use: depression; **Tofranil** also used to treat enuresis in children.
MONOAMINE OXIDASE INHIBITORS (MAO): Inhibit the enzyme monoamine oxidase, which breaks down norepinephrine and serotonin increasing the concentration of these neurotransmitters.		
Isocarboxazid (**Marplan**): PO Phenelzine sulfate (**Nardil**): PO Tranylcypromine (**Parnate**): PO	Drowsiness, insomnia, dryness of mouth, urinary retention, hypotension. Adverse reactions: tachycardia, tachypnea, agitation, tremors, seizures, heart block, hypotension.	1. Potentiate many drug actions: narcotics, barbiturates, sedatives, and atropine-like medications. 2. Have a long duration of action; therefore, 2 - 3 weeks must go by before taking another drug while on an MAO inhibitor. 3. Interact with specific foods and drugs (ones containing tyramine or sympathomimetic drugs). May cause a severe hypertensive crisis characterized by marked elevation of blood pressure, increased temperature, tremors, and tachycardia. Foods to avoid: coffee, tea, cola beverages, aged cheeses, beer and wine, pickled foods, avocados, figs, and many over-the-counter cold preparations, hayfever medications, and nasal decongestants. 4. Monitor for bladder distention by checking urinary output. 5. Have a lag time of 2-4 weeks before notice effects. 6. **Parnate:** Most likely to cause hypertensive crisis and onset of action is more rapid. **Use:** primarily psychotic depression and depressive episode of bipolar affective disorder.

Appendix 6-3:
ANTIDEPRESSANT MEDICATIONS

MEDICATIONS	SIDE EFFECTS	NURSING IMPLICATIONS
MISCELLANEOUS ANTI-DEPRESSANTS		
Trazodone (**Desyrel**): PO	Sedation, orthostatic hypotension, nausea, vomiting, can cause priapism (prolonged, painful erection of the penis).	1. See general nursing implications on previous page.
Bupropion (**Wellbutrin**): PO	Weight loss, dry mouth, dizziness.	

Appendix 6-4:
ANTIPSYCHOTIC (NEUROLEPTIC) MEDICATIONS

❖GENERAL NURSING IMPLICATIONS❖
— Use cautiously in elderly adults.
— Give daily dose 1-2 hours before betime.
— When mixing for parenteral use, do not mix with other drugs.
— Inject deep IM - client should stay in reclined position 30 - 60 minutes after dose.
— Caution against driving a car or operating machinery.

MEDICATIONS	SIDE EFFECTS	NURSING IMPLICATIONS
PHENOTHIAZINES: Block dopamine receptors and also thought to depress various portions of the reticular activating system; have peripherally exerting anticholinergic properties (atropine-like symptoms, dryness of mouth, stuffy nose, constipation, blurring of vision).		
Aliphatic types— Chloropromazine hydrochloride (**Thorazine**): PO, IM, IV suppository Promazine hydrochloride (**Sparine**): PO, IM, IV Piperazine types— Prochlorperazine (**Compazine**): PO, IM, IV, suppository Fluphenazine hydrochloride (**Prolixin**): PO, IM Trifluoperazine (**Stelazine**): PO, IM Piperidine types— Thioridazine (**Mellaril**): PO Mesoridazine besylate (**Serentil**): PO, IM	***Extrapyramidal (movement disorder):*** occurs early in therapy and is usually managed with other drugs *acute dystonia* - spasm of muscles of the tongue, face, neck, or back, oculogyric crisis (upward deviation of the eyes), opisthotonus. *Parkinsonism* - muscle tremors, rigidity, spasms, shuffling gait, stooped posture, cogwheel rigidity. *akathisia* -motor restlessness, pacing. ***Tardive dyskinesia:*** (occurs late in therapy -symptoms are often irreversible) slow worm-like movements of the tongue is earliest symptom, later -fine twisting, writhing movements of the tongue and face, grimacing, lip smacking, involuntary movements of the limbs, toes, fingers, and trunk. ***Neuroleptic malignant syndrome:*** rare problem, fever (> 41°C), "lead-pipe" muscle rigidity, agitation, confusion, delirium, respiratory and acute renal failure. **Endocrine:** amenorrhea, increased libido in women, decreased libido in men, delayed ejaculation, increased appetite, weight gain, hypoglycemia, and edema. ***Dermatologic:*** photosensitivity. ***Hypersensitivity reaction:*** jaundice, agranulocytosis.	1. Check blood pressure prior to administration; to avoid postural hypotension, encourage client to rise slowly from sitting or lying position. 2. Be aware of the antiemetic effect of the phenothiazines; may mask other pathology such as drug overdose, brain lesions, or intestinal obstruction. 3. Client teaching: protect skin from sunlight; wear long-sleeved shirts, hats, and sunscreen lotion when out in the sunlight. 4. Explain importance of reporting any signs of sore throat, fever, or symptoms of infection. 5. Encourage periodic liver function studies to be done. 6. Teach that drug may turn urine pink or reddish brown. 7. Extrapyramidal symptoms treated with anti-cholinergics, (i.e., **Cogentin**). 8. ***Uses:*** severe psychoses; schizophrenia; manic phase of bipolar affective disorder; personality disorders; and severe agitation and anxiety; also an adjunct to preoperative anesthesia (e.g., **Compazine, Phenergan)**. 9. Long term use of phenothiazines requires assessment of involuntary movement (AIMS testing).
OTHER ANTIPSYCHOTIC DRUGS:		
Haloperidol (**Haldol**): PO, IM	Significant extrapyramidal effects; low incidence of sedation, orthostatic hypotension; does not elicit photosensitivity reaction.	1. May reduce prothrombin time. 2. Often used as the initial drug for treatment of psychotic disorders. ***Uses:*** tics, vocal disturbances, and psychotic schizophrenia.
Risperidone (**Risperdal**): PO	Anxiety, somnolence, extrapyramidal symptoms, dizziness, constipation, GI upset, rhinitis	1. **Risperdal** most frequently prescribed antipsychotic due to lack of serious side effects.

phytonadione mephyton
(Vit. K)

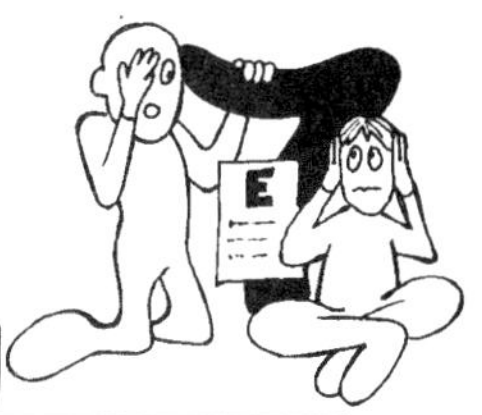

Sensory

PHYSIOLOGY OF THE EYE

A. Structures of the eyes (Figure 7-1).
 1. Sclera - tough, protective covering of the outside of the eye.
 2. Cornea - transparent tissue over the pupils.
 3. Ciliary muscle - muscular body that allows the eye to focus through contraction and relaxation.
 4. Iris - controls the amount of light; gives the eye the characteristic color.
 5. Retina - contains millions of nerve cells to coordinate and transmit signals to the opposite nerve.
 6. Aqueous humor - fluid that fills anterior and posterior chambers; circulates through the pupil and empties into canal of Schlemm.
 7. Vitreous humor - fluid that fills the cavity posterior to the lens.
 8. Crystalline lens - provides for the convergence and refraction of light rays and images onto the retina; enables vision to be focused.
 9. Optic nerve - leaves the eyeball through the retina at the location of the optic disc.

B. Eyelids - protective coverings of the eye.
 1. Conjunctiva - inner lining of the eyelid.
 2. Lacrimal gland - excretes lacrimal fluid (tears) to lubricate, clean, and protect the outer surface of the eye.

Data Collection

A. External data collection.
 1. Assess position and alignment of the eyes.
 2. Evaluate for presence of ptosis.
 3. Inspect lids and conjunctiva for discharge or inflammation.
 4. Assess color of sclera.
 5. Evaluate size and equality of pupils.
 6. Evaluate pupillary reaction to light.

B. Evaluate history.
 1. Eye pain and headaches.
 2. Decrease or blurred vision.
 3. Eye infections.
 4. Floating or "dots" in field of vision.
 5. Chronic illnesses and medications
 6. Surgical procedures.

C. Evaluate visual acuity (Appendix 7-1).

DISORDERS OF THE EYE

NURSING PRIORITY: *Important to teach client to report any of the following symptoms: progressive dimming of vision, "floaters" or specks, partial/complete loss of vision which may signal an acute attack of glaucoma, retinal detachment or side effects of drugs or other diseases.*

Geriatric Priority: *Age related macular degeneration is found mostly in adults older than age 65 and accounts for a large percentage of diminished central vision in the older adult. There is no known treatment or prevention of this process.*

Glaucoma

❑ **Glaucoma is a group of conditions characterized by an increase in intraocular pressure and progressive loss of vision. It is a chronic condition and a leading cause of blindness.**

A. Aqueous humor flows between the iris and the lens, then flows out the anterior chamber. When pressure increased there is damage to the optic nerve.

B. Intraocular pressure is determined by the rate of production of aqueous humor, the resistence to flow, and the pressure in the anterior eye veins.

C. Majority of clients with glaucoma have the open angle type, which develops more slowly and is chronic.

Data Collection

 1. Risk factors.
  a. Familial tendency.
  b. Over 40 years of age.
  c. Diabetic.
  d. History of injury or eye surgery.
  e. Ocular problems (cataract surgery).
  f. Damage to vision is permanent.
  g. Extended use of systemic steroids
 2. Diagnostics - increased intraocular pressure. (above 22 mm Hg) (Appendix 7-1).
 3. Clinical manifestations of chronic open-angle glaucoma.
  a. Gradual loss of peripheral vision (i.e., tunnel vision).
  b. Vague headache.
  c. Halos around lights.
  d. Transient blurred vision.

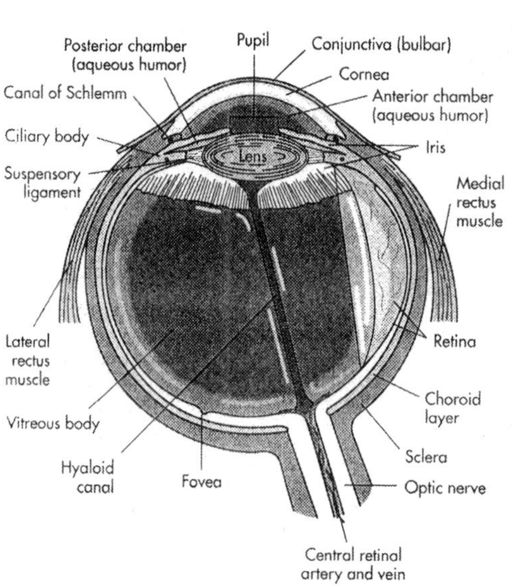

Figure 7-1: Structures of the eye
Reprinted with permission: Phipps, WJ, Sands, JK, & Marek, JF (1999). *Medical Surgical Nursing: Concepts & Clinical Practice,* 6th ed. Philadelphia: Mosby, p. 1812

e. Blindness will eventually occur if untreated.

f. Generally painless, symptoms occur late.

Treatment

1. Medications (Appendix 7-2).
   a. Topical miotics.
   b. Topical beta-blockers (ophthalmic).
2. Surgical intervention.
   a. Laser trabeculoplasty—usually done outpatient with a topical anesthetic.
   b. Glaucoma filtering procedures.

NCLEX ALERT: *Assist client to compensate for a sensory impairment. (Decease hearing, sight, etc.)*

Nursing Intervention

✦ *Goal: to teach client and significant others about the problems of increased intraocular pressure, treatment to control problem, and consequences of failure to follow prescribed regime.*

1. Correct instillation of prescribed eye medications; client must remain on medication in order to control disease.
2. Importance of continual follow-up medical care.
3. Importance of wearing a medical alert identification.
4. Show client correct administration of eye medication and have client demonstrate.
5. Damage to current vision cannot be corrected. Focus of care is to prevent further damage to vision.

***NURSING PRIORITY:** Decreased visual acuity usually occurs when there is irreversible damage to the optic nerve.*

✦ *Goal: to decrease intraocular pressure.*

1. Client should avoid straining at stool, lifting, stooping, and sneezing.
2. Administer antiemetic properly, as vomiting causes increased intraocular pressure.
3. Any medication that causes pupillary dilatation (atropine) will cause increased intraocular pressure.
4. Provide emotional support.
   a. Orient clients to objects within visual field.
   b. Encourage verbalization regarding fear of blindness and loss of independence.

Self-Care

1. Teach how to instill eye drops.
2. Stress importance for lifelong medical treatment and eye exams.
3. Advise all care givers of condition.
4. Review with ophthalmologist all across the counter drugs prior to taking them

NCLEX ALERT: *Instruct client about managing his/her health condition.*

Cataract

❑ **A complete or partial opacity of the lens is known as a *cataract.* It may occur at birth (congenital cataract); however, it occurs most commonly in adults past middle age (senile cataracts).**

Data Collection

1. Clinical manifestations.
   a. Painless.
   b. Gradual decrease in visual acuity.
   c. Pupil appears gray to milky white.
   d. Decreased perception of colors.
2. Diagnostics (Appendix 7-1).
   a. Decrease in visual acuity.
   b. Ophthalmoscopic exam.
   c. Slit lamp examination.

Treatment

1. Surgical treatment is only method of correcting problem; surgery is usually performed when client begins to experience problems in activities of daily living.
2. Since the lens was removed, the client must have some type of replacement lens. Lens implant is usually done at time of surgery.

Nursing Intervention

✦ *Goal: to provide appropriate nursing care in preoperative phase.*

1. Administer medication - mydriatic (dilating drops) are administered at intervals approximately one hour prior to surgery.
2. Provide emotional support by encouraging verbalization of fears and concerns.
3. General preoperative and postoperative teaching according to anticipated activities and care.

✦ *Goal: to ensure that client does not experience postoperative complications; most cataract surgery is done under local anesthesia.*

1. Administer medications, teach client how to administer medications (Appendix 7-2).
   a. Antibiotics.
   b. Steroids.
2. Assess for hemorrhage characterized by sudden ocular pain and subconjunctival hemorrhage.
3. Eye patch is usually worn for 24 hours to prevent client from rubbing eye.
4. *Report to RN immediately any sudden, severe ocular pain.*
5. Instruct client regarding signs of infection and complications.
   a. Pain.
   b. Purulent drainage.
   c. Decrease in vision.
   d. Increased redness and subconjunctival hemorrhage.

Box 7-1: Elderly Care Focus
Promoting Independent Activities of Daily Living for the Client with Diminished Vision

MEDICATIONS

Use different shapes of containers with lids (square, round, triangular) when client has to take medications more than once a day.

Obtain medication boxes with raised letters or numbers on them for the days of the week.

Obtain a "talking clock" which states the time.

SAFETY

NCLEX ALERT: *Use interventions to protect client from injury. Review client environment for safety features.*

Remove throw rugs.

Use nonbreakable dishes, cups, and glasses.

Keep appliance cords short and out of walkways.

Avoid footstools in favor of recliner with a built-in footrest.

Cleansers, cleaning fluids, and caustic chemicals should be labeled with large, raised lettering.

Have hand grips installed in bathrooms.

Put nonskid stripping on tub floor surface.

Encourage use of an electric razor.

Wear protective eyeware when there is a risk of injury or contamination of the eyes.

COMMUNICATION

Use telephones that have programmed, automatic dialing features. Be sure to include emergency phone numbers, such as fire department, police, relatives, friends, and 911 (or whatever emergency number is available).

DAILY LIVING CONSIDERATIONS

Provide information on "Meals on Wheels" for assistance in having cooked, ready to eat meals delivered.

Find out which local grocery stores provide a "shop by phone" or delivery service.

Encourage use of a microwave for cooking, as it is safer than using a standard stove.

Encourage the use of large-print books, newspapers, and magazines for reading. Also, many of these books, etc. are available on audiotape at local libraries and vision aid services.

NCLEX ALERT: *Assist in activities of daily living. Provide physical care that meets special needs of the older adult client.*

Self-Care

1. Eye patch may be worn on affected eye for 24 hours after surgery. May be worn at night after 24 hours to prevent client from rubbing eyes.
2. If redness and discharge occur, client should clean eye with a soft damp washcloth.
3. Promote independent activities of daily living (Box 7-1).
4. Notify doctor if "floaters," pain, flashing lights, decrease in vision, or increased redness occurs.
5. Vision is usually stabilize withing 6-10 weeks and vision correction will be done.
6. Client should wear sun glasses because the operative eye will be light sensitive.

Retinal Detachment

❑ **A separation of the two layers of the retina is called *retinal detachment.***

Data Collection

1. Risk factors.
   a. Severe myopia.
   b. Diabetic retinopathy.
   c. Trauma.
   d. Degenerative changes in the retina.
   e. Previous cataract surgery.
2. Diagnostics.
   a. Ophthalmoscopic examination.
3. Clinical manifestations.
   a. Sudden onset, no pain.
   b. Flashes of light in visual field.
   c. Sensation of a veil or cobwebs over the eye.
   d. Floating spots.
   e. May experience area of blank vision.
   f. Eventually results in loss of vision.

Treatment

Principle of treatment is to seal the hole by creating an inflammatory reaction that will promote scar adhesion.

1. Vitreretinal surgery to attempt to promote readherence of retinal layers.
2. Scleral buckling - traction on the retina to promote contact of detached retinal layers.

Nursing Intervention

✦ *Goal: to prevent further deterioration of vision.*

1. Position client so area of detachment is in dependent position.
2. Have client avoid jerky head movements (brushing hair and teeth, shaving).
3. Have client avoid coughing.

✦ *Goal: to keep client from experiencing complication of scleral buckling (see Nursing Intervention to prevent further deterioration of vision).*

1. Prevent nausea and vomiting.
2. Avoid activities that increase intraocular pressure: bending, lifting, sneezing, coughing, vomiting

Self-Care

1. Reading and activity may be restricted for several weeks postoperative.
2. Eye pads may be worn for comfort or they may be worn at night to prevent rubbing of the eyes.
3. No heavy lifting or heavy work for at least six weeks.
4. Client may be more comfortable in dark glasses.

Conjunctivitis

❑ **Inflammation or infection of the conjunctiva.**

Data Collection

A. Type types.

1. Allergic conjunctivitis—burning, tearing, itching, and vascular injection (redness).
2. Mucopurulent bacterial conjunctivitis ("pink eye")—conjunctival edema, tearing, thick, purulent drainage (eyelids stick together).

Treatment

1. Ophthalmic antibiotic eye ointment for bacterial infection.

Nursing Intervention

✦ *Goal: to prevent transmission.*

1. Teach client not to rub eyes.
2. Encourage frequent good hand washing.
3. Cleanse eyelids with warm saline compresses to remove crusts before administering eye medications.
4. Common for infection to spread to unaffected eye.
5. Teach client how to avoid contamination of tip of medication tube.
6. Good hand washing by client and everyone in contact with client.

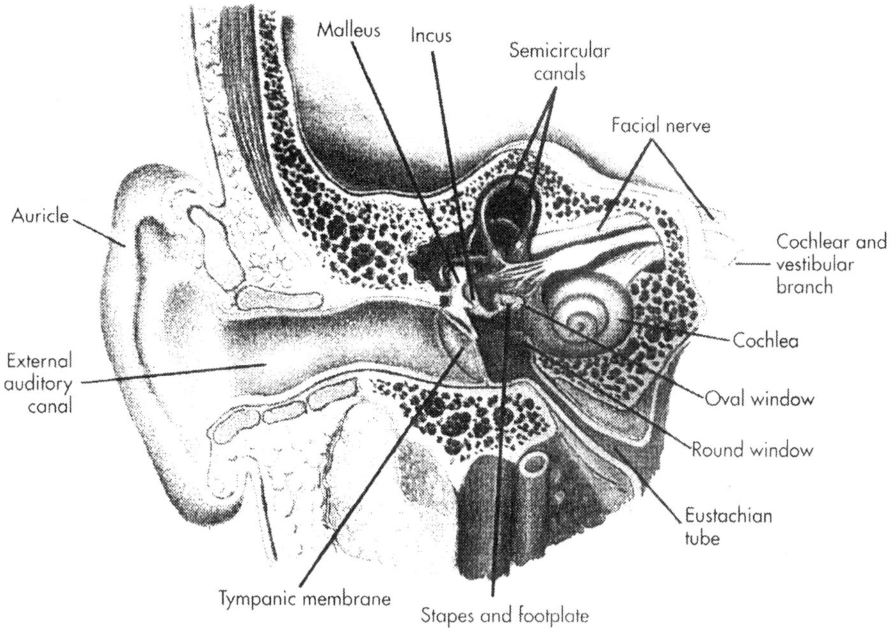

Figure 7-2: Structures of the ear
Reprinted with permission: Phipps, WJ, Sands, JK, & Marek, JF (1999). *Medical Surgical Nursing: Concepts & Clinical Practice,* 6th ed. Philadelphia: Mosby, p.1852.

PHYSIOLOGY OF THE EAR

A. External ear (Figure 7-2).

1. Auricle or pinna - the cartilage and connective tissue forming the outside of the ear.
2. External auditory canal - function is to collect the transmitted sound waves to the tympanic membrane; outer half of canal secretes cerumen (wax) which provides a protective function.
3. Tympanic membrane - a tough membrane separating the external and middle ear; transmits vibrations from external ear to the malleus of the middle ear.

B. Middle ear.

1. Contains three small articulating bones - malleus, incus, stapes.
2. The eustachian tube in infants and young children is shorter and wider than in adults.
3. Problems in the external and middle ear cause conductive hearing loss.

C. Inner ear.

1. Bony labyrinth - concerned with maintaining equilibrium.
2. Cochlea - contains organ of Corti, which is the receptive end organ for hearing.
3. Pathology of the inner ear or nerve pathway can result in sensorineural hearing loss.

Data Collection

A. External assessment of the ear.

1. Assess placement of the ears - low -set ears may be indicative of congenital anomalies.
2. Movement of the ear lobe should not elicit pain.
3. Note presence of any discharge in the external ear canal.

DISORDERS OF THE EAR

Acute Otitis Media

❑ **This is an acute infection of the middle ear. Infants and young children are predisposed to the development of otitis media because the eustachian tube is shorter, wider, and straighter than in the adult ear. Common organisms are: *H.influenza, streptococcus, and staphylococcus.***

Data Collection

1. Risk factors.
   a. Age.
   b. History of upper respiratory infection.
2. Clinical manifestations.
   a. Pain from pressure in the middle ear.
      (1) Infants - irritable, pull at their ears, sucking aggravates pain.

Box 7-2: Elderly Care Focus
Improving Communication with Hearing Impaired Clients

- Standing in front of client at eye level to speak with light on your face helps with speech reading, (i.e., reading lips).
- Get client's attention by raising your hand or arm.
- Do not walk back and forth in front of client while speaking.
- Speak clearly and in an even tone; do not shout.
- Do not chew gum, cover mouth, or smile excessively while talking.
- Because clients rely on visual cues, watch your facial expressions.
- Encourage professional counseling in speech and sign language.
- Assist client in obtaining hearing aid, if appropriate.
- Promote social interaction appropriate for elderly adult.

(2) Young children verbally complain of severe ear pain.

b. Fever varies greatly.

c. Nasal congestion.

d. If tympanic membrane ruptures, purulent drainage may be present in the outer ear; pain will decrease temporarily.

e. Hearing loss with recurrent rupture.

Treatment

1. Medications.

a. Antibiotics.

NURSING PRIORITY: *Teach the parents to give the child all of the antibiotic.*

b. Analgesics (topical, i.e., **Auralgan**).

c. Antipyretics (**Tylenol**).

d. Decongestants.

e. Ear drops (antibiotic and steroid combination).

2. Surgical - Myringotomy for recurrent cases which do not respond to medication; drainage of the middle ear with insertion of myringotomy tubes.

Nursing Intervention

✦ *Goal: to enable parents of clients to describe problem, handle medication schedule, and cope with home care.*

1. Recurrent infections cause an increased risk of permanent hearing loss.
2. Antibiotics should be given around the clock, and the complete prescribed amount should be given.
3. Administer acetaminophen or ibuprofen for pain and fever.
4. Decongestants may be administered to decrease fluid collection, thereby decreasing incidence of infection and discomfort.
5. Decreased incidence of milk pooling around eustachian tube.

a. Hold, or elevate child's head while feeding.

b. Do not prop bottle and allow child to fall asleep.

c. Encourage juice or water prior to sleeping.

6. Child should not go swimming or get water in the ears.
7. Teach that myringotomy tubes usually come on their own within 3-12 months.

Hearing Loss

❑ **Hearing loss results from an impairment of the transmission of sound waves.**

1. Conductive - results from an impairment in transmission of sound from the outer or middle ear or both. Client will be able to benefit from a hearing aid.
2. Sensorineural (perceptive) - results from a problem in the inner ear, or a nerve pathway. Incoming sound cannot be analyzed correctly. Client will not benefit from a hearing aid.
3. Mixed conductive and sensorineural.
4. Impacted cerumen can lead to hearing loss; occurs often in the elderly.

Data Collection

1. Risk factors.

a. Age related changes, increased incidence in clients over 65.

b. Prolonged exposure to high intensity sound waves.

NURSING PRIORITY: *Ear plugs should be worn when the potential for loud noise exists.*

c. Repeated, chronic ear infections.

d. Prenatal problems of rubella and eclampsia.

e. Premature birth.

f. Ototoxic medications.

2. Diagnostics (Appendix 7-1).

a. Audiogram.

b. Weber and Rinne tests to differentiate between conductive and sensorineural loss.

3. Clinical manifestations.

a. Speech problems - deterioration of present speech, or delayed speech development.

b. General indifference to sound.

c. Social withdrawal.

d. Decreased self-confidence.

e. Responds more to facial expressions than to verbal ones.

f. Inappropriate emotional response.

Treatment

1. Hearing aid, if conductive loss.
2. Speech therapy.
3. Sign language.
4. Stapedectomy for otosclerotic lesions.

NCLEX ALERT: *Modify care for client who has a prosthesis. Provide care for client who uses assistive devices. Hearing loss is very common in older adult clients*

Nursing Intervention

✦ *Goal: to promote communication and socialization of the hearing-impaired client (see Box 7-2).*

1. Provide information concerning a TDD (telephone device for the deaf) which transmits typed words over the phone line.
2. Suggest light-activated devices rather than sound-activated devices—connecting doorbell, smoke, and security alarms to an electrical device which causes lights to flicker on and off.
3. Avoid crowded, noisy environments (such as restaurants) especially if a hearing aid is used, since it amplifies the background sound.
4. Teach how to care for hearing aid (Box 7-3).
5. Teach client how to remove ear wax, if impacted cerumen is a problem; may need an ear irrigation (Appendix 7-3).

✦ *Goal: to ensure that client who undergoes stapedectomy will not experience complications postoperatively.*

1. Appropriate preoperative teaching regarding postoperative activities.
2. Assess for dizziness.
3. Maintain safety measures when client is dizzy.
4. Instruct client not to blow nose.
5. Instruct client that hearing may not improve for several weeks because of edema in the operative area.

Self-Care

1. Avoid washing hair for about two weeks; after that, avoid getting water in the ears.
2. Avoid flying and swimming for several months.

> **Box 7-3:** Elderly Care Focus
> ***Hearing Aid Care***
>
> - Keep the hearing aid dry; do not wear it while bathing, swimming, or allow it to get wet during a rain shower.
> - Avoid using hair spray, cosmetics, or oils around the ear.
> - Always keep extra batteries on hand.
> - When not using hearing aid, turn it off and remove the battery to store it.
> - Avoid dropping the hearing aid (has delicate electronics) or exposing it to extremes in temperatures (i.e., leaving it on a window ledge in the sunlight).
> - Clean ear mold part with a mild soap and water; do not get it excessively wet.
> - Clean any debris or, cerumen from the hole in the middle part that goes in the ear by using a toothpick or pipe cleaner
> - If the hearing aid does not work, change the battery or check the on-off switch, check the connection between the ear mold and receiver, clean it using the steps described above, or take it in to an authorized hearing aid service center.

3. Report unusual sensations or "sloshy" feelings in the ear.
4. Avoid contact with people with upper respiratory infections.

Ménière's Disease

❑ **Ménière's Disease is a problem occurring in the inner ear.**

Data Collection

1. Clinical manifestations.

   a. Severe vertigo.

   b. Tinnitus (ringing in the ears).

   c. Sensorineural hearing loss.

   d. Violent paroxysmal attacks may occur, lasting 10 minutes or up to several hours.

   (1) Severe nausea, vomiting.

   (2) Loss of balance.

   (3) No pain or loss of consciousness.

   e. Client may proceed normally between attacks.

   f. Condition frequently gets progressively worse, with attacks occurring more frequently and lasting longer.

   g. Progressive hearing loss.

Treatment

1. Medications.

   a. Valium (to control vertigo).

   b. Antiemetics.

c. Antihistamines.

d. Meclizine (**Antivert**).

2. Diet - low sodium or low salt.
3. Surgical - labyrinthectomy.

Nursing Intervention

✦ *Goal: to provide emotional and physical support during an acute attack.*

1. Maintain bed rest in a quiet, dimly lit room.
2. Client may assume a position of comfort.
3. Disturb or move the client only when necessary. Avoid unnecessary nursing procedures.
4. May need to administer medications parenterally if client is nauseated.
5. Keep side rails up to protect client from falling.

Self-Care

✦ *Goal: to teach client measures to prevent or to cope with problem at home.*

1. Take medications as directed.
2. Stop smoking.
3. Avoid alcohol.
4. Maintain a low-sodium diet.
5. Cope appropriately with hearing loss.

Study Questions—Sensory

1. A client has scratched the cornea of the left eye. The edema does not allow the left eyelid to close completely. What measure would be appropriate to protect the eye?

① cover both eyes and lower room lights.
② use artificial tears and cover left eye with a patch.
③ have the client use sun glasses while ambulating.
④ do eye exercises with the nonaffected eye.

2. What is appropriate plan for care with a client who has glaucoma?

① preventing secondary infection.
② having the eyes examined for reading glasses.
③ covering the eye to relieve pressure.
④ controlling intraocular pressure.

3. What is a common finding obtained during a nursing assessment on a client with Ménière's disease?

① severe vertigo.
② sloshy feeling in ears.
③ watery drainage from ears.
④ low grade temperature.

4. What is the therapeutic response of a mydriatic eye medication?

① constriction of the pupil.
② dilatation of the pupil.
③ increase intraocular pressure.
④ decrease intraocular pressure.

5. A infant has a history of frequent otitis media. What would be important teaching information to tell the mother?

① avoid the use of decongestants.
② encourage formula prior to sleeping.
③ stop antibiotics as soon as the fever subsides.
④ hold and elevate the infant's head while feeding.

6. The nurse is instructing the client on administration of eye drops. What nursing observation would indicate the client understands how to administer the drops?

① Positions himself on his left side to administer drops in the left eye.
② Instills the drops into the lower conjunctival sac.
③ Blows his nose prior to administering drops.
④ Cleans the tip of the applicator with a tissue prior to administering.

7. The nurse would teach the client which of the following about glaucoma?

① the lens of the eye becomes cloudy.
② there is an increase of pressure in the eyeball.
③ the cornea becomes stretched causing blurred vision.
④ the pupil becomes constricted allowing minimal vision.

8. Which of the following is not considered a risk factor for hearing loss?

① prenatal problem of rubella.
② repeated, chronic ear infections.
③ taking penicillin and cephalosporin medication.
④ exposure to high intensity sound waves.

9. In teaching an elderly client about the care of his hearing aid, it would be important for the nurse to include in the teaching plan which of the following?

① always keep extra batteries on hand.
② clean ear mold part by soaking in alcohol.
③ always leave hearing aid turned on when out of the ear.
④ continue to wear hearing aid it, even while sleeping.

10. A client has a diagnosis of glaucoma. Which of the following medications are contraindicated?

① atropine sulfate (**Atropisol**).
② pilocarpine (**Pilocar**). TX
③ meperidine (**Demerol**).
④ fentanyl (**Duragesic**).

11. After a client's eye has been anesthetized, what would the nurse instruct the client to do?

① not to watch television for at least one day to reduce strain.
② not to rub the eye for 15 to 20 minutes.
③ to irrigate the eye every hour till sensation is felt.
④ to wear an eye patch for two days.

12. A client comes to the clinic with decreased hearing. Examination of the ear canal reveals a large amount of ear wax. The nurse prepares for removal of the wax by:

① forceps.
② normal saline irrigation.
③ D/5/W irrigation.
④ cotton swab applicator.

13. To improve communication with the hearing impaired, it is important to include all the following except:

① have a writing pad available.
② raise your voice slightly.
③ use short sentences or phrases with frequent pauses in the conversation.
④ stand directly in front of the client to allow them to see your face.

14. A nurse is teaching a family about the use of a hearing aid. The nurse bases her response on the knowledge that the hearing aid does which of the following?

① provides mechanical training for the damaged part of the ear.
② amplifies sound but does not improve the ability to hear.
③ amplifies sound and improves the ability to hear.
④ assists to heal the damaged part of the ear.

15. The nursing management of a client with Ménière's disease includes which of the following?

① place the bed in a semi-Fowler's position.
② increase fluid intake by 2000cc per day.
③ increase sodium in the diet.
④ avoid sudden movements.

16. What is the procedure used to correct otosclerosis?

① irrigation of the inner ear with antibiotics.
② placement of myringotomy drainage tubes.
③ stapedectomy.
④ mastoidectomy.

17. What is the most common cause of loss of central vision in the older adult?

① retinal detachment.
② glaucoma.
③ macular degeneration.
④ cataract.

Appendix 7-1:
OPHTHALMIC AND HEARING DIAGNOSTICS

OPHTHALMIC DIAGNOSTICS

SNELLEN CHART is used in screening for visual acuity problems. Client is placed 20 feet from the chart and visual acuity is expressed in a ratio of what he/she **should** see at 20 feet to what he/she **can** see at 20 feet. A ratio of 20/50 means that the client can see at 20 feet what he/she should see at 50 feet.

TONOMETER TESTS
Non-contact Tonometer—a puff of air is directed toward the cornea, which causes indentation and allows measurement of intraocular pressure. Normal pressure is 12-22 mm HG. pressure.

DIRECT OPHTHALMOSCOPY is performed with a handheld ophthalmoscope.

BIOMYCROSCOPY (slit-lamp exam) is used for assessment of the anterior eye for problems of the cornea, iris, lens, and to evaluate the depth of the anterior chamber.

REFRACTIVE ERROR EVALUATION determines what refractive errors have occurred because light is not correctly focused on the retina. Conditions that occur in refractive errors are:
(a) **myopia** (nearsightedness)— trouble seeing at a distance
(b) **hyperopia** (farsightedness)— trouble seeing up close
(c) **presbyopia**— leads to poor accommodation for near vision (common in older adults)
(d) **astigmatism**— when there is an uneven curvature of the cornea

HEARING DIAGNOSTICS

AUDIOGRAM is a graphic outline of an individual's hearing ,as measured by various tones. Tones introduced into the external auditory opening will measure air conduction. Tones introduced over the mastoid bone will measure appropriate nerve conduction.

RINNE TEST is conducted by holding a vibrating tuning fork over the mastoid bone until the client can no longer hear it.

WEBER TEST is conducted by placing a vibrating tuning fork on top of the client's head or in the middle of the forehead, the sound should be heard equally well in each ear.

OTOSCOPY is the examination of the external ear and the tympanic membrane utilizing an otoscope.

Appendix 7-2: OPHTHALMIC MEDICATIONS

❖ GENERAL NURSING IMPLICATIONS ❖

— To decrease systemic absorption, teach client to apply gentle pressure to the lacrimal sac (tear duct) during and immediately following instillation of drops.
— Instruct client or family in proper administration of eye drops or ointment,(i.e., maintain sterile technique and prevent dropper contamination, and store away from heat).
— Expect some blurriness from ointments and apply at bedtime, if possible, to avoid safety problems from diminished vision.
— Instruct client to report changes in vision, blurring, difficulty breathing, or flushing.

MEDICATIONS	SIDE EFFECTS	NURSING IMPLICATIONS
CARBONIC ANHYDRASE INHIBITORS: Restricts actions on enzyme necessary for production of aqueous humor.		
Acetazolamide **(Diamox)** po	GI disturbances Increased urination Loss of K Loss of bicarbonate	1. Use with caution in clients with acidosis, diabetes. 2. Assess for hypokalemia. 3. Administer drug in AM because of diuretic effect. 4. Increased lethargy.
Dorzolamide **(Trusopt)** topical Brinzolamide **(Azopt)**	Allergic reaction on eye and lid Blurred vision, tearing, eye dryness.	
MIOTICS: Contraction of ciliary muscle (pupillary constriction), thus increasing flow of aqueous humor.		
Pilocarpine **(Pilocar, Isopto Carpine)**, 0.5% to 4% solutions, topical	Sustained constriction of ciliary muscle - miosis. Blurred vision.	1. Contraindicated in inflammatory eye conditions. 2. Used in treatment of glaucoma
BETA-BLOCKERS: Reduces intraocular pressure by decreasing formation of aqueous humor.		
Timolol maleate (**Timoptic**)	Eye irritation Bradycardia, hypotension,	1. A decrease in the resting heart rate may occur if there is systemic absorption. 2. Overdose an/or systemic absorption may cause cardiac problems and bronchospasm.
Betaxolol HCl (**Betoptic**)	Insomnia Bradycardia	
MYDRIATICS: Blocks response of sphincter muscle of iris, produces dilation of pupil; may cause paralysis of accommodation.		
Atropine sulfate (**Atropisol**): 0.25 percent to 2 percent solution, topical Tropicamide (**Mydriacyl**)	Stinging. Flushing, dry mouth, dizziness	1. Contraindicated in glaucoma client. 2. Dark glasses may be worn to decrease discomfort from photophobia. 3. Use only ophthalmic preparations.
Phenylephrine	Transient burning, stinging, blurred vision	1. Precautions to prevent systemic absorption.
DIAGNOSTICS: Surface of eye absorbs dye, thus demonstrating corneal abrasions.		
Fluorescein sodium (**Fluoresite, Fluor-I-strip**)	Stinging, burning sensation. Blurred vision Photophobia	1. Avoid touching eye with tip of dropper. 2. Used to diagnose corneal lacerations in clients with eye trauma. 3. Aqueous humor will stain green, indicating a leak from the anterior chamber.
ADRENERGICS (Sympathomimetics): Decreases production of aqueous humor and enhances outflow.		
Dipivefrin HCl (**Propine**) Epinephrine	Transient burning and stinging.	1. May increase heart rate. 2. Instruct client to prevent systemic absorption. 3. Used in treatment of glaucoma.

Appendix 7-3:
NURSING PROCEDURE ■ **EAR IRRIGATION** ■

COMMON SOLUTIONS
Warm tap water or normal saline
2-4% boric acid
0.8% bicarbonate of soda
Glycerine and water.

✓ Key Points: Irrigation

- Temperature of irrigating solution should be near body temperature (37°C, approximately 98°F). If too cold or hot, can cause dizziness and nausea.
- To soften cerumen, add a few drops of warm mineral oil or hydrogen peroxide to the ear.
- Use an ear syringe, or a bulb syringe may be used.
- Use no more than 2-3 ounces of irrigating fluid at a time.
- Gently insert the tip of the syringe into the ear, than repeatedly pump the solution into and out of the ear canal.
- Turn the client on his side to allow ear canal to drain.
- Teach the client how to irrigate his own ears.

NCLEX ALERT: *Explain/teach client about treatments/procedures.*

Congestive Heart failure is a core measure
pneumonia is a core measures
myocardial Infarction is a core measure

8 Endocrine System

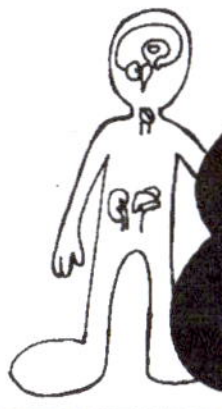

THYROID GLAND

A. Located in the anterior portion of the neck.

B. Disorders of the thyroid gland result in hyperfunction and hypofunction or simple enlargement of the gland.

C. Anterior portion of the pituitary gland controls secretions of the thyroid stimulating hormone (TSH).

D. Thyroid gland responds to levels of TSH in regulating body metabolism.

E. Disorders of the thyroid gland are result in hyperfunction or hypofunction of the gland, or there may be a simple enlargement of the thyroid.

Data Collection

A. Assess changes in weight and appetite — (↑ or ↓).

B. Assess for intellectual development and mental changes - increased irritability, excitability, nervousness, altered mood and affect, confusion, and coma.

C. Assess for changes in hair and skin, altered general appearance, and sexual dysfunction.

DISORDERS OF THE THYROID GLAND

Hyperthyroidism

❑ **Other names for this condition are Graves' disease, toxic goiter and thyrotoxicosis. The condition is characterized by excessive output of thyroid hormones.**

Data Collection

1. More prevalent in women 30 - 40 years of age.
2. Intolerance to heat.
3. Significant weight loss despite increased appetite and food intake.
4. Tachycardia.
5. Increase in systolic blood pressure.
6. Visual problems.
   a. Exophthalmos (bulging eyeballs).
   b. Changes in vision.
   c. Eyelid retraction (lidlag).
7. Increased peristalsis leading to diarrhea.
8. Diagnostics (Appendix 8-1) - increase in T_3, T_4, and decrease in TSH.
9. Mood fluctuations
10. Amenorrhea.

Treatment

1. Surgical - thyroidectomy for cancer of the thyroid.
2. Medical.
   a. Reduce or destroy thyroid tissue - irradiation of thyroid gland with radioactive iodine, eventually resulting in absence of thyroid tissue and no production of thyroxin.
   b. Antithyroid medications (Appendix 8-2).

Complications: Thyroid Storm

1. May occur after surgery or treatment with radioactive iodine.
2. Data collection
   a. Systolic hypertension.
   b. Tachycardia.
   c. Fever.
   d. Increased agitation, anxiety.
   e. Gastrointestinal symptoms.

Nursing Intervention

✦ *Goal: to decrease effects of excess thyroid.*

1. Maintain client in quiet environment, try to eliminate additional stress.
2. Cool environment.
3. Sedatives if appropriate.
4. Well-balanced meals (high in calories and high in vitamins), small meals served four to six times per day.
5. Protect the client's eyes if exophthalmos is present.
   a. Moistening drops or ointments.
   b. Assess for excess tearing, an indication of dry cornea.

✦ *Goal: to maintain homeostasis in client experiencing thyroid storm or crisis.*

1. Decrease body temperature and heart rate.
   a. Hypothermia blanket.
   b. Acetaminophen to decrease fever.
   c. Medications to reduce tachycardia.
2. Supplemental oxygen to meet increased metabolic demands.
3. Administer antithyroid medications and/or iodine preparations to decrease thyroxin output.

Figure 8-1: Glands of the Endocrine System
Reprinted with permission: Phipps, WJ, Sands, JK, & Marek, JF (1999). *Medical Surgical Nursing: Concepts & Clinical Practice*, 6th ed. Philadelphia: Mosby, p.1033.

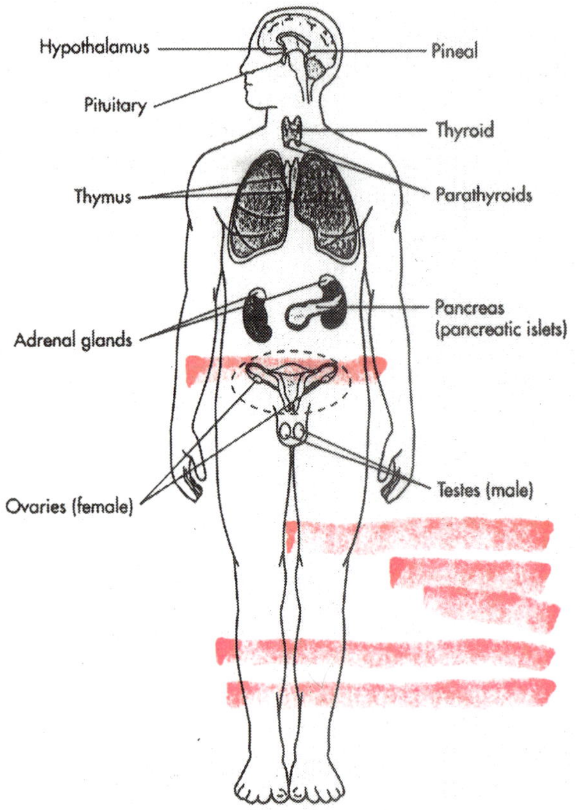

✦ *Goal: to provide appropriate preoperative nursing measures if surgery is indicated.*

1. Decrease environmental stimulus.
2. Demonstrate to client how to provide neck support postoperatively (use hand to support back of head when moving).

✦ *Goal: to maintain homeostasis postoperative thyroidectomy.*

1. Maintain semi-Fowler's position to avoid tension on the suture line.
2. Analgesics for pain.
3. IV fluids until nausea and swallowing difficulty subside.
4. *Check dressings on the side and back of the neck for bleeding and report any bleeding to RN.*
5. Assess for hematoma around the wound.
6. Check calcium lèvels for potential damage to parathyroids during surgery.
7. Support head and neck when changing position.
8. Ice collar for edema and comfort.

NCLEX ALERT: *Safe care (airway, nutrition, hemorrhage) of the hyperthyroid and thyroidectomy client is frequently an area tested.*

✦ *Goal: to prevent complications of respiratory distress following thyroidectomy.*

1. *Assess client frequently for noisy breathing and increased restlessness and report to RN.*
2. Voice changes and increasing hoarseness may be indicative of laryngeal edema. *Report findings to RN immediately.*
3. Keep tracheotomy set readily available.

✦ *Goal: Decrease radiation exposure in the client being treated with radioactive iodine.*

1. Urine is the most highly contaminated body secretion. Either flush commode 2-3 times after client urinates, or store urine in containers in the room until radioactivity decreases.
2. Advise family and client to avoid oral contact for 2-3 days, saliva is contaminated.
3. For any body fluid spills (urine, vomitus, etc) contact Radiation Safety Officer for the facility. Do not clean up the spill.
4. General guideline is to maintain 1 meter (a little over 3 feet) distance from client unless direct contact is necessary.
5. Infants and pregnant women should avoid contact with client for approximately 2-3 days.
6. Specific guidelines are established by the Radiation Safety Officer and determined by the amount of medication the client received.

Self-Care

1. Make sure client understands the implications of taking the thyroid medication every day and advising health care provider of any changes in their condition.
2. Client will be on thyroid replacement for life.

NCLEX ALERT: *Instruct client about managing his/her health condition.*

Hypothyroidism (Myxedema)

❑ **This condition is characterized by a slow deterioration of thyroid function. It occurs primarily in older adults and five times more frequently in women than in men.**

Data Collection

1. Extreme fatigue and apathy.
2. Menstrual disturbances.
3. Hair loss, brittle nails, and dry skin.
4. Intolerance to cold.

5. Anorexia.
6. Constipation.
7. Bradycardia.
8. Weight gain.
9. Decrease in T_3, T_4 and increase in TSH.
10. Previous treatment for hyperthyroid condition and poor compliance with replacement therapy.

Treatment

1. Replacement of thyroid hormone.
2. Low-calorie diet to promote weight loss.
3. Decrease in cholesterol intake.

Nursing Intervention

✦ *Goal: to assist the client to return to hormone balance.*

1. Begin thyroid replacements and evaluate client response.
2. Provide a warm environment.

> ***NURSING PRIORITY**: Administer sedatives and hypnotics with caution due to increased susceptibility. These medications tend to precipitate respiratory depression in the hypothyroid client.*

3. Prevent constipation.
4. Assess progress.
   a. Decrease in body weight.
   b. Intake and output balance.
   c. Decrease in visible edema.
   d. Energy level and mental alertness should increase in two to fourteen days and continue to rise until normal.
5. Need for lifelong thyroid drug therapy.

PARATHYROID GLAND

A. Four small parathyroid glands are located near or embedded in the thyroid gland.

B. The hormone secreted is parathyroid hormone (PTH), which is primarily involved in the control of serum calcium levels.

Data Collection

A. History of problems of calcium metabolism.

B. Assess for changes in mental or emotional status.

C. Evaluate reflexes and neuromuscular response to stimuli.

D. Evaluate serum calcium levels.

DISORDERS OF THE PARATHYROID

Hyperparathyroidism

❑ **This condition is characterized by an excessive secretion of parathyroid hormone (PTH), resulting in hypercalcemia. Decalcification occurs in the bones as the calcium moves from the bones into the serum, resulting in an increase in the serum calcium.**

Data Collection

1. Bone cysts and pathologic fractures.
2. Renal calculi.
3. CNS problems drowsiness, fatigue, lethargy.
4. GI symptoms of constipation, nausea and vomiting, epigastric discomfort.
5. Increase in serum calcium

Treatment

Depends on cause and overall condition of client.

1. Surgical removal of the parathyroid gland.
2. Decrease level of circulating calcium.
3. Increase in circulating volume to dilute calcium.

Nursing Intervention

✦ *Goal: to decrease level of serum calcium.*

1. High fluid intake to dilute serum calcium and urine calcium levels.
2. Encourage mobility, as immobility increases demineralization of bones.
3. Limit foods high in calcium.

✦ *Goal: to assess client's tolerance of and response to increased parathyroid hormone.*

1. Monitor for cardiac arrhythmias.
2. Assess for renal involvement.
   a. Strain urine for stones.
   b. Evaluate for low back pain (renal).
   c. Check for hematuria.
   d. Check for renal and urinary tract infections.

✦ *Goal: to provide appropriate preoperative and post-operative measures if surgery is indicated (Chapter 3).*

Postoperative care of parathyroidectomy client is same as for a thyroidectomy client.

Hypoparathyroidism

❑ **This condition is characterized by a decrease in parathyroid hormone (PTH), resulting in hypocalcemia. Severe hypocalcemia results in tetany.**

Data Collection

1. May occur with inadvertent removal of parathyroid gland during thyroidectomy or radical neck dissection.
2. Muscle weakness and cramps.
3. Numbness and tingling around lips and in hands and feet.
4. Overt/acute tetany (potentially fatal).
   a. Bronchospasm, laryngospasm.
   b. Seizures.
5. Decrease in serum calcium and PTH.

Treatment

1. Chronic.
   a. Oral calcium.
   b. High doses of vitamin D to enhance calcium absorption.
   c. Increased calcium in the diet.

> ***NURSING PRIORITY:** Hypocalcemia may precipitate a life-threatening situation. Carefully evaluate any client with calcium imbalance and report to RN.*

2. Acute.
   a. Calcium through slow IV drip (calcium gluconate, calcium chloride).
   b. Sedatives, anticonvulsants.
   c. Parathyroid hormone IM.

Nursing Intervention

✦ *Goal: to assist client to increase serum calcium levels.*

1. Administer calcium preparations.
2. Evaluate increases in serum calcium and decreases in serum phosphate.

✦ *Goal: to prevent complications of neuromuscular irritability.*

1. Quiet environment.
2. Low lights.
3. Seizure precautions.

✦ *Goal: to help client avoid complications of respiratory distress.*

1. Bronchodilators.
2. Tracheotomy set easily available.
3. Frequent assessment of respiratory status. *Report any changes immediately to RN.*

PANCREAS

A. The pancreas is located in the upper left aspect of the abdominal cavity.

B. The pancreas produces the enzymes, trypsin, amylase, and lipase which are secreted into the duodenum and are necessary for the digestion and absorption of nutrients.

C. Located within the pancreas are the Islets of Langerhans which contain beta cells. These cells are responsible for the production of insulin. Insulin is necessary in maintaining adequate carbohydrate metabolism.

Data Collection

1. Evaluate changes in weight, particularly increase in weight in the adult, and decrease in weight in a child.
2. Evaluate alterations in fluid balance.
3. Evaluate changes in mental status.
4. Evaluate serum glucose levels.
5. Evaluate pancreatic enzyme studies.
6. Evaluate the abdomen for epigastric pain and abdominal discomfort.

DISORDERS OF THE PANCREAS

Diabetes Mellitus

❑ **A complex, multi-system disease characterized by the absence of or a severe decrease in the production of insulin.**

A. Pathophysiology.

1. The primary function of insulin is to facilitate utilization of carbohydrates, thereby controlling the blood glucose level.
2. Insulin is secreted by the beta cells in the islets of Langerhans in the pancreas.
3. The body uses carbohydrates for energy.
4. If carbohydrates are not available to be utilized for energy, the cell will begin to break down the fats and protein stores.
   a. Breakdown of the fat results in the production of ketone bodies which may cause acidosis.
   b. Protein is wasted during insulin deficiency.

5. When the circulating glucose cannot be utilized for energy, the level of the serum glucose will increase (hyperglycemia).

B. Classification.

1. Type I diabetes.
   a. Characterized by beta cell destruction which usually results in absolute insulin deficiency.
   b. Onset frequently in early childhood, most often before age 15.
   c. Previously called juvenile diabetes.
   d. Client will remain Type I diabetic for rest of his life.
   e. Client will require insulin injections for control of blood sugar.
2. Type II diabetes.
   a. Insulin deficiency caused by defects in insulin production, or by excessive demands for insulin; client may not be dependent on insulin administration for survival.
   b. Onset predominately in adults, generally over age 40, but may occur at any age.
   c. Previously called adult onset diabetes (AODM).
   d. Associated with obesity, all overweight people require more insulin.
   e. May require insulin for control.
3. Impaired fasting glucose (IFG).
   a. Intermediate stage of impaired glucose homeostasis between normal glucose levels and diabetes.
   b. Fasting glucose > 100 mg/dL but < 126 mg/dL.
4. Impaired glucose tolerance (IGT).
   a. Intermediate stage defined by oral glucose tolerance test (OGTT).
   b. OGTT of > 140mg/dL but < 200 mg/dL.
5. Gestational Diabetes.
   a. Develops during pregnancy.
   b. May not occur in future pregnancies, but client is at high risk for developing Type II diabetes as an older adult.
   c. Infant may be large for gestational age and may experience hypoglycemia shortly after birth.

Data Collection

1. Types I and II (common symptoms).
   a. Three Ps.
      (1) Polyphagia — excessive hunger.
      (2) Polydipsia — excessive thirst.
      (3) Polyuria — excessive urine.
   b. Fatigue.
   c. Increased frequency of infections.
   d. Fasting blood glucose is above 126 mg/dL on at least two occasions.
   e. Random or causal blood glucose of 200 mg/dL or greater, plus classic signs and symptoms.
   f. Oral glucose tolerance test at 2 hours is above 200mg/dL.
   g. Urine is positive for glucose and ketones.
   h. Diagnosis is based on two or more lab test, with two or more values outside the normal range. Lab values have to be consistently abnormal.

***NURSING PRIORITY:** Normal fasting glucose is **less than** 110 mg/dL or a 2 hr pp (post prandial) is **less than** 120 mg/dL.*

2. Type I.
   a. Weight loss.
   b. Excessive thirst.
   c. Bed-wetting.
   d. Onset is rapid, generally over a few weeks.
3. Type II.
   a. Weight gain (obese).
   b. Visual disturbances.
   c. Onset is slow, may occur over months.
   d. Classic signs may be overlooked as signs of aging.

Treatment

1. Medications
   a. Insulin—all clients. Primary function of insulin is to transport glucose into the muscle and fat cells. (Table 8-1).
   b. Oral hypoglycemia agents—(Appendix 8-2).
   c. Medication interactions and diabetic control—diuretics, glucocorticoids, and beta-blockers may cause hyperglycemia.
2. Exercise—needs to be planned, not sporadic.
3. Diabetic diet (See Chapter 3).
   a. Decrease calories for weight loss.
   b. Diet to meet nutritional needs and maintain optimum glucose level and weight.

NCLEX ALERT: *Metabolic effects of exercise: Reduces insulin needs; increases utilization of glucose; less extreme fluctuation of glucose levels.*

Table 8-1: PROFILE OF INSULINS

TYPE	ONSET OF ACTION	PEAK ACTION	DURATION OF ACTION	NURSING IMPLICATIONS
RAPID ACTING				
Insulin lispro (**Humalog**): SQ	< 15 min	1 hr	3-5-4.5 hr	***NURSING PRIORITY:*** *Because of quick onset of action, client must eat immediately.*
Regular insulin[R] (**Humulin R, Novolin R**) SQ, IV	1/2 to 1 hr	2 to 4 hrs	6 to 8 hrs	***NURSING PRIORITY:*** *Administer injections - 1. May mix regular insulin with other insulins. 2. Only regular insulin may be given IV.*
INTERMEDIATE ACTING				
Isophane insulin suspension [NPH] (NPH, Lente, Novolin N, Purified Pork NPH): SQ	1 to 2 hr	6 to 12 hrs	18 to 24 hrs	1. Hypoglycemia tends to occur in mid-to late-afternoon. 2. Never give IV. 3. May be mixed with regular insulin.
LONG ACTING				
Insulin zinc suspension [L] (Ultralente): SQ	1 to 3 hrs	6 to 12 hrs	18 to 24 hrs	1. Slow onset may require readjustment of carbohydrate intake. 2. Prolonged action may require more between-meal and bedtime snacks. 3. May be mixed with regular insulin.
MIXTURE				
NPH 70u and regular insulin 30 u (**Humulin 70/30, Novolin 70/30**):SQ	1/2 hr	2 to 12 hrs	24 hrs	1. Eliminates problem of mixing different types. 2. Do not give IV. 3. NPH 70/30 - regular insulin will peak in 2-4 hours, NPH in 6-12 hours, the overlap of the two types is 4-6 hours after administration. 4. Response to insulin mixtures vary with individuals.
NPH 50u and regular insulin 50u (**Humulin 50/50**):SQ	1/2 hr	3-5 hrs	24 hrs	

NCLEX ALERT: *Identify/intervene to control hypo/hyperglycemia. Know various insulins and nursing implications. Specifically, know when to anticipate reaction and what to teach the client about his insulin.*

NURSING PRIORITY: *It is important to give the diabetic client very specific written guidelines regarding exercise. The client must understand that exercise will reduce the need for insulin; dosages must be calculated according to specific need.*

Complications—Insulin Therapy

1. Hypoglycemia (Table 8-2).
2. Lipodystrophy (tissue atrophy and hypertrophy).
   a. Associated with administration of cold insulin and poor rotation of injection sites.
   b. Injection of insulin into lipodystrophic tissue may result in poor absorption of the insulin, requiring increased dosages.
   c. If injection site is changed, client may be at increased risk for developing insulin reaction because of the increased utilization. Dosage may need to be reduced.
   d. Primarily a problem with beef and pork insulin, less problem with **Humulin** insulin.

Complications—Associated with poorly controlled diabetes

1. Diabetic ketoacidosis (DKA) (Table 8-2).
   a. A severe increase in the hyperglycemia state.
   b. Occurs predominately in Type I, (IDDM).
2. Clinical manifestations of diabetic ketoacidosis (Table 8-2).
   a. Onset.
      (1) May be acute or occur over several days.
      (2) May result from stress, infection, surgery, or lack of effective insulin control.
      (3) Results from poorly controlled diabetes.
   b. Severe hyperglycemia (300 mg/dL or greater).

Table 8-2: Comparison Of Dka And Hypoglycemia

	DKA	Hypoglycemia
Age	All ages	All ages
GI	Anorexia, nausea, vomiting, diarrhea	Normal
Mental state	Dull, confusion increasing to coma	Difficulty in concentrating, coordinating; eventually coma
Temperature	Possible increase due to dehydration	Normal
Pulse	Tachycardia	Tachycardic to bradycardic as coma develops
Breathing	Initially deep and rapid; leads to Kussmaul	Normal
Breath odor	Fruity, acetone	Normal
Lab Values - Serum		
Glucose	High, 300 to 1,500 mg/dl	Below 70 mg/dl.
Ketones	High/large	Normal
pH	Acidotic (below 7.35)	Normal
Hematocrit	High due to dehydration	Normal
Lab Values - Urine		
Sugar	High	Negative
Ketones	High	Negative
Onset	Slow	Rapid
Classification of diabetes	IDDM, primarily NIDDM - in severe distress	IDDM NIDDM

c. Presence of metabolic acidosis.
d. Urine ketones and sugar are increased.
e. Excessive weakness, increased thirst.
f. Abdominal pain, nausea, vomiting.
g. Fruity (acetone) breath.
h. Kussmaul respirations.
i. Decreased level of consciousness.
j. Dry mucous membranes.
k. Increased temperature due to dehydration.
l. Hyperkalemia

3. Poorly controlled diabetes
   a. Increase in glycosylated hemoglobin levels.
   b. Excessive weight gain, or loss.
   c. Problems with peripheral circulation, visual acuity as well as other vascular complications.
   d. Frequent urinary tract infections.

Complications—Long term diabetes

1. Angiopathy - premature degenerative changes in the vascular system.
2. Peripheral vascular disease - decreased circulation to lower extremities.
3. Eye disorders - blurred vision, retinopathy, cataracts.
4. Nephropathy — involves the kidneys; will often lead to renal failure.
5. Kidney disease - pyelonephritis, diabetic nephropathy (damaged blood supply to the kidney).

NCLEX ALERT: *Identify neurological changes in client.*

6. Peripheral neuropathy - may cause general pain and tingling ; may progress to painless neuropathy.
7. Infections.

NURSING PRIORITY: *Painless peripheral neuropathy is a very dangerous situation for the diabetic. Severe injury may occur to the lower extremities and the client will not be aware of it. Clients must be taught to visually inspect their feet and legs.*

Clinical Implications of Diabetes in Pregnancy

1. During the second and third trimester, the normal response is for the insulin needs to increase.

2. Increased tendency toward the development of metabolic acidosis.
3. Tendency to intensify the existing complications of diabetes.
4. If client is Type II diabetic, medication will be changed to insulin injections for duration of pregnancy.

Nursing Intervention

(All types)

✦ *Goal: to return serum glucose to normal level.*

1. Initially administer regular insulin on a sliding scale basis according to need (Table 8-3).
   a. Rotate injection sites - abdomen area of highest absorption.
   b. Intrasite rotation - several injections within one site, but one inch apart.
   c. Sliding scale used most often when client's insulin needs are changing - surgery, infection, etc.
2. Maintain adequate fluid intake.
3. Evaluate serum electrolytes, especially serum potassium levels.
4. *Evaluate for clinical manifestations of hypoglycemia and hyperglycemia and report to RN.*
5. After client's health status begins to stabilize, insulin needs or oral hypoglycemic agents will be reevaluated.
6. 6. Begin therapeutic diet (decreased simple carbohydrates, limited caloric intake)

NURSING PRIORITY: *Evaluate intake; do not give an NPO client insulin, unless IV is in place.*

Self-Care

1. Assess current level of knowledge regarding diabetes and nutrition.
2. Administration of insulin (Table 8-3).
   a. Correct injection techniques.
   b. Rotate injection sites.
   c. Signs and symptoms of hypoglycemia.
   d. Check expiration date on the insulin.
   e. Duration and peak action of prescribed insulin.
   f. Allow for ample practice time.
   g. Administer at the same time each day; do not skip medication.
3. Oral hypoglycemia agents.
   a. Take medication as scheduled.
   b. Do not skip or add dose.
4. Exercise.

Table 8-3:
IMPLICATIONS IN THE ADMINISTRATION OF INSULIN

1. Do not administer cold insulin; it increases lipodystrophy and pain at site.
2. A 10 ml vial of unrefrigerated insulin should be discarded after 30 days, regardless of how much was used.
3. Regular, NPH, and lente insulin does not need refrigeration if kept away from heat and sunlight.
4. Insulin pens (NPH and 70/30) should be discarded after one week of storage at room temperature. Regular cartridges, which don't contain preservatives, may be left unrefrigerated for up to one month.
5. Extreme temperatures (less than 36°F or greater than 86°F) should be avoided.
6. Shaking the vial (especially NPH and lente) decreases the risk of an inconsistent concentration of insulin, because rolling the vial does not adequately mix the suspension .
7. Rotate injection sites - rotation within one anatomic site is preferred; injection sites should be one inch apart. Each site should not be reused for several days.
8. Abdomen is area for most rapid insulin absorption, followed by the arms, and then slower in the thighs and buttocks.
9. Use only insulin syringes to administer insulin.
10. Check expiration date on insulin bottle.
11. When drawing up regular insulin with a long acting insulin, draw up the regular (clear) before the longer acting (cloudy) insulin.
12. Regular insulin is used for administration by sliding scale and periods when blood sugar is unstable and difficult to control.
13. Insulin may be injected through lightweight clothing.

   a. Establish an exercise program.
   b. Avoid sporadic exercise.
5. Diet.
   a. Regularly scheduled mealtimes.
   b. Teach and reinforce understanding of food groups and balanced nutrition.
6. Infection control.
   a. Report infections promptly to health care provider.
   b. Insulin requirements may increase with severe infections.
   c. Increased problems with vaginitis and skin irritation.
7. Avoid injury.
   a. Decreased healing capabilities, especially in lower extremities.
   b. Maintain adequate blood supply to extremities - avoid tight-fitting clothing around the legs.
   c. Proper foot care (Chapter 11: PVD).
8. Understanding of "sick day" directions (Table 8-4)

Table 8-4:
"SICK DAY" GUIDELINES

1. If you do not feel well (not eating regularly, fever, lethargy, nausea and vomiting, etc.), call your health care provider.
2. Check your blood glucose every 2 hours and urine ketones when voiding.
3. Increase your intake of fluids that are high carbohydrate; every hour drink fluids that replace electrolytes - fruit drinks, sports drinks, regular soft drinks (not diet beverages).
4. If you cannot eat and you have replaced 4 to 5 meals with liquids, notify your health care provider.
5. Get plenty of rest; if possible, have someone stay with you.
6. Do not omit or skip your insulin injections or oral medications unless specifically directed to do so by your health care provider.
7. Follow your health care provider's instructions regarding blood glucose levels and insulin or oral hypoglycemics.
8. Stay warm, stay in bed and do not overexert yourself.

✦ *Goal: to identify clinical manifestations characteristic of DKA; to assist client to return to homeostasis.*

1. Frequent monitoring of vital signs.
2. Frequent urine checks for sugar and acetone.
3. Hourly urine measurements.
4. Monitor blood glucose levels frequently.
5. *Report to RN any changes in serum electrolytes (particularly potassium) or glucose.*

Hypoglycemia (Insulin Reaction)

❑ **Hypoglycemia is a condition characterized by decreased serum glucose levels, which in turn results in decreased cerebral function.**

Data Collection

1. Lability of mood.
2. Emotional changes, confusion.
3. Headache.
4. Impaired vision.
5. Tachycardia.
6. Nervousness, tremors.
7. Diaphoresis.
8. Serum glucose below 50 mg/dl.
9. Negative urine acetone.

Treatment

1. Administer carbohydrates by mouth if client is awake.
   a. Milk preferred in children with a mild reaction; it provides immediate lactose as well as protein and fat for prolonged action.

Box 8-1: Elderly Care Focus
Diabetic Care

***NURSING PRIORITY:** Symptoms of polydipsia, polyuria, and polyphagia may present as dehydration, confusion, delirium, incontinence, weight loss, and anorexia.*

- Determine mental status and manual dexterity to handle injections.
- Determine that client has visual acuity adequate to read syringe and insulin labels.
- Determine if client can access the injection sites.
- Is client alert and mentally capable of making judgements on medications?
- Determine if the client can pay for supplies.
- What is the client's attitude about needles and injections?
- Assess how many other medications is the client taking; problems with "polypharmacy" (too many medications).
- Determine family's or client's ability to accurately perform serum glucose testing.
- What is the client's support system?

   b. Administer simple sugars (orange juice, honey, candy), but if client does not eat within 1-2 hours, need to follow with complex carbohydrates like milk, cheese, crackers.

2. *If client is unconscious, report to RN immediately and prepare to give glucagon.*

Nursing Intervention

✦ *Goal: to increase serum glucose level.*

1. Administer glucose/carbohydrate preparations as indicated.

NCLEX ALERT: *Intervene to control hypo/hyperglycemia When in doubt of diagnosis of hypoglycemia versus hyperglycemia, administer carbohydrates -severe hypoglycemia can result in permanent brain damage.*

2. Thorough assessment of the diabetic client for the development of hypoglycemia.

✦ *Goal: to assist client to demonstrate an understanding of the precipitating causes of hypoglycemia and identify activities to prevent development.*

NCLEX ALERT: *Instruct client about managing his/her health condition.*

1. Instruct the diabetic client to always carry simple carbohydrates.
2. Administer between-meal snacks at the peak action of the insulin.
3. Between-meal snacks should limit simple carbohydrates and increase complex carbohydrates and protein.
4. Client should carry some type of carbohydrates when he exercises.

Pancreatitis

❑ **Pancreatitis is an inflammatory condition of the pancreas. Results in autodigestion of the pancreas by its own enzymes.**

Data Collection

1. Severe abdominal pain.
   a. Radiates to the back or the flank area.
   b. Aggravated by eating.
2. Persistent vomiting.
3. Abdominal distention, decrease in bowel sounds; bluish discoloration of flank and around umbilicus.
4. Tachycardia.
5. Impaired glucose tolerance (increased blood sugar)
6. Jaundice, fever, steatorrhea.
7. Increase in serum amylase and lipase.

Treatment

1. Medications.
   a. Analgesics - Meperidine (**Demerol**). Morphine is avoided because it is associated with pancreatic spasm.
   b. Smooth muscle relaxants.
   c. Anticolinergics
   d. Antacids.
   e. Antibiotics.
2. Decrease pancreatic stimulus.
   a. NPO, IV fluids.
   b. Bed rest.
   c. Begin with bland diet.
      (1) High carbohydrate, low fat, low protein.
      (2) Decrease in stimulants such as spices, alcohol, tea and coffee.
   d. Eliminate precipitating cause (i.e., biliary tract obstruction, medications) if possible.
   e. Pancreatic enzyme replacement.

Nursing Intervention

✦ *Goal: to relieve pain and decrease pancreatic stimulation.*

1. Administer analgesics.
2. Position on side or in semi-Fowler's.
3. Bed rest.
4. Maintain NPO initially.
5. Maintain nasogastric tube to suction.
6. Small, frequent feedings when food is allowed.
7. Diet (see treatment).

✦ *Goal: to prevent complications.*

1. Assess for hyperglycemia.
   a. Monitor serum glucose.
   b. Administer insulin as indicated.
2. Maintain adequate hydration.
3. Assess for normal bowel function.
4. Maintain cardiovascular status - evaluate for hypotension.
5. Observe for the development of fever.
6. Assess for respiratory complications and need for respiratory support.
7. *Identify electrolyte imbalances, especially hypocalcemia and dehydration, and report to RN.*

Cancer of the Pancreas

❑ **The majority of tumors occur in the head of the pancreas. Tumors in the body of the pancreas frequently do not cause symptoms until growth is advanced. Cancer of the pancreas has a poor prognosis; the five-year-survival rate is low.**

Data Collection

1. Dull, aching abdominal pain.
2. Abdominal pain is aggravated by eating.
3. Nausea, vomiting, anorexia.
4. Progressive weight loss.
5. Jaundice.
6. Fluctuations in serum glucose - hyperglycemia

Treatment

1. Surgery - Whipple's procedure: an extensive abdominal resection and removal of organs involved in the malignancy.
2. Radiation therapy.

Nursing Intervention

✦ *Goal: to maintain homeostasis (see nursing intervention for pancreatitis).*

✦ *Goal: to provide appropriate preoperative nursing measures if surgery is indicated.*

1. Maintain adequate hydration and nutrition.
2. Evaluate for bleeding problems; administer vitamin K supplement as indicated.
3. Control hyperglycemia.

✦ *Goal: to promote comfort, prevent complications, and assist to maintain homeostasis postoperative Whipple's.*

1. General postoperative care (Chapter 3).
2. Evaluate for bleeding tendencies.
3. *Monitor for fluctuation in serum glucose levels and report to RN.*
4. Maintain NPO and nasogastric suction until peristalsis returns.
5. Encourage adequate nutrition when appropriate.
   a. Decrease fats, increase carbohydrates.
   b. Small, frequent feedings.
   c. Control nausea and vomiting.
   d. Evaluate for digestion problems.

Self-Care

1. Evaluate for bouts of anxiety and depression due to severity of illness and prognosis.
2. Assist client in setting realistic goals.
3. Encourage ventilation of feelings.
4. Determine ability to maintain adequate nutrition.

ADRENAL GLANDS

A. The adrenal glands are located at the top of each kidney.

B. Adrenal medulla - secretes epinephrine and norepinephrine; under the influence of the sympathetic nervous system. Essential for maintenance of normal blood pressure.

***NURSING PRIORITY:** In clients experiencing problems of the adrenal medulla, anticipate severe fluctuations in blood pressure.*

C. Adrenal cortex - main body of the adrenal gland; responsible for the secretion of glucocorticoids, mineralocorticoids, and adrenal sex hormones; adrenalcorticoid function is essential for life.

D. Function of the adrenal cortex is controlled by the negative feedback mechanisms regulating hormone release; pituitary gland secretes ACTH, which in turn regulates hormone release of the adrenal cortex.

Data Collection

A. Adrenal medulla.
1. Evaluate changes in blood pressure.
2. Assess for changes in metabolic rate.

B. Adrenal cortex.
1. Evaluate changes in weight.
2. Evaluate changes in the skin color and texture, and in presence and distribution of body hair.
3. Assess cardiovascular system for instability as evidenced by a labile blood pressure and cardiac output.
4. Evaluate GI discomfort.
5. Assess status of potassium and sodium
6. Assess for changes in glucose metabolism.
7. Assess for changes in reproductive system and in sexual activity.
8. Evaluate changes in muscle mass.

DISORDERS OF ADRENAL GLANDS

Addison's Disease

❑ **This disorder is caused by a decrease in secretion of the adrenal cortex hormones.**

Data Collection

1. Weakness, fatigue.
2. Anorexia and weight loss
3. Emotional disturbances
4. Gastrointestinal disturbances.
5. Bronze pigmentation of the skin.
6. Postural hypotension.
7. Hypoglycemia.
8. Changes in distribution of body hair.
9. Adrenal crisis.
   a. Profound fatigue.
   b. Dehydration.
   c. Vascular collapse, severe hypotension.
   d. Renal shutdown.
   e. Severe decrease in serum sodium and increase in serum potassium.
   f. Decreased levels of circulating ACTH.

Treatment

Replace corticosteroids (ACTH).

Nursing Intervention

✦ *Goal: to assist client experiencing an adrenal crisis to return to homeostasis.*

1. Monitor IV infusion of normal saline.
2. Client will receive large doses of corticosteroids IV.
3. *Frequent evaluation of vital signs; report changes to RN.*
4. Assess daily weights and level of edema for sodium and water retention.
5. Evaluate serum potassium levels.
6. Keep client immobilized and quiet.

> ***NURSING PRIORITY:*** *If any client is experiencing difficulty with maintaining adequate blood pressure, do not move him unless absolutely necessary. Avoid all unnecessary nursing procedures until the client is stabilized.*

✦ *Goal: to maintain optimum hormone levels and be free of drug side effects (See Appendix 5-7).*

1. Administer PO steroid preparations with food or an antacid.
2. Evaluate for edema and fluid retention.
3. Assess serum sodium and potassium levels.
4. Check daily weight.
5. Increase protein and carbohydrates.
6. Evaluate for hypoglycemia.
7. Observe for Cushingoid symptoms.

Self-Care

1. Lifelong steroid therapy may be necessary.
2. Infection, diaphoresis, and injury will necessitate an increase in the need for steroids and may precipitate a crisis state.
3. Do not stop taking the medication; if the client cannot take the medication due to illness, contact the doctor.
4. Report gastric distres; it may be due to steroids.
5. Carry a medical identification card.

Cushing's Syndrome

❑ **This disorder occurs as a result of excess levels of adrenal cortex hormones.**

> ***NURSING PRIORITY:*** *The most common cause of Cushing's syndrome is the long term use of steroid therapy in treatment of chronic conditions. The symptoms of the syndrome are the same regardless of the origin of the problem.*

Data Collection

1. Marked change in personality.
2. Changes in appearance.
   a. Moon face.
   b. Deposit of fat on the back.
   c. Thin skin, purple striae.
   d. Thin extremities.
   e. Bruises and petechiae.
3. Carbohydrate intolerance
4. GI distress.
5. Mood changes.
6. Increased susceptibility to infection.
7. Sodium and fluid retention.
8. Changes in secondary sexual characteristics.
   a. Loss of menses.
   b. Facial hair on women, loss of pubic hair.
   c. Enlarged breasts in men.
9. Osteoporosis, pathologic fractures.

Treatment

Depends of the etiology of the problem.

Nursing Intervention

✦ *Goal: to provide support and assist client's return to hormone balance.*

1. Restrict sodium and water intake.
2. Monitor fluid and electrolyte levels.
3. *Evaluate for hyperglycemia and report blood sugar levels to RN*
4. Assess for GI disturbances.
5. Protect from infection.

✦ *Goal: to identify problem early and prevent complications.*

1. *Excessive sodium and water retention - monitor for edema, hypertension, CHF, and report to RN.*
2. *If potassium depletion occurs, report to RN.*
3. Evaluate client's ability to cope with change in body image.
4. Predisposed to fracture; promote weight bearing; monitor for joint and bone pain.

Self-Care

1. Stress the need for continuous health care.
2. Encourage continuation of activities.
3. Assist client to identify methods of coping with problems of therapy.

Study Questions—Endocrine

1. A client with diabetic ketoacidosis would present with what type of respiratory pattern?

① rapid and deep respirations.
② rapid and shallow respirations.
③ normal with sleep apnea.
④ Cheyne-Stokes respirations.

2. A client in the ER is diagnosed with insulin shock. The nurse would anticipate which medication to be ordered?

① NPH insulin.
② metformin (**Glucophage**).
③ regular insulin.
④ glucagon.

3. A client is placed on insulin sliding scale. What type of insulin would be used?

① Ultralente insulin.
② regular insulin.
③ NPH insulin.
④ Novolin L.

4.While gathering information on a diabetic client, the nurse smells a sweet, fruity odor. What would be important for the nurse to check?

① serum blood sugar.
② blood urea nitrogen.
③ ketosis in the urine.
④ urinary output.

5. A client has an order for a glycosylated hemoglobin to be done. What is the purpose of this test?

① to determine the glucose levels over the past 120 days.
② to evaluate the blood sugar after a 24 hour fasting.
③ to determine the level of insulin present in the body.
④ to evaluate the function of the pancreas.

6. The client is directed by the nurse to use intrasite rotation for insulin injection sites. What is the purpose of this rotation?

① to prevent convulsions from a hypoglycemic reaction.
② to maintain an equal rate of absorption of insulin.
③ to prevent anaphylactic reaction from insulin.
④ to decrease confusion in remembering injection site.

7. A diabetic client comes into the emergency room with a diagnosis of diabetic ketoacidosis. The nurse would anticipate what symptoms with this client?

① shallow respirations, bradycardia, confusion.
② pallor, diaphoresis, and tachycardia.
③ low blood pressure, diaphoresis, nausea and vomiting.
④ rapid deep respirations, tachycardia, confusion.

8. Which client would be most likely to be able to control their diabetes through diet and exercise?

① a 10 year old child.
② a 30 year old woman with onset at age 11 years.
③ a 1 year old child.
④ a 60 year old woman with onset at age 45 years.

9. When a client returns to his room post-thyroidectomy, what equipment is important for the nurse to have easily available?

① oral airway.
② tracheotomy tray and suction.
③ paper and pencil.
④ a small cassette tape recorder.

10. A client experiences a "thyroid storm" after the removal of his thyroid gland. What is the cause of this complication?

① release of calcium from parathyroid glands.
② thyroid hormones moving into the blood during thyroid surgery.
③ sudden increase of parathyroid hormone into the endocrine system.
④ calcification of the thyroid gland and related structures.

11. What would be noted on the assessment of a client with hyperthyroidism?

① dry skin, bradycardia, and hypertension.
② difficulty staying awake, increased appetite, and weight gain.
③ marked weight gain, hypertension, and tachycardia.
④ increased activity, difficulty sleeping, and weight loss.

12. The nurse is caring for a client who is 8 hours post thyroidectomy. What is important postoperative nursing care?

① have the client speak every 5-10 minutes to determine level of hoarseness.
② provide a high calcium diet to replace calcium lost during procedure.
③ evaluate behind the neck for presence of blood from incision.
④ assist client to do range of motion neck exercises to prevent contractures.

13. A client is admitted with a diagnosis of Cushing's syndrome. What is an important consideration for the nurse to make in caring for this client?

① he is going to be intolerant of heat, his pulse and blood pressure will be increased.
② due to decreased inflammatory response, he will be at increased risk for infection.
③ it is important to maintain strict intake and output due to hypovolemia.
④ due to his activity intolerance, he will be kept on bed rest and a high sodium diet.

14. What would be important to include in the diet of a hyperthyroid client?

① carbohydrates, protein, fiber.
② low calories, low carbohydrates, fiber.
③ high fats, low calories, fiber.
④ minerals, high calories, vitamins.

15. The nurse is caring for a client during the immediate postoperative period following a thyroidectomy. What is a serious complication that may occur as a result of damage to the parathyroid gland during surgery?

① tetany.
② headache.
③ heart block.
④ pitting edema.

16. The nurse is admitting a client with a diagnosis of acute pancreatitis. What is important nursing care for this client?

① assess for edema and weight gain
② initiate measures to control temperature.
③ control hypertension and tachycardia.
④ implement measures to control vomiting.

17. Clients with hyperthyroidism may experience a problem with bulging eyes. What nursing care is important in caring for this problem?

① daily assessment for development of infection.
② frequent eye drops and ointment for eyes at night.
③ eye irrigations with normal saline every 6 hours.
④ check the visual acuity every four hours.

18. The nurse is caring for a client who has Addison's disease. How will the nurse evaluate the client for complications associated with this condition?

① evaluate client for presence of fluctuating blood pressure.
② assess for development of fever and purulent drainage.
③ frequent respiratory checks for decreased movement of air.
④ strict intake and output to determine compromised renal function.

Appendix 8-1: ENDOCRINE DIAGNOSTICS

DIAGNOSTIC TEST	CLINICAL/NURSING IMPLICATIONS
THYROID:	
• Thyroxine (T_4) • Triiodothyronine (T_3 uptake) • Thyroid-stimulating hormone (TSH)	1. Increased values are associated with hyperthyroidism. 2. Decreased values are associated with hypothyroidism. 3. Heparin will cause false elevation of T_4. 4. TSH is decreased in hyperthyroidism and is elevated in hypothyroidism.
PANCREAS:	
• **Serum:** Oral glucose tolerance test	1. Test is timed to rule out diabetes by determining rate of glucose absorption from serum. 2. Insulin and oral hypoglycemics should not be administered before test. 3. Normal value: 1 hour less than 150mg, at 2 hour, less than 120mg.
• Glycosolated hemoglobin (HbA_{1c})	1. More accurate test of diabetic control, because it measures glucose attached to hemoglobin (indicates overall control for past 120 days which is the lifespan of the RBC). 2. Nondiabetic usually 2-8%. 2-6% considered good diabetic control. >8% is considered poor diabetic control.
• Fasting blood sugar (FBS)	1. Maintain client in fasting state 12 hours until blood drawn. 2. If client is a known diabetic and experiences dizziness, weakness and fainting, and draw the blood sugar at that time. 3. Normal value < 110mg or 70 -100 mg/dl.
• Postprandial blood sugar (2 hr p.p.)	1. Involves measuring the serum glucose two hours after a meal. 2. Normal is less than 120m; level is significantly increased in diabetic.
• **Urine:** Sugar (Clinistix, Clinitest, Labstix)	1. Use fresh double-voided specimen. 2. A rough indicator of serum glucose levels. 3. Results may be altered by various medications.
• Serum amylase and lipase	1. Used to evaluate pancreatic cell damage. 2. Elevated in pancreatitis and pancreatic cancer.

Appendix 8-2:
MEDICATIONS USED IN ENDOCRINE DISORDERS

MEDICATIONS	SIDE EFFECTS	NURSING IMPLICATIONS
ANTITHYROID: Inhibits production of thyroid hormone; does not inactivate thyroid in circulating blood.		
Propylthiouracil (**PTU**):*PO* Methimazole (**Tapazole**): *PO*	Agranulocytosis; abdominal discomfort; nausea, vomiting, diarrhea, crosses placenta (Same; crosses placenta more rapidly)	1. May increase anticoagulation effect of heparin and oral anticoagulants. 2. May be combined with iodine preparations. 3. Monitor CBC. 4. Store **Tapazole** in light-sensitive container. 5. May be used prior to surgery or treatment with radioactive iodine.
Lugol's solution: *PO* Saturated solution of potassium iodide (**SSKI**): *PO*	Inhibits synthesis and release of thyroid hormone	1. Administer in fluid to decrease unpleasant taste. 2. May be used to decrease vascularity of thyroid gland prior to surgery.
RADIOACTIVE IODINE: Accumulates in the thyroid gland; causes partial or total destruction of thyroid gland through radiation.		
Iodide, I^{131}	Discomfort in thyroid area; bone marrow depression; permanent hypothyroidism.	1. Check that antithyroid drugs are discontinued 2 to 4 days prior to administering I^{131}. 2. Radiation precautions on body secretions—3 days. 3. Client should avoid contact with women who are pregnant and small children. 4. Increase fluids immediately after treatment, as radioactive isotope is excreted in the urine.(See Chp 2 for radiation safety).
THYROID REPLACEMENTS: Replacement of thyroid hormone.		
Levothyroxine sodium (**Levothyroid, Levoxyl, Synthroid**): *PO, IM, IV* Liothyronine (**Cytomel**)	Overdose may result in symptoms of hyperthyroidism: tachycardia, heat intolerance, nervousness	1. Be careful in reading exact name on label of medications; micrograms and milligrams are used as units of measure. 2. Generally taken once a day before breakfast. 3. Within 3-4 days begin to see improvement, maximum effect in 4-6 weeks.
PANCREATIC ENZYMES: Replacement enzyme to aid in digestion of starch, protein and fat.		
Pancreatin: *PO* Pancrelipase (**Pancrease, Cotazym, Vioplase**), *PO*	GI upset and irritation of the mucous membranes.	1. Client is usually on a high-protein, high-carbohydrate, low-fat diet. 2. Enteric-coated tablets should not be crushed or chewed. 3. Pancreatin may be given before, during, or within one hour after meals. 4. Pancrelipase is given just before or with each meal or snack.
ANTIHYPOGLYCEMIC: Increases plasma glucose levels and relaxes smooth muscles.		
Glucagon: *IM, IV, SQ*	None significant.	1. Watch for symptoms of hypoglycemia and treat with food *first, if conscious.* *2. Client usually awakens in 5-20 min. after receiving glucagon.* *3. If client does not respond, anticipate IV glucose to be given.*

Appendix 8-2:
MEDICATIONS USED IN ENDOCRINE DISORDERS

MEDICATIONS	SIDE EFFECTS	NURSING IMPLICATIONS
ORAL HYPOGLYCEMIA AGENTS (See Table 8-1 for Insulin)		
❖ GENERAL NURSING IMPLICATIONS ❖ — Dose should be decreased for elderly. — Use with caution in clients with renal and hepatic impairment. — All oral hypoglycemics are contraindicated in pregnant clients. — All clients should be carefully observed for symptoms of hypo- and hyperglycemia. — Medications should be taken in the morning.		
SULFONYLUREAS: stimulate the pancreas to make more insulin		
Glipizide (**Glucotrol**): PO Glyburide (**Micronase, Diabeta**): PO Glimepriride (**Amaryl**): PO Tolbutamide (**Orinase**): PO Tolazamide (**Tolinase**): PO	Hypoglycemia, , jaundice, GI disturbance, skin reactions	1. Tolbutamide has shortest duration of action, requires multiple daily doses. 2. Glyburide has a long duration of action. 3. Interacts with: calcium channel blockers, oral contraceptives, glucocorticoids, phenothiazines, thiazide diuretics.
BIGUANIDES: decrease sugar production in the liver and help the muscles use insulin to breakdown sugar		
Metformin (**Glucophage**): PO	Dizziness, nausea, back pain, possible metallic taste	1. Metformin is administered with meals. 2. Metformin has a beneficial effect on lowering lipids. 3. Weight gain may occur.
ALPHA-GLUCOSIDASE INHIBITORS: slow down how the body absorbs sugar after eating		
Acarbose (**Precose**): PO Miglitol (**Glyset**): PO	Flatulence, diarrhea, abdominal pain	1. Take acarbose with meals; not effective on an empty stomach. 2. Acarbose is contraindicated in clients with inflammatory bowel disease.
MEGLITINIDES: lowers glucose levels by stimulating release of insulin.		
Repaglinide (**Prandin**): PO	Hypoglycemia	1. Client should eat within 30 minutes of taking medication. 2. Peaks in 1 hour.

Notes

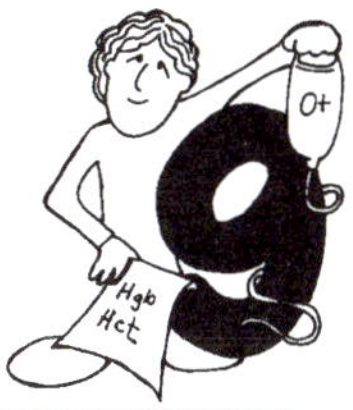

Hematologic System

PHYSIOLOGY OF THE BLOOD

A. Functions of the blood.
  1. Transports oxygen from the lungs to the tissues and carbon dioxide from the tissues to the lungs.
  2. Transports nutrients from intestine to body cells.
  3. Transports waste products to kidney for excretion.

B. Components .
  1. Plasma - 90 percent water; accounts for about half of the total blood volume.
  2. Formed elements (cells); account for about half of the volume.
    a. Erythrocytes (red cells).
    b. Leukocytes (white cells).
    c. Thrombocytes (platelets).

C. Characteristics of plasma.
  1. Plasma is clear, straw colored, and does not contain cellular elements.
  2. Globulins - primary function is prevention of infection.
  3. Fibrinogen - necessary element in normal clot formation; produced in the liver.
  4. Prothrombin -necessary element for normal coagulation.
    a. Produced in the liver.
    b. Normal production is dependent on availability of adequate vitamin K.

D. Characteristics of erythrocytes (red blood cells).
  1. Formed in the red bone marrow; erythropoiesis is the production of red blood cells.
  2. Vitamin B_{12} and folic acid are necessary for the production of normal erythrocytes.
  3. Hemoglobin is the primary component of the red cell.
  4. Primary function is transportation of oxygen and carbon dioxide.
  5. The fraction of the blood occupied by the erythrocytes is called the hematocrit.

E. Characteristics of the leukocytes (white blood cells).
  1. Function is to protect the body against invading microorganisms.
  2. Leukocytosis refers to an overall increase in the leukocytes; leukopenia refers to an overall decrease in the leukocytes.

F. Characteristics of thrombocytes (platelets).
  1. Function - primarily involved with hemostasis. When vessel wall is damaged platelets adhere to the area and eventually form a platelet plug to decrease bleeding.
  2. Thrombocytosis refers to a marked abnormal increase in thrombocytes; thrombocytopenia refers to a marked abnormal decrease in thrombocytes.

G. Blood classification.
  1. Major blood groups - A, B, AB, and O.
  2. Rh factor.
    a. Rh factor is present on the red cell.

Box 9-1: Elderly Care Focus
Age Related Findings for the Hematologic System

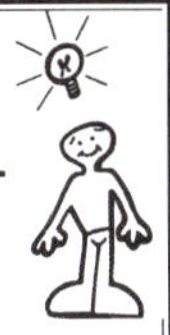

Assessment Area	*Hematologic System Findings*	*Elderly Changes & Significance*
Nail beds (check for capillary refill)	Pallor, cyanosis, and decreased capillary refill is often noted in hematologic disorders.	Nails are typically thickened and discolored. Need to use another body area, such as the lips to assess capillary refill.
Hair distribution	Thin or absent hair on trunk and extremities may indicate poor oxygenation and blood supply to area.	Older adults are losing body hair, but often in an even pattern distribution that has occurred slowly over time.
Skin moisture and color	Skin dryness, pallor, and jaundice may occur with anemia, leukemia, etc.	Dry skin is a normal aspect of aging and thus becomes a unreliable indicator of skin moisture. Pigment loss and skin changes along with some yellowing occurs with aging. Pallor may be noted in older adults that is not associated with anemia, as they tend not to go outdoors as often as younger adults and get exposed to sunlight.

b. Rh is positive or factor is present in 85 percent to 95 percent of the population.

System Data Collection

A. Evaluate history.

1. History of disease of bone marrow or organs affecting production of blood.
2. History of treatment which depressed bone marrow activity (especially chemotherapy or radiation therapy).
3. Family history of problems (inheritance pattern).

B. Bleeding problems occurring during pregnancy, labor and delivery, or immediately after birth in both mother and infant.

C. Presence of disorders, aging, or disease processes other than the hematologic disorders (Box text 9-1).

D. Evaluate effect hematologic disorder has on client's life style and daily living (ADL).

1. How long has client experienced symptoms?
2. What are current activities and metabolic requirements of the client?
3. Presence or absence of bleeding episodes.
4. Ability to control pain.

E. Assess client's current nutritional status.

F. Evaluate current blood values.

G. Evaluate status of respiratory and cardiovascular systems in maintaining homeostasis.

DISORDERS OF THE HEMATOLOGIC SYSTEM

Anemias

❑ ***Anemia* is characterized by a low red cell count and ↓ hemoglobin and hematocrit.**

NCLEX ALERT: *Modify client's care based on the results of laboratory test.*

A. **Iron-deficiency anemia** - characterized by poor dietary habits and poor iron intake.

1. Common in older infants (whose primary diet is milk), teenage girls and pregnant women.
2. Decreased hemoglobin and hematocrit.
3. Lethargy to severe fatigue.
4. Headache.
5. Pale mucous membranes.
6. Treatment:
   a. Iron replacement in the diet.
   b. Increased intake of folic acid.

B. **Pernicious anemia** - condition characterized by lack of intrinsic factors secreted by gastric cells; intrinsic factors are necessary for the utilization of vitamin B_{12} (cyanocobalamin).

1. More common in elderly.
2. Smooth, sore, red tongue.
3. Weak, listless, pale.
4. Confusion.
5. Paresthesia in the extremities.
6. Loss of sense of balance.
7. Treatment: lifelong injections of vitamin B_{12}

C. Aplastic anemia - characterized by depression of the bone marrow in production of red cells.

1. Medications may precipitate aplastic anemia - chemotherapeutic agents and antibiotics.
2. Radioactive therapy may lead to aplastic anemia.
3. Weakness, pallor.
4. Dyspnea.
5. Fever.
6. Infections.
7. Thrombocytopenia leading to bleeding problems.
8. Treatment: bone marrow transplant.

Nursing Intervention

For clients with anemia.

✦ *Goal: to assist in establishing a diagnosis.*

1. Complete nutritional evaluation.
2. History of possible causes.

✦ *Goal: to decrease body oxygen needs.*

1. Assess client's tolerance to activity.
2. Provide diversional activities, but provide for adequate rest.
3. May need supplemental oxygen.

✦ *Goal: to prevent infections.*

1. Decrease exposure.
2. Prompt evaluation of temperature elevations.
3. Observe for leukocytosis.
4. Maintain adequate hydration.

✦ *Goal: to assess for complications of chronic anemic state.*

1. Evaluate ability of cardiovascular system to maintain adequate cardiac output.
2. B/P
3. Pulse

4. Urine output
5. Alert and oriented, no excessive lethargy
6. Evaluate for symptoms of hypoxia (Chapter 10).

✦ *Goal: to assist client to understand implications of disease and measures to maintain health.*

1. Medical treatment.
2. Importance of continuing medical follow-up.
3. Side effects of medications.
4. Identify foods high in iron and folic acid.

Sickle Cell Anemia

❑ **Sickle Cell Anemia is a problem which is characterized by a sickling effect of the erythrocytes.**

A. Predominantly a problem of children - condition is hereditary. Child may be asymptomatic between crises.

B. Sickling problem is not apparent until infant is four to six months old. The increased levels of fetal hemoglobin up to that age prevent serious sickling problems.

C. Conditions precipitating sickling effect.
  1. Dehydration.
  2. Decreased oxygen and acidosis.

D. Pathologic changes of sickle cell disease result from:
  1. Increased blood viscosity.
  2. Increased red cell destruction.
  3. Increased viscosity eventually causes ischemia and tissue necrosis due to capillary stasis and thrombosis.

Data Collection

1. Weakness, anorexia, vomiting.
2. Enlarged spleen and liver.
3. Hematuria.
4. Decreased ability to concentrate urine.
5. Vaso-occlusive crisis - hand-foot syndrome involving infarctions of the short tubular bones in the hand and feet; precipitates severe pain and swelling of the hands and feet.
6. CNS - stasis, thrombosis, and ischemia precipitating a CVA.
7. Blood - increased hemolysis of red cells; chronic anemia.

Treatment

1. Prevention of the sickling problem.
   a. Adequate hydration.
   b. Adequate oxygenation.
   c. No specific medication; clients generally do not require iron.
   d. Daily folic acid supplement when red blood cells are low.
2. Treatment of sickle cell crises.
   a. Bed rest.
   b. Hydration.
   c. Analgesic for pain.
   d. Antibiotics.
   e. Adequate oxygenation.
   f. Transfusions (Appendix 9-3).
3. Surgery - splenectomy.

Nursing Intervention

✦ *Goal: to prevent Sickle Cell Disease.*

1. Participate in community screening and education programs.
2. Refer parents who are trait carriers to genetic counseling.

✦ *Goal: to prevent sickling crisis.*

1. Maintain adequate hydration.
2. Promote tissue oxygenation.
3. Prevent infection.

✦ *Goal: to control pain.*

1. Assessment of involved area.
2. Appropriate analgesics.
3. Position for comfort.
4. Apply warmth to area involved.
5. Maintain bed rest.

***NURSING PRIORITY:** Care of the child with sickle cell disease frequently centers around hydration and pain control. Review pain control in Chapter 3, hydration in Chapter 5.*

✦ *Goal: to maintain adequate hydration and oxygenation.*

1. Evaluate for adequate hydration.
2. Encourage fluid intake.
3. Monitor IV fluid carefully.
4. Evaluate electrolyte balance.
5. Administer O_2 as indicated.
6. Good pulmonary hygiene.

Self-Care

1. Encourage fluid intake to maintain adequate hydration.
2. Report temperature elevations, vomiting, diarrhea, pain.

3. Encourage normal growth and developmental activities as tolerated by the child.
4. Client with sickle cell disease should avoid situations which may precipitate hypoxia.
   a. Traveling to high-altitude areas.
   b. Flying in an unpressurized aircraft.
   c. Participating in strenuous exercise or contact sports.
5. Assist parents to understand implications of the disease and measures to maintain health.

Leukemias

❑ **Leukemia is an uncontrolled proliferation of abnormal white cells.**

A. Three primary consequences of leukemia.
   1. Anemia from red cell destruction and bleeding.
   2. Infection from decreased production of healthy white cells (neutropenia).
   3. Bleeding tendencies due to decreased platelets.

B. Types of leukemia.
   1. Acute lymphocytic leukemia (ALL, blast or stem cell).
      a. Primarily in children with peak occurrence around four years of age.
      b. Favorable prognosis with chemotherapy.
      c. Leukemic cells will infiltrate the meninges precipitating increased intracranial pressure.
      d. Onset may be acute to chronic.
   2. Acute myelogenous leukemia (AML).
      a. Affects all age groups; incidence increases with age.
      b. Onset is generally slow.
      c. Prognosis is poor, even with chemotherapy.
   3. Chronic.
      a. Chronic myelogenous (CML).
      b. Chronic lymphocytic (CLL).

Data Collection

1. Anemia, infection and bleeding tendencies occurring together.
2. Anorexia, weight loss.
3. Fatigue, lethargy.
4. Increased CNS irritability, headache, confusion.
5. Petechiae, bruises easily.
6. Complaints of bone and joint pain.
7. Bone marrow aspiration to evaluate cell production.
8. Enlarged liver and spleen.

Table 9-1: BLEEDING PRECAUTIONS

Use: Clients with leukemia or hemophilia, receiving anticoagulants or thrombolytic medications.

✦ Limit number of venipunctures and IM injections. Guaiac stools as necessary.

✦ Oral hygiene -
—discourage flossing
—soft toothbrush or no toothbrush, may need to use Q-tips while gums are friable.
—avoid harsh mouthwashes
—frequent mouth rinse with mild mouthwash.

✦ Electric razor for shaving.

✦ Assess perianal area for fissures and bleeding.

✦ Discourage client from blowing his nose.

✦ Avoid aspirin products, evaluate NSAIDs for bleeding properties.

✦ Avoid catheters when possible - urinary and suctioning.

✦ Avoid overinflation of blood pressure cuff or leaving cuff inflated for prolonged period of time.

✦ Provide safe environment and prevent injury according to age (pad siderails, soft toys, houseshoes, etc).

✦ Monitor for bleeding episode - nosebleed, hematuria, increased bruising

NCLEX ALERT: *Implement interventions to manage potential client circulatory complications (hemorrhage, embolus, shock, etc.).*

Treatment

1. Medications.
   a. Corticosteroids.
   b. Chemotherapy.
2. Bone marrow transplant.
3. Red cell, platelet transfusions.

Nursing Intervention

✦ *Goal: to prevent infection.*

NCLEX ALERT: *Identify signs and symptoms of an infection.*

1. Assess for evidence of systemic infection - fever, inflammation, pain.
2. Monitor temperature elevation closely, contact doctor for temperature of 100°F orally or above.
3. Meticulous skin care, especially oral hygiene and around perianal area.
4. Protect client from exposure to infection; degree of restriction depends on immunosuppression.

5. Isolate child from communicable childhood diseases, especially chicken pox.
6. Live virus vaccinations are not administered to a client who is receiving immunosuppressive therapy or who is already immunosuppressed.
7. Live virus vaccinations may be done during a remission.
8. Avoid urinary catheterizations

NURSING PRIORITY: *A remission is characterized by absence of leukemia cells and disorders, and disappearance of all disease symptoms.*

9. Maintain adequate hydration.
10. Decrease bacteria in foods - thoroughly wash fresh fruits and vegetables or cook them.
11. Women should avoid use of tampons.
12. Discourage cleaning cat litter boxes or bird cages.
13. Discourage live plants and flowers in the home.

✦ *Goal: to prevent or limit bleeding episodes.*

1. Use local direct pressure measures to control bleeding.
2. Restrict strenuous activity.
3. Involve client in evaluating level of activity; decrease activity when platelet counts are low.

✦ *Goal: to provide pain relief.*

1. Use acetaminophen rather than aspirin.
2. Maintain environment conducive to rest.
3. Position carefully; may coordinate with analgesics.
4. Evaluate effectiveness of pain relief; administer analgesic prior to pain becoming severe.

✦ *Goal: to decrease effects of chemotherapy(Table 2-4).*

NCLEX ALERT: *Observe for effects of medications.*

✦ *Goal: to prevent complications of transfusions (Appendix 9-3).*

NCLEX ALERT: *Instruct client about managing his/her condition.*

Hemophilia

❑ **Hemophilia is a defect in the clotting mechanism. The disease is usually diagnosed during the toddler stage when the child begins to walk.**

Data Collection

1. Large, spreading bruises.
2. Bleeding into joints (hemarthrosis).
3. Recurring joint bleeding leads to severe restriction of joint mobility.
4. Intracranial hemorrhage may be fatal.
5. Hemorrhage into the gastrointestinal tract may precipitate obstruction.
6. Sex-linked family inheritance pattern.
7. Platelet and prothrombin counts are frequently within normal limits.

Treatment

1. Fresh frozen plasma.
2. IV administration of deficient factor.
   a. Cryoprecipitate.
   b. Concentrated AHF.
3. Treatment may be carried out at home.

Nursing Intervention

✦ *Goal: to prevent spontaneous bleeding episodes Table 9-1).*

1. Decrease risk of injury.
   a. Make environment as safe as possible without hampering motor development.
   b. Avoid contact sports.
2. Good dental care, since mucous membranes bleed easily.
3. Maintain normal weight; increased weight causes increased strain on the joints.
4. Avoid any aspirin compounds; NSAIDs should be evaluated regarding bleeding tendencies.
5. Administer clotting factors prior to invasive medical procedures.

NCLEX ALERT: *Implement interventions to manage potential client circulatory complications (hemorrhage, embolus, shock, etc.).*

✦ *Goal: to recognize and treat bleeding episodes.*

1. Apply pressure to the area.
2. Immobilize and elevate the joints involved.
3. Apply cold pack to promote vasoconstriction.

✦ *Goal: to prevent permanent joint degeneration.*

1. Elevate joint and immobilize during acute bleeding.
2. Initiate passive range of motion after acute phase.
3. Physical therapy after the acute phase.
4. Maintain pain relief during physical therapy.

Study Questions—Hematologic

1. What is the most common cause of death in a client with leukemia?

① hemorrhage.
② congestive failure.
③ heart block.
④ infection.

2. What is the primary treatment for a client with pernicious anemia?

① vitamin B12.
② anticoagulants.
③ vitamin A.
④ ferrous sulfate.

3. What is the purpose of administering Vitamin K to a newborn?

① to supplement the poor intake of the vitamin.
② to enhance the function of the gastrointestinal cells.
③ to increase resistence to infection.
④ to prevent bleeding episodes.

4. A client has received chemotherapy for cancer of the lung. What type of anemia is associated with this treatment?

① sickle cell anemia.
② iron deficiency anemia.
③ pernicious anemia.
④ aplastic anemia.

5. Which disease is characterized by abnormally shaped red blood cells that clog the small capillaries?

① sickle cell anemia.
② Hodgkin's disease.
③ hemophilia.
④ hemolytic anemia.

6. What problem frequently contributes to bleeding/coagulation problems?

① aplastic anemia.
② hemoglobin abnormalities.
③ low platelet counts.
④ decreased red blood cells.

7. What are the characteristics of a client who has hemophilia?

① muscle pain and vomiting.
② joint pain and bleeding.
③ nausea and fever.
④ petechia and tachycardia.

8. What medication might be used to stimulate bone marrow to produce red blood cells in the renal client?

① heparin therapy.
② dexamethasone (Decadron).
③ epoetin alfa (Epogen).
④ vitamin B12.

9. The nurse is caring for a client with a hemoglobin of 8.2 gm/dl. What are important nursing measures?

① increase fluids and ambulate at tid.
② assess for tachycardia, keep warm.
③ monitor for bleeding tendencies.
④ assess for bradycardia and fever.

10. A child is recovering from a sickle cell crisis. What is important to promote the health in order of this child after discharge?

① maintain good hydration status.
② avoid active virus vaccinations.
③ avoid contact with peers.
④ increase intake in high caloric foods.

11. What are considered the primary signs and symptoms of iron deficiency anemia?

① hyperactivity with periods of depression.
② increased urinary output and restlessness.
③ fatigue and pallor.
④ decreased respirations and pulse.

12. A child has a severe laceration on his finger and it is bleeding profusely. What is the best nursing action?

① put an ice bag on the finger.
② apply pressure at the site.
③ apply pressure at the brachial artery.
④ prepare injection of Vitamin K.

13. A client has been placed on bleeding precautions. What is important to include in the nursing care?

① draw blood studies tid to determine clotting factors.

② encourage house shoes and soft toothbrush.

③ encourage increased intake of iron rich foods.

④ catheterize the client to determine renal bleeding.

14. What laboratory test is used to measure the amount of red blood cells, white blood cells, and platelets?

① Prothrombin time (PT).

② Partial thromboplastin time (PTT).

③ White blood count (WBC).

④ Complete blood count (CBC).

Appendix 9-1: HEMATOLOGIC DIAGNOSTICS

TEST	NORMAL	CLINICAL AND NURSING IMPLICATIONS
Bone Marrow Aspiration or Biopsy	All formed cell elements within normal range (erythrocytes, leukocytes, and platelets).	1. Report indicates presence, absence, or ratio of cells characteristic of a suspected disease. 2. Preferred site is posterior iliac crest. 3. Appropriate client preparation: - local anesthetic used. - feeling of pressure when bone marrow is entered; pain occurs as marrow is being withdrawn. 4. Post test: - observe for bleeding at site. - apply pressure to site. - bed rest for approximately 30 minutes afterward. - analgesics as indicated.
Sickle Cell Test (Sickledex))	No hemoglobin S present.	1. Routine screening test for sickle cell trait or disorder; does not distinguish between them. 2. False negative in infants under 3 months. 3. False positive can occur for up to four months after a transfusion of red cells that are positive for the trait.
COMPLETE BLOOD COUNT:		
Platelets	150,000 - 400,000mm^3	1. Decreased platelets (thrombocytopenia) associated with bleeding.
Red blood cell count (RBC)	4.0 - 6.0mm^3	1. Decreased in clients with bone marrow depression and anemias.
Hemoglobin	Female: 15 - 16 gm/100dL Male: 14 - 18 gm/100dL Newborn: 14 - 20 gm/100cc	1. Components of the red cell responsible for oxygen transport. 2. Decreased in anemias, chronic and acute blood loss, and bone marrow depression.
Hematocrit	Female: 37% - 47% Male: 40% -54% Newborn: 52% - 62%	1. Values reflect the volume of red cells found in 100cc of whole blood. 2. Low levels in anemias, bone marrow depression. 3. An effective indicator of hydration status. An increase in hematocrit may be indicative of a decrease in fluid volume resulting in hemoconcentration.
White blood cell count (WBC)	Adults: 5,000 to 10,000mm^3 Child: (2 years) 6,000 to 17,000mm^3	1. White blood cells are an important component in the body's defense against infection. 2. Elevated levels (leukocytosis) is associated with infection. 3. Decreased levels (leukopenia) is associated with diseases of the blood and bone marrow depression.

Appendix 9-2:
HEMATOLOGIC MEDICATIONS

MEDICATIONS	SIDE EFFECTS	NURSING IMPLICATIONS
IRON PREPARATIONS: Replacement		
Ferrous fumarate (**Feostat, Femiron**): IM, PO Ferrous gluconate **(Fergon, Ferralet)** Ferrous sulfate **(Feosol, Fer-in-sol)** Iron dextran injection **(InFed, DexFerrum)** : IV, IM	GI irritation Nausea Constipation Toxic reactions: Fever Urticaria	1. Absorbed better on empty stomach; however, may cause GI upset. 2. Liquid preparations should be diluted and given through a straw to prevent staining of the teeth. 3. Tell client stool may be black. 4. If given IM, use Z- tract method to prevent tissue staining and trauma. 5. Eggs, milk, cheese and antacids inhibit oral iron absorption. 1. Parenteral iron used only if oral iron is not effective. 2. Parenteral iron preparations have higher incidence of anaphylactic reaction.
VITAMIN K: Necessary for normal prothrombin activity		
Vitamin K (**Aquamephyton**): PO, SQ, IM, IV	GI upset, rash Hypersensitivity reaction if given IV; rash, urticaria	1. Pain, hematoma formation at injection site. 2. Protect medication from light. 3. Antidote for **Coumadin**. 4. Administered at birth to prevent hemorrhagic disease of the newborn.
GLYCOPROTEIN HORMONE: Stimulates production of red blood cells.		
Epoetin alfa (erythropoietin) **(Epogen)**:IV, SQ	Allergy to albumin Hypertension	1. Use: treat anemia secondary to renal failure and anemia associated with chemotherapy 2. Monitor hematocrit and hemoglobin levels every two weeks when desired level is reached, maintenance dose begun. 3. Monitor BP, since renal clients have problems with hypertension.

Appendix 9-3:
GUIDELINES FOR MONITORING BLOOD TRANSFUSIONS

GENERAL NURSING IMPLICATIONS:

NCLEX ALERT: *Monitor administration of blood or blood products.*

1. The practical nurse should be familiar with the Nurse Practice Act of the individual state and hospital policies regarding the administration of blood and blood products.

2. When blood is brought to the patient care unit from the blood bank, it should be started immediately. Blood should never be stored in a unit refrigerator or allowed to sit at room temperature.

3. Never add any medication to blood products or to the infusion line of a blood product.

4. The usual rate of infusion in an adult is 1 unit of blood over 3 to 4 hours, depending on the condition of the client. The RN should set the initial rate.

5. Determine if client has a history of allergy, specifically a previous reaction to transfused blood.

6. Baseline vital signs must be obtained immediately prior to handling the blood. *Notify the RN if the client's temperature is above 101°*F or increases more than 2°F, if any other vital signs have changed significantly from previous readings. Check vital signs q1h during and 1 hour after transfusion.

7. The client is most likely to experience a reaction during the first 50 cc of blood infused. Monitor for reaction.

8. Blood deteriorates rapidly after 2 hours of exposure to room temperature. Blood should not hang longer than 4 hours.

TRANSFUSION REACTIONS:

Hemolytic Transfusion Reaction:

1. Fever, chills, temperature elevation of 2°.
2. Headache.
3. Low back pain.
4. Flushing
5. Tachycardia.
6. Hypotension.
7. Dyspnea.
8. Immediate onset.

Allergic Reaction:

1. Urticaria (hives).
2. Pruritus.
3. Facial flushing.
4. Wheezing.
5. No fever.

Nursing Implications:

1. Stop transfusion immediately and *notify the RN.*
2. Change the IV tubing; do not allow blood in the tubing to infuse into the client.
3. Maintain vein open with normal saline.
4. Monitor vital signs.
5. Obtain first voided urine specimen to test for blood in the urine.
6. Anticipate blood samples to be drawn by the lab.
7. If client has a history of allergic reaction, antihistamines may be given prior to starting the infusion.

Respiratory System

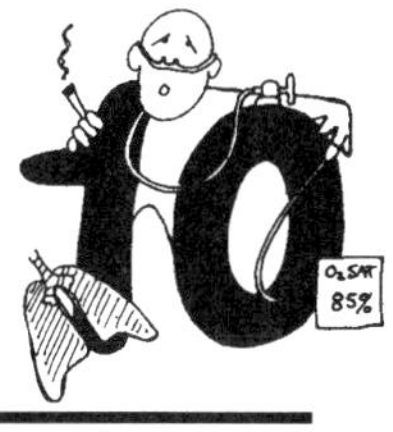

❑ The respiratory unit focuses on pathophysiologic conditions which interfere with gas exchange. The conditions or diseases are grouped according to similarities of the condition, as well as similarities of nursing care. When problems of gas exchange occur, regardless of the precipitating cause, a hypoxic state is frequently the result. A thorough understanding of hypoxia and appropriate nursing interventions for the hypoxic client are necessary for an understanding of the disease processes and ensuing nursing interventions.

PHYSIOLOGY OF THE RESPIRATORY SYSTEM

Organs of the Respiratory System

A. Larynx.
   1. Lies in the middle of the neck.
   2. Controls airflow and prevents foreign objects from entering the airway.
   3. Vocal cords are located in the lower aspect of the larynx.
   4. Glottis - the opening of the vocal cords and the narrowest portion of the laryngeal cavity.
   5. Epiglottis - the area immediately above the glottis.

B. Trachea.
   1. Extends from the larynx downward into the thoracic cavity.
   2. Contains cartilage rings to maintain patency of the airway to the lungs.

C. Bronchial tree (Figure 10-1).
   1. Trachea divides into the right and left mainstem bronchi; which extend into the lung.
   2. The right mainstem bronchus is shorter and wider than the left; therefore, foreign objects are more likely to enter the right side.
   3. Terminal bronchioles - branches from the secondary bronchi.

D. Lungs (organs of respiration).
   1. Lungs are located within the thoracic cavity.
   2. Mediastinum is the area between the lungs; it contains: heart, thoracic aorta, vena cava, pulmonary artery and veins, trachea, esophagus.
   3. Pleura - the transparent serous membrane around the lungs.
      a. Each lung is sealed within its own compartment by the pleura.
      b. Visceral pleura - adheres to the surface of the lung.
      c. Parietal pleura - covers the inner wall of the chest.
      d. Pleural cavity - potential space between the pleura membrane; normally, pleura layers are in close contact.
   4. Lungs.
      a. Divided into lobes.
         (1) Right lung - three lobes.
         (2) Left lung - two lobes.
      b. Each terminal bronchus branches into respiratory bronchiole.
      c. The alveolar ducts are located at the end of the terminal respiratory bronchioles.
      d. Alveoli - area of gas exchange; diffusion of O_2 and CO_2 between the blood and the lungs occurs across the alveolar membrane.
      e. Surfactant is produced in the alveoli; primary function is to facilitate alveolar expansion and to prevent collapse.
   5. Premature infants frequently have inadequate production of surfactant.
   6. Blood supply to the lungs.
      a. Pulmonary arteries to pulmonary capillaries to alveoli, where exchange of gas occurs.
      b. Bronchial arteries supply the nutrients to the lung tissue and do not participate in gas exchange.

Physiology of Respiration

External respiration is a process by which gas is exchanged between the circulating blood and the inhaled air.

A. Atmospheric pressure - that pressure exerted on all body parts by surrounding air.

B. Intrapulmonic pressure - the pressure within the bronchial tree and alveoli.

C. Gases flow from an area of high pressure to an area of low pressure; pressure below atmospheric pressure is designated as negative pressure.

D. Inspiration.
   1. Stimulus to the diaphragm and the intercostal muscles by way of the CNS.

2. Through the airways the lungs are open to atmospheric pressure. Air will flow into the lungs to equalize that of atmospheric pressure.

E. Expiration.

1. Diaphragm and intercostal muscles relax and return to a resting position, therefore lungs recoil and capacity is decreased.
2. Air will flow out until intrapulmonic pressure is again equal to atmospheric pressure.

F. Compliance describes how elastic or how easily the lungs can be inflated. When compliance is decreased, the lungs are more difficult to inflate.

G. Control of respiration.

1. Movement of the diaphragm and accessory muscles of respiration are controlled by the respiratory center located in the brain stem (medulla and pons). The respiratory center will control respirations by way of the spinal cord. The diaphragm and intercostal muscles are innervated by the nerves which come from the spinal cord.
2. The medulla contains chemoreceptors responsive to changes in CO_2 blood levels.
3. Carotid and aortic bodies are responsive to changes in the arterial O_2 levels.

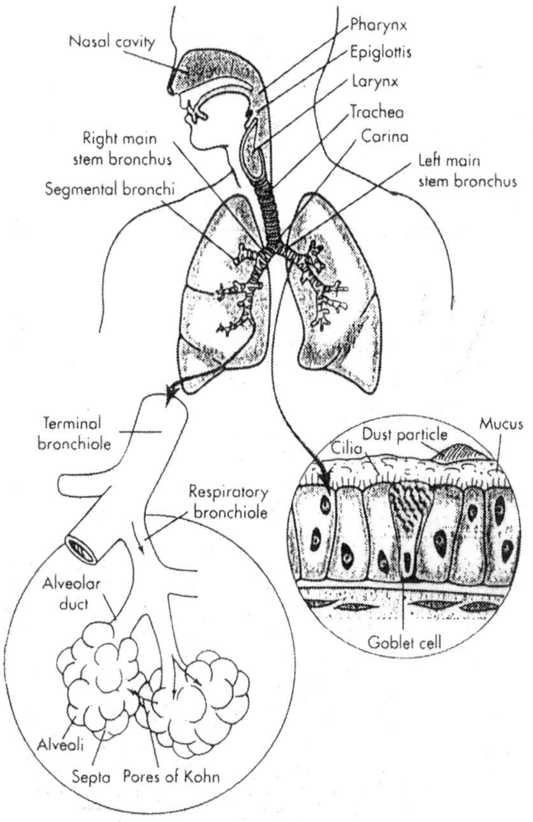

Figure 10-1: Respiratory System
Reprinted with permission: Phipps, WJ, Sands, JK, & Marek, JF (1999). *Medical Surgical Nursing: Concepts & Clinical Practice*, 6th ed. Philadelphia: Mosby, p. 838

Table 10-1: NORMAL ARTERIAL BLOOD GAS VALUES

Acidity index	pH	7.35 -7.45
Partial pressure of dissolved O_2	PO_2	80 to 100 mm Hg
Percentage of Hgb saturated with O_2	O_2 saturation	95 percent or above
Partial pressure of dissolved CO_2	PCO_2	35 to 45 mm Hg
Bicarbonate	HCO^{3-}	22 to 28 mEq/L

a. Primary function is to monitor arterial O_2 levels; maintain little control over normal ventilation.
b. When arterial O_2 decreases to below 60 mm mercury pressure, stimulation to breathe is initiated by this area.
c. In a person whose primary stimulus to breathe is hypoxia, this becomes the mechanism of ventilatory control.

System Data Collection

A. History.

1. Status of immunizations.
   a. Tuberculin skin test.
   b. DPT.
   c. Polio.
   d. Pneumovax for clients over age 65 or high-risk clients.
2. History of medication.
3. Occupation and occupational environment.
4. Habits - smoking, alcohol intake.

B. Physical data collection.

NCLEX ALERT: *Identify progressive changes in respiratory status - primary indicators of respiratory disorders are sputum production, cough, dyspnea, hemoptysis, chest pain and wheezing.*

1. Initially observe client's resting position.
   a. Does client appear comfortable and not in distress?
   b. Assess client's respiratory status in the sitting position if possible.
2. Evaluate vital signs (Table 10-2).
   a. Are they appropriate for age level?
   b. Establish data base and compare with previous data.
   c. Assess client's overall response.
      (1) Normal vital signs vary greatly from one individual to another.

(2) A blood pressure of 90/60 may be normal for one person, but may be hypotensive for another person.

3. Assess upper airway passages and patency of the airway.
4. Inspect the neck for symmetry: check to see if the trachea is in midline and observe for jugular vein distention.
5. Assess the lungs.
   a. Visually evaluate the thoracic cavity.
      (1) Do both sides move equally?
      (2) Observe characteristics of respirations and presence of retractions.
   b. Palpate chest for tenderness, masses, and symmetry of motion.
   c. Auscultate breath sounds; begin at posterior base and compare each area side to side. Breath sounds should be present and equal bilaterally.
6. Assess cough reflex and sputum production.
   a. Is cough associated with pain?
   b. What precipitates coughing episodes?
   c. Is cough productive or nonproductive?
   d. Characteristics of sputum.
      (1) Consistency.
      (2) Amount.
      (3) Color (should be clear).
   e. Presence of hemoptysis.
      (1) Duration.

TABLE 10-2: Normal Vital Signs

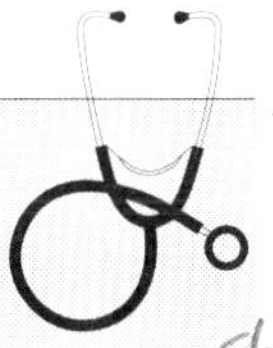

Neonate:	
Respiration	30 to 60
Pulse	110 to 160
Child 2 to 4 years:	
Respiration	24 to 32
Pulse	90 to 130
Child 6 to 10 years:	
Respiration	20 to 26
Pulse	100
Blood Pressure	80/40 to 110/80
Adult:	
Respiration	12 to 18
Pulse	60 to 100
Blood Pressure	90/60 to 140/90

NCLEX ALERT: *Determine if client vital signs are abnormal.*

Table 10-3: EFFECTIVE COUGHING

- Increase activity prior to coughing - walking, or turning from side to side.
- Place client in sitting position, preferably with feet on the floor.
- Client should turn his shoulders inward and bend his head slightly forward.
- Take a gentle breath in through the nose and breathe completely.
- Take two deep breaths through the nose and mouth and hold for 10-15 seconds.
- On the third deep breath, cough to clear secretions.
- Sips of warm liquids (coffee, tea, or water) may stimulate coughing.
- Demonstrate to client how to splint chest or incision during cough to decrease pain.
- Incentive spirometry will promote lung expansion and alveolar inflation.

NCLEX ALERT: *Plan interventions to minimize anticipate side effects and expected symptoms. Plan and implement interventions to prevent complications of respiratory status.*

(2) Amount.

NURSING PRIORITY: *When mucus is retained and pools in the lungs, gas diffusion may be affected and infection may occur.*

7. Assess for abnormal respiratory pattern.
   a. Hyperventilation-increased rate and depth of respiration often associated with loss of CO_2
   b. Tachypnea-rapid, shallow breathing which may be associated with CO_2 retention.
   c. Bradypnea-slow, regular breathing, may be drug- induced (narcotics).
   d. Cheyne-Stokes-apnea episodes alternating with hyperventilation found in heart failure, anemia, and brain damage (severe anoxia).
   e. Kussmaul's-rapid, deep breathing associated with diabetic ketoacidosis.
8. Assess for and evaluate dyspnea.
   a. Onset of dyspnea.
   b. Presence of orthopnea.
   c. Presence of expiratory and inspiratory wheezes.
   d. Presence of noisy expiration.
   e. Level of tolerance of activity.
   f. Correlation of vital signs with dyspnea.
   g. Presence of cyanosis.

NCLEX ALERT: *Determine oxygenation status of client. Identify progressive changes in respiratory status.*

9. Assess for and evaluate chest pain.
   a. Location of pain.
   b. Character of pain.
   c. Pain associated with cough.
   d. Pain either increased or decreased with breathing.
10. Evaluate extremities for clubbing (characteristic of clients with chronic respiratory disorders).
11. Evaluate lab data.
   a. Hemoglobin and hematocrit (presence of polycythemia or anemia).
   b. Electrolyte imbalances.
   c. Arterial blood gases (Table 10-1).

NCLEX ALERT: *Modify client's care based on the results of diagnostic/lab test*

RESPIRATORY DISORDERS

Hypoxia

❑ **Hypoxia is a condition characterized by an inadequate amount of oxygen available for cellular metabolism.**

Box Text 10-1: Geriatric Considerations in Respiratory Assessment

Body Changes	*Respiratory Changes*
Kyphosis	Decrease ability to cough and deep breath effectively.
Decreased chest expansion	Decreased O2 levels, increased risk for atelectasis.
Decreased ability to handle secretions and infection.	Increased risk for aspiration, infection, atelectasis.
Decreased chest expansion	Decreased oxygenation, and increased risk for hypoventilation.
Altered pulmonary function	Decreased breath sounds, deceased vital capacity, increased residual volume.

Table 10-4: SYMPTOMS OF RESPIRATORY DISTRESS AND HYPOXIA

Early Symptoms	Late Symptoms
Restlessness	Extreme restlessness to stupor
Tachycardia	Dyspnea
Tachypnea, Exertional	Depressed respiration
Dyspnea	Bradycardia
Anxiety	Cyanosis
Diaphoresis	
Poor judgment	
Disorientation	
Confusion	
Headache	

Specific to Pediatrics: flaring nares, subcostal and sternal retractions, expiratory grunting, inspiratory stridor, feeding difficulty, head bobbing while sleeping

NURSING PRIORITY: *Immediately notify RN of any changes in the client's respiratory status.*

NCLEX ALERT: *Identify progressive changes in respiratory status.*

A. Hypoxemia - ↓ oxygen saturation of the blood.
   1. Mild hypoxemia is when the PaO_2 falls below 80mmhg, severe hypoxemia is when PaO_2 falls below 50mm Hg.
   2. Disorders causing respiratory obstruction and alveolar hypoventilation.

B. Hypoxia may be precipitated by inadequate circulation.
   1. Shock.
   2. Cardiac failure.

C. Anemia precipitates hypoxia due to decrease in oxygen-carrying capacity of the blood.
   1. Inadequate red cell production.
   2. Deficient or abnormal hemoglobin.

Data Collection

1. Risk factors/etiology.
   a. Chronic hypoxia.
      (1) COPD.
      (2) Cystic fibrosis.
      (3) Cancer of the respiratory tract.
      (4) CHF.
      (5) Chronic anemia.
   b. Inflammatory problems affecting alveolar surface area, and membrane integrity (pneumonia).
   c. Acute hypoxia.

Table 10-5: PREVENTION OF ASPIRATION

- Have suction equipment available.
- Position in semi to high Fowler's.
- Put dentures in, if available.
- Place food on unaffected side of face.
- Do not rush client, allow adequate time to chew and swallow.
- Remove drinking straws unless otherwise indicated.
- Encourage thick liquids and soft foods.
- Examine client's mouth for residual food.
- Maintain client in semi to high Fowler's position for 30 minutes after eating.

Clients At High Risk For Aspiration:

- CVA with facial and tongue weakness.
- Laryngectomy.
- Tracheotomy.
- Seizures.
- Increased sedation after surgery.
- Elderly clients without their dentures.
- Infants with facial or palate birth defects.
- Post procedure that requires depression of gag reflex: gastroscopy and bronchoscopy.

NCLEX ALERT: *Identify potential for aspiration related to client status. Intervene to improve respiratory status.*

(1) Acute respiratory failure.

(2) Sudden airway obstruction.

(3) Conditions affecting pulmonary expansion (i.e., respiratory paralysis).

(4) CHF.

(5) Hypoventilation (sedation, anesthesia, etc.).

2. Clinical manifestations - underlying respiratory problem either chronic or acute (Table 10-4).
3. Diagnostics.
   a. ABGs.
   b. Pulmonary function tests.
   c. Hemoglobin and hematocrit levels.
   d. Clinical manifestations.
   e. History of chronic problems.
   f. Pulse oximetry

Nursing Intervention

✦ *Goal: to maintain good pulmonary hygiene and prevent hypoxic episode (Box 10-1).*

1. Position client to maintain patent airway.
   a. Unconscious client - position on side with the chin extended, head slightly elevated.
   b. Conscious client - elevate the head of the bed and position on side, or semi-Fowler's.
2. Encourage coughing and deep breathing.
3. Suction client as indicated by amount of sputum and ability to cough.

Box 10-2: Elderly Care Focus

Respiratory Care Priorities

- Provide adequate rest periods between activities, such as bathing, going for treatments, eating, etc.
- Use semi to high Fowler's as tolerated for feeding client to prevent aspiration.
- Have chairs and other supports for client in easy reach when ambulating, so client may sit to rest.
- Encourage annual flu shot for individuals over age 65 and determine if older adult has received pneumococcal vaccination.

4. Maintain adequate fluid intake to keep secretions liquefied - 3000 to 4000cc daily (unless contraindicated by cardiac or renal problems).
5. Encourage exercises and ambulation as indicated by condition.
6. Administer expectorants.
7. Administer O_2 as indicated.
8. Prevent aspiration (Table 10-5).

✦ *Goal: to assess and implement nursing measures appropriate to current level of hypoxia.*

1. Assess patency of airway (first priority).
   a. Can client speak? If not, initiate emergency procedures. (Appendix 10-3).
   b. If speaking is difficult because of level of hypoxia, call for immediate assistance, but remain with client.
   c. If client is able to speak in sentences and is coherent, continue with assessment of the problem.
   d. Is client working hard to maintain respiration?
   e. Evaluate amount of secretions and ability to cough; suction if indicated.
2. Maintain calm approach, as increasing anxiety will potentiate hypoxia. Remain with the client who is experiencing severe dyspnea.

***NURSING PRIORITY:** Increasing anxiety will accelerate the dyspnea in a client who is experiencing severe difficulty breathing.*

3. Position adult and older children in semi-Fowler's if not contraindicated.

***NURSING PRIORITY:** Position a dyspneic client with a pillow lengthwise behind his back and head. Do not flex his head forward or backward.*

4. Infants

a. Place infant in an infant seat, or elevate the mattress.

b. Cyanosis that increases with crying is usually cardiac in origin; cyanosis that decreases with crying is usually respiratory in origin.

c. Cyanosis of the mucous membranes in the mouth, inner aspect of the lips and gums and mottling of extremities are usually indicative of pathological problems.

5. Assess color, presence of retractions, and diaphoresis.
6. Evaluate vital signs: are there significant changes from previous readings?
7. Evaluate presence of and level of tachycardia.
8. Evaluate chest movements: are they symmetrical?
9. Evaluate breath sounds.
10. Assess client for chest pain with dyspnea.
11. *Notify RN of significant assessment findings.*
12. Remain with client experiencing acute dyspnea or hypoxic episodes.

Pneumothorax

❑ **Air in the pleural cavity results in the collapse of atelectasis of that portion of the lung. This condition is known as *pneumothorax.***

A. Tension pneumothorax - the development of a pneumothorax that allows excessive buildup of air in the pleural space.

1. Causes a shift in the mediastinum toward the unaffected side.
2. A tension pneumothorax can very rapidly become an emergency situation.

Data Collection

1. Risk factors/etiology.

a. Ruptured bleb on lung surface (spontaneous).

b. Thoracentesis.

c. Trauma and fractured ribs pierce the pleura.

2. Clinical manifestations.

a. Dyspnea, tachypnea.

b. Tachycardia.

c. Sudden, sharp pleural pain, especially on inspiration.

d. Anxiety, increasing restlessness.

e. Asymmetrical chest wall expansion.

f. Decreased breath sounds on affected side.

g. Possible development of a tension pneumothorax.

(1) Decreased cardiac filling - leading to decreased cardiac output.

(2) Tracheal shift from midline toward unaffected side.

(3) Increasing problems of hypoxia.

3. Diagnostics.

a. Chest X-ray.

b. Clinical manifestations.

Treatment

Placement of chest tubes connected to water-sealed drainage (Appendix 10-4).

Nursing Intervention

✦ *Goal: to recognize problem and prevent severe hypoxic episode (see Nursing Intervention, Hypoxia).*

1. *Notify RN of deterioration of client's respiratory status.*
2. Put client to bed in semi-Fowler's position and begin oxygen.
3. Prepare client for insertion of chest tubes.

✦ *Goal: to reinflate lung without complications.*

1. Have client cough and deep breathe every two hours.
2. Encourage exercise and ambulation.
3. Establish and maintain underwater-seal chest drainage (Appendix 10-4).

Chest Trauma

❑ **Open chest wound - an open or "sucking" chest wound may be caused by a penetrating injury of the chest.**

1. Assessment

a. An accident resulting in a chest wound with evidence of air moving in and out via the wound.

b. Accidental removal of a chest tube.

2. Treatment

a. Have client take a deep breath and hold it while applying an occlusive dressing.

b. Prepare for insertion of a chest tube.

A. Flail Chest - loss of the stability of the chest wall with respiratory impairment due to multiple rib fractures on the same side, generally caused by motor vehicle accidents.

1. Assessment

a. Paradoxical respirations - movement of fractured area in opposite direction of other areas of the chest wall.

b. Hypoxia

2. Diagnostics.

a. X-ray of chest wall

b. ABGs

3. Treatment

a. Maintain patent airway.

b. If pulmonary function is compromised, endotracheal intubation and mechanical ventilation are done to provide internal stabilization.

Nursing Intervention

✦ *Goal: to improve ventilation in client with chest trauma.*

1. Ongoing assessment for hypoxia.
2. Monitor oxygen administration and ABGs.
3. Ongoing assessment for presence of pneumo thorax and tension pneumothorax.
4. Maintain calm atmosphere and assist client to decrease anxiety.
5. Medications as indicated for pain control.

Pulmonary Emboli

❑ **A pulmonary embolus is the obstruction of a pulmonary blood vessel, most often due to the presence of air, fat, amniotic fluid, or a mobilized thrombus.**

A. The severity of the problem depends on the size and number of emboli.

B. The majority of emboli arise from thrombi in the deep veins of the legs and pelvic area.

C. A pulmonary embolus must originate from the venous circulation or the right side of the heart.

NCLEX ALERT: *Implement interventions to manage potential client circulatory complications. Identify progressive changes in respiratory status.*

Data Collection

1. Risk factors/etiology.

a. Conditions predisposing to venous stasis (surgery, immobility).

b. Thrombophlebitis.

c. Pregnancy.

d. Obesity.

2. Clinical manifestations.

a. Dyspnea.

b. Sudden, sharp, chest pain aggravated by breathing.

c. Coughing, frequently with hemoptysis.

d. Tachycardia.

e. Symptoms of hypoxia (Table 10-4).

f. May result in sudden death if pulmonary vessel involved is large.

3. Diagnostics.

a. Pulmonary angiogram.

b. Lung scan.

c. EKG (nonspecific).

d. Chest X-ray (nonspecific).

e. ABGs(nonspecific).

Treatment

1. Bed rest.
2. Oxygen.
3. Anticoagulants (Heparin) to prevent further thrombus formation.
4. Analgesics for severe chest pain.
5. IV fluids.

Nursing Intervention

✦ *Goal: to identify and prevent development of pulmonary emboli.*

1. Elderly clients are at higher risk for deep vein thrombosis.

NCLEX ALERT: *Implement interventions to promote venous return*

2. Clients who are immobilized are high risk. (Chp 3)

a. Postoperative

(1) orthopedic surgery such as knee, and hip replacements

(2) gynecological surgery

(3) Clients with fractures

(4) Clients with conditions requiring bed rest - CHF, myocardial infarction

✦ *Goal: to identify problem and implement nursing measures to alleviate hypoxia (see Nursing Intervention, Hypoxia).*

NURSING PRIORITY: *Prevention of venous stasis is critical in preventing the development of pulmonary emboli in the immobilized client.*

Croup

❑ **The term *croup* describes a group of conditions characterized by edema and inflammation of the respiratory tract.**

A. Acute epiglottitis - a severe infection of the epiglottis, characterized by rapid inflammation and edema of the area.
  1. Generally occurs in children two to four years old; may rapidly cause airway obstruction.
  2. Clinical manifestations (Table 10-4- Hypoxia).
    a. Triad of symptoms: spontaneous cough, presence of drooling, and agitation.
    b. Sore throat, swallowing difficulty.
    c. Symptoms of increasing respiratory obstruction.
      (1) Characteristic position - sitting with the neck hyperextended and mouth open, drooling.
      (2) Inspiratory stridor (crowing).
      (3) Retraction.
      (4) Increased restlessness.
      (5) Onset is usually rapid occurring over several hours.
    d. High fever (above 102°F).
  3. Treatment - oxygen, artificial airway (either endotracheal tube or tracheotomy) and antibiotics
B. Acute laryngotracheobronchitis (LTB) - inflammation of the vocal cords, subglottal tissues, trachea.
  1. Occurs primarily in children under 5 years old.
  2. Clinical manifestations
    a. Onset over several days
    b. Frequently preceded by upper respiratory infection.
    c. May get worse at night.
    d. Respiratory distress.
      (1) Inspiratory stridor.
      (2) Retractions.
      (3) Restlessness.
    e. Slight temperature elevation (usually below 102°F.).
  3. Treatment - cool mist, IV fluids if child cannot maintain PO intake, and bronchodilators.

Nursing Intervention

✦ *Goal: to maintain patent airway in hospitalized child.*
  1. Tracheotomy set readily available.

> ***NURSING PRIORITY:*** *Do not examine child's throat, as it may precipitate airway spasm - especially in epiglottitis.*

  2. Suction airway as indicated with tracheotomy or endotracheal tube.
  3. If child is in severe respiratory distress, do not leave unattended.

✦ *Goal: to evaluate and maintain adequate ventilation.*
  1. Assess for increasing hypoxia.
  2. Maintain child in humidified oxygen.
  3. Conserve energy and promote rest.
  4. Child may assume a position of comfort, generally sitting.
  5. *Notify RN of increasing respiratory difficulty.*

> ***NURSING PRIORITY:*** *Early signs of impending airway obstruction are the same as early signs of hypoxia.*

✦ *Goal: to maintain hydration and nutrition.*
  1. Do not give PO fluid until danger of aspiration is past.
  2. IV fluids during acute episodes.
  3. High caloric liquids when danger of aspiration is over.

> ***NURSING PRIORITY:*** *Administer fluids very cautiously to a client who is having difficulty breathing. Begin with small sips of water to determine if he can swallow effectively. Do not begin with fluids that contain any fat (milk) due to the increased risk of the client aspirating.*

Respiratory Syncytial Virus (RSV)

❑ **Most common cause of bronchiolitis and lower respiratory tract infections in infants and young children.**
  1. Most common in winter and spring in children under 2 years old.
A. Transmitted by direct contact with respiratory secretions.
  1. Clinical manifestations.
    a. Tachypnea, chest retractions.
    b. Paroxysmal wheezy cough, dyspnea.
    c. Diminished breath sounds.
    d. Rhinorrhea, copious amounts of secretions.
    e. Can progress to obstructed bronchioles and severe respiratory distress (Table 10-4 Hypoxia).
    f. Extremely contagious, infant should be isolated from other children.
  2. Treatment
    a. Rest, fluids and humidified oxygen.
    b. Mist therapy via ultrasonic nebulizer
    c. Antiviral agents.

✦ *Goal: to decrease transmission.*
  1. Good hand washing
  2. Wear gloves and gown.

3. Maintain respiratory isolation, prevent cross contamination by care givers.

Tonsillitis

❏ Tonsillitis is an inflammation and infection of the palatine tonsils.

Data Collection

1. Risk factors/etiology.
   a. Viral.
   b. Beta hemolytic streptococcus.
   c. Infection is seasonal; peaks in winter.
2. Clinical manifestations.
   a. Edematous, enlarged tonsils.
   b. Difficulty swallowing and breathing.
   c. Mouth breathing.
   d. Frequently precipitates *otitis media*.
   e. Fever.
3. Diagnostics.
   a. Confirm by visualization of the oral pharynx.
   b. Throat culture to identify organism, beta hemolytic streptococcus is the most common .

Treatment

1. Appropriate antibiotic for identified organism.
2. Surgery - tonsillectomy for severe repeated episodes of tonsillitis.

Nursing Intervention

✦ *Goal: to assist parents to understand disease process and to promote comfort and healing in home environment.*

1. Soft or liquid diet.
2. Cool mist vaporizer to maintain moisture to mucous membranes.
3. Antibiotics - important to give child all of the medication prescribed in order to prevent reoccurrence.
4. Analgesics, antipyretic (acetaminophen).

✦ *Goal: to provide preoperative nursing measures as appropriate if surgery is indicated (Chapter 3).*

✦ *Goal: to maintain patent airway and evaluate for bleeding postoperative tonsillectomy.*

NCLEX ALERT: *Implement interventions to prevent aspiration by client. The tonsillectomy client should be positioned on the side or on the abdomen with the knee flexed to prevent aspiration from bloody drainage or vomitus.*

1. Restrict fluids until child is fully awake; administer cool, clear liquids initially.
2. Evaluate for frequent or continuous swallowing, tachycardia, and pallor due to bleeding,
3. Suction equipment should be available.
4. Check the throat with a flashlight.
5. Ice collar to decrease edema.
6. Evaluate voice for increasing hoarseness.
7. Aspirin is contraindicated.

Self-Care

1. Child will have sore throat for seven to ten days.
2. Symptoms of bleeding, especially significant on the fifth to tenth postoperative days when tissue sloughing occurs.
3. Maintain adequate hydration; avoid citrus, acid, coarse or spicy foods for 5-7 days.
4. Child may return to school seven to ten days postoperatively.

Pneumonia

❏ Pneumonia is an inflammatory process in the lung caused by an infectious organism. The exudate produced by the infectious process will precipitate obstruction in the bronchiole and a decrease in gas exchange at the alveolar level.

A. Pneumonia is generally classified according to causative organism - either viral or bacterial.
B. Aspiration pneumonia occurs when foreign material or gastric contents are aspirated into the lung.

NCLEX ALERT: *Identify signs and symptoms of infection. Intervene to improve respiratory status.*

Data Collection

1. Predisposing conditions.
   a. Chronic upper respiratory infection.
   b. General anesthesia.
   c. Immobility.
   d. Smoking.
   e. Decreased immune state.
   f. Most frequent cause of death in clients over 65 years old.
2. Clinical manifestations.
   a. Fever, chills.
   b. Tachycardia.
   c. Tachypnea, dyspnea.
   d. Productive cough.
      (1) Thick, dark, purulent or rusty colored sputum.

e. Pleuritic chest pain.
f. Malaise.
g. Respiratory distress (Table 10-4:Hypoxia).
h. Diminished breath sounds.

Geriatric Priority: *An elderly client may initially present with mental confusion and volume depletion rather than with respiratory symptoms and fever.*

3. Diagnostics.
   a. Culture of organism from sputum.
   b. Chest X-ray.

Treatment

1. Antibiotic according to organism identified (Appendix 5-10).
2. Bronchodilators

NURSING PRIORITY: *Obtain specimens from clients - do not start antibiotics until a good sputum specimen has been collected. An accurate culture and sensitivity cannot be done if client has already been started on the antibiotics.*

3. Inhalation therapy.
   a. Cool oxygen mist.
   b. Postural drainage.
   c. Bronchodilators.

Nursing Intervention

✦ *Goal: to decrease infection and remove secretions to facilitate oxygen and carbon dioxide exchange.*

1. Have client turn, cough, and deep breathe.
2. Liquify secretions.
   a. Adequate hydration.
   b. Cool mist inhalation.
3. Evaluate changes in sputum.
4. Employ nursing measures to prevent and evaluate levels of hypoxia (see Nursing Interventions, Hypoxia).
5. Maintain comfort with analgesics.

Self-Care

1. Plan activity around rest periods.
2. Take all of antibiotics prescribed.
3. Return to doctor for:
   a. Return or increase in fever and chills
   b. Chest pain.
   c. Hemoptysis
4. Maintain high fluid intake.
5. Assess elderly for confusion and lethargy.

Geriatric Priority: *The immobilized geriatric client is at a high risk for the development of pneumonia.*

Tuberculosis (TB)

❑ **Tuberculosis is a bacterial infection in the lungs. It may also involve the kidneys, bones, lymph nodes, and meninges.**

A. Characteristics.

1. Organism is primarily transmitted through respiratory droplets. It is inhaled and will implant on alveolar surface.
2. Characteristic tissue reaction is the formation of a tubercle in the lung.
3. The tubercle may never erode but calcify and remain dormant after the initial infection. However, the tubercle may contain living bacilli that can reactivate several years later.
4. Primary tubercles heal over a period of months. These lesions may contain living bacilli that can reactivate after many years. Clients are asymptomatic during this time.
5. Tuberculosis is transmitted in the small droplets of moisture (aerosolization) from the respiratory tract. The infected droplets are then inhaled by a susceptible person.
6. Increased incidence of TB in AIDS clients due to their debilitated state.

Data Collection

1. Predisposing conditions.
   a. Frequent close contact with infected individual, who frequently has not been diagnosed.
   b. Debilitating conditions and diseases: HIV-positive, elderly, alcoholics, children under age 5.
   c. Poor nutrition and crowded living conditions.
2. Etiology—Mycobacterium tuberculosis, a gram-positive, acid-fast bacillus.
3. Clinical manifestations (client may be asymptomatic).
   a. Fatigue, malaise.
   b. Anorexia, weight loss.
   c. May have a chronic cough progressing to more frequent and productive cough.
   d. Low-grade fever in the late afternoon.
   e. Night sweats.
   f. Hemoptysis and chronic productive cough.
4. Diagnostics (Appendix 10-1).
   a. Tuberculin skin testing.

(1) Positive reaction means the individual has been infected or has developed a sensitivity to the protein; does not differentiate between active or dormant infection.

(2) A positive reaction to a TB skin test means that the person has at some time been exposed to the TB bacillus and has developed antibodies. It does not mean that the person has an active TB infection, or is free of tuberculosis.

(3) After exposure to bacilli, it is usually 2-6 weeks before sensitivity develops and results in a positive skin test.

b. Chest X-ray - may demonstrate presence of calcified lesions.

c. Bacteriologic studies to identify acid-fast bacilli (Appendix 10-1).

NCLEX ALERT: *Apply principles of infection control. Respiratory precautions for tuberculosis client.*

Treatment

1. Chemotherapy (Appendix 10-2).
   a. Medical regimen usually involves simultaneous administration of three or more medications; this is done to increase the therapeutic effect of medication and to decrease development of resistant bacteria.
   b. Course of treatment may be from 6 to 24 months.
   c. Approximately two to four weeks after the client has been on TB medications, his sputum will be negative; thereafter, the risk of transmitting the disease is minimal.
2. Decreased activity.
3. Client will most often be followed and treated on an outpatient basis.

Nursing Intervention

✦ *Goal: to prevent transmission of the disease.*

1. Hospitalized client
   a. When caring for the client, the nurse should wear a HEPA respirator mask.
   b. The client should be placed on respiratory precautions, in a private room that has special ventilation to prevent spread of airborne bacteria.
2. Teach client to cover mouth and nose when sneezing or coughing.
3. Teach client careful handwashing routine.
4. TB is more likely to be spread by clients who have active, undiagnosed TB.

✦ *Goal: to maintain good pulmonary hygiene and prevent hypoxic episodes (see Nursing Intervention, Hypoxia).*

Self-Care

1. Teach client importance of taking all of prescribed medications.
2. Client should use measures at home to decrease contamination with pulmonary secretions: cover his nose and mouth when coughing or sneezing, dispose of tissue in plastic bags.
3. Respiratory isolation usually not necessary at home, as family members have already been exposed. All family members should be evaluated for active disease.
4. Client should wear a mask when he is in contact with other people.
5. Instruct client regarding the importance of adequate nutrition.
6. Discuss with client problems he may experience regarding decreased physical strength and stamina.
7. Stress importance of good handwashing routine.
8. Stress importance of returning to doctor for sputum checks.

COPD or CALD

❑ **COPD or Chronic Air Flow Limitation Disorder (CALD) is a group of respiratory diseases characterized by chronic obstruction of airflow.**

Data Collection

1. Risk factors/etiology.
   a. Cigarette smoking.
   b. Chronic infections.
   c. Inhaled irritants.
2. Clinical manifestations.
   a. Exertional dyspnea or dyspnea at rest.
   b. Chronic cough.
      (1) Non-productive or absent in emphysema.
      (2) Excessive sputum and chronic coughing in chronic bronchitis.
   c. Wheezing.
   d. Frequent respiratory infections.
   e. Pursed-lip breathing.
   f. Prolonged expiration with diminished breath sounds.
   g. Easily fatigued.
   h. Use of accessory muscles of respiration.
   i. Digital clubbing.
   j. Barrel chest.

k. Orthopnea.

3. Diagnostics.(Appendix 10-1).
   a. Pulmonary function studies.
   b. ABGs (See Table 10-1).

Treatment

1. Prevention or treatment of respiratory infections.
2. Medications: bronchodilators, mucolytics and expectorants, steroids (see Appendix 10-2).
3. Chest physiotherapy (postural drainage and nebulized bronchodilators.
4. Breathing exercises.
5. Low flow oxygen.
6. Decrease in pulmonary irritants (smoking).

***NURSING PRIORITY:** The optimum amount of oxygen is the concentration that reverses the hypoxemia without causing adverse side effects.*

Nursing Intervention

✦ *Goal: to improve ventilation.*

1. Assist client to balance activities and increasing dyspnea; schedule active exercise after respiratory therapy.
2. Humidified oxygen at 1 to 3 liters per minute via nasal cannula.
   a. Attempt to maintain a PO_2 of at least 65mmHg.
   b. A significant increase in PO_2 may decrease respiratory drive.
   c. The risk of inducing hypoventilation should not prevent the administration of oxygen in low levels to the COPD client experiencing respiratory distress.

NCLEX ALERT: *Administer prescribed oxygen therapy to client, determine oxygenation status of client. Monitor client receiving oxygen therapy.*

3. Prolonged, planned rest periods.
4. Avoid cough suppressants.
5. High-Fowler's or sitting position.
6. Maintain adequate hydration to facilitate removal of secretions.

NCLEX ALERT: *Observe for effects of medications. Administer narcotics, tranquilizers and sedatives with caution as they will depress the respiratory center.*

✦ *Goal: to maintain adequate nutrition.*

1. Soft, high-protein, high calorie diet, may supplement diet with high calorie liquid supplements.
2. Postural drainage at least 45 minutes prior to meals.
3. Good oral hygiene after postural drainage and prior to meals.
4. Small frequent meals.
5. May use oxygen via nasal prongs or cannula during meals.

Self-Care

1. Encourage client and family to verbalize feelings about condition and lifelong restriction of activities.
2. Include client in active planning for home care.
3. Instruct client regarding medication schedule and side effects of prescribed medications.
4. Teach the client to recognize signs and symptoms of upper respiratory infection and when to call physician.
5. Avoid contact with people with upper respiratory infections.
6. Evaluate support system in home.

Asthma or RAD

❑ **Asthma or Reactive Airway Disorder (RAD) is an intermittent, reversible, obstructive airway problem. It is characterized by exacerbations and remissions.**

A. Intermittent narrowing of the trachea and bronchial tissue caused by:
   1. Constriction of the smooth muscles
   2. Excessive mucus production.
   3. Mucosal edema of the respiratory tract.

B. Exercise-induced asthma - initially after exercise there is an improvement in the respiratory status, followed by a significant decline; occurs in the majority of asthmatic clients.

C. Between attacks the client is generally asymptomatic.

D. *Reactive airway disease* is term used to describe asthma in children when onset is before age 3.

E. Emotional factors are known to play an important role in precipitating childhood asthma attacks. Family interactions frequently contribute to the overall pattern of the child's asthma attacks.

Data Collection

1. Risk factors/etiology.
   a. Familial tendencies.

b. Hypersensitivity.

c. Non-allergic asthma in adults usually occurs after a respiratory infection and is more prominent in people over age 35.

d. In children, frequently a history of chronic bronchitis, eczema or pneumonia.

2. Diagnostics.

a. History of hypersensitivity reactions.

b. Clinical manifestations.

c. ABGs.

d. Pulmonary function tests.

3. Clinical manifestations.

a. Paroxysmal cough.

b. Shortness of breath, tachypnea.

c. Expiratory wheezing.

d. Symptoms of hypoxia.

e. Retractions.

f. Tachycardia.

g. Increased anxiety, restlessness.

h. Exercise intolerance

4. Complications - Status asthmaticus: severe asthma, unresponsive to initial treatment.

***NURSING PRIORITY:** If the symptoms of asthma do not respond to the client's usual method of treatment, he should seek medical attention. Status asthmaticus can be a life-threatening situation.*

Treatment

1. Medications (appendix 10-2).

2. Respiratory therapy.

a. Supplemental oxygen.

b. Cool mist inhalation.

c. Chest physiotherapy - postural drainage and percussion and suctioning if necessary after the acute attack.

Nursing Intervention

(See Nursing Intervention, Hypoxia)

✦ *Goal: to relieve asthmatic attacks.*

1. Position in high-Fowler's or sitting with chest forward.

2. Assess breath sounds.

a. Pediatrics - inspiratory wheezing indicates a serious problem; wheezing on inspiration and expiration in less severe episodes; a *decrease* in wheezing indicates situation is worsening.

b. Adults - inspiratory and expiratory wheezing common, monitor for improved airway clearance and increased breath sounds.

3. Respiratory therapy: supplemental oxygen, cool mist, and aerosol bronchodilators.

4. Maintain calm, reassuring manner.

5. Maintain adequate fluid intake, sometimes lukewarm fluids are more soothing and liquify secretions

***NURSING PRIORITY:** Do not give PO fluids to a severely dyspneic client.*

6. Determine if adult client has any history of cardiac problems - respiratory medications may put increased strain on diseased heart.

Self-Care

1. Assist family to identify sources of stress (i.e., problems with discipline, fear of asthma attacks); refer for counseling as appropriate.

2. Educate regarding avoidance of allergens - household dust, mold, animal dander, cigarette smoke.

3. Implement therapeutic measures before asthma attack becomes severe.

4. Administer bronchodilators prior to postural drainage.

5. Encourage bronchodilators and good warm-up exercises prior to exercise to assist in preventing exercise induced asthma.

6. Avoid upper respiratory infections and teach client good hand washing techniques.

7. Schedule opportunity for client and family to learn how to perform chest physiotherapy at home.

NCLEX ALERT: *Reinforce explanation of respiratory interventions to client and family.*

Cystic Fibrosis

❑ **This disorder is a generalized dysfunction precipitated by an obstruction of the exocrine gland ducts. The factor responsible for the multiple clinical manifestations of the disease process is the mechanical obstruction caused by thick mucus secretions.**

A. Organs affected by disease process.

1. Pancreas - decreased excretion of pancreatic enzymes, which are essential components in the digestion and absorption of fats and proteins.

Pancreatic damage predisposes client to glucose intolerance.

2. GI tract - decreased absorption of nutrients.
3. Liver - biliary obstruction and fibrosis, eventually causing cirrhosis.
4. Pulmonary system - bronchial obstruction by thick mucus, causing atelectasis. The thick mucus provides excellent medium for bacterial growth and secondary respiratory infections.

B. Condition is usually diagnosed in early childhood, many CF clients are adults and lead a very productive active life.

Data Collection

1. Risk factors/etiology: inherited as an autosomal recessive trait.
2. Clinical manifestations.
   a. Wide variation in severity and extent of manifestations as well as period of onset.
   b. GI tract - steatorrhea or fatty, foul smelling stools.
   c. Decreased weight due to poor absorption of nutrients.
   d. Respiratory tract - chronic cough, increasing problems with hypoxia and upper respiratory infections due to excessive mucus/sputum production.
   e. Excessive salt on the skin: "salty taste when kissed."
3. Diagnostics.
   a. Family history.
   b. Sweat chloride test.
   c. Pancreatic enzymes - decreased or absent
4. Complications.
   a. Cor pulmonale (right-sided heart failure).
   b. Frequent pulmonary infections.
   c. Respiratory failure.
   d. Glucose intolerance is common in adult clients.

Treatment

1. Diet - high calorie, high protein, fats as tolerated or decrease in fats, increased salt intake.
2. Vitamin K may be given in cases of liver involvement.
3. Pancreatic enzyme replacement (Appendix 8-2).
4. Pulmonary therapy.
   a. Physical therapy: postural drainage - percussion and vibration, breathing exercises.
   b. Aerosol therapy: nebulization in conjunction with postural drainage.
   c. Expectorants (Appendix 10-2).
5. Antibiotics prophylactically and when there is evidence of infection.
6. Encourage child/client to be involved and responsible for health care as much as possible.

Nursing Intervention

✦ *Goal: to maintain nutrition.*

1. Balanced diet from all food groups - may have some fats to promote compliance; if restriction is necessary it frequently is in the fat intake.
2. Maintain adequate salt intake.
3. Pancreatic enzymes with meals and snacks.
4. Good oral hygiene after postural drainage.
5. Postural drainage one to two hours prior to meals.

✦ *Goal: to maintain ventilation.*

1. Assist client to mobilize secretions.
   a. Postural drainage, breathing exercises, nebulization treatments.
   b. Encourage daily active exercises appropriate to child's capacity and developmental level.
2. Prevent respiratory infections.
3. Maintain adequate PO fluid intake.

✦ *Goal: to promote independence in ADL's*

1. Encourage children to be responsible for own medications and treatments.
2. Teach children how to avoid upper respiratory infections in school.
3. Genetic counseling should be available to young adults.

Pulmonary Edema

❑ **This condition is caused by an abnormal accumulation of fluid in the lung.**

A. Pulmonary congestion occurs when the pulmonary capillary bed becomes engorged with blood. The left side of the heart is unable to pump the blood to the systemic circulation and that pressure backs up into the pulmonary vascular bed.

B. The right side of the heart continues to pump blood into the pulmonary circulation. This type of pulmonary edema is cardiac in origin.

C. An increase in circulating blood volume from poor renal function, cardiac disease, and/ or IV fluid overload will decrease the diseased heart's ability to pump the increased load.

NCLEX ALERT: *Identify and intervene to life threatening situation.*

Data Collection

1. Sudden onset of dyspnea.
2. Severe anxiety, apprehension.
3. Cool, moist skin.
4. Tachycardia.
5. Orthopnea.
6. Severe coughing.
7. Noisy, wet respirations that do not clear with coughing.
8. Frothy, blood-tinged sputum.

> ***NURSING PRIORITY:** Pulmonary edema can become a medical emergency very rapidly.*

Treatment

1. O_2 in high concentration.
2. Diuretics - rapid-acting IV.
3. Bronchodilator.
4. Digitalis.
5. Intubation with mechanical ventilation

Nursing Intervention

✦ *Goal: to assess and implement nursing measures appropriate to level of hypoxia (see Nursing Intervention, Hypoxia).*

> ***Geriatric Priority:** Increased fluid intake in geriatric clients may precipitate a cardiac overload. Carefully monitor client's respiratory response to increased PO and IV fluids.*

✦ *Goal: to improve ventilation.*

1. Position in high-Fowler's with legs dependent.
2. Administer O_2.
3. Evaluate level of hypoxia and dyspnea.
4. *The RN may administer morphine by IV push.*
   a. It is essential that the client be sedated to a point that he no longer fights or resists the treatment.
   b. The fear of not being able to breathe is so strong that the client cannot cooperate.
5. Bronchodilators may be given by IV infusion to decrease respiratory distress.
6. Assist RN to monitor client's respiratory status.

✦ *Goal: to reduce circulating volume and cardiac workload.*

1. Diuretics (Appendix 11-5) to decrease circulating volume.
2. Digitalis (Appendix 12-2), catecholamines (Appendix 11-6) to increase cardiac output .
3. Carefully monitor all IV fluids and continuous evaluation of overall hydration status.

✦ *Goal: to provide psychological support and decrease anxiety.*

1. Approach client in a calm manner.
2. Explain procedures.
3. Remain with client in acute respiratory distress.

✦ *Goal: to prevent recurrence of problem.*

1. Recognize early stages.
2. Maintain client in semi-Fowler's position.
3. Decrease levels of activity.
4. Extreme precaution in administration of fluids.
5. Monitor daily weights and assess weight gain and fluid balance.

Cancer of the Larynx

❑ **A malignancy of the vocal cords or some other part of the larynx.**

Data Collection

1. Risk factors/etiology.
   a. More common in men 50 to 65 years old.
   b. Smoking increases incidence.
   c. Vocal straining.
   d. Chronic laryngitis.
2. Clinical manifestations (may be asymptomatic).
   a. Voice change, hoarseness.
   b. Dysphagia.
   c. Foul breath.
   d. Weight loss.
   e. Dyspnea.
   f. Hemoptysis
3. Diagnostics - direct laryngoscopic examination and biopsy of the lesion involved.

Treatment

(Varies with the extent of the malignancy.) See Cancer, Chapter 2.

1. Radiation - generally over several weeks; most successful when cancer is diagnosed early.
2. Chemotherapy - initial response is favorable; however, remissions tend to occur.
3. Surgical intervention.
   a. Partial laryngectomy - preserves the normal airway; speech may be altered. If a tracheotomy is performed, it is removed after the risk of swelling and airway obstruction have subsided.

b. Total laryngectomy - requires a permanent tracheotomy for breathing and an alternative method of speaking.

4. Speech therapy
   a. Esophageal speech - the techniques may be taught to the client within about a week of surgery. Requires compression of air in the esophagus and expelling it to form words.
   b. Electric larynx - a battery powered apparatus that projects sound into the oral cavity. Advantage is that it may be used soon after surgery, but has a very mechanical sound to the voice
   c. Tracheoesohageal puncture - a one way valve is placed in the stoma to divert air into the esophagus and out the mouth. A voice prostheses is fitted into the valve. This method most closely resembles normal speech.

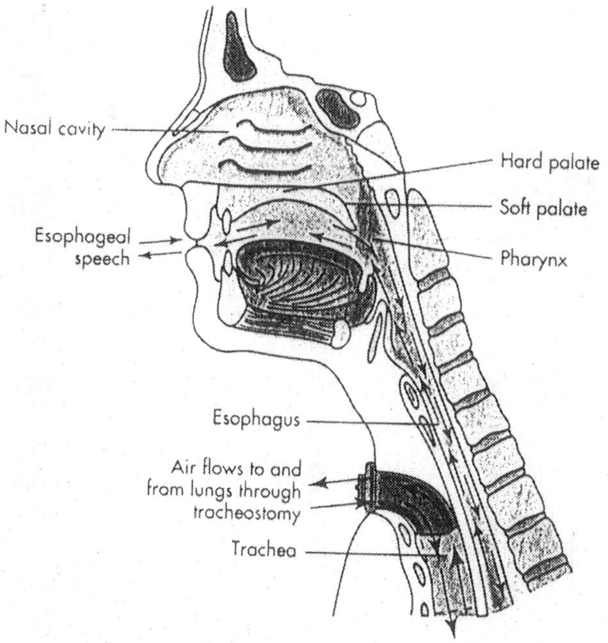

Figure 10-2: Permanent Tracheostomy.
Reprinted with permission: Phipps, WJ, Sands, JK, & Marek, JF (1999). *Medical Surgical Nursing: Concepts & Clinical Practice*, 6th ed. Philadelphia: Mosby, p. 892.

Nursing Intervention

✦ *Goal: to prepare client for surgery.*

1. General preoperative preparation (Chapter 3).
2. The surgeon should discuss with the client the method of postoperative airway control (temporary or permanent tracheotomy).
3. Follow-up discussion with the client regarding information for the temporary trach or permanent trach as indicated by the physician.
4. Encourage ventilation of feelings regarding a temporary or a permanent loss of voice postoperatively.
5. If total laryngectomy is anticipated, schedule a visit from the speech pathologist or member of the laryngectomy club to reassure client of rehabilitation potential.
6. Establish a method of communication for immediate postoperative period.
7. With a total laryngectomy, the sense of smell will be lost.

✦ *Goal: to prevent aspiration and maintain patent airway.*

NCLEX ALERT: *Provide tracheostomy care to client*

1. If tracheotomy is not performed, evaluate for hematoma and increasing edema of the incisional area precipitating respiratory distress.
2. Position in semi-Fowler's.
3. Observe for signs and symptoms of hypoxia.
4. Avoid analgesics that depress respiration.
5. Promote good pulmonary hygiene and prevent respiratory complications.
6. If tracheostomy is present, suction as indicated (See Appendix 10-6).
7. Coughing and deep breathing to mobilize secretions.
8. If tracheostomy is present, oxygen with humidification.
9. Maintain adequate hydration.

✦ *Goal: to promote postoperative nutrition.*

1. Method of nutritional intake depends on the extent of the surgical procedure.
2. Nasogastric feeding tubes are frequently utilized until the suture line begins to heal.
3. Oral intake may be started when temporary tracheotomy tube is still in place.
   a. Start with non pourable pureed foods.
   b. Liquids are not offered until swallowing has been relearned.
   c. Aspiration is at high risk for the partial laryngectomy client.
4. Good oral hygiene.
5. Treat nausea quickly to avoid vomiting.
6. Soft, nonirritating foods if oral intake is resumed.

✦ *Goal: to assist client and family to identify resource people in the community for speech rehabilitation postoperative laryngectomy.*

1. If some of the vocal cord is left, client will have gradual improvement in voice; generally allowed to begin whispering two to three days postoperative.
2. Follow-up visit from laryngectomy club member, if appropriate.
3. Assist client to identify appropriate community resources for speech therapy depending on type of speech.

NCLEX ALERT: *Provide support to client with changes in body image.*

Self-Care

1. Encourage client to begin own suctioning and caring for the tracheostomy prior to leaving the hospital.
2. Assist the client and family in obtaining equipment for home use.
   a. System for humidification of air in home environment.
   b. Suction equipment necessary for tracheostomy care.
   c. Equipment for care of the tracheostomy.
3. Use a shower shield over stoma during showering.
4. Shield the airway during the day with a protective cover or stoma guard.
5. Clean the stoma with mild soap and water; lubricate edges of stoma with a non-oil-based lubricant to prevent drying.
6. Activities are encouraged, but excessive fatigue should be avoided.
7. Client should carry appropriate identification.

Cancer of the Lung (Bronchogenic carcinoma)

❑ **This is a tumor arising from within the lung. It may represent the primary site or may be a metastatic site from a primary lesion elsewhere. Frequently advanced by the time of diagnosis; therefore, the overall survival rate is low.**

Data Collection

1. Risk factors.
   a. Smoking.
   b. Occupational exposure and inhalation of irritants.
2. Clinical manifestations.
   a. Cough or change in a chronic cough.
   b. Change in respiratory pattern -wheezing, dyspnea.
   c. Hemoptysis - blood- streaked to frank blood.
   d. Chest or shoulder pain or tightness.
   e. Hoarseness, dysphagia
   f. Common sites of metastasis.
      (1) Lymphatics.
      (2) Bone, brain, and other lung.
3. Diagnostics.
   a. Chest x-ray.
   b. Cytologic exam of early morning sputum.
   c. Bronchoscopy and biopsy.

Treatment

See Cancer, Chapter 2.
(Varies with extent of the malignancy.)

1. Radiation.
2. Surgery.
   a. Lobectomy - removal of one lobe of the lung.
   b. Pneumonectomy - removal of the entire lung.
3. Chemotherapy.
4. Palliative - may include radiation to shrink tumor, care directed toward airway, pain management, and comfort.

Nursing Intervention

✦ *Goal: to prepare client for surgery.*

1. General preoperative preparations (Chapter 3).
2. Improve quality of ventilation prior to surgery.
   a. No smoking.
   b. Bronchodilator.
   c. Good pulmonary hygiene.
3. Discuss anticipated activities in the immediate postoperative period.
   a. Chest tubes and thoracic incision.
   b. Pain control.
   c. Shoulder exercises.
4. Encourage ventilation of feelings regarding diagnosis and impending surgery.
5. Establish baseline data for comparison postoperatively.
6. Orient client to the intensive care unit, if indicated.

✦ *Goal: to maintain patent airway and promote ventilation postoperative thoracotomy.*

1. Removal of secretions from tracheobronchial tree either by coughing or suctioning.
2. Have client cough frequently and deep breathe.

3. Close evaluation of vital signs, auscultation of breath sounds.
4. Closely observe pulse oximetry, *notify RN if consistently changing or dropping.*
5. Supplemental O_2 as indicated.
6. Control of pain so client can take deep breaths and cough.
7. If in stable condition, position in semi-Fowler's to promote optimum ventilation.
8. Check with physician for positioning after surgery - positioning is based on extent of resection.
9. Encourage ambulation as soon as possible.
10. Maintain water-seal drainage system (See Appendix 10-4).
11. The pneumonectomy client will not have chest tubes, since no lung is left in the pleural cavity.
12. Sometimes a tube is placed to remove excessive fluid that collects in the pleural cavity.

✦ *Goal: to assess and support cardiac function postoperative thoracotomy.*

1. Monitor for tachycardia.
2. Evaluate cardiac output; cardiac arrhythmias from hypoxia or mediastinal pressure will decrease cardiac output.
3. Evaluate hourly urine output.
4. Administer fluids and transfusions with extreme caution; client is very susceptible to development of pulmonary edema.
5. *Notify RN of any significant changes in vital signs, activity tolerance, or respiratory status.*
6. Shoulder and arm exercises to maintain mobility.
7. Encourage progressive ambulation.

Self-Care

1. No more smoking; avoid respiratory irritants.
2. Discuss positions that enhance breathing.
3. Continue activities and exercises; stop any activity that causes shortness of breath, chest pain, or undue fatigue.
4. Avoid lifting heavy objects until complete healing has occurred.
5. Notify the doctor for any changes in breathing, difficulty swallowing, or increasing hoarseness.
6. Return for follow-up care as indicated.

Study Questions—Respiratory

1. What is a non-invasive procedure to measure arterial oxygen levels?

① pulse oximetry.
② spirometry.
③ blood gases.
④ venogram.

2. Chronic pulmonary clients are usually on low dose oxygen via nasal cannula. What problem would occur if these clients received too high an oxygen concentration?

① hyperventilation.
② tachypnea.
③ hypoventilation.
④ increased snoring.

3. A thoracentesis procedure is to be done in the client's room. The nurse would place the client in which position?

① prone position with feet elevated.
② sitting with upper torso over bedside table.
③ lying on left side with right knee bent.
④ semi-Fowler's with lower torso flat.

4. What nursing assessment finding indicates the development of pneumonia as a complication?

① diminished breath sounds.
② use of accessory respiratory muscles.
③ dry hacking cough at night.
④ bradypnea and lethargy.

5. A client has thick pulmonary secretions. The nurse would anticipate which classification of drug to be ordered?

① antihistamine.
② mucolytic.
③ decongestant.
④ bronchodilator.

6. Why should a client with a history of increased blood pressure be cautious about using a decongestant?

① may cause a problem with urinary frequency.
② bradycardia is an common untoward effect.
③ increases vascular vasoconstriction.
④ frequently causes a headache.

7. What assessment findings would indicate a positive response in the client who is being treated for an acute asthmatic problem?

① respiratory rate of 18.
② pulse oximetry of 90%.
③ pulse rate of 110.
④ non-productive cough.

8. What potential complication may occur with each of these conditions: immobility, estrogen therapy, and a fractured femur?

① renal damage.
② hypertension.
③ osteoporosis.
④ pulmonary embolus.

9. A client is experiencing progression of his chronic pulmonary condition. What would be the characteristic data found on the assessment of this client?

① increased temperature and headache.
② hyperventilation and bradycardia.
③ dyspnea with increasing cough and fatigue.
④ production of sputum and frequent cough.

10. What condition is caused by abnormally low levels of oxygen in the blood?

① hypoxemia.
② septicemia.
③ hyperventilation.
④ hypercapnia.

11. What is important for the nurse to anticipate in providing care a client who is 2 days post op total laryngectomy?

① he will have a hoarse voice and difficulty speaking.
② the tracheotomy stoma will require cleansing and protection.
③ he will experience respiratory fatigue with activity.
④ hourly suctioning will be required to reduce secretions.

12. A client is three days postoperative from a thoracotomy. What would be a normal finding on assessment of the chest tube?

① dark drainage with no fluctuation of the fluid in the tubing.
② bubbling in the collection chamber on expiration.
③ 300cc daily of serosanguineous drainage.
④ moderate amount of bright red drainage in tubing.

13. The nurse auscultates the upper lung fields of a client with asthma and hears wheezing bilaterally. What causes the wheezing sounds?

① tachypnea and bradycardia.
② increased thickness of mucus.
③ movement of air through narrowed airways.
④ the sound of oxygen delivered via nasal cannula.

14. What statement is correct regarding the procedure for suctioning a client through a tracheotomy?

① catheter is inserted into the tracheotomy tube, intermittent suction is applied until there are no further secretions present.
② the nose and upper airway are suctioned, then the tracheotomy is suctioned.
③ with suction applied, the catheter is inserted into the tracheotomy tube until resistence is met, then catheter is withdrawn. .
④ catheter is inserted into tracheotomy until slight resistence is met, suction is applied as the catheter is withdrawn.

15. What complication might occur in a client who is experiencing increasing broncho spasm?

① metabolic alkalosis.
② hypertension.
③ respiratory arrest.
④ pneumonia.

16. What would create an increased risk of pulmonary infection in the client with chronic pulmonary disease?

① fluid imbalance with pitting edema.
② pooling of respiratory secretions.
③ increase in anterior posterior chest diameter.
④ decreased activity and dehydration.

17. The nurse is assigned to work with a client with active tuberculosis. What assessment findings would the nurse anticipate to be present?

① cough, low grade fever, and night sweats.
② tachycardia, oliguria, night sweats.
③ upper body rash, night sweats, coughing.
④ dyspnea, pleural edema, lack of appetite.

18. A client's forearm has a raised red area about 16mm in diameter after 72 hours. What is the correct interpretation of this Mantoux skin test?

① a negative skin reaction.
② an allergy to the serum.
③ active tuberculosis is present.
④ exposure to the tubercle bacillus.

19. A client is one day postoperative thoracotomy. What nursing observations would indicate the chest tubes are working correctly?

① good bilateral breath sounds, fluctuation of fluid level in drainage tube.

② bubbling in the water sealed chamber with each expiration.

③ bloody drainage in the drainage chamber of the collection device.

④ no drainage or fluctuation of fluid level in tubing coming from the client.

20. How should a sputum specimen for culture and sensitivity be collected?

① collect specimen prior to beginning antibiotics.

② specimen should be collected in the morning.

③ have client rinse his mouth with mouthwash before collecting specimen.

④ collect the specimen at the end of the day to get a concentrated sample.

Appendix 10-1:
PULMONARY DIAGNOSTICS

- CHEST X-RAY:
An x-ray of the lungs and chest wall; no specific pre -or- post care.

- SPUTUM STUDIES:
Culture and Sensitivity (C & S): obtained in order to determine presence of pathogenic bacteria; also determines to which antibiotic the specific organism is sensitive.
Nursing Implications: Obtain the specimen for the culture prior to administering the antibiotics.
Acid-Fast Bacilli : sputum collection and analysis when tuberculosis is suspected.
Cytology: tumors in pulmonary system may slough cells into the sputum; these cells may then be identified.

- BRONCHOSCOPY:
Provides for direct visualization of larynx, trachea, bronchi; client is generally NPO for six hours prior to the exam; preoperative medication is given and the client's upper airway is anesthetized topically. Client is frequently placed in a sitting position and is awake throughout the procedure.
Nursing Implications: Before the test administer sedation and remove dentures and any oral prosthesis. If biopsy is done, carefully assess client for bleeding; do not give anything by mouth until the gag reflex returns. Evaluate respiratory status for signs of distress. After the exam, evaluate the client for return of cough reflex before allowing any PO intake.

- PULMONARY FUNCTION STUDIES:
Purpose:(1) evaluation of the lungs to maintain ventilation; (2) evaluation of response to bronchodilator therapy; (3) differential diagnosis of pulmonary disease, (4) determine progress of client with chronic pulmonary disease. The client must be alert and cooperative, he/she should not be sedated. The client is taken to the pulmonary function laboratory and is asked to breathe into a cylinder from which a computer interprets and records data in specific values. The client must be able to follow directions.
Nursing Implications: client should not smoke for several hours prior to the test. The nurse should determine if the Bronchodilators need to be withheld or given prior to the test.

- LUNG SCAN:
(V/Q Scan): a nuclear medicine procedure to assess the integrity of the pulmonary vessels; particularly useful in the client suspected of having a pulmonary embolus or a ventilation/perfusion problem. A radioactive dye is injected and the specific uptake is recorded on x-ray film; client is not sedated nor on dietary restrictions for the exam.

- OXIMETRY:
An indirect method of measuring the ratio of oxygenated hemoglobin to the total amount of hemoglobin, or the level of oxygen saturation ($Sa0_2$). Measurement is made by placing a sensor on the finger or ear lobe; a beam of light passes through the tissue. Provides a method for continuously evaluating the oxygen saturation levels. It is non-invasive and there are no pre- or- post oximetry preparations. A 90% oxygen saturation (SaO_2) can be compared to a PaO_2 of 55mm Hg; SaO_2 at 90% or below should be immediately evaluated; normal values are 95-100 % SaO_2.

- PULMONARY ANGIOGRAPHY:
Contrast material is injected into the pulmonary arteries and the angiography permits visualization of the pulmonary vasculature. Provides a definitive diagnosis for pulmonary emboli. Client may be NPO for several hours prior to test and may be sedated. Exam is conducted in the x-ray department under fluoroscopic visualization.
Contraindications: (1) dye allergies, (2) unstable client, (3) uncooperative clients.
Complications: (1) cardiac dysrhythmias, (2) anaphylactic reaction to dye (3) hematoma at injection site.
- COMPUTED TOMOGRAPHY (CT)
Lungs are scanned in layers to provide images of a cross sectional view of the chest. Contrast agents may be used.
Nursing Implications: All metal should be removed from the client's body and the client is required to lie still while the machine rotates taking pictures.

- THORACENTESIS:
A large needle is inserted into the pleural cavity; fluid and air are removed. It is utilized for diagnostic as well as therapeutic purposes.
Nursing Implications:
1. Explain procedure to client; it is important that he is very still during the procedure.
2. Position client sitting on the side of the bed with the arms and head over the bedside table. If unable to assume sitting position, place on affected side with the head of the bed slightly elevated. Area containing fluid should be dependent.
3. Support and reassure the client during the procedure.
4. Closely monitor vital signs and general appearance during procedure.
4. After the procedure position the client in a semi-Fowler's position.
5. Evaluate for development of hypoxia secondary to a pneumothorax.
6. Anticipate a chest x-ray after completion to check for possible pneumothorax.
7. *Report respiratory changes to RN.*

Appendix 10-1: PULMONARY DIAGNOSTICS

- ARTERIAL BLOOD GAS STUDIES (ABG):
Measurement of the pH and partial pressures of dissolved gases (O_2, CO_2) of the arterial blood; requires approximately 3 cc of arterial blood obtained through an arterial puncture. If client's O_2 concentration or ventilatory settings have been changed, or if a client has been suctioned, then ABGs should not be drawn for at least 30 minutes (see Table 10-1 Normal ABG Values). Pressure should be maintained at the puncture site for a minimum of 5 minutes. The arterial blood sample should be tightly sealed and placed on ice.
Nursing Implications: Observe puncture site for hematoma development.

- MANTOUX SKIN TEST:
An intradermal skin test; it does not determine if a client has active tuberculosis. A positive result indicates that the client has been exposed to the tubercle bacillus and has developed antibodies (sensitized).
Nursing Implications:
1. Intradermal injection - a small needle (25-27 gauge) is used to inject 0.1 cc of purified protein derivative (PPD) under the skin. The needle is inserted bevel up just below the skin surface, a raised area or "wheal" will form under the skin.
2. The most common area for injection is the inner aspect of the forearm.
3. The client should be given specific directions to return, or plans should be made to read the test in 48 to 72 hours.
4. Interpretation: The largest area of induration is measured, not the area of erythema or inflammation.
   a. 5mm induration or more is positive in immunosuppresed clients, or people who have been recently exposed to active TB.
   b. 10mm induration is positive for people who are at increased risk of infection. This includes IV drug abusers, chronic medical conditions, children under 4 years, institutionalized people.
   c. 15mm induration is positive for people who do not meet any of the other criteria.
5. A chest X-Ray or prophylactic medication follow-up to determine if there is dormant TB, active TB, or the person was exposed and has an adequate immune response. It is also important to determine when and where the person came in contact with the TB bacillus.

NCLEX ALERT: *Modify clients care based on results of diagnostics/lab test. Monitor client during or after a procedure. Explain/teach about scheduled treatments/procedures.*

Appendix 10-2: RESPIRATORY MEDICATIONS

MEDICATIONS	SIDE EFFECTS	NURSING IMPLICATIONS
BRONCHODILATORS: Relax smooth muscle of the bronchi, promoting bronchodilation and reducing airway resistance. Also inhibits the release of histamine.		
❖GENERAL NURSING IMPLICATIONS❖ — Metered Dose Inhalers (MDI) - hand-held pressurized devices that deliver a measured dose of drug with each "puff." When two "puffs" are needed, one minute should lapse between the two "puffs." A spacer should be used to increase the delivery of the medication. —Dry Powder Inhalers (DPI) deliver more medication to lungs, does not require coordination as with MDI, one minute should lapse between "puffs." — Bronchodilators - beta-$_2$ agonists and theophylline are given with caution in the cardiac client, since tachydysrhythmias and chest pain may occur. — Aerosol delivery systems have less side effects and are more effective.		
Epinephrine (**Adrenaline**): aerosol, SQ, IV	Headache Dizziness Hypertension Tremors Dysrhythmias	1. Do not use in clients with hypertension or dysrhythmias. 2. Primarily used to treat asthma attacks and anaphylactic reactions.
Theophylline (**Aminophylline**): PO, rectal, IV	Tachycardia Hypotension Nausea/vomiting Seizures	1. Theophylline blood levels should be drawn for long term use; therapeutic levels between 10-20 mcg/ml; above 20mcg/ml are toxic. 2. IV administration may cause rapid changes in vital signs. 3. Considered to be a third line drug for use with asthma.
***NURSING PRIORITY:** Monitor blood levels of medications.*		
RAPID ACTING		
BETA-$_2$ AGONIST: Albuterol (**Proventil,** **Ventolin**): MDI, DPI, PO Terbutaline (**Brethine**): aerosol, PO Pirbuterol (**Maxair**) MDI		1. Used for short term relief of acute reversible airway problems. 2. Not used on continuous basis in absence of symptoms. 3. Client teaching regarding proper use of MDI and DPI.
ANTI-CHOLINERGIC: Ipratropium bromide (**Atrovent**) aerosol		1. Frequently used for COPD clients and severe asthmatics for treatment of acute airway problems. 2. Therapeutic effects begin within 30 seconds
LONG ACTING CONTROL		
CORTICOSTERIODS: Beclomethasone (**Beclovent**) MDI Triamcinolone acetonide (**Azmacort**) MDI	Oropharyngeal candidiasis, hoarseness	1. Works well with seasonal and exercise-induced asthma (EIA). 2. Prophylactic use decreases number and severity of attacks 3. May be used with beta-$_2$ agonist. 4. Gargle after each dose and use a spacer to decrease candidiasis.
NONSTERIODAL ANTIFLAMMATORY: Cromolyn sodium (**Intal**) MDI	Throat irritation, bad taste, cough	1. Prophylactic use decreases number and severity of attacks. 2. Prevents bronchoconstriction before exposure to known precipitant (e.g. exercise) 3. Administered via MDI - not for an acute attack.
Nedocromil sodium (**Tilade**)	Minimal side effects	
LEUKOTRIENE MODIFIERS Montelukast (**Singular**) PO		1. Given to children over 6 years old. 2. Maximal effects develop within 24 hours.
Zafirlukast (**Accolate**) PO		1. Administer within 1 hour before or 2 hours after eating.

Appendix 10-2: RESPIRATORY MEDICATIONS

MEDICATIONS	SIDE EFFECTS	NURSING IMPLICATIONS
ANTITUBERCULAR: Broad-spectrum antibiotic specific to tubercle bacilli.		
❖GENERAL NURSING IMPLICATIONS❖ — Client is not contagious when sputum culture is negative. — Respiratory isolation when sputum is positive for bacilli. — Treatment includes combination of medications for about 6 to 8 months. — Monitor liver function studies for clients on combination therapy. — Medications may be administered once daily or on a twice weekly schedule. — Teach clients they should not stop taking the medications when they begin to feel better. — Advise client to return to the doctor if he notices any yellowing of his skin or eyes, or begins to experience pain or swelling in joints, especially the big toe.		
Isoniazid (**INH**): PO, IM	Peripheral neuritis Hypersensitivity Hepatotoxicity Gastric irritation	1. Administer with (pyridoxine) Vitamin B_6 to prevent peripheral neuritis. 2. Primary medication used in prophylactic treatment of tuberculosis.
Rifampin (**Rifadin**): PO	Peripheral neuropathy Hypersensitivity Gastric upset Hepatitis	1. Medication most commonly used with isoniazid. 2. May negate the effectiveness of birth control pills. 3. Body secretions may turn orange - urine, perspiration, tears.
Ethambutol (**EMG** or **Myambutol**): PO	Skin rash Gastric upset Peripheral neuritis Optic neuritis Increased uric acid levels	1. Frequently administered with rifampin and **INH**.
Pyrazinamide (**PZA Pyrazinamide, Fibrazid**): PO	Hepatotoxicity Increased uric acid levels	1. Should be taken concurrently with another antituberculosis agent.
DECONGESTANTS: Produces decongestion by acting on sympathetic nerve endings to produce constriction of dilated arterioles.		
Ephedrine hydrochloride (**Bronkotabs, Tendral, Mini-Thins**): PO	Tremors Tachycardia Palpitations Nervousness Headache GI upset	1. Caution client regarding use of OTC medications (cough syrup, cold medications, allergy medications) as ephedrine is a common ingredient in all of these. 2. Cardiac and hypertensive clients should check with their physician prior to taking the medication. 3. May be abused by people seeking the increased CNS stimulation.
Phenylephrine hydrochloride (**Sinex, NEO-Synephrine, Rhinall, Sinarest Nasal**): PO, SQ, intra-nasal	Increased blood pressure Tachycardia Palpitations Trembling Light headedness	1. With intranasal preparations, rebound congestion may occur.
Phenylephrine PO, nasal aerosol spray Pseudoephedrine: PO, nasal aerosol spray (**Sudafed**)	CNS stimulation, anxiety, insomnia	1. Will cause rebound congestion; caution clients to limit use of aerosol nasal sprays to 3 to 5 days. 2. Medications are frequently found in OTC combination decongestants.

NCLEX ALERT: *Evaluate client's use of home remedies and over-the-counter medications.*

Appendix 10-2:
RESPIRATORY MEDICATIONS

MEDICATIONS	SIDE EFFECTS	NURSING IMPLICATIONS
ANTIHISTAMINE: Blocks histamine release at H_1 receptors.		
Diphenhydramine HCL (**Benadryl**): PO, IV, IM Clemastine (**Tavist**): PO Chlorpheniramine (**Chlortrimeton): **PO Loratadine (**Claritin**): PO Fexofenadine (**Allegra**): PO	Sedation Dysrhythmias Dry mouth	1. Used to treat mild allergic disorders. 2. Loratadine and terfenadine are non-sedating. 3. Antihistamines should not be taken during the third trimester of pregnancy. 4. May be found in numerous OTC combination medications. 5. Due to excessive drying effect, asthmatic clients should take medications only on recommendation of physician.
EXPECTORANT: Stimulates secretions. Reduces the viscosity of the mucus.		
Guaifenesin (**Robitussin**): PO	Nausea GI upset	1. Increase fluid intake for effectiveness.
ANTIVIRAL: Antiviral use for treatment of severe RSV in hospitalized children.		
Ribavirin (**Virazole**): aerosol	Anemia, increased respiratory problems	1. Should not be used with infants on mechanical ventilation. 2. Carefully monitor respiratory status of child. 3. Pregnant nurses should not have direct contact with medication.

Appendix 10-3:
SUDDEN AIRWAY OBSTRUCTION

NCLEX ALERT: *Identify and intervene in life-threatening client situations.*

✦ *GOAL: To identify respiratory obstruction.*

1. If the victim can speak or cry, there is probably adequate air exchange.
2. If the victim cannot speak or cry but is conscious, proceed to implement abdominal thrusts to clear the obstructed airway.
3. If the victim is unconscious:
    a. Open the airway and evaluate breathing.
    b. If no evidence of breathing, attempt to ventilate via mouth to mouth or mouth to nose and mouth.
    c. If air does not enter the lungs, check for the patency of the airway and attempt to ventilate again.
    d. If still unable to ventilate, initiate procedure for relieving obstructed airway.

✦ *GOAL: To clear obstructed airway: Adult (conscious and unconscious).*

NURSING PRIORITY: *If the adult client is coughing forcefully, do not interfere with attempts to cough and expel the foreign body. Do not administer any forceful blows to the back.*

ADULT AND CHILD:

1. Conscious: Heimlich maneuver until obstruction is removed or victim becomes unconscious.
2. Unconscious: Evaluate airway and attempt to ventilate. If unable to ventilate, then proceed with steps for removal of foreign body.
    a. The rescuer kneels astride the victim's thighs; with the heel of the hand, apply forceful upward thrust to the abdomen well below the xiphoid and above the umbilicus.
    b. Administer 5 abdominal thrusts, return to the victim's head, evaluate the airway, attempt to ventilate. A blind sweep of the mouth may be done in adult with airway obstruction.
    c. If the above procedure does not relieve the airway, the steps for removal should be repeated until an open airway is established.
    d. Back blows are no longer recommended for relief of airway obstruction in the adult.

NURSING PRIORITY: *The procedure to remove airway obstruction is not effective in the child with epiglottitis or sudden airway obstruction due to inflammation of upper airways.*

✦ *GOAL: To clear obstructed airway: Infant (conscious and unconscious).*

1. Straddle the infant over the forearm with the head dependent.
2. Deliver 4 forceful back blows between the shoulder blades.
3. Supporting the head,, turn the infant back over and administer four chest thrusts (lower one-third of the sternum,, approximately one finger breadth below the nipple line).
4. Attempt to remove foreign body if it can be visualized.

NURSING PRIORITY: *Do not do a blind sweep of the infant or child's mouth. The foreign body should be visualized before attempting to sweep the mouth.*

Appendix 10-4:
WATER-SEALED CHEST DRAINAGE

PURPOSE:

1. To remove air and fluid from the pleural cavity.
2. To restore negative pressure in the pleural cavity and promote re-expansion of the lung.

PRINCIPLE OF WATER-SEALED CHEST DRAINAGE:

The water seal serves as a one-way valve; it prevents air, under atmospheric pressure, from re-entering the pleural cavity. On inspiration, air and fluid leave the pleural cavity via the chest tube. The water-seal keeps the air and fluid from re-entering. Both chest bottles and Pleur-Evac work on the same principle of water-sealed drainage systems.

***NURSING PRIORITY:** There must be a water-seal between the client and the atmospheric pressure. In the bottle setup, the chest tube from the client must go under water before being exposed to the atmospheric pressure. In the Pleur-evac system, there is a water-sealed chamber between the client and the atmospheric pressure.*

EQUIPMENT:

Pleur-evac - a type of molded, plastic system that provides a three-chamber system. There is a waterseal chamber, a collection chamber, and a suction control chamber. When suction is applied, there should be a continuous, gentle bubbling in the suction control chamber.

One-bottle system - chest tube from client goes through underwater seal and drainage is accomplished by gravity. It is the simplest water-sealed system. Prior to the chest tube being connected, approximately 300 cc of normal saline is poured into the bottle. The chest tube is connected to the bottle opening that has a glass or plastic tube that extends approximately 2 cm under water. The amount of saline should be carefully marked on the bottle. The chest bottle serves both as the collection reservoir and as the underwater seal. A positive pressure in the pleural space will force air and fluid out the chest tube; the air will bubble out, but the water-seal prevents air from being drawn back into the pleural cavity.

NURSING IMPLICATIONS:

Assessment
1. Evaluate character of respirations.
2. Evaluate for hypoxia.
3. Assess for symmetrical chest wall expansion.
4. Evaluate breath sounds bilaterally.
5. Palpate around insertion site for subcutaneous emphysema.

Intervention
1. Range of motion of the affected arm and shoulder.
2. Encourage coughing and deep breathing every two hours.
3. Encourage ambulation if appropriate.
4. Pain medications as indicated.
5. Low-or semi-Fowler's position.

Observe drainage system for proper functioning.
1. Water level in tubing from the client should fluctuate (tidal): rise on inspiration and fall on expiration.
2. Continuous bubbling should not occur in the fluid where water-seal is maintained; continuous bubbling indicates an air leak; continuous bubbling should occur only in the system that maintains a third chamber for suction control.
3. Initial bubbling may occur with coughing or with deep respiration as air is moved out of the pleural cavity.
4. Place a piece of tape on the outside of the drainage collection bottle to monitor amount of drainage. Be sure to indicate initial water added to bottle to establish water-seal.

Appendix 10-4:
WATER-SEALED CHEST DRAINAGE

Maintain water-sealed system.

1. Keep all drainage equipment below level of client's chest.
2. Evaluate for dependent loops in the tubing; this increases the resistance to the drainage. All extra tubing should be coiled in the bed and flow in a straight line to the system.
3. Tape all connections.
4. Note characteristics and amount of drainage. Mark level on the drainage system PRN and every eight hours.
5. Vigorous "milking" or stripping chest tubes is controversial. Stripping or milking may be done when the chest tube becomes occluded with a clot, most often in the immediate postoperative time. Stripping should not be done routinely on all clients.
6. Change collection chamber when approximately half full. The increased volume in the collection chamber increases resistance to flow of drainage. It is institution policy whether the nurse can change the collection chamber.

Figure 10-3: Water Sealed Chest Drainage
Reprinted with permission: Phipps, WJ, Sands, JK, & Marek, JF (1999). *Medical Surgical Nursing: Concepts & Clinical Practice*, 6th ed. Philadelphia: Mosby, p.956.

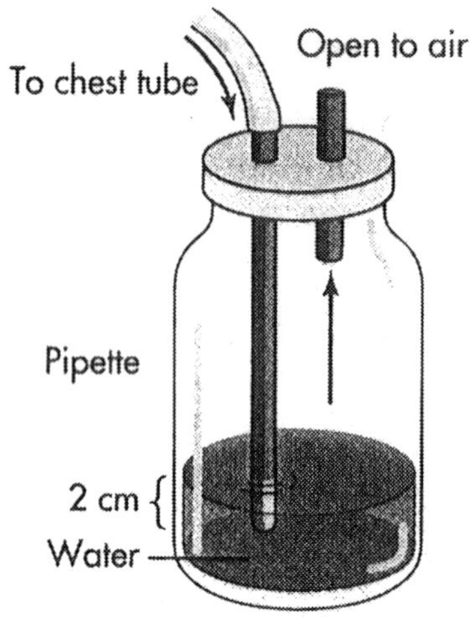

One-Bottle setup

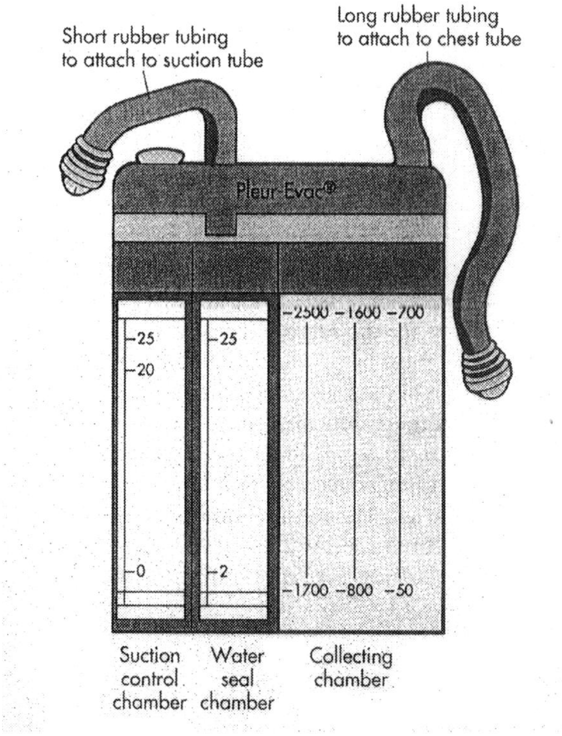

Pleuravac System

Appendix 10-4:
WATER-SEALED CHEST DRAINAGE

NCLEX ALERT: *Maintain patency of client tubes to prevent complications. Monitor client drainage for each tube. Position tubes to promote drainage. Identify progressive changes in respiratory status.*

Chest tube removal.

1. Criteria for removal of the tube:
   a. Minimum or no drainage.
   b. Fluctuations stop in the water-seal chamber.
   c. Chest X-ray reveals expanded lung.
   d. Client is breathing comfortably.
2. Procedure.
   a. Obtain equipment.
   b. Generally, the physician will want the client in a low-or semi-Fowler's position unless contraindicated.
   c. The physician will ask the client to exhale and hold it or to exhale and bear down. Either of these procedures will increase the intrathoracic pressure and prevent air from entering the pleural space.
   d. With the client holding his breath, the physician will quickly remove the tube and place an occlusive bandage over the area; client can then breathe normally.
   e. Assess the client's tolerance of the procedure; a chest X-ray should be done to determine that the lungs remain fully expanded.

Appendix 10-5:
ARTIFICIAL AIRWAYS

❑ **ENDOTRACHEAL INTUBATION: Placement of an endotracheal (ET) tube through the mouth or nose into the trachea.**

✦ *GOAL: To provide an immediate airway; to maintain a patent airway; to facilitate removal of secretions.*

Nursing Interventions:

1. Provide warm, humidified oxygen at designated level.
2. Establish method of communication since the client cannot speak; child cannot cry.
3. Maintain safety measures.
   a. Prevent client from removing tube inadvertently.
   b. Secure ET tube to the face.
   c. Child with an ET tube requires continuous attendance.
4. Assess for symmetrical expansion of chest wall and bilateral breath sounds. If tube slips farther into the trachea, it may pass into the right mainstem bronchus, obliterating the left mainstem bronchus.
5. Provide oral hygiene; assess for pressure areas on the nose or the mouth.
6. If the client is on assisted ventilation through a ventilator or is receiving a respiratory treatment via a positive pressure machine, the cuff on the ET tube must be inflated. If the client has adequate spontaneous respirations and is not on assisted ventilation, the cuff is left deflated.
7. Maintain the client in a semi-Fowler's position.
8. Suction as indicated (see Appendix 10-6).

Appendix 10-5:
ARTIFICIAL AIRWAYS

❑ **TRACHEOSTOMY: A surgical opening into the trachea.**

✦ *GOAL: To maintain airway over an extended period of time and to facilitate removal of secretions.*

Nursing Interventions:

1. Maintain warm, humidified oxygen at designated level.
2. Establish method of communication since client cannot speak; child is unable to cry.
3. Maintain safety measures.
   a. Secure tracheal tube to the client's neck.
   b. Prevent clothing or bedcovers from occluding area of trachea opening.
   c. Child with a tracheostomy requires continuous attendance.
4. Assess for symmetrical expansion of chest wall and bilateral breath sounds.
5. Provide oral hygiene.
6. Cuff must remain inflated if client is on a volume ventilator or receiving a respiratory treatment. If the client has adequate spontaneous respiration, the cuff is usually left deflated.
7. Suction as indicated (see Appendix 10-6).
8. The tracheal tube obturator should be taped to the head of the bed. If the tracheostomy tube is accidentally removed, the obturator is necessary for replacing the tube.

With both types of artificial airways, frequent nursing assessment of respiratory status is imperative.

NCLEX ALERT: *Provide tracheostomy care.*

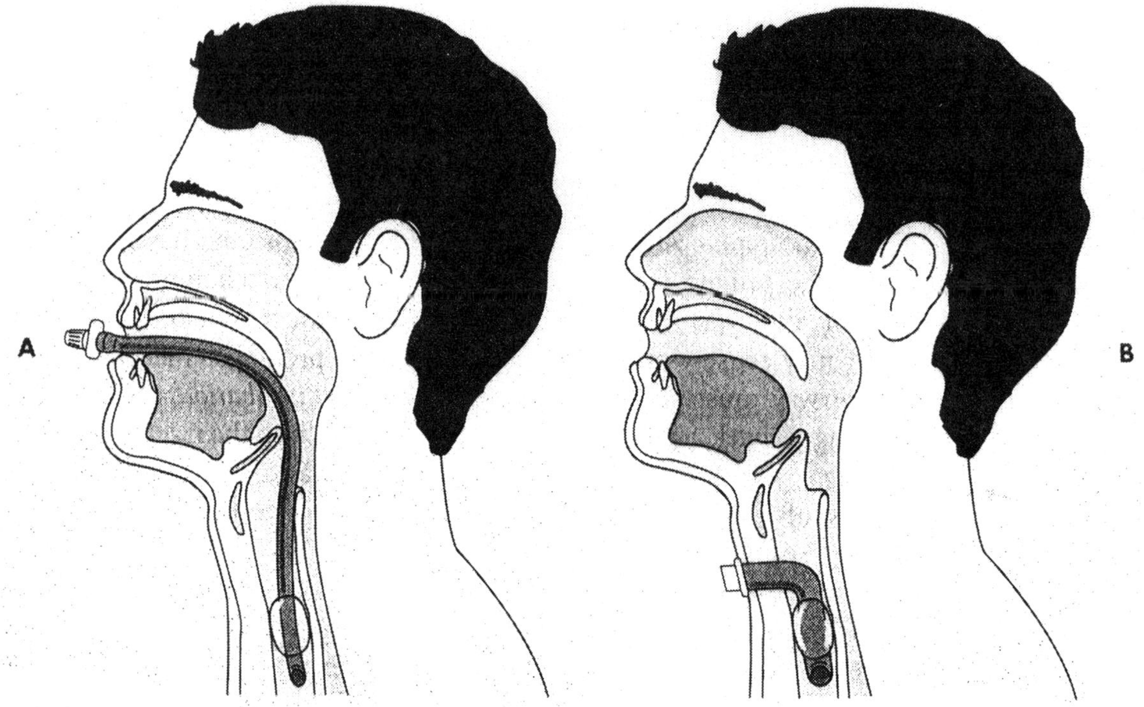

Figure 10-4: Position For Endotracheal/ Tracheostomy Tube.
Reprinted with permission: Phipps, WJ, Sands, JK, & Marek, JF (1999). *Medical Surgical Nursing: Concepts & Clinical Practice*, 6th ed. Philadelphia: Mosby, p.904

Appendix 10-6:
SUCTIONING THROUGH ARTIFICIAL AIRWAYS

NURSING PRIORITY: *Suctioning the endotracheal tube or the tracheostomy is done to remove excess secretions and to maintain patent airway. The client should always be suctioned prior to deflating a cuff.*

1. Determine that the client needs to be suctioned.
   a. Auscultate lungs to detect presence of secretions.
   b. Observe client to see if he/she is coughing and experiencing difficulty with removal of secretions.
2. Explain procedure if client is not familiar with it, or simply indicate to client that you are going to assist him/her with the removal of the secretions.
3. All equipment introduced into the trachea or the endotracheal tube should be sterile.
4. Prepare the equipment. Attach the suction catheter to the suction source while maintaining sterile glove and suction catheter.
5. If client is not in immediate danger of airway occlusion, hyperoxygenate with 100% O_2 for five to six minutes, or at least three hyperinflations.
6. Gently insert sterile catheter into the opening without suction being applied. Insert catheter to the point of slight resistance, then pull catheter back one to two centimeters.
7. Apply intermittent suction as you gently rotate the catheter on removal.
8. Each suctioning pass should not exceed 10 to 15 seconds in duration.
9. Reconnect client to oxygen source and evaluate if one suctioning episode was sufficient to remove secretions.
10. Hyperoxygenate client for 1-5 minutes after suctioning; assess vital signs and O_2 saturation, values should return to normal or to the previous or higher levels prior to suctioning.
11. Avoid suctioning client prior to blood gases being drawn. Client should stabilize for approximately 30 minutes prior to blood gases being drawn.

Complications of Suctioning:

1. Hypoxia - preoxygenate with high % of O_2 prior to and after suctioning.
2. Dysrhythmias - limit suctioning to 10-15 seconds, monitor rhythm during suctioning. If bradycardia develops, discontinue suctioning immediately .
3. Bronchospasm - try to time the suctioning with client's own cycle, insert tube during inspiration.
4. Airway trauma - maintain suction level below 120mm Hg.
5. Infection - use sterile technique; assess the color and quantity of sputum suctioned.
6. Atelectasis -use suction catheters that are approximately 1/3 or less of diameter of tube.

NCLEX ALERT: *Intervene to improve respiratory status (insert oral airway, suction, etc.).*

Appendix 10-7: OXYGEN

Methods Of Administration:	1. ***Low flow systems*** - nasal cannula, standard mask, non-rebreather mask. Oxygen is measured in liters per minute flow (LPM). 2. ***High flow systems*** - Venturi mask, nebulizer mask, and volume ventilators. Oxygen is measured in fractions of inspired oxygen (FIO_2) in concentrations from 24% to 100%.
Humidification:	1. Adds water vapor to inspired gas. 2. Prevents drying and irritation of respiratory membranes. 3. Loosens thick secretions, allowing them to be more easily removed.
Indications for Oxygen Use:	1. A decrease in oxygen in the arterial blood (hypoxemia). 2. An increase in the work of breathing. 3. To decrease the cardiac workload.
Safety Precautions For Oxygen Administration:	1. Properly ground all electrical equipment. 2. Do not permit any smoking by anyone in the area. 3. Use water-base, not oil-base lubricants.

COMPLICATIONS OF OXYGEN THERAPY

Oxygen Toxicity:	A medically induced condition produced by inhalation of high concentrations of oxygen over a prolonged period of time. 1. Tracheal irritation. 2. Dyspnea and increasing cough. 3. Decrease in vital capacity. 4. The PaO_2 continues to decrease, even with an increasing FIO_2.
Atelectasis:	Alveoli collapse with increased oxygen concentrations; there is a decrease in the production of surfactant.
Retinal Damage:	High concentrations of oxygen over a prolonged period of time in the adult client can precipitate changes in the lens and cornea. Retrolental fibroplasia occurs in infants who require high concentrations of oxygen.

NCLEX ALERT: *Administer prescribed oxygen therapy. Determine oxygenation status of client. Monitor client receiving oxygen therapy.*

Appendix 10-8: NURSING PROCEDURE ■ SPUTUM SPECIMEN COLLECTION ■

✦ Test analyzes sputum samples (material expectorated from client's lungs and bronchi during deep coughing) to diagnose respiratory disease, identify the cause of pulmonary infections, identify abnormal lung cells, and assist in managing pulmonary disease.

✓ Key Points: Specimen Collection

- Encourage client to increase fluid intake the night before to assist in collecting specimen.
- Collect the specimen early in the morning, as bacteria is most concentrated at this time.
- No mouth wash prior to collection of specimen.
- Aerosal mist will assist to decrease thickness of sputum and increase effectiveness of coughing.
- Maintain strict asepsis and standard precautions in collecting and transporting specimen; utilize a sterile specimen collection container.
- Cytology specimens and acid-fast bacillus — may need to obtain several consecutive morning specimens.
- Culture and sensitivity — initial specimen should be obtained before administering antibiotics.

Clinical Tips for Problem Solving

If client experiences pain while coughing,

❑ Support/splint painful area with roll pillows to minimize pain and discomfort.
❑ Encourage client to take several deep breaths prior to beginning (Table 10-3). This assists in triggering the cough reflex and aerates the lungs.

If client is unable to obtain sputum specimen,

❑ Attempt procedure early in the morning; when mucus production is greatest.
❑ Notify physician to obtain orders for a bronchodilator or nebulization therapy.

NCLEX ALERT: *Collect client specimen according to policies/procedures. Explain procedures for specimen collection.*

Notes

Vascular System

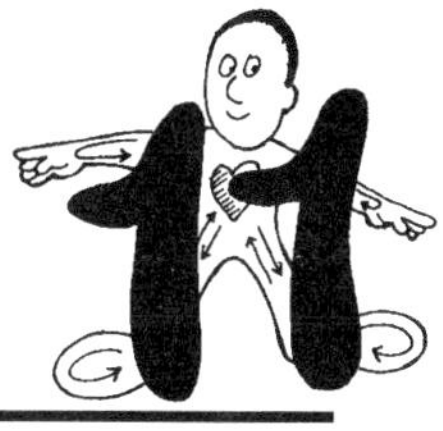

PHYSIOLOGY OF THE VASCULAR SYSTEM

Vessels

A. Arteries.

1. Primary function is to transport nutrients and oxygen to the cellular level.
2. Arterial vascular system is a high pressure system with a rapid blood flow.

B. Capillaries.

1. Small microscopic vessels at the cellular level.
2. Capillary bed is the area of circulation where the arterioles branch into capillaries and exchange between the circulating volume and the interstitial fluid occurs.

C. Veins.

1. Primary function of the veins is to return blood to the heart.
2. Veins contain valves to maintain direction of blood flow and to prevent the backflow of blood. prevent the back flow of blood and maintain direction of blood flow.
3. Venous system is a low pressure system.

D. Circulatory systems.

1. Systemic circulation - the flow of blood from the heart into the aorta and through the arteries to the capillary bed, where cellular nutrition and oxygenation occur.
2. Pulmonary circulation - the flow of blood from the right ventricle through the pulmonary artery into the lungs, then through the capillary beds of the lungs, where the blood picks up oxygen and releases carbon dioxide and returns back into the left ventricle through the pulmonary veins.
3. Hepatic-portal circulation - the flow of blood from the venous system of the stomach, intestines, spleen, and pancreas into the portal vein and through the liver for removal of foreign material; venous blood leaves the liver through the hepatic vein and into the inferior vena cava for return to the heart.

E. Lymphatic system - primary function is to return fluid and protein to the blood from the interstitial fluid.

Mechanics of Blood Flow

A. Blood flow is controlled by:

1. The diameter of the vessel.
2. The length of the vessel.
3. The pressure at either end of the vessel.
4. The viscosity of the blood.

B. Physiological control.

1. Autoregulation - the ability of tissue to control its own blood flow. Autoregulatory system enables blood supply to vital organs (brain, kidney, heart) to remain relatively constant, even though blood pressure may fluctuate within normal ranges.
2. Nervous system control.
   a. Parasympathetic nervous system — influence on blood flow is the regulation of the heart rate by the vagus nerve.
   b. Sympathetic nervous system.
      (1) Primary influence of sympathetic system is on arterioles for dilation and constriction of the vessels in order to maintain peripheral resistance and vasomotor tone.
      (2) Peripheral resistance is resistance of arterioles to flow of blood.
      (3) Dilation decreases peripheral resistance, thereby decreasing blood pressure; vasoconstriction increases peripheral resistance, thereby increasing blood pressure.

Blood Pressure

A. Systolic blood pressure represents the ejection of the blood from the heart. The systolic pressure is determined primarily by the amount of blood ejected.

B. Diastolic pressure represents the pressure remaining in the arteries at the end of systole. Diastolic pressure depends on the ability of the arteries to stretch and handle the blood flow.

C. Pulse pressure is the difference between the systolic and diastolic pressures.

D. Decreased renal blood flow will precipitate an increase in blood pressure.

DISORDERS OF THE VASCULAR SYSTEM

Arteriosclerosis

❑ ***Arteriosclerosis* is the most common disease of the *arteries*. The word means "hardening of the arteries."**

A. Atherosclerosis - most common classification of arteriosclerosis; characterized by stenosis and obstruction in the lumen of the vessel. (Fig. 11-1)

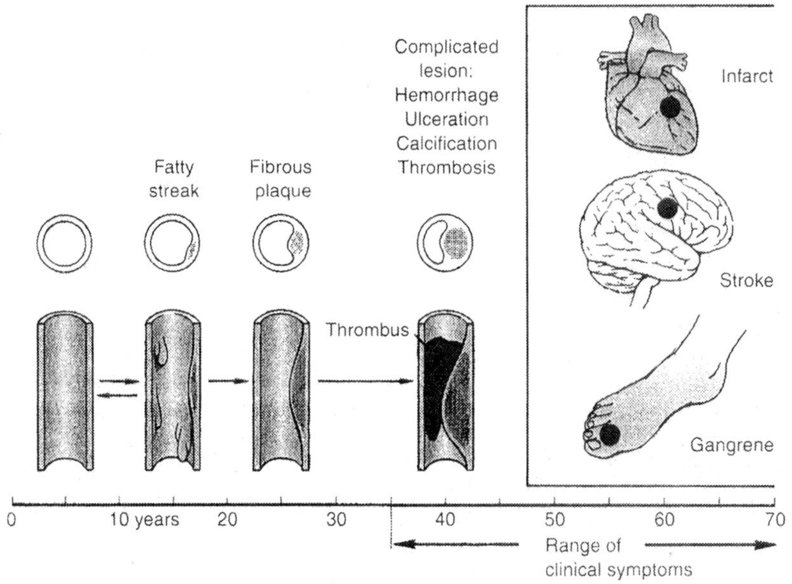

Fig 11-1: Schematic Concept of the Progression of Atherosclerosis.
Reprinted with permission: Smeltzer, SC, Bare, BG, *Brunner and Suddarth's Textbook of Medical Surgical Nursing,* 9th ed. Lippincott: Philadelphia, p. 689.

1. Process is slow; generally no evidence of problems until a major artery is affected and there is severe decrease in blood supply to tissue supplied by artery involved.
2. Arteries commonly affected by atherosclerosis and ensuing problems.
   a. Coronary arteries - myocardial infarction.
   b. Cerebrovascular arteries - cerebrovascular accident.
   c. Aorta-aortic aneurysm, peripheral occlusive disease.
   d. Large peripheral arteries - peripheral occlusive disease.

Data Collection

1. Modifiable risk factors.
   a. Diet high in saturated fats (cholesterol).
   b. Smoking.
   c. Obesity.
   d. Decreased activity.
   e. Stress.
2. Non-modifiable risk factors.
   a. Familial tendencies.
   b. Age.
3. Conditions accelerating atherosclerotic development.
   a. Diabetes mellitus.
   b. Hypertension.
   c. High cholesterol levels with high triglyceride levels
4. Clinical manifestations - depend on artery involved.
5. Diagnostics.
   a. Clinical manifestation of specific area involved.
   b. Increased serum triglycerides, lipids, and cholesterol.

Treatment

1. Decrease cholesterol diet.
2. Decrease risk factors as appropriate.
3. Anti-hyperlipidemic medications (Appendix 11-2).
4. Peripheral vasodilating medications.
5. Vascular surgery.

Nursing Intervention

See Nursing Intervention for specific areas involved.

Hypertension

❑ ***Hypertension* is a persistent increase in blood pressure.**

A. Classification.
   1. Essential (primary, benign, idiopathic) - etiology unknown; accounts for approximately 85 to 95 % of hypertensive clients.
   2. Secondary - accounts for approximately 10 to 15 percent of hypertension cases; the sustained elevation is due to an identifiable cause.

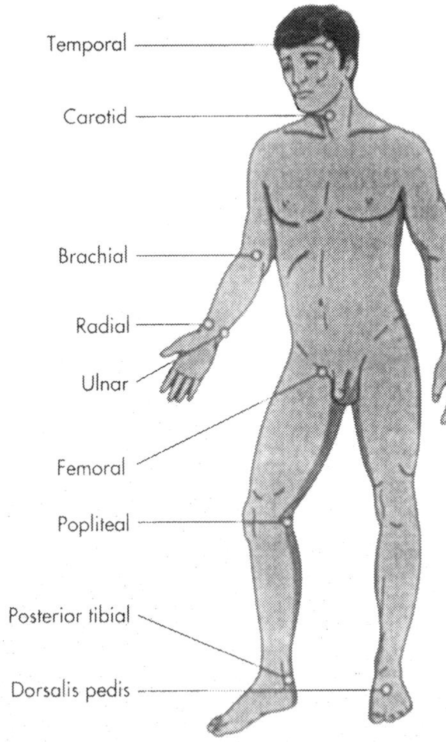

Figure 11-2: Body Sites for Peripheral Pulses.
Reprinted with permission: Phipps, WJ, Sands, JK, & Marek, JF (1999). *Medical Surgical Nursing: Concepts & Clinical Practice*, 6th ed. Philadelphia: Mosby, p. 619.

a. Increased intracranial pressure.
b. Renal disease.
c. Pregnancy- induced hypertension (toxemia).
d. Cushing's syndrome.
e. Thyrotoxicosis.

3. Malignant hypertension - a sustained increase in the diastolic pressure which is unresponsive to treatment.
4. Hypertensive crisis - when the degree of hypertension is a life-threatening situation.

Data Collection

1. Risk factors in essential hypertension (See Table 11-2).
2. Clinical manifestations of essential hypertension.
   a. Increase in blood pressure.
   b. Headache.
   c. Dizziness.
   d. Palpitations.
   e. Increase in the rate of atherosclerosis.
3. Clinical manifestations of malignant hypertension.
   a. Diastolic pressure usually above 120 mm Hg.
   b. More critical in clients with previously compromised cardiovascular system.

Box 11-1: Elderly Care Focus
Evaluation of Blood Pressure

- If a client has been hypertensive for a long period of time, the client's "normal" blood pressure may need to be higher to maintain adequate blood flow and allow client to perform ADL.
- For clients over 65, high blood pressure may be defined as systolic over 160mm Hg and diastolic over 95mm Hg.
- Increased problems with orthostatic hypotension; teach client how to avoid.
- Obtain blood pressure standing, lying, and sitting. Make sure client has not had any nicotine or coffee for about an hour prior to taking blood pressure.
- Compliance problems occur when client has to take several medications for B/P, as well as cope with other chronic health problems.

   c. Blood pressure is unresponsive to medications.
   d. May be a complication of essential and secondary hypertension.
   e. May precipitate a hypertensive crisis.

NCLEX ALERT: *Compare current data to client baseline data (e.g. vital signs). Determine if vital signs are abnormal*

4. Diagnostics.
   a. Increase in blood pressure, especially diastolic pressure on two separate occasions at least 2 weeks apart.
      (1) Diastolic of 90mmHg or higher.
      (2) Systolic of 140mmHg or higher.
   b. Diagnostics to rule out problem of secondary hypertension.

Geriatric Priority: *For clients over 65, high blood pressure may be defined as systolic over 160mmHg and diastolic over 95mmHg.*

5. Complications.
   a. Coronary artery disease.
   b. Cerebral vascular disease (Chapter 15).
      (1) Transient ischemic attacks (TIA).
      (2) Cerebrovascular accident (CVA).
   c. Nephrosclerosis - ischemia of the intrarenal vessels.
   d. Retinal damage - ischemia of the arterioles in the retina.
   e. Hypertensive crisis.

Table 11-1: Risk Factors in Essential Hypertension

NONMODIFIABLE FACTORS	*MODIFIABLE FACTORS*
Age	Obesity
Sex	Stress
Ethnic group	Cigarette smoking
Family history	Excess sodium intake Elevated lipids

NCLEX ALERT: *Review with client understanding of health promotion behaviors.*

Treatment

1. Diet.
   a. Low sodium.
   b. Weight reduction, client should be within 0% of ideal weight.
   c. Decreased cholesterol and saturated fats.
2. Regular exercise.
3. Antihypertensive medications (See Appendix 11-4, Table 11-2).
4. Diuretics to decrease circulating volume (See Appendix 11-5).

NCLEX ALERT: *Assist client with prescribed dietary modifications.*

5. Limit alcohol intake to 1-2 ounces per day.
6. Assist client to cope effectively with stress.
7. Stop smoking.

Nursing Intervention

✦ *Goal: to identify the high-risk individual, and educate public regarding disease process.*

1. Encourage client to participate in community blood pressure screening programs.
2. Educate public regarding risk factors.
3. Identify health promoting behavior for high-risk individuals. See Table 11-3

✦ *Goal: to reduce blood pressure and assist client to maintain control.*

1. Assess response to medication.
   a. Antihypertensives (See Appendix 11-4).
   b. Diuretics (See Appendix 11-5).

Table 11-2: Lifestyle Modifications for Hypertension Prevention and Control

- Lose weight if over weight
- Limit alcohol intake
- Increase aerobic physical activity (30-45 minutes 3-4 days a week.
- Reduce sodium intake, 2.4 sodium, 6g sodium chloride per day.
- Maintain daily potassium intake.
- Maintain adequate intake of dietary calcium and magnesium
- Stop smoking
- Reduce intake of dietary saturated fat and cholesterol

NCLEX ALERT: *Review client/family understanding of health promotion behaviors.*

2. Evaluate blood pressure in a lying down, sitting, and then a standing position.
3. Maintain low-sodium diet.
4. Assess changes in weight with regard to low-sodium intake and diuretics.
5. When blood pressure is initially decreased, evaluate client's tolerance to decrease.
   a. Presence of postural hypotension.
   b. Urinary output.
   c. Change in energy level.
   d. Changes in level of consciousness.
6. *Notify the RN of significant changes in BP. Maintain client on bedrest until RN can evaluate situation.*

***NURSING PRIORITY:** Obtain hemodynamic measurements - the BP of a hypertensive person should be measured lying down, sitting, and then standing. It is measured in both right and left arms.*

Self-Care

1. Continue low-cholesterol, low-sodium diet.
2. Decrease weight if appropriate.
3. Assist to identify an appropriate, consistent, regular exercise program.
   a. A gradually increasing exercise program.
   b. Episodic strenuous activity should be avoided.
   c. Walking, swimming, slow jogging.
   d. Avoid weight lifting and heavy isometric exercises.

NCLEX ALERT: *Identify side effects and adverse reactions of medications*

4. Take prescribed medications.
   a. Take medication at regular times.
   b. Know the names and common side effects of the medications.
   c. Side effects of the medication.
   d. Poor relationship between client and health care providers may cause non-compliance.
   e. Instruct about medications for self-administration.
5. Avoid hot baths, steam rooms, spas (increases vasodilating effect of medications).
6. Decrease problems of orthostatic hypotension.
   a. Get up slowly, sit at the bedside to regain equilibrium, then stand slowly.
   b. Wear elastic support hose.
   c. Lie or sit down when dizziness occurs.
   d. Do not stand or sit for prolonged periods of time.
7. Side effects of medication are frequently temporary.
8. If sexual problems or impotence develop, contact physician. Do not stop taking medication.

Peripheral Vascular Disease (PVD)

❑ ***PVD*** **primarily involves narrowing and obstruction of the *arteries* of the extremities, especially the lower extremities. The atherosclerotic lesion causes chronic arterial obstruction, which leads progressively to decreased oxygen delivery to the tissue.**

A. Lesions are predominantly found in the lower aorta, from below the renal arteries extending through the popliteal area.
B. By the time symptoms occur, the artery is approximately 85 to 95 percent occluded.
C. The femoral, popliteal, and iliac are the most common sites affected.

NCLEX ALERT: *Recognize client with conditions resulting in insufficient vascular perfusion.*

Data Collection

1. Risk factors (see also those for atherosclerosis).
   a. More common in males.
   b. Generally occurs during the fifth or sixth decade of life.
   c. Familial tendency.
   d. Diabetics.
2. Clinical manifestations.
   a. Intermittent claudication (pain with activity, relieved by rest).
   b. Ischemic pain at rest (increasing severity).
   c. Paresthesia of the feet.
   d. Pallor of the extremities.
   e. Decreased or absent peripheral pulses. (Fig. 11-2)
      (1) Pedal.
      (2) Popliteal.
      (3) Femoral.
   f. Poor healing of injuries on the extremities.
   g. Changes in the skin.
      (1) Cool to touch.
      (2) Shiny, fragile, poor turgor.
      (3) Dry, scaly.
      (4) Loss of hair on the lower leg.
   h. Brittle, thick toenails.
   i. Dependent rubor - dusky, purplish discoloration of extremity when in dependent position.

NURSING PRIORITY: *Identify symptoms of deep vein thrombosis - the clinical manifestations of PVD are the same for any client experiencing arterial vascular circulation problems (cardiac catheterization, compression under a cast, etc.).*

Treatment

1. Medical.
   a. Vasodilating medications.
   b. Decrease progression of atherosclerosis.
   c. Prevent and control infections.
   d. Decrease dietary cholesterol intake.
   e. Exercise program as tolerated.
2. Surgical - procedures are done when intermittent claudication interferes with the client's activities of daily living or when the circulation must be restored in order to salvage the limb.
   a. Endarterectomy - removal of plaque within the artery.
   b. Bypass graft.
   c. Excision of affected area with graft replacement.
   d. Sympathectomy.
3. Percutaneous transluminal angioplasty - utilization of a balloon catheter to compress the plaque against the arterial wall.

Nursing Intervention

✦ *Goal: to evaluate level of involvement of the extremity.*

1. Assess peripheral pulses; compare quality of pulses in the lower extremities.
2. Evaluate skin on the affected extremity.
   a. Color, warmth.
   b. Capillary refill.
   c. Condition of the skin and nailbeds.
   d. Presence of ulcers or lesions.
3. Assess tolerance to activity; at what point pain occurs.

NCLEX ALERT: *Review assessment of peripheral pulses. Notify supervisor of signs of potential complications*

✦ *Goal: to prevent injury and infection.*

1. Avoid vigorous rubbing of the extremity.
2. Prevent skin breakdown at pressure sites - heel, ankle, and knees.
3. Heel covers and bed cradle to prevent pressure on the toes and heel.
4. Maintain good skin hygiene and proper care of toenails.
   a. Do not trim the toenails.
   b. Do not trim callouses or corns.
   c. *Advise RN if client has ingrown toenails.*
5. Teach client to always wear shoes.

NCLEX ALERT: *Identify client methods for preventing complications associated with illness. Identify factors that affect wound healing.*

✦ *Goal: to increase arterial supply and decrease venous congestion to the extremity.*

1. Encourage moderate exercise, (i.e., walking).
2. Active postural exercises (Buerger-Allen exercises).
3. Maintain constant warm temperature; do not use hot water bottles or heating pads.
4. Avoid pressure in the posterior popliteal area.
   a. Do not raise knee gatch on the bed without raising the foot of the bed to eliminate the pressure behind the knee.
   b. When the client is sitting in a chair, make sure the feet are flat on the floor to decrease the pressure from the edge of the chair behind the knee.
   c. Teach client to avoid clothing that is tight and restricts circulation to the lower extremities (knee-high hose, girdles, etc.).
5. If there are ulcers on the legs or feet the client may be maintained on bedrest until areas are healed.
6. Prevent vasoconstriction
   a. Decrease caffeine intake.
   b. Stop smoking.
   c. Avoid chilling.

✦ *Goal: to assist client to control chronic diseases precipitating problems with peripheral vascular disease.*

1. Diabetes.
2. Hypertension.

***NURSING PRIORITY:** In planning nursing intervention to prevent complications in the diabetic client, the problem of peripheral vascular disease must be included.*

✦ *Goal: to provide appropriate preoperative care (See Chapter 3).*

✦ *Goal: to evaluate and promote circulation in affected extremity postoperative vascular surgery.*

1. Extremity circulation checks - initially every 15 minutes, then hourly, then every four hours. *Notify RN immediately of any changes in pulses*
2. Encourage movement of the extremity as soon as client is awake.
3. Encourage client to be out of bed and ambulate as soon as indicated, pulse checks when client returns to bed.
4. Do not raise the knee gatch of the bed.
5. Avoid flexion in the area of the graft (femoral or popliteal areas).
6. Assess client's response to anticoagulants, maintain bleeding precautions (Chpater14).
7. Continue measures to protect the feet.
8. 6. Assess for development of dependent edema, may require compression dressings or diuretic.

✦ *Goal: to provide general postoperative care as indicated (See Chapter 3).*

Self-Care

1. Decrease weight if appropriate.
2. Avoid:
   a. Standing or sitting for prolonged periods of time.
   b. Constrictive clothing.
   c. Smoking.
3. Avoid trauma to the extremities.

4. Inspect extremities daily for:
   a. Discolored areas.
   b. Breaks in the skin.
   c. Infection.
5. Do not apply direct heat to the legs.
6. Exercise as tolerated, stop if pain occurs.
7. Very careful, consistent care of the feet.
   a. Do not go barefoot.
   b. Do not put lotion on open ulcers or sores.
   c. Elevate feet if they are swelling.
   d. Check feet daily.
8. Maintain good nutrition.

NCLEX ALERT: *Review client adaptations to illness and/or disease. Assist client tn identifying behaviors that could impact health.*

Thromboangiitis obliterans (Buerger's Disease)

❑ **An inflammatory, thrombotic problem of the distal *arteries*; starts distally and progresses upward.**

Data Collection

1. Intermittent claudication.
2. Pain is predominant symptom
3. Cyanosis and redness of the extremity.
4. Increased sensitivity to cold in the extremity.
5. Decreased sensation.
6. Peripheral pulses may be diminished or absent.
7. Smoking aggravates the problem.

Treatment

No cure; treatment is based on symptoms.

Nursing Intervention

✦ *Goal: to evaluate level of involvement of the extremity and increase circulation to the extremity.*

1. Encourage client to decrease or stop smoking.
2. Evaluate tolerance to activity.
3. Inspect feet for vascular changes.
4. Have client perform postural exercises to decrease venous congestion.
5. Circulatory checks of the affected extremity.

NURSING PRIORITY: *The vascular problem has a direct relationship to cigarette smoking. The client should understand that in order for the condition to be controlled, he must quit smoking.*

✦ *Goal: to assist client to understand implications of the disease and measures to maintain health (see PVD Goal to assist client to understand implications of the disease).*

Raynaud's Disease

❑ **A disease characterized by episodic spasms of the *small cutaneous arteries*. It occurs primarily in the fingers.**

Raynaud's phenomena

A. Intermittent episodic spasms of the arterioles of the extremities. Spasms are not necessarily correlated with other peripheral vascular problems.

B. Condition usually occurs in the hands and is bilateral and symmetrical.

Data Collection

1. Increased incidence in females age 20 to 49.
2. Symptoms are precipitated by:
   a. Exposure to cold.
   b. Emotional upset.
   c. Smoking.
3. Initially, there is pallor or cyanosis due to the vasospasm, causing numbness and tingling. As digits warm, there is redness, warmth, and throbbing as hyperemia occurs.
4. Involvement generally is bilateral.
5. Pulses may remain adequate.
6. Attacks are usually intermittent.

Treatment

1. No cure; treatment is based on symptoms.
2. Vasodilating medications.

Nursing Intervention

✦ *Goal: to assist client to understand disease implications and measures to increase arterial circulation.*

1. Decrease or quit smoking.
2. Evaluate client's response to activities.
3. Circulatory checks of the affected extremity.
4. Visual inspection of the skin of the affected extremity.

Aneurysm

❑ **A dilation or sac formed on the wall of an *arterial vessel.***

A. Abdominal aortic aneurysm (AAA) - occurs primarily in the abdominal aorta below the renal arteries.

B. Thoracic aortic aneurysm - located on the aorta in the thoracic area.

C. Factors common to aneurysms.

1. Increase in size of the vessel due to continuous pulsation of blood.
2. Eventual rupture.

D. Dissecting aneurysm.

1. Characterized by destruction of small muscle and elastic tissue of artery.
2. Bleeding between the layers of the vessel wall occurs.
3. Aortic aneurysm dissection is usually accompanied by severe back, abdominal, or chest pain.
4. Dissection precedes rupture of the artery, however, symptoms may not be recognized.

Data Collection

1. Clinical manifestations - abdominal aortic aneurysm.
   a. May be asymptomatic.
   b. Complaints of back, flank, or abdominal pain.
   c. Epigastric discomfort.
2. Diagnostic (See Appendix 11-1).
   a. X ray.
   b. Aortography.
   c. Sonography.
3. Complications - rupture, hemorrhage, and renal failure.

Treatment

Directed toward prevention of rupture; surgical resection of the aneurysm.

Nursing Intervention

✦ *Goal: to prepare client and family for anticipated surgery.*

NCLEX ALERT: *Determine if client is prepared for surgery. Monitor client after surgery.*

1. Provide appropriate preoperative care (See Chapter 3).
2. Identify other chronic health problems.
3. Evaluate characteristic of pulses in the lower extremities, mark them and document status of circulation for evaluation postoperative.
4. Do not vigorously palpate the abdomen.
5. Evaluate for indications of dissection.
   a. Constant intense pain.
   b. Symptoms of hemorrhagic shock.
   c. Abdomen may remain soft.
6. Keep blood pressure at lowest level for client tolerance.

✦ *Goal: to promote graft patency and optimum circulation postoperative aneurysm resection.*

1. General postoperative care as indicated (See Chapter 3).
2. Maintain adequate blood pressure to facilitate tissue perfusion and filling of the graft.
3. IV fluids and blood components as indicated.
4. Initially, hourly checks of peripheral circulation - characteristics of pulses in lower extremities.
5. Evaluate urine output hourly.
6. Evaluate BUN and serum creatinine levels to assess renal function.
7. *Immediately report to the RN any changes in the status of circulation of a client's extremity.*

NCLEX ALERT: *Recognize client conditions result ing in insufficient vascular perfusion, review assessment of peripheral pulses of client. Pulse checks are critical in the vascular surgery client. The nurse should compare the peripheral pulses in the lower extremities. (See PVD).*

✦ *Goal: to maintain homeostasis and prevent infection postoperative aneurysm resection.*

1. Maintain adequate body warmth in initial postoperative period.
2. Prophylactic antibiotics.
3. Assess for and evaluate elevation of temperature.
4. Evaluate for return of GI function.
   a. Bowel sounds.
   b. Distention.
   c. Passage of flatus.
   d. Diarrhea.
5. Nasogastric suction generally utilized in immediate postoperative period.

✦ *Goal: to assist client to understand implications of the disease and measures to maintain health postoperative aneurysm resection (See PVD Goal to assist client to understand implications of the disease).*

Shock (Severe Hypotension)

❑ ***Shock* is characterized by inadequate blood flow and tissue perfusion.**

A. For adequate circulation to occur, all parts of the circulatory system must function effectively together.
 1. Vascular tone to maintain normal resistance of the vessels.
 2. Ability of the heart to maintain cardiac output.
 3. Adequate amount of total blood volume.

B. The initial problems precipitating shock and the specific treatment of the problems are very different. However, regardless of the precipitating cause of shock, the underlying problem is inadequate tissue perfusion.

C. Classification of shock.
 1. Hypovolemic shock.
  a. Reduced venous return due to reduced blood volume; 15 to 25% reduction in volume.
  b. Conditions.
   (1) Hemorrhage.
   (2) Burns.
   (3) Severe fluid loss.
 2. Cardiogenic shock.
  a. Heart is unable to effectively circulate the intravascular volume.
  b. Conditions.
   (1) Dysrhythmia.
   (2) MI.
   (3) CHF.
 3. Distributive shock.
  a. An increase in the blood volume on the venous side with a decrease in the venous return to the heart.
  b. Conditions.
   (1) Neurogenic - spinal cord shock, loss of nerve supply to blood vessels.
   (2) Septic - vasodilation from severe infection.
   (3) Anaphylactic - vasodilation secondary to histamine release (allergic reactions).
 4. Obstructive shock.
  a. Physical impediment to the mainstream of blood flow.
  b. Conditions.
   (1) Pulmonary embolism.
   (2) Vena cava compression.
   (3) Tension pneumothorax

NCLEX ALERT: *Implement interventions to manage potential client circulatory complications. Be able to recognize clients at increased risk, early symptoms of shock and initiate protective and preventive action.*

Data Collection

Signs and symptoms of shock are essentially the same regardless of the precipitating cause.

 1. Risk factors.
  a. Increased incidence in the very young and in the very old.
  b. Increased incidence in clients with chronic progressive disease states.
  c. Trauma.
  d. Postoperative hemorrhage.
 2. Clinical manifestations.
  a. Early (compensatory) body's compensatory mechanisms are able to maintain cardiac output and tissue perfusion.
   (1) Oriented.
   (2) Restless, increased anxiety, apprehensive.
   (3) Increase in pulse rate
   (4) Skin cool to touch.
   (5) Normal blood pressure.
   (6) Increased respiratory rate.
   (7) Urinary output may be slightly decreased, but within normal range; may occur even with a normal blood pressure.

NCLEX ALERT: *Identify client factors that could interfere with elimination. Decreased urinary output is often an early observable sign of decreased renal perfusion secondary to decrease in cardiac output.*

  b. Decompensated- body can no longer compensate to maintain blood pressure and tissue perfusion decreases.
   (1) Decreasing sensory perception.
   (2) Nausea and vomiting.
   (3) Cool, moist skin.
   (4) Rapid, shallow respirations.
   (5) Skin color pallor to cyanotic.
   (6) Decrease in urine to oliguria levels.
   (7) Tachycardia, pulse may be weak and thready.
   (8) Decrease in blood pressure.
  c. Progressive - the cycle of inadequate tissue perfusion continues.

(1) Progressively decreasing level of consciousness.
(2) Cool, moist skin (clammy).
(3) Cyanosis.
(4) Labored, irregular respirations.
(5) Tachycardia to bradycardia.
(6) Anuria.
(7) Continued decrease in blood pressure.

3. Diagnostics - based on the clinical manifestations and history of underlying problems.

Treatment

Depends on the underlying problem.

Nursing Intervention

✦ *Goal: to identify and correct cause of shock.*

✦ *Goal: to maintain ventilation and prevent hypoxia (see Chapter 10).*

✦ *Goal: to correct acid-base imbalance (see Chapter 5).*

✦ *Goal: to assess and support the cardiovascular and respiratory systems.*

1. Monitor blood pressure closely in individuals at increased risk.
2. Evaluate cardiac output in response to dysrhythmias.
3. Maintain bedrest.
4. Supine position with legs elevated (do not position in Trendelenburg).
5. Evaluate rate and quality of respirations.
6. Evaluate ABGs for hypoxia and development of acidosis.
7. Provide supplemental oxygen as indicated.
8. Maintain airway patency.
9. Hypovolemic shock requires an increase in the circulating volume.

✦ *Goal: to evaluate renal response to decrease in cardiac output.*

1. Maintain Foley catheter.
2. Take hourly urine measurements.
3. Carefully assess renal response to increase in IV fluids.

✦ *Goal: to maintain homeostasis and decrease effects of shock.*

1. Evaluate neuro status hourly and PRN.
2. Continue to orient client.
3. Decrease unnecessary sensory stimuli.
4. Maintain NPO; provide oral hygiene.
5. Evaluate for bowel sounds and distention due to intestinal ischemia.
6. Keep client comfortably warm; do not allow chilling.
7. Do not administer medications PO, IM, or subcutaneous because of decreased tissue perfusion. *(RN will administer medications IV push.)*
8. Provide emotional support; continue to talk with client and describe procedures before they are done.
9. Avoid unnecessary nursing procedures.

Varicose Veins

❑ ***Varicose veins* occur when *veins* in the lower trunk and extremities become congested and dilated because of incompetent valves in the vessels, as well as loss of elasticity of the vessel wall. As venous pressure increases, the muscle around the vein fails to constrict effectively, and there is increased congestion and decreased venous return.**

Data Collection

1. Risk factors.
   a. Congenital weakness of the vein walls.
   b. Obesity.
   c. Pregnancy.
2. Clinical manifestations.
   a. Dilated, tortuous subcutaneous veins.
   b. Cosmetic appearance of the vein is objectionable.
   c. Pressure or pain after prolonged standing.
   d. Pain is generally relieved by elevating the extremity.
3. Complications — venous stasis.

Table 11-1: Nursing Measures To Decrease Venous Stasis

✦ Encourage mobility; even standing at the bedside promotes venous tone.

✦ Elastic stockings:
—Hospitalized clients should wear them all the time.
—Removed for bath, but replaced prior to getting out of bed.
—Home clients generally wear them during the day, should be put on before getting out of bed; and removed when they go to bed.
—Do not allow stockings to bunch up behind the knee.
—Don't hang feet dependent when putting stockings on; elevate or put them parallel on the bed.

✦ Teach client to elevate legs for about 20 minutes every four or five hours.

✦ Avoid prolonged sitting; walk around every 1-2 hours.

✦ Don't cross legs when sitting

✦ Do not wear restrictive clothing.

✦ Maintain good fluid intake, avoid dehydration.

a. Thrombophlebitis.
b. Pulmonary emboli.

Treatment

1. Medical.
   a. Rest with feet elevated.
   b. Elastic support hose.
   c. Walking exercises.
2. Surgical
   a. Scleropathy - injection of sclerosing agents into affected vein.
   b. Surgical ligation of the veins, may be combined with vein stripping as well.

NCLEX ALERT: *Implement interventions to promote client venous return. Plan interventions to prevent client complications of cardiovascular system.*

Nursing Intervention

✦ *Goal: to identify client at high risk and prevent development of varicosities.*

1. Encourage client to avoid sitting or standing for prolonged period.
2. Prevent injury to extremity.
3. Encourage client to avoid constrictive clothing.
4. Teach client to avoid rubbing extremities.

NCLEX ALERT: *Identify complications of immobility, Monitor client responses to interventions for preventing complications from immobility. With any condition that causes an increase in venous stasis or inflammation to a vein, there is a significant increased risk for the development of thrombosis and an embolus.*

✦ *Goal: to assist client to understand implications of the disease and measures to maintain health.*

1. Elastic hose should be put on before getting out of bed in the morning.
2. Maintain good skin care of lower extremities.
3. Decrease weight if appropriate.
4. Avoid prolonged standing or sitting in the work environment.
5. Avoid constrictive clothing

Thrombophlebitis

❑ **This disease which is also referred as venous disease/deep vein thrombosis or DVT begins with an inflammation of the *vein*. The inflammatory process initiates clot formation. Thrombi occurring in the deep veins are of particular concern because there is increased incidence of embolus formation.**

A. Thrombosis is the development of a clot in the vein; thrombophlebitis is the inflammation of the vein. Sometimes it is difficult to determine which problem occurred first.
B. When a client experiences a problem with thrombophlebitis in a deep vein, there is permanent damage to the vessel. This increases the risk of the client developing the problem again.
C. The thrombus formation generally occurs as a result of:
   1. Venous stasis.
   2. Increased coagulability of the blood.
   3. Damage to the wall of the vessel.
D. Thrombi arise from the deep veins of the legs, pelvis, and abdomen.

Data Collection

1. Risk factors.
   a. Venous Stasis.
      (1) Surgery.
      (2) Pregnancy.
      (3) Obesity.
      (4) Congestive heart failure.
   b. Increased blood coagulation.
   c. Injury to vessel wall.
   d. Acute myocardial infarction.

NCLEX ALERT: *Implement measures to manage potential circulatory complications. Due to the multiple types of conditions that precipitate the circulatory complications, questions may be incorporated into the care of the surgical client, the obstetric client, or any client with problems of circulation.*

2. Clinical manifestations.
   a. Area around the vein is tender to touch, reddened, and warm.
   b. Deep thrombosis.
      (1) Swollen extremity.
      (2) Pain.
      (3) Warm, cyanotic skin.
      (4) Increased temperature.
   c. Positive Homan's sign - this is no longer considered an accurate indicator of thrombophlebitis.
3. Diagnostics - clinical manifestations.

4. Complication - thrombus formation with risk of pulmonary embolus.

Treatment

1. Medical (primary method of treatment).
   a. Bedrest.
   b. Elevate extremity.
   c. Warm, moist heat.
   d. Anticoagulant (Appendix 11-3).
   e. Elastic stocking if edema is present after client is ambulatory.
   f. Elastic stocking on *unaffected leg* during period of bed rest.
   g. Range of motion on *unaffected leg* during bed rest.
2. Surgical intervention - done to prevent pulmonary emboli.
   a. Venous thrombectomy.
   b. Vena cava ligation.
   c. Umbrella filter device in the vena cava .

Nursing Intervention

✦ *Goal: to prevent problem of thrombophlebitis in clients at high risk.*

> ***NURSING PRIORITY:** The best way to prevent the development of a pulmonary emboli is to prevent the development of DVT or thrombophlebitis. It is much easier to prevent the problem than it is to treat it.*

1. Prophylactic measures for the surgical client (See Chapter 3).
2. Prevent complications of immobility (See Chapter 3).
3. Prophylactic anticoagulation may be utilized in the high-risk client (hip and prostate surgery).
4. Nursing measures to increase venous return Table 16-6).
   a. Do not cross legs in the bed or while sitting.
   b. Do not place a pillow under the knees.
   c. Do not stand or sit in one position for prolonged period of time.
   d. Isometric exercises of the calf and thigh muscles.

✦ *Goal: to decrease inflammatory response and prevent emboli formation.*

1. Bedrest with feet elevated.
2. Warm, moist soaks to dilate arteries and veins and to decrease lymphatic congestion and promote healing.
3. Observe client for adverse reactions to anticoagulants (See Appendix 11-3).
4. Elastic stockings if client's legs become edematous after ambulating.
5. Do not use pillow under the knees or elevate the knee gatch of the bed.
6. Measure circumference of calf daily to determine changes.
7. Utilization of pneumatic compression devices or sequential compression devices to facilitate venous return in immobilized clients.

Self-Care

1. Avoid oral contraceptives.
2. Decrease/stop smoking.
3. Avoid constrictive clothing.
4. Exercise regularly.
5. Decrease weight if appropriate.
6. Decrease sodium in diet if edema is present.
7. Follow instruction regarding anticoagulation therapy at home.
8. Measures to increase venous return (Table 16-6.)
9. Report: increased pain, swelling, redness or skin changes.

> **NCLEX ALERT:** *Implement interventions to promote client venous return. Review client teaching about health risks.*

Study Questions—Vascular

1. What would be the long-term effect of hypertension on the heart?

① left ventricular hypertrophy, congestive heart failure.
② coronary artery disease, myocardial infarction, angina.
③ cardiac murmurs and rubs, edema, varicose veins.
④ diabetes, atrophy of the ventricles, pericarditis.

2.What is a complication of long-term, poorly controlled hypertension on the central nervous system?

① increased pressure of cerebral spinal fluid.
② migraine headache and vertigo.
③ damage to cerebral vessels.
④ damage to the optic nerve.

3. A client complains of dizziness after standing up. The nurse retakes the client's blood pressure and notices a substantial drop in the systolic pressure. What problem has occurred?

① orthostatic hypotension.
② rebound hypertension.
③ postural hypertension.
④ syncope.

4. The nurse is administering Heparin. What is the correct procedure for administration of this medication?

① check the prothrombin time and administer the medication if it is below 30 seconds.
② use a 22 gauge, ½ inch needle and inject the medication subcutaneously.
③ inject the medication into the deltoid and rub carefully to disperse medication.
④ with a 25 gauge, 5/8 inch needle, inject the medication into the abdomen.

5. What are considered to be contributing factors in the development of essential hypertension?

① obesity, drug abuse, smoking.
② obesity, smoking, history of cancer in the family.
③ sedentary lifestyle, obesity, vegetarian diet.
④ sedentary lifestyle, obesity, smoking.

6. A hypertensive client is concerned about her medications. She asks the nurse how long she will have to take medication. What is the best nursing response?

① she will return to her doctor in two months, the medications may be discontinued at that time.
② when her blood pressure returns to normal for a period of 6 months, her medication will be discontinued.
③ to maintain stable control of her blood pressure, she will remain on the medication indefinitely.
④ the medication may be adjusted every month, she needs to talk with the doctor.

7. What is the primary goal of treatment for the client with peripheral vascular disease?

① promote venous blood return.
② control pain and maintain vascular integrity.
③ control seizures and maintain mobility.
④ improve blood supply to the extremities.

8. A client has a peripheral arterial disorder. What would the nursing assessment reveal?

① diminished pedal pulses.
② 3+ edema bilaterally.
③ dusky gray color of the feet.
④ muscle spasms in the feet.

9. The nurse is assessing a client who is 12 hours postoperative for a repair of his aortic aneurysm. The nurse would immediately report which findings?

① total urinary output of 110 cc since surgery.
② no bowel sounds in any of the four quadrants.
③ legs and feet cool to touch bilaterally.
④ pulses weak and equal in both extremities.

10. What is included in the nursing management of a client with deep vein thrombosis?

① activities as tolerated.
② passive range of motion to affected extremity.
③ foot of bed elevated and bed rest.
④ ambulate in hall twice daily.

11. A client has been diagnosed with left leg thrombophlebitis. Which findings would not be typical of this condition?

① pain and tenderness in the left leg.
② warmth over infected area.
③ redness over infected area.
④ decreased quality of pulse in left leg.

12. An elderly client has occasional pain in the legs while ambulating, but the pain is not present when the client is at rest. What is this type of pain called?

① arterial-venous shunting.
② thrombosis.
③ intermittent claudication.
④ angina.

13. What client profile indicates a high risk for the development of peripheral vascular disease?

① a 76-year-old with hypertension and diabetes mellitus.
② a 65-year-old with a history of hypertension and alcohol abuse.
③ a 25-year-old athlete with a family history of diabetes.
④ a 35-year-old with family history of cardiovascular disease.

14. A client has a diagnosis of deep vein thrombosis. What is a typical assessment finding?

① coldness to the extremity with edema.
② swollen red extremities.
③ thready pulse and slow capillary return.
④ pain with swelling in affected part of leg.

15. A client is to be discharged, what is the most common anticoagulant therapy the client will continue using at home?

① urokinase (**Abbokinase**).
② sodium heparin (**Heparin**)
③ dipyridamole (**Persantine**).
④ warfarin sodium (**Coumadin**).

16. The nurse is caring for a client following a thoracotomy. What assessment finding would be present if the client is experiencing hypovolemic shock from excessive bleeding?

① urine output below 30cc per hour.
② jugular vein distention with head elevated.
③ chest tube drainage of 50cc per hour for 4 hours.
④ blood pressure of 100/70, pulse at 100.

17. The intake of which of these items would affect the control of a client with high blood pressure?

① caffeine, sugar, milk products.
② chocolate, tea, caffeine.
③ caffeine, amphetamines, nicotine.
④ fruits, sugar, amphetamines,

18. A client is taking a diuretic for treatment of his hypertension. What foods would the nurse encourage the client to eat?

① orange juice and apricots.
② cranberry juice and dairy products.
③ leafy green vegetables and apple juice.
④ grains, legumes, and fish.

19. Orthostatic hypotension is most prominent in what age group?

① elderly clients.
② children.
③ teenagers.
④ middle-aged adults.

20. What are the symptoms of a client who is experiencing postural hypotension?

① slow pulse and muscle cramping with activity.
② lightheadedness and syncope when standing up.
③ headaches and restlessness after a meal.
④ lightheadedness and syncope when lying down.

Appendix 11-1: VASCULAR DIAGNOSTICS

WHOLE BLOOD CLOTTING TIME	NORMAL VALUE	THERAPEUTIC VALUE	
SERUM STUDIES			
Prothrombin time (PT)	11-18 sec. range	1 - 2 ½ times normal	See Nursing Implications for clients on anticoagulant medications (Appendix 11-3). Range of values are dependent on reagents used in individual laboratories. Serum levels should be reported with the "control level" in order to evaluate results of study.
Partial thromboplastin time (PTT) (traditional)	Normal: 60 -90 sec.	1 ½ to 2 ½ times normal	
Activated partial thromboplastin time (aPTT)	Activated: 30 -45 sec.	1 ½ to 2 ½ times normal	
International normalizing ratio (INR)	Mathematically calculated depending on laboratory's methods	2.0 to 4.0	
INVASIVE STUDIES			
• Peripheral arteriography (angiography)	Involves injection of a radiopaque dye into either the artery or the vein; x-rays are taken to identify atherosclerotic plaques, occlusions, traumatic injury or presence of aneurysms.	1. Explain procedures to client; mild sedative may be indicated. 2. After procedure: a. Circulatory checks distal to the puncture site. b. Observe client for allergic reactions to the dye.	
• Venography (phlebography)			

Appendix 11-2: ANTIHYPERLIPIDEMIC MEDICATIONS

MEDICATIONS	SIDE EFFECTS	NURSING IMPLICATIONS
ANTIHYPERLIPIDEMIC MEDICATIONS: Decreases LDL cholesterol, but preferably does not decrease the HDL cholesterol. First line of treatment for increased cholesterol is dietary therapy to reduce cholesterol intake.		
Cholestyramine (**Questran**): PO Colestipol (**Colestid**): PO	GI disturbances Constipation	1. Supplemental fat soluble vitamins in long-term therapy. 2. Mix powder with several ounces of fluid for administration.
Nicotinic acid (**Niacin, Nicolar**): PO	Flushing Hyperglycemia Hyperuricemia GI disturbances	1. Used with caution in clients with gallbladder disease, diabetes and gout. 2. Flushing occurs in almost all clients, will diminish over several weeks.
Gemfibrozil (**Lopid**): PO Lovastatin (**Mevacor**): PO	Rashes, GI disturbances, hepatoxic	1. Should not be given to clients with pre-existing gall bladder disease. 2. Will potentiate warfarin derivative anticoagulants (**Coumadin**).

Appendix 11-3: ANTICOAGULANTS

MEDICATIONS	SIDE EFFECTS	NURSING IMPLICATIONS
ANTICOAGULANTS: Prolong coagulation by inactivation of clotting factors (heparin) and by decreasing synthesis of clotting factors (Coumadin).		
Heparin: IV, sq	Hemorrhagic tendencies: hematuria, bleeding gums, frank hemorrhage	1. Check the aPTT for normal levels vs therapeutic levels. 2. Protamine sulfate is the antidote. 3. Will not dissolve established clots. 4. May not be given PO. 5. Effective immediately after administration. 6. Anticoagulation effect is short. 7. Identify if heparin is being used to treat thromboembolic problem or as prophylaxis for thromboembolic problems.
Enoxaparin (**Lovenox**) SQ		1. Use: prophylaxis for coagulation in high-risk clients (hip or knee replacement) 2. Dosage is not interchangeable with heparin.
Coumarin Derivatives: Warfarin (**Coumadin**): PO, IV (**Dicumarol**): PO		1. Check the PT and INR to evaluate level of anticoagulation. 2. Vitamin K is the antidote. 3. Client teaching for home care: bleeding precautions advise all health care providers of medication not recommended if pregnant or lactating maintain routine checks on coagulation studies 4. Utilized for long-term anticoagulation. 5. Check drug literature when administering with other medications; drug interactions are common. 6. Should not be administered to clients at high-risk for hemorrhagic problems. 7. Oral contraceptives may decrease effectiveness.

NCLEX ALERT: *Observe for effects of medications. Review the nursing implications associated with administration of anticoagulants.*

Appendix 11-4:
ANTIHYPERTENSIVE MEDICATIONS

❖ GENERAL NURSING IMPLICATIONS ❖

— Advise client that postural hypotension may occur and how to decrease effects.
— Client should be instructed regarding sedation; hazardous activities should be avoided.
— Hypotension may be increased by hot weather, hot showers, hot tubs, and alcohol ingestion.
— Client should not abruptly discontinue medication or change dosage without consulting health care provider.
— Encourage a low sodium diet and weight maintenance or reduction.
— Encourage to stop smoking.
— Have client report unpleasant side effects related to sexual dysfunction.

NCLEX ALERT: *Observe for effects of medications. Evaluate client's use of medications.*

MEDICATIONS	SIDE EFFECTS	NURSING IMPLICATIONS
VASODILATORS: Acts directly on vascular smooth muscle to produce vasodilation.		
Hydralazine HCl (**Apresoline**): PO, IM, IV	Tachycardia Angina palpitations Anorexia Headache	1. Advise client that postural hypotension may occur. 2. Medication may precipitate myocardial ischemia. 3. May be used in combination with other antihypertensive medications.
Nitroprusside (**Nipride**): IV	Nausea Vomiting Headache Diaphoresis Abdominal pain	1. Generally used to treat hypertensive crisis. 2. Solution must be prepared immediately prior to use and protected from light during administration. 3. Should be given via infusion pump to insure accurate flow rate. 4. Should be used with caution in clients with liver and renal impairment. 5. Client should be closely monitored; preferably in a critical care setting.
CENTRALLY ACTING SYMPATHOLYTICS (ALPHA AGONISTS): Decreases sympathetic effect (norepinephrine) on BP and decreases sympathetic tone which leads to dilation of both arterioles and veins.		
Clonidine (**Catapres**): PO, patch Methyldopa (**Aldomet**): PO, parenteral	Dry mouth & nasal mucosa, drowsiness, impotence, postural hypotension	1. If withdrawn abruptly, may precipitate a hypertensive crisis. 2. More prolonged problems with postural hypotension and impotence.
ANGIOTENSIN-CONVERTING-ENZYME INHIBITORS (ACE): Reduce peripheral vasculature resistance without increasing cardiac output, rate, or contractility; angiotension antagonist.		
Captopril (**Capoten**): PO Enalapril (**Vasotec**): PO	Postural hypotension, GI distress, hyperkalmia, insomnia, potential aggravating nonproductive cough.	1. Instruct client to stay in bed for 3-4 hours after initial dose. 2. Monitor BP closely after the first dose for pronounced hypotension. 3. Monitor electrolytes; this medication causes retention of potassium. 4. Elderly client is at highest risk for postural hypotension.
BETA ADRENERGIC BLOCKERS: See Appendix 12-2		
CALCIUM CHANNEL BLOCKERS - see Appendix 12-2		

Appendix 11-5:
DIURETICS

❖GENERAL NURSING IMPLICATIONS ❖

— Evaluate daily weights for fluid loss or gain.
— Maintain intake and output records.
— Monitor for hypokalemia.
— Advise client of foods that are potassium-rich.
— Administer medications in the morning.
— Teach clients how to decrease effects of postural hypotension.
— Monitor blood pressure response to diuretics.
— Interactions:
  Digitalis action is increased in presence of hypokalemia.
  Lithium levels may be increased in presence of hyponatremia.

NCLEX ALERT: *Monitor effects of medications. Maintain special diet for client based on diagnosis/nutritional needs.*

MEDICATIONS	SIDE EFFECTS	NURSING IMPLICATIONS
LOOP DIURETICS: Block sodium and chloride reabsorption,, which causes water and solutes to be retained in the nephron. Prevention of reabsorption of water back into the circulation causes an increase in excretion of the water, therefore diuresis.		
Furosemide (**Lasix**): PO, IM, IV Ethacrynic acid (**Edecrin**): PO, IV Bumetanide (**Bumex**)	Dehydration, hypotension; excessive loss of potassium, sodium, chloride, hyperglycemia, hyperuricemia.	1. Strong diuretic that provides rapid diuresis. 2. Use with caution in the elderly.
THIAZIDE DIURETICS:		
Chlorothiazide (**Diuril**): IV, PO Chlorthalidone (**Hygroton**): PO Hydrochlorothiazide (**Hydrodiuril, Esidrex**): PO	Dehydration, hypotension; excessive loss of potassium, sodium, chloride, hyperglycemia, hyperuricemia.	1. Frequently used as first line drug to control essential hypertension.
POTASSIUM SPARING DIURETICS: Blocks the effect of aldosterone on the renal tubule.		
Spironolactone (**Aldactone**): PO Triamterene (**Dyrenium**): PO	Menstrual irregularities, impotence, hypotension	1. May be used in combination with other diuretics to reduce potassium loss. 2. Potassium-sparing effects may result in hyperkalemia.
OSMOTIC DIURETIC: Increases osmotic pressure of the fluid in the renal tubule, thus preventing reabsorption of sodium and water		
Mannitol (**Osmitrol**): IV	Pulmonary edema, CHF, tissue dehydration, nausea, vomiting	1. Stop infusion if client begins to show symptoms of CHF, pulmonary edema. 2. Use an IV filter to prevent infusion of crystals.

Appendix 11-6: MEDICATIONS USED FOR TREATMENT OF SHOCK

❖GENERAL NURSING IMPLICATIONSV

— Most often limited to critical care settings; constant monitoring is required.
— Most often administered in diluted solution by IV drip.
— Careful frequent observation and evaluation of blood pressure.
— Continuous EKG monitoring; observe client closely for cardiac dysrhythmias.
— Monitor urinary output every hour.
— Frequent and close monitoring of IV infusion site; leakage into tissue may cause tissue sloughing.
— Medications should not be administered to clients receiving MAO inhibitors.

ADRENERGIC AGONIST / CATECHOLAMINE: Increases myocardial contractility, thereby improving cardiac output.

MEDICATIONS	SIDE EFFECTS	NURSING IMPLICATIONS
Dopamine (**Intropin**)	Dysrhythmias (tachycardia), angina, hypertension, headaches	1. In low doses, enhances renal blood flow. 2. If extravasation occurs, stop infusion immediately and infuse area with an antagonist/antidote.
Dobutamine (**Dobutrex**)		
Amrinone (**Inocor**)		
Isoproterenol (**Isuprel**)	Tachycardia	1. May also be used as a bronchodilator when administered by inhalation. 2. Generally not utilized in hypotension where tachycardia is a problem. 3. Utilized to maintain cardiac output in clients with AV heart block prior to pacemaker insertion.
Epinephrine hydrochloride (**Adrenalin**): IV		1. Be sure to read label correctly and utilize correct strengths. 2. Observe for cardiac dysrhythmias. 3. Use in treatment of anaphylactic shock and cardiac arrest.
Norepinephrine (**Levophed**)		1. If extravasation occurs, infiltrate the area with phenotolamine (**Regitine**).

Appendix 11-7: VASCULAR ACCESS LINES

Central Line - a line inserted into the venous system and progressed into the thoracic cavity. Most common insertion site is the subclavian or jugular vein with the end of the line being in the superior vena cava or the right atrium. There are several different types of venous catheters on the market that can be classified as central lines. A central line is necessary for a central venous pressure reading, and for hyperalimentation solutions.

Tunneled ports (Hickman, Broviac) -Requires surgical placement, has an external port. The distal tip of the catheter lies in the superior vena cava, just above the right atrium.

Implanted ports (Mediport, Port A Cath) port is implanted under the skin; activities are not restricted. Skin must be punctured to access the catheter. Client should avoid wearing constrictive clothing over site.

NCLEX ALERT: *Provide care for client with central venous access device.*

Flushing - routine flushing may be required after administration of medications. Flushing usually done with normal saline.

Accessing - Gloves are worn and appropriate skin preparation done for implanted ports; on external ports the connectors are cleansed prior to accessing.

Dressing changes - Implanted sites require cleansing after exit, but do not require a dressing. External sites require ad dressing, either gauze or transparent.

Notes

Cardiac System

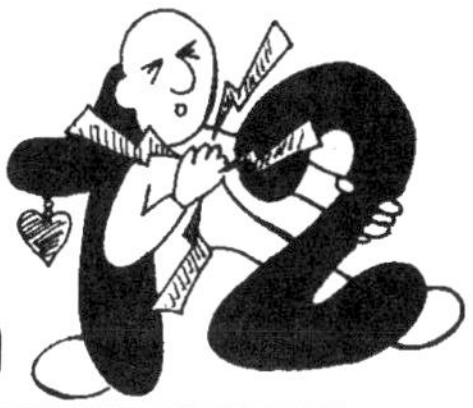

PHYSIOLOGY OF THE CARDIAC SYSTEM

A. The heart is located in the mediastinal space of the thoracic cavity.

B. The apex of the heart points downward and to the left and comes in contact with the chest wall at about the fifth to sixth intercostal space; in the normal individual, the point of maximum impulse (PMI) may be palpated here; this is also the area to auscultate and evaluate the apical heart rate.

C. Myocardial wall.
  1. Epicardium - the outer surface.
  2. Myocardium - the middle layer of cardiac muscle.
  3. Endocardium - the lining of the inner surface of the cardiac chambers.

D. Cardiac chambers (Figure 12-1).
  1. Four chambers are located within the heart; these chambers represent two pumps.
    a. Right side pump - right atrium and right ventricle, separated by the tricuspid valve.
    b. Primary function of the right side of the heart is to receive blood from the vascular system and to pump the blood through the lungs.
    c. Left side pump - left atrium and left ventricle, separated by the mitral valve.
    d. Primary functions of the left side of the heart is to receive oxygenated blood from the lungs and to pump the blood through the systemic circulation.
  2. Both atria are the receiving chambers; both ventricles are the ejecting chambers.
  3. The atrioventricular septum separates the respective chambers.
  4. The right side of the heart has a thinner myocardium than the left side and is a low-pressure system.
  5. The left ventricle is composed of a thicker muscle, is a high-pressure system, and is capable of generating enough force to eject blood through the aortic valve and through the systemic circulation.
  6. Pericardium - a fibroserous sac that surrounds the heart.

E. Cardiac valves - maintain the directional flow of blood through the heart chambers.

F. Direction of blood flow through the heart structure (See Figure 12-1).
  1. From the venous system, the blood enters the right atrium via the superior vena cava; through the tricuspid valve into the right ventricle; ejected through the pulmonic valve into the pulmonary artery; to the lungs for oxygenation.
  2. Oxygenated blood returns to the left atrium via the pulmonary veins; through the mitral valve into the left ventricle; ejected through the aortic valve into the aortic arch; into the systemic circulation.
  3. The pulmonary artery is the only artery in the circulatory system to carry unoxygenated blood; the pulmonary vein is the only vein in the circulatory system to carry oxygenated blood.

G. Cardiac Function.
  1. One complete cardiac cycle consists of contraction of the myocardium (systole) and subsequent relaxation of the myocardium (diastole).
  2. The amount of blood ejected from the ventricle is the stroke volume.
  3. Cardiac output.
    a. The heart pumps approximately 5 liters of blood every minute.
    b. The heart rate increases with exercise; therefore, cardiac output increases.
    c. The cardiac output will vary according to the amount of venous return.

H. Myocardial blood flow.
  1. Coronary arteries supply the heart muscle with oxygenated blood.
  2. Collateral circulation.
    a. There are no direct connections between the large coronary arteries.
    b. With gradual occlusion of large coronary vessels by ASHD, the smaller vessels increase in size and provide alternative blood flow.
    c. Because of the development of the circulation, coronary artery disease may be well-advanced before the client experiences symptoms.

System Data Collection

A. Health history.
  1. Identify presence of risk factors for the development of arteriosclerotic disease (Table 12-1).
  2. Respiratory.
    a. History of difficulty breathing.
    b. Medications taken for respiratory problems.
    c. Determine normal activity level.

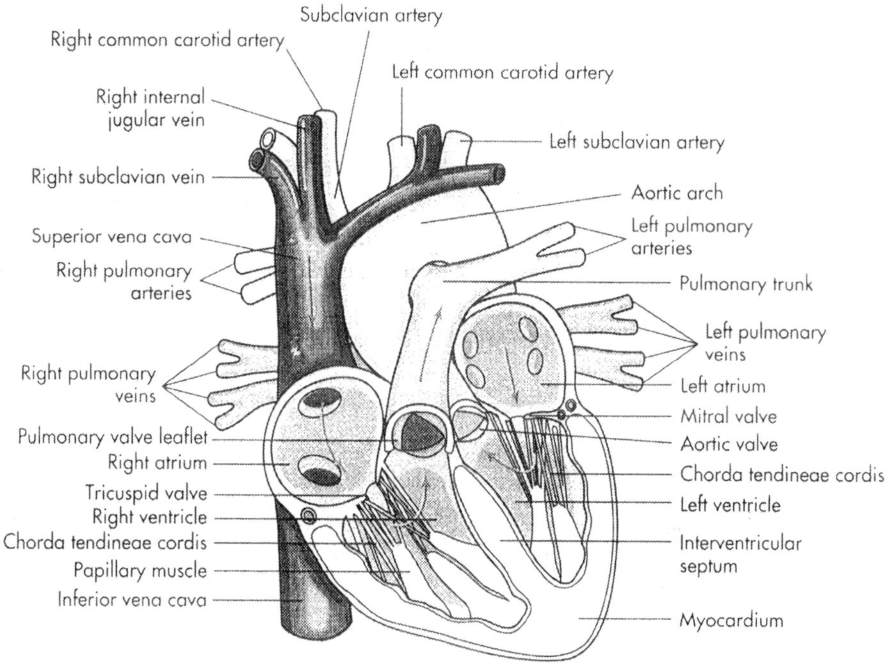

Figure 12-1: Circulation of Blood Through Chambers
Reprinted with permission: Phipps, WJ, Sands, JK, & Marek, JF (1999). *Medical Surgical Nursing: Concepts & Clinical Practice*, 6th ed. Philadelphia: Mosby, p. 604.

3. Circulation.
   a. History of chest discomfort.
   b. History of edema, weight gain.
   c. History of syncope.
   d. Medications taken for the heart or for high blood pressure.

B. Physical assessment.

1. What is the overall general appearance of the client: any evidence of distress; what is the level of orientation and ability to think clearly?
2. Evaluate blood pressure.
   a. Pulse pressure - the difference between the systolic and diastolic pressures.
   b. Assess for postural hypotension - decrease in blood pressure when the client stands.
3. Evaluate character of pulse
   a. Rate, rhythm
   b. Regularity, presence of irregular beats.
   c. Pulse deficit - the difference in the rate of the pulse at the radius and at the apex (or apical rate).
   d. Pulse quality - the amplitude or quality of the pulse. Should be evaluated bilaterally.
      (1) +1- thready, weak, rapid pulse.
      (2) +2 - diminished pulse, cannot be obliterated.
      (3) +3 - easy to palpate, full, cannot obliterated.
      (4) +4 - strong bounding pulse, may be abnormal.
   e. Palpitations - client describes a feeling or sensation of rapid, bounding, or irregular heartbeat.
4. Assess quality and pattern of respirations and evidence of respiratory difficulty.
5. Apical heart rate - listen for the apical pulse and count the apical rate at the fifth intercostal space, mid-clavicular line.
6. Evaluate peripheral pulses and for presence of peripheral edema.
7. Weight gain - 3 or more pounds in 24 hours represents fluid gain.
8. Evaluate for presence of chest discomfort.
   a. Location.
   b. Intensity of pain.
   c. Precipitating causes.
9. Determine client's activity level; increasing fatigue with mild exercise occurs with cardiac clients.

DISORDERS OF THE CARDIAC SYSTEM

ARTERIOSCLEROTIC HEART DISEASE

❑ **Arteriosclerotic heart disease (ASHD, coronary artery disease) occurs as a result of the buildup of plaque or fatty material in the coronary artery causes a narrowing of the lumen of the artery and results in a decreased blood supply to the heart muscle (see Chapter 11).**

Table 12-1: RISK FACTORS IN ASHD

MODIFIABLE RISK FACTORS:
Elevated serum cholesterol/triglyceride levels
High blood pressure
Cigarette smoking
Sedentary lifestyle
Obesity
Type A personality (high-pressure lifestyle, competitive)
Diabetes mellitus

NON-MODIFIABLE RISK FACTORS:
Genetic predisposition
Positive family history of heart disease
Increasing age
Gender -occurs more often in men

NCLEX ALERT: *Review client/family understanding of health promotion behaviors/activities.*

Angina Pectoris

❑ **This is a syndrome characterized by transient anterior chest pain.**

A. Pain occurs when oxygen demands of the heart muscle exceed the ability of the coronary arteries to deliver it.

B. Temporary ischemia does not cause permanent damage of the myocardium. Pain frequently subsides when the precipitating factor is removed.

Data Collection

1. Risk factors/etiology.
   a. Arteriosclerotic heart disease (Table 12-1).
   b. Cardiac ischemia.
   c. Increased cardiac demands.
      (1) Exercise.
      (2) Emotional stress.
      (3) Heavy meals.
2. Clinical manifestations.
   a. Pain in varying levels of severity - frequently described as mild to moderate.
   b. Pain generally located in substernal area.
   c. Pain may radiate to left shoulder and upper arm.
   d. Client may describe pain as squeezing, choking, constricting, or as a vague feeling of pressure and indigestion.
   e. Anginal pain usually lasts short period of time - five minutes or less. Anginal pain precipitated by a heavy meal or anger may last longer.
   f. Typical exertion-pain-rest- relief pattern is classic for anginal pain.
   g. Diaphoresis.
   h. Severe apprehension.
   i. Frequently will deny seriousness of the pain.
   j. Most often correlates with increased activity, and increased cardiac demands.

Geriatric Priority: *In the elderly client, dyspnea, not angina, may be the presenting symptom of myocardial ischemia.*

3. Diagnostics (Appendix 12-1).
   a. Clinical manifestations.
   b. EKG.
   c. Stress test.
   d. Cardiac catheterization.

Treatment

1. Medication (Appendix 12-2).
2. Cardiac interventional procedures.
   a. Percutaneous transluminal angioplasty -a balloon is passed into the affected coronary artery to the area of obstruction. The balloon is inflated in an attempt to compress the atherosclerotic area and re-establish blood flow to the myocardium.
   b. Intracoronary stents - a tube is placed in the coronary vessel to maintain patency.
3. Restricted activity.
4. Supplemental oxygen.
5. Decreased cholesterol diet.
6. Decreased intake of stimulants (coffee, tea).
7. Control of modifiable risk factors.

Complications

1. Arrhythmias.
2. Myocardial infarction.

Nursing Intervention

✦ *Goal: to decrease pain and increase myocardial oxygenation.*

1. Maintain bed rest. Position client in reclining position with head elevated.
2. Notify the RN immediately of a client's chest pain.
3. Begin supplemental O2.
4. Administer medications.
   a. Nitroglycerin sublingual (Table 12-2).
   b. Narcotic analgesics (Morphine).
5. Maintain calm, reassuring atmosphere.
6. Evaluate vital signs.

Table 12-2: CLIENT EDUCATION FOR ADMINISTRATION OF NITROGLYCERIN

1. Keep in a tightly closed, dark glass container.
2. Carry supply at all times.
3. Fresh tablets should cause a slight burning/tingling under the tongue.
4. Purchase a new supply of medication every four to six months.
5. Take nitroglycerin prophylactically to avoid pain - sexual intercourse, exercise, walking, etc.
6. Take nitroglycerin when pain begins, and stop all activity.
7. If pain is not relieved in three to five minutes, take another nitroglycerin. Repeat procedure if still no relief.
8. If after taking a total of three nitroglycerin, there is no pain relief, seek medical attention immediately.
9. Side effects of nitroglycerin are headache, dizziness, and flushing.

NCLEX ALERT: *Evaluate client's use of medications. Monitor client's use of medications. Review client/family teaching on self-administration of medications.*

7. If client's pain is severe, remain with the client.

✦ ***Goal: to evaluate characteristics of anginal pain and client's overall response.***

1. Does pain increase with breathing? (anginal pain is generally not affected by breathing or changes of position.)
2. Assess activity tolerance or precipitating factor.
3. Assess characteristics of pain.
   a. Length.
   b. Onset - gradual or sudden.
   c. Response of pain to nitroglycerin.
   d. Client's description of pain.
4. Evaluate response of pain to treatment or progression to more severe level.
5. Assess respiratory status and response to pain.
6. Assess for presence of irregular heartbeats and document as indicated.

NURSING PRIORITY: *To relieve chest pain and to decrease cardiac damage resulting from an inadequate blood and oxygen supply to the myocardium, there must be an immediate reduction in the workload of the heart that results in a decrease in the oxygen requirements.*

7.

✦ *Goal: to provide care post cardiac interventional therapies.*

1. Monitor for chest pain and hypotension, reocclusion is primary complication.
2. Frequent reassessment of status of circulation distal to area of cannulation.
3. A sheath may be left in place, monitor area for bleeding. If bleeding occurs, put manual pressure on the area and *notify the RN.*
4. Prevent flexion of affected extremity and maintain bed rest for 6-8 hours.
5. Avoid heavy lifting; may return to work in 1-2 weeks.
6. *Notify RN of any bleeding at site and of chest pain or syncope.*

Self-Care

1. Education regarding ASHD.
   a. Will be able to identify personal risk factors and appropriate health practices to decrease risk factors.
   b. Will be able to identify factors precipitating pain.
2. Avoid activities that precipitate pain - large meals, smoking, strenuous exercise, extremes in weather.
3. Understand medication (Table 12-2), activity and diet regimen.
4. If pain persists and is not relieved by medication, client will call physician and or go to closest emergency room.

Myocardial Infarction

❑ **A *myocardial infarction* (MI, coronary occlusion, heart attack) is a total occlusion of a portion of a coronary artery. Immediately following the occlusion, there is myocardial ischemia. In the hours following, the tissue becomes necrotic.**

A. Most common site of infarction is the left ventricle.

B. The severity of the situation depends on the area of the heart involved, as well as the size of the infarction.

C. The presence of pre-established collateral circulation will assist in decreasing the size of the necrotic area.

NURSING PRIORITY: *Danger of death from an MI is greatest during the first two weeks. It is particularly increased in the first 24 to 48 hours.*

Data Collection

1. Risk factors/etiology.
   a. ASHD.
   b. May be precipitated by exercise or increased stress.
   c. Frequently no precipitating factors.

2. Clinical manifestations.
   a. Typical pain is severe, substernal, crushing, and unrelieved by nitroglycerin.
   b. Denial of the seriousness of the pain.
   c. Pain may radiate down the arm or up to the jaw.
   d. Dyspnea.
   e. Syncope.
   f. Nausea, vomiting.
   g. Onset is usually sudden.
   h. Diaphoresis.
   i. Extreme weakness.
   j. Decrease in blood pressure.
   k. Dysrhythmias - tachycardia, irregular rhythm.
3. Diagnostics (Appendix 12-1).

NCLEX ALERT: *Determine if client's vital signs are abnormal. Recognize client with conditions resulting in insufficient vascular perfusion.*

Treatment

1. Thrombolytic therapy (Appendix 12-2)- are effective if administered immediately or within the first three to six hours after the MI.
2. Supplemental oxygen.
3. IV line for medications.
4. Medications (Appendix 12-2) and Aspirin.
5. Dietary restrictions.
   a. Initially NPO or on a liquid diet.
   b. Progress to diet as tolerated - low sodium and low cholesterol.
   c. Decrease intake of stimulants (coffee, tea).
6. Pain control - pain increases cardiac workload.
7. Open heart surgery for myocardial revascularization.

Complications

1. Cardiogenic shock.
2. Dysrhythmias.
3. Congestive heart failure.

NCLEX ALERT: *Plan and implement intervention to prevent client complications of cardiovascular system.*

Nursing Intervention

✦ *Goal: to decrease pain and increase myocardial oxygenation (See related goal, Angina).*

✦ *Goal: to evaluate characteristics of cardiac pain and client's overall response (See related goal, Angina).*

NCLEX ALERT: *Check client discomfort and pain levels. Check client response to interventions.*

✦ *Goal: to maintain homeostasis and decrease effects of MI.*

1. Maintain IV access.
2. Maintain bed rest initially
3. Evaluate urinary output and renal response to changes in circulation.
4. Frequent assessment of cardiac rate and rhythm - dysrhythmias are major cause of death after an MI.
5. Assess respiratory system for increasing dyspnea and pulmonary congestion.
6. Evaluate peripheral circulation; assess for dependent edema.
7. Frequent assessment of vital signs.
8. Frequent assessment of chest pain.
9. NPO initially, then clear liquid to progressive diet.
10. Promote normal bowel pattern.
    a. Stool softeners.
    b. Bedside commode.
    c. Caution against straining at stool.
11. Decrease anxiety.
    a. Administer pain medication promptly.
    b. Keep client informed regarding progress and immediate plan of care.
    c. Decrease sensory overload.
    d. Encourage verbalization of concerns and fears.
    e. *Advise RN immediately regarding client's chest pain.*
12. Monitor for changes in neurological status - confusion, disorientation, etc.
13. Monitor progressive activity.
    a. Early activities should not increase heart rate greater than 25% of resting rate.
    b. Assess heart rhythm, fatigue, B/P after each activity.
    c. Resting tachycardia is a contraindication to activity.

Self-Care

1. Participate in organized cardiac rehabilitation program.

a. Monitored exercise.
b. Dietary modifications.
c. Continued education regarding ASHD and decreasing personal risk factors.

2. Understand medication regimen (Table 12-2).
3. Teach client how to check his radial pulse for rate and regularity.
4. Teach client how to evaluate response to increased exercise.
5. Exercise in climate controlled areas.
6. Call the doctor for increased pain not controlled by nitroglycerine, significant changes in pulse rate, decrease in activity tolerance, syncope, increase in dyspnea.
7. Sexual intercourse generally is resumed 4-6 weeks post MI, or when client can climb one flight of stairs without difficulty.
   a. Do not drink alcohol or eat a large meal prior to sexual activity.
   b. Take nitroglycerine prior to sexual activity.
8. Return to physician for regular check-ups.

NCLEX ALERT: *Reinforce teaching with client/family regarding managing health problems.*

Heart Failure

❑ ***Heart failure*** **is the inability of the heart to pump adequate amounts of blood into the systemic circulation in order to meet tissue metabolic demands**

Physiology of heart failure

A. Left-sided failure (congestive heart failure - CHF).
1. Results from failure of the left ventricle to maintain adequate output.
2. Blood backs up into the left atrium and into the pulmonary veins.
3. Increasing pressure in the pulmonary capillary bed causes lungs to become congested, resulting in respiratory distress.
4. Increasing pulmonary pressure results in increased pressure on right side of heart.

B. Right-sided failure (cor pulomonale).
1. Results from failure of the right ventricle to maintain adequate output.
2. Blood backs up into the systemic circulation and causes peripheral edema.

C. Both sides of the heart are dependent on the other for adequate function.
1. Left-sided failure results in pulmonary congestion; this causes increase in pulmonary pressure, which puts increased workload on the right side of the heart and precipitates right sided failure.
2. Although origin of problem may begin solely on one side, the majority of clinical situations involve failure on both sides.

D. In infants and young children, the problem is not due to an impaired left ventricle, but due to a defect that produces a large shunt.

NURSING PRIORITY: *If the situation does not differentiate between right and left sided failure, consider the client to be in congestive failure that involves both sides of the heart.*

Data Collection

1. Risk factors/etiology.
   a. Valvular disease.
   b. Myocardial disease.
   c. Congenital heart disease.
   d. Fluid overload.
2. Clinical manifestations.

NCLEX ALERT: *Determine changes in cardiovascular status. Determine if client vital signs are abnormal.*

a. Impaired cardiac function.
   (1) Tachycardia evaluated according to age level (see Table 10-2).
   (2) Enlarged heart from dilatation and hypertrophy.
   (3) Poor perfusion - cool extremities, weak pulses, poor capillary refill.
   (4) In infants, a failure to thrive and gain adequate weight.

b. Pulmonary congestion (left sided failure).
   (1) Dyspnea and cough.
   (2) Orthopnea, tachypnea.
   (3) Paroxysmal nocturnal dyspnea (PND) occurs while client is asleep.
   (4) Symptoms of respiratory distress and hypoxia (see Table 10-4).
   (5) Hemoptysis
   (6) Congested breath sounds.
   (7) Feeding difficulties in infants due to dyspnea and decreased exercise tolerance.

c. Systemic congestion (right sided failure).
   (1) Hepatomegaly (enlarged liver) - may be an early sign in children.

(2) Peripheral edema.

(3) Dependent edema or generalized in infants; evaluate by weight gain.

(4) Ascites.

(5) Increase in CVP.

Treatment

1. Treatment of the underlying problem.
2. Prevention.
   a. Adequate treatment of hypertension.
   b. Early treatment of dysrhythmias.
3. Oxygen.
4. Bed rest, semi or high Fowler's position.
5. Medications (Appendix 12-2).
6. Decrease sodium diet.
7. Fluid restriction -adults and older children. Infants seldom need fluid restrictions due to feeding difficulty.

NURSING PRIORITY: *The goals for therapeutic intervention in adult clients with congestive failure are:*
**Improve cardiac output - digitalis and oxygen.*
**Decrease the workload - decrease activity, administer ACE inhibitors.*
**Decrease the circulating volume - diuretics, decrease sodium and fluid intake, place client in semi-Fowler's position.*

Nursing Intervention

✦ *Goal: to decrease cardiac demands and improve cardiac function.*

1. Early identification and treatment of dysrhythmias.
2. Limit physical activity.
3. Maintain normal body temperature; avoid chilling.
4. Provide supplemental oxygen.
5. Provide uninterrupted sleep when possible.
6. Monitor urinary output - assess for any correlation of decreased urine output with decreased cardiac output.
7. Minimize crying in children and infants.
8. Maintain normal body temperature in infants; chilling increases oxygen consumption.
9. Decrease stress and anxiety; encourage parents to remain with child.
10. Carefully assess vital signs and compare with other physical assessment data.

NURSING PRIORITY: *In any client receiving digitalis and diuretics, it is very important to monitor the serum potassium level. A severe decrease in the serum potassium may affect cardiac rhythm, and may precipitate digitalis toxicity.*

✦ *Goal: to decrease circulating volume.*

1. Diuretics (Appendix 11-5).
2. Decreased sodium diet.
3. Calculate fluids carefully; client frequently on fluid restriction.
4. Evaluate fluid retention by accurate daily weight.
5. Accurate intake and output.

✦ *Goal: to reduce respiratory distress and promote gas exchange.*

1. Position.
   a. Adult in semi-Fowler's or in an armchair, do not elevate client's legs as this increases venous return.
   b. Infants and small children may breathe better side-lying with the knees drawn up to the chest.
   c. Infants may be placed in an infant seat.
   d. Make sure diapers are loosely pinned and safety restraints do not hinder maximum expansion of the chest.
2. Administer humidified oxygen.
3. Decrease exposure to upper respiratory infection.
4. Evaluate breath sounds.
5. Bed rest to gradual activity. Determine client's respiratory response to increased activity.

✦ *Goal: to monitor for development of hypoxia (Chapter 10).*

Pediatric Priority: *Cyanosis that decreases with crying is associated with respiratory function; cyanosis that increases with crying is associated with cardiac function.*

✦ *Goal: to maintain nutrition.*

1. Due to dyspnea, eating is sometimes difficult.
2. Small, frequent feedings; allow client adequate time.
3. Infants may need to be gavaged, due to increased work of sucking.
4. Infants generally not on fluid restriction, due to decreased intake from dyspnea.
5. Do not prop the bottle and burp the infant frequently.

NCLEX ALERT: *Plan and implement interventions to prevent client complications of cardiovascular conditions.*

Rheumatic Carditis

❑ **Rheumatic carditis occurs in about 40% of clients with rheumatic fever, it primarily affects the cardiac valves.**

A. Usually preceded by a group A *beta hemolytic* streptococcal infection.

NURSING PRIORITY: *Prevention and adequate treatment of streptococcal infections prevents the development of rheumatic fever.*

B. Myocardial involvement is characterized by an inflammatory response, causing scarring of the cardiac valves. Mitral valve is the most common area affected.

Data Collection

1. Clinical manifestations rheumatic carditis.
   a. Carditis - murmur, pericarditis, tachycardia.
   b. Precordial pain.
2. Clinical manifestations rheumatic fever.
   a. Polyarthritis.
   b. Carditis and fever.
   c. Chorea - CNS involvement characterized by involuntary purposeless movement, no residual damage occurs.
   d. Possible rash.
   e. Subcutaneous nodules.

Treatment

1. Prevention: Adequate treatment of streptococcal.
2. Bed rest to decrease cardiac workload.
3. Salicylates to control inflammatory process.
4. Prophylactic treatment.
   a. Initiated after acute therapy.
   b. Administration of penicillin over extended period of time.
   c. Administration of prophylactic penicillin before and after invasive medical procedures which increase risk factor of infection (GU procedures, dental work, etc.).

Complications

1. Severe valvular damage precipitates the development of congestive heart failure and may require open heart surgery for replacement of diseased valve.

Nursing Intervention

(Child is generally cared for in the home environment).

✦ *Goal: to assist parents and family to provide home environment conducive to healing and recovery.*

1. Decrease activity; bed rest if pulse rate is increased or if febrile.
2. Encourage routine activities within the home.
3. Friends may visit for short periods; child is not contagious.
4. Arrange for school work to be continued at home as appropriate.
5. Maintain adequate nutrition and hydration.
6. Administer analgesics for joint pain.

✦ *Goal: to assist client to understand need for long-term prophylactic antibiotic therapy.*

1. Importance of preventing recurring infections.
2. Importance of prophylactic therapy prior to invasive medical procedures.
3. Continued medical follow-up for the development of valvular problems as child grows.

Endocarditis (Bacterial, Infective)

❑ ***Endocarditis* is an infection of the valves and inner lining of the heart.**

A. Organism may enter from any site of localized infection.

B. Organism grows on the endocardium and produces a characteristic lesion consisting of vegetation, fibrin deposits, collagen; the lesion then may invade adjacent valves.

C. Lesion is fragile and may break off and form an embolus.

Risk Factors

1. Congenital heart disease.
2. Prosthetic valve replacement.
3. IV drug abuse.

Data Collection

1. Onset is gradual with nonspecific symptoms.
   a. Intermittent fever, high or low grade.
   b. Anorexia, weight loss.
   c. Joint pain.
   d. Petechiae (common).
2. Cardiac murmur.
3. Symptoms secondary to emboli.
   a. Spleen - splenomegaly, upper left quadrant pain.
   b. Kidney - flank pain, hematuria.

c. Brain - hemiplegia, decreased level of consciousness.

d. Pulmonary - dyspnea, chest pain, hemoptysis.

Treatment

1. Identification of infectious organism and appropriate antibiotic therapy (Appendix 5-10).
2. Bed rest if high fever or if evidence of cardiac damage.
3. Prophylactic antibiotics for 3-5 years, especially in children with history of rheumatic fever or congenital abnormalities.

NCLEX ALERT: *Identify signs and symptoms of infections. Plan and implement interventions to prevent complications.*

Nursing Intervention

✦ *Goal: to assist parents to understand need for long-term prophylactic therapy in high-risk children (See related Goal, rheumatic fever).*

✦ *Goal: to maintain homeostasis and prevent complications over long-term hospitalization.*

1. Maintain pattern of decreased activity, assess activity tolerance.
2. Evaluate for complications of emboli and congestive heart failure.

Self-Care

1. Explain the purpose of long-term antibiotic therapy.
2. Inform dentist and doctors prior to any invasive procedure - tooth extraction, cystoscopy, etc. Antibiotics will be ordered prophylactically.
3. Monitor temperature daily, report fever, chills, malaise, increasing fatigue, weight loss to the physician.
4. Progressive activity schedule until client is back to previous level of activity.

Pericarditis

❑ ***Pericarditis* is an inflammation of the pericardium.**

Data Collection

1. Chest pain aggravated by breathing, swallowing.
2. Pericardial friction rub caused by myocardium rubbing against inflamed pericardium.
3. Fever.
4. Dyspnea, tachypnea.
5. Restlessness, irritability, anxiousness.
6. May occur after an MI.

Treatment

1. Acute.
   a. Treat underlying problem.
   b. Bed rest.
   c. Anti-inflammatory medications

Nursing Intervention

✦ *Goal: to maintain homeostasis and promote comfort.*

1. Assess characteristics of pain; administer appropriate analgesics.
2. Upright position, with client leaning forward may relieve the pain.
3. Decrease anxiety as client often associates problem with an MI; assist client to distinguish the difference.
4. In clients with chronic pericarditis, evaluate for symptoms of heart failure and initiate appropriate nursing intervention.

Cardiovascular Disease in Pregnancy

❑ **Rheumatic heart disease and congenital heart defects account for the greatest incidence of cardiac disease in pregnancy. Of these, mitral valve stenosis is by far the most common.**

A. Normal physiological alterations of pregnancy that increase cardiovascular stress.
   1. Increase in oxygen requirements.
   2. Increase in cardiac output.
   3. Weight gain.
   4. Hemodynamic changes during delivery.

B. As normal pregnancy advances, cardiovascular system is unable to maintain adequate output to meet increasing demands.

Data Collection

Clinical manifestations indicative of cardiac decompensation are those of impending cardiac failure.

1. Frequent cough.
2. Progressive general edema.
3. Progressive dyspnea.
4. Excessive fatigue for level of activity.
5. Dysrhythmias.
6. Congested breath sounds.

7. Cardiac decompensation increases with length of gestation; increased incidence at 28-32 weeks gestation.

Treatment

1. Management of the pregnant client.
   a. Good nutritional intake; may require decrease in calories to avoid excessive weight gain.
   b. Limited activity, frequent rest periods.
   c. Iron supplement.
   d. Fluid and sodium are usually not restricted.
   e. Diuretics only if cardiac disease is severe.
   f. If severe, may be hospitalized at 28 to 32 weeks, due to impending cardiac failure.
   g. Prophylactic penicillin to prevent infection - especially important in women with mitral valve disease from rheumatic fever.
2. Management of the client during intrapartum.
   a. Vaginal low forceps delivery is common.
   b. Regional or local anesthesia generally utilized for delivery.
   c. Continuous monitoring of fetus and mother.
   d. Supplemental oxygen.
3. Management of the client during postpartum.
   a. Because of dramatic changes in the hemodynamic system, the postpartum period is another time of increased risk for cardiac failure in the mother.
   b. Client is treated symptomatically according to status of cardiovascular system.

NCLEX ALERT: *Provide care for client experiencing complications of pregnancy.*

Nursing Intervention

✦ *Goal: to assist client to maintain homeostasis during pregnancy.*

1. Written information regarding nutritional needs.
2. Nursing assessment to identify early symptoms of cardiac failure.
3. Frequent rest periods; activity may be severely restricted the last trimester.
4. Decrease stress by keeping client informed of progress.

✦ *Goal: to maintain homeostasis in postpartal period.*

1. Assessment of pulmonary and cardiac adaptation to changes in hemodynamics.
2. Maintain semi-Fowler's position or left lateral position with the head elevated.
3. Gradual progression of activities depending on cardiac status as indicated by:
   a. Pulse rate.
   b. Respiratory status.
   c. Activity tolerance.
4. Progressive ambulation as soon as possible to prevent venous thrombosis.
5. Assist mother and family to prepare for discharge.

CONGENITAL HEART DISEASE

A. Clinical manifestations depend on the severity of the defect and the adequacy of pulmonary blood flow.

B. Classifications.
1. Cyanotic
   a. Infant or child becomes cyanotic due to unoxygenated blood being pumped into the circulation.
   b. Occurs as a result of a left to right shunt in the heart.
2. Acyanotic
   a. Infant or child does not become cyanotic, but there is an increased workload on heart due to the cardiac defect.
   b. Occurs as a result of right-to-left shunt in the heart.

C. Physical consequences of congenital defects.
1. Retarded physical growth.
   a. Failure to gain weight, which often is due to inability to take in adequate calories.
   b. Tachycardia and tachypnea precipitate an increase in caloric requirements.
2. Excessive fatigue, especially during feedings.
3. Frequent upper respiratory infections.
4. Dyspnea.
5. Tachycardia.
6. Tachypnea.
7. Cyanosis (cyanotic defect).
8. Clubbing (cyanotic defect).

D. Diagnostics (Appendix 12-1).
1. Cardiac catheterization.
2. Chest x-ray.
3. Echocardiogram.
4. Predisposing maternal history.
5. Clinical manifestations.

Nursing Intervention

✦ *Goal: to evaluate infant's response to cardiac defect.*

1. Determine what infant's Apgar score was at birth.
2. Evaluate adequacy of weight gain.
3. Assess feeding problems.
   a. Poor sucking reflex.
   b. Poor coordination of sucking, swallowing, breathing.
   c. Fatigues easily during feeding, may result in inadequate intake.
4. Frequency of upper respiratory infections.
5. Cyanosis at rest or precipitated by activity.
6. Presence and quality of pulses in extremities.
7. Bacterial endocarditis is a primary concern prior to and after correction of congenital defect.

✦ *Goal: to assist parents in adjusting to diagnosis.*

1. Allow family to grieve over loss of perfect infant.
2. Evaluate parents' level of understanding of the child's problem.
3. Foster early parent-infant attachment; encourage touching, holding, and general physical contact.
4. Assist the family to develop relationship which foster optimum growth and development of all family members. (See Chapter 3 for psychosocial aspect of chronically ill children.)

Study Questions—Cardiac

1. The nurse is preparing a client for a cardiac catheterization. What is important for the nurse to explain to the client regarding his care after the test?

① it will be important for you to lie flat for several hours.
② it will be necessary for you to ambulate soon after the test.
③ you will be very sleepy, let the nurse know if you are hurting.
④ there will be a catheter in your bladder because you cannot get up.

2. A cardiac catheterization is scheduled for a client. In considering allergic reactions to the dye used in the procedure, an allergic reaction to what food would cause the nurse the most concern?

① eggs.
② milk products.
③ shellfish.
④ penicillin.

3. Cardiac isoenzymes are ordered on a client who possibly had an myocardial infarction. What will this test assess?

① presence of myocardial tissue damage.
② the possibility of GI involvement.
③ contractility of the heart muscle.
④ fluid build-up in the pericardium.

4. The nurse is assessing the apical heart rate on a client. Where on the chest wall should the nurse place the stethoscope?

① midline and to the left of the mediastinum.
② mid-clavicular line, fifth intercostal space on the left.
③ fifth intercostal space, left mid-axillary line.
④ right of mediastinum, anterior to the axillary area.

5. A client with bacterial endocarditis is being discharged. What is important to teach this client?

① begin exercise regime in about two weeks.
② increase your fluid intake of fruit juices.
③ keep taking your antibiotic.
④ return weekly for an electrocardiogram.

6. What is the rationale for a low sodium diet in the client with congestive heart failure?

① decrease fluid retention and improve cardiac output.
② increase fluid retention and increase cardiac output.
③ decrease high potassium levels.
④ increase serum sodium levels.

7. The nurse is administering nitroglycerine to a client who is complaining of chest pain. What is a common side effect of this medication?

① tachycardia.
② hypertension.
③ nausea and vomiting.
④ headache.

8. A client has left sided heart failure and the nurse notes he has is experiencing increasing dyspnea and tachycardia. What is the immediate nursing care?

① determine when he last had his anticoagulants.
② assess the stressors in his home life.
③ assess adequacy of urinary output.
④ position in high Fowler's with feet dependent.

9. What is important to teach a client who is starting sublingual nitroglycerin tablets?

① take it with a full glass of water.
② keep it in a clear container.
③ remember it has a rapid onset action of 2 to 5 minutes.
④ take it at the first onset of chest pain.

10. The congestive heart failure client has digoxin ordered. What would the nurse expect to find when evaluating for the therapeutic effectiveness of the drug?

① improved respiratory status and increased urinary output.
② increased heart rate and blood pressure.
③ diaphoresis with decreased output.
④ increased heart rate with increased respirations.

11. As edema decreases in a client with heart failure, what is the expected physiological response?

① increased body weight.
② rales across all lung fields.
③ increased respiratory rate.
④ urinary output increases.

12. A client is 2 days post myocardial infarction. Which nursing goal would be inappropriate in planning the care for this client?

① encourage client to express fears about the heart attack.
② relieve chest pain.
③ slowly increase activity with isometric exercises.
④ provide a low sodium diet.

13. A nurse notices jugular vein distention in the cardiac client. This is an early sign of the development of what complication?

① dehydration.
② left-sided heart failure.
③ right-sided heart failure.
④ cardiovascular accident.

14. What assessment finding in a client with a myocardial infarction would cause the most immediate concern?

① decreased urinary output.
② jugular vein distention.
③ shooting pain in the left upper thigh.
④ tachycardia with pedal edema.

15. What is a common side effect of nitroglycerin?

① tachycardia.
② increased blood pressure.
③ decreased urine output.
④ postural hypotension.

16. A client arrives at the emergency room complaining of severe chest pain and states that he had a heart attack two years ago. The nurse anticipates which analgesic will be given?

① hydromorphone hydrochloride (**Dilaudid**).
② morphine sulfate.
③ fentanyl (**Duragesic**).
④ oxycodone (**Percodan**).

17. What is considered a modifiable risk factor for coronary artery disease?

① age.
② race.
③ diet.
④ heredity.

18.What is considered an invasive cardiac diagnostic test?

① exercise stress test.
② cardiac MRI.
③ echocardiogram.
④ cardiac catheterization.

19. A client has been on digitalis for several months. The nurse is preparing to administer the daily dose of digitalis. What is an important nursing consideration?

① monitor for bleeding precautions.
② check for any nausea and vomiting.
③ assess breath sounds.
④ monitor for first degree heart block.

20. Why is the client placed on a firm surface to perform CPR?

① the heart is compressed between the sternum and the spine.
② it is easier to establish and maintain an open airway.
③ promotes venous return back to the central system.
④ decreases the potential for damage to the xiphoid process.

Appendix 12-1: CARDIAC DIAGNOSTICS

SERUM LABORATORY STUDIES:

Cardiac Enzymes:
Enzymes are drawn to evaluate myocardial damage and to identify myocardial infarction.

Nursing Implications:
1. Enzymes must be drawn on admission and obtained in a serial manner thereafter. There is a characteristic pattern to the increases and decreases of the enzyme response in the client with a myocardial infarction.
2. The larger the infarction; the larger the enzyme response.
3. Increased levels of CPK are significant; however, due to the rapid rise and subsequent decrease the pattern may be missed.
4. IM injections, medications, other disease entities, and tissue injury will affect enzyme changes; however, isoenzymes help discriminate myocardial tissue damage from other tissue injury.
5.CPK-MB increases within 4 - 6 hours after an MI, peaks in 18 - 24 hours (sometimes peaks at levels 6 times the normal value), returns to normal in 3 - 4 days.
6. Troponin level elevated in 4-6 hours after an MI, peaks within 10-24 hours.

NONINVASIVE DIAGNOSTICS:

Electrocardiogram (EKG, ECG):
A graphic representation of the electrical activity of the heart, generally conducted utilizing a twelve-lead format. Test to identify conduction in rhythm disorders and the occurrence of ischemia, injury, or death of myocardial tissue.

Holter Monitor:
Client is connected to a small portable EKG unit with recorder which records the client's heart activity for approximately 24 hours. The client is supposed to keep a log of activity, pain, or palpitations. Tell the client to bathe prior to being placed on monitor. The client should not shower or bathe after the monitor is in place. The recording is then analyzed, comparing it to client's activity log.

Exercise Stress Test:
This test involves the client exercising, usually on a treadmill, which increases with speed and incline to increase the heart rate. EKG leads are attached to the client and the response of the heart to exercise is evaluated.

Nursing Implications:
1. Appropriate pretest client education.
2. Client should:
   a. Avoid smoking and eating immediately prior to test.
   b. Avoid stimulants, eating, and extreme temperature changes immediately after test.
3. Blood pressure is monitored periodically during the test.
4. Reasons for terminating an exercise stress test: chest pain, greatly increased heart rate, serious cardiac dysrhythmias, severe hypertension, severe dyspnea, sudden loss of coordination, EKG changes -significant ST segment depression
   - If any of the above changes occur and the test is terminated, it is said to be a positive stress test.

Echocardiogram:
An ultrasound procedure to evaluate function and structure and valvular function of the heart. These sound waves are displayed on a graph and interpreted.

Magnetic Resonance Imaging:
A magnetic field and radio waves are used to detect and define the differences between healthy tissue and diseased tissue. Provides images in three dimensions. The client should not have any metal on his/her body, remove all jewelry, hair clips. Clients with permanent metal implanted in the body (pacemakers, implanted clips and wires, insulin pumps) are not candidates for MRI.

Positron Emission Tomography (PET)
Provides information regarding the perfusion and metabolism of an area of the heart. The procedure takes about 2-3 hours and a radioactive dye is injected.

INVASIVE DIAGNOSTICS:

Cardiac Catheterization:
This is an invasive procedure where a catheter is passed through an artery or vein into the heart. Cardiac catheterization will provide data regarding status of the coronary arteries, as well as cardiac muscle function, valvular functions, and left ventricular function (ejection fraction).

Right side catheterization—provides information regarding the function and structure of the right atrium, ventricle, pulmonic valve, and tricuspid valve.

Left side catheterization—provides information regarding the function and structure of the left atrium, ventricle, aortic valve, and mitral valve. The catheter is manipulated through the aorta and dye is injected into the coronary arteries (coronary angiogram).

Appendix 12-1: CARDIAC DIAGNOSTICS

Nursing Implications:

1. Pretest preparation
   a. NPO six hours before test.
   b. Check for dye allergy, especially iodine.
2. Posttest.
   a. Evaluate catheterization site for hematoma formation.
   b. Evaluate circulatory status and pulses distal to catheterization site.
   c. *Notify RN immediately of any changes in circulatory status of the extremity post cardiac catheterization.*
   d. Assess for arrhythmias.
   e. Avoid flexion of joint in immediate proximity of catheterization site.

Nursing Implications:

1. Pretest preparation.
   a. NPO six hours before test.
   b. Check for dye allergy, especially iodine and shellfish.
   c. Appropriate client education (flush feeling when dye is injected).
2. Posttest.
   a. Evaluate catheterization site for hematoma formation.
   b. Evaluate circulatory status of pulses distal to catheterization site.
   c. Assess for dysrhythmias.
3. Avoid flexion of joint at catheterization site.
4. Keep head of bed elevated at 30° or less.
5. Fluids will be encouraged to flush the dye out of the body.

NCLEX ALERT: *Physical preparation, client education, and nursing implications for clients undergoing treatments and procedures. Monitor client during and after procedure.*

Appendix 12-2: CARDIAC MEDICATIONS

MEDICATIONS	SIDE EFFECTS	NURSING IMPLICATIONS
NITRATES: Increases blood supply to the heart by dilating the coronary arteries; cardiac workload is reduced due to decrease in venous return because of peripheral vasodilation.		
Isosorbide dinitrate (**Isordil, Sorbide**): *PO* Nitroglycerin (**NTG, Nitrostat**): *sublingual* Nitroglycerin (**Nitro-Bid, Nitrol**): *topical*	Headaches (will diminish with therapy), postural hypotension, syncope, blurred vision, dry mouth, reflex tachycardia	1. Advise client that alcohol will potentiate postural hypotension. 2. Educate client regarding self-medication. (Table 12-2). 3. Report to physician continuous headaches, blurred vision, or dry mouth. 4. Topical application is used for sustained protection against anginal attacks. 5. Avoid skin contact with topical form; remove all previous applications when applying topical form.
CALCIUM CHANNEL BLOCKERS: Blockade of calcium channel receptors in the heart causes decreased cardiac contractility and a decreased rate of sinus and A-V node conduction.		
Diltiazem (**Cardizem**): *PO, IV* Nifedipine (**Procardia**): *PO* Verapamil (**Calan, Isoptin**): *IV, PO*	Constipation, exacerbation of CHF, hypotension, bradycardia, peripheral edema	1. ***Uses:*** chronic stable angina, hypertension, and supraventricular dysrhythmias. 2. Nifedipine is less likely to exacerbate pre-existing cardiac conditions; is not effective in treating dysrhythmias. 3. Intensifies cardiosuppressant effects of beta blocker medications

Appendix 12-2: CARDIAC MEDICATIONS

MEDICATIONS	SIDE EFFECTS	NURSING IMPLICATIONS
BETA-ADRENERGIC BLOCKING AGENTS: Blockade of beta $_1$ receptors in the heart causes: decreased heart rate, decreased force of contraction, and decreased rate of AV conduction.		
Nadolol (**Corgard**): PO Propranolol (**Inderal**): PO, IV Metoprolol (**Lopressor**): PO, IV Timolol (**Blocadren**): PO Atenolol (**Tenormin**)	Bradycardia, CHF, hypotension, depression, lethargy and fatigue	1. Evaluate client for precipitation of and/or increase of CHF, or dysrhythmia involving heart block. 2. May increase effectiveness of calcium channel blockers. 3. ***Uses:*** angina, hypertension, and cardiac dysrhythmias. 4. Teach clients how to decrease effects of postural hypotension 5. Teach clients not to stop taking medication when they feel better. 6. Bradycardia is common adverse effect. 7. Check pulse prior to administering. 8. If diabetic, monitor blood glucose levels, hypoglycemic symptoms may be blocked.

ANTIDYSRHYTHMIC MEDICATIONS: Decreases cardiac excitability, delays cardiac conduction either in the atrium or ventricle. Atropine is cardiac stimulant for bradycardia.

❖GENERAL NURSING IMPLICATIONS❖

— Assess client for changes in cardiac rhythm and impact on cardiac output.
— Evaluate effect of medication on dysrhythmia and resulting effects on cardiac output.
— Client should be on bed rest and cardiac monitor for IV administration.
— Have atropine available for cardiac depression resulting in symptomatic bradycardia.
— All cardiac depressant medications are contraindicated in clients with sinus node or AV node blocks.
— Digitalis will enhance cardiac depressant effects.
— Closely monitor for dysrhythmias that are precipitated by the treatment.

MEDICATIONS	SIDE EFFECTS	NURSING IMPLICATIONS
Quinidine sulfate (**Quinidine Sulfate, Quinidex**): *PO*	Vertigo, nausea, vomiting and diarrhea; progressive AV block, cinchonism-tinnitus, visual problems, headache	1. Use: supraventricular dysrhythmias and to convert client to sinus rhythm. 2. Medication is not recommended to be administered parenterally.
Disopyramide (**Norpace**): *PO*	Anticholinergic - urinary retention, dry mouth, constipation, bradycardia, hypotension	1. High incidence of urinary retention. 2. Contraindicated for use in clients with CHF. 3. ***Use:*** ventricular dysrhythmias.
Lidocaine hydrochloride (**Xylocaine**): *IV*	Drowsiness, confusion, seizures, severe depression of cardiac conduction.	1. ***Use:*** ventricular dysrhythmias
Tocainide (**Tonocard**) PO	Nausea, tremors	1. Use: to prevent/control ventricular dysrhythmias.
Mexiletine (**Mexitil**) PO	Nausea/vomiting, CNS- tremors, dizziness	1. Use: To prevent/control ventricular dysrhythmias.
Amiodarone hydrochloride (**Cardarone**) PO, IV	Nausea/vomiting, pulmonary toxicity	1. Use: treatment of ventricular fibrillation and tachycardia that do not respond to other medications. 2. Hypertension is not uncommon, keep clients on bed rest during treatment.
Procainamide (**Pronestyl**): *PO, IV*	Systemic lupus erythematosus-like syndrome, blood dyscrasias, hypotension, prolonged QT interval.	1. ***Uses:*** short- and long-term control of ventricular and supraventricular dysrhythmias. 2. If joint pain and inflammation occur, client should contact physician.
Propranolol Hydrochloride (**Inderal**)	(See previous discussion of beta adrenergic blockers)	

Appendix 12-2:
CARDIAC MEDICATIONS

MEDICATIONS	SIDE EFFECTS	NURSING IMPLICATIONS
ANTIDYSRHYTHMIC MEDICATIONS: *Continued*		
Atropine sulfate: IV, PO, SQ, IM	Dry mouth Blurred vision Dilated pupils	1. Used to block cardiac stimulation, primarily for bradycardias that are hemodynamically significant, or PVCs related to slow heart rate. 2. Carefully assess client's cardiac output in response to the bradycardic episode.

THROMBOLYTIC MEDICATIONS: Binds to fibrin in a thrombus and initiates fibrinolysis to break up a clot. Converts the circulating plasminogen to plasmin to begin fibrinolysis; is not clot specific.

❖GENERAL NURSING IMPLICATIONS❖

— Therapy should begin as soon as the myocardial infarction is diagnosed, or when there is history of prolonged angina.
— Bleeding precautions (Table 9-1).
— Streptokinase should be administered with an IV filter.

MEDICATIONS	SIDE EFFECTS	NURSING IMPLICATIONS
Streptokinase (**Streptase**):IV	Bleeding and hypotension	1. Client with recent (1 year) history of streptococcal infection or previous treatment with streptokinase will have antibodies against medication and it will not be as effective.
Anteplase (**Activase**): IV Reteplase (**Retavase**) IV		1. ***Uses:*** clients with history of streptococcal infection or previous treatment with streptokinase.

CARDIAC GLYCOSIDES (Digitalis): Increases myocardial contractility and cardiac output; decreases conduction of impulses through the AV node.

❖GENERAL NURSING IMPLICATIONS❖

— Take the apical pulse for a full minute, if the rate is below 60 in an adult, below 90 in a child, hold the medication and notify the physician.
— Evaluate for tachycardia, bradycardia, and irregular pulse. If there is significant change in rate and rhythm, hold the medication and notify the physician.
— Evaluate serum potassium levels and response to diuretics, hypokalemia potentiates action of digitalis. Gastrointestinal symptoms are frequently the first indication of digitalis toxicity.
— Teach client not to increase or double dose for missed doses.
— Quinidine and verapamil both increase plasma levels of digitalis.
— To achieve maximum results rapidly, a loading dose is administered, then reduced to a maintenance dose.

MEDICATIONS	SIDE EFFECTS	NURSING IMPLICATIONS
Digoxin (**Lanoxin**) PO, IV	Anorexia, nausea, vomiting, visual disturbances, fatigue, drug induced dysrhythmias	1. Therapeutic plasma levels of digoxin are 0.5-2.0 ng/ml. 2. First sign of toxicity is usually GI symptoms. 3. ***Uses:*** supraventricular tachycardia, CHF
Digitoxin (**Crystodigen**): PO		1. Effects of medication last much longer than digoxin, more difficult to adjust.

Geriatric Priority: *Elderly clients are more sensitive to digitalis and are more likely to experience digitalis toxicity.*

Appendix 12-3:
CARDIOPULMONARY RESUSCITATION (CPR)

❑ **The American Heart Association has established standards for cardiopulmonary resuscitation. For further delineation of the procedure, consult the American Heart Association Cardiopulmonary Resuscitation Guidelines. The American Heart Association defines a child as 1 year to approximately 8 years and infant as birth to one year. Basic cardiac life support involves the ABCs of CPR - Airway, Breathing, and Circulation.**

1. **Airway.**
   - Identify that victim is unconscious.
   - Activate the EMS system or code blue protocol.
   - Place client in position to open airway.
   - Open the airway: head tilt, chin lift.
   - Determine if victim is breathing. (Look, listen, and feel for breaths.)
   - If victim is breathing, place in recovery position.
   - If victim is not breathing, initiate rescue breathing.
2. **Breathing.**
   - Maintain the open airway.
   - Pinch nostrils closed.
   - Give 2 full breaths utilizing mouth-to-mouth technique (mouth-to-nose and mouth may be utilized in small children and infants).
3. **Check the pulse.** After giving two full breaths, check the pulse. On the adult and child, check the carotid; on the infant, check the pulse on the inside of the upper arm midway between the elbow and shoulder. If the pulse is present, continue rescue breathing.

   Adult: 1 breath every 5 seconds or 12 per minute.
   Child and Infant: 1 breath every 3 seconds or 20 per minute.
   If pulse is absent, begin external cardiac compressions.

NURSING PRIORITY: *Do not check the pulse prior to establishing ventilation. An open airway and rescue breathing must be established before continuing any further in the CPR sequence.*

Pediatric Priority: *Be careful not to hyperextend the infant's head, it may block the airway. Don't pinch the nose shut on an infant, cover the nose with your mouth. Breathe slowly, just enough to make the chest rise.*

4. **External cardiac compression.**
   - Place the victim on a firm surface. If the client is in the bed, put a cardiac board behind the victim. DO NOT attempt to remove the victim from the bed.
   - Locate the lower half of the sternum in the adult and the child. For the adult, place one hand over the lower sternum; place the other hand on top of the previous hand. For a child, utilize the heel of one hand. For an infant, locate the nipple line; the area for compression is one finger's width below the line; use two fingers for compression.
   - Depress the sternum $1\frac{1}{2}$ to 2 inches in the adult; children depress 1 to $1\frac{1}{2}$ inches; infants depress $\frac{1}{2}$ to 1 inch.
   - Compression and relaxation should be of equal duration.

Adult:
One rescuer and 2 rescuers -- 15 compressions (rate to maintain compression at approximately 100 per minute) to 2 ventilations.
Two rescuers (if client is intubated) - 5 compressions (rate of 80 to 100 per minute) to 1 ventilation.

Infant and Child:
One rescuer - 5 compressions (rate greater than 100 per minute) to 1 ventilation.

5. **Do not interrupt CPR for more than 5 seconds.**
6. **Termination of CPR: The nonphysician individual should continue resuscitation efforts until one of the following occurs:**
   - Spontaneous circulation and ventilation have been restored.
   - Resuscitation efforts are transferred to another equally responsible person who continues the resuscitation procedure.
   - A physician, or physician-directed person, assumes responsibility for resuscitation procedure.
   - The victim is transferred to an emergency medical service (i.e., paramedics and ambulance).
   - The rescuer is exhausted and unable to continue resuscitation.

NCLEX ALERT: *Identify and intervene in life-threatening client situations. Notify primary health care provider about unexpected response/emergency situation of client.*

Appendix 12-4:
CARDIAC DYSRHYTHMIAS

❑ **A *dysrhythmia* (arrhythmia) is defined as an interruption in the normal conduction of the heart, either in the rate or the rhvthm.**

CHARACTERISTICS OF NORMAL SINUS RHYTHM:

Rate - 60 to 100
Rhythm - regular
P waves - present, precede each QRS
P-R interval - .12 to .20 seconds
QRS - present and under .10 second

Dysrhythmias may be classified according to rate, either bradycardia or tachycardia. They are also classified according to their origin - atrial or ventricular. Ventricular dysrhythmias are more life-threatening than atrial dysrhythmias.

Nursing Implications:

1. Evaluate client's tolerance of the dysrhythmia.
   Level of consciousness, increased lethargy
   Hypotension or postural hypotension
   Pulse rate - tachycardiac/bradycardic
   Urinary output
2. Maintain adequate cardiac output - keep client on bedrest until parameters of dysrhythmia are determined.

NCLEX ALERT: *Intervene to control cardiovascular status (initiate protocol to manage cardiac dysrhythmia.*

Appendix 12-5:
PACEMAKERS

Permanent - an internal generator is inserted into soft tissue of upper chest or abdomen and electrodes are positioned according to the pacing mode; procedure planned and conducted under fluoroscopy and optimal conditions. Pacemakers are used in persistent chronic heart block or sustained bradycardia.

Pacing Modes

Demand - the heart is stimulated to beat when the client's pulse rate falls below a set value or rate (majority of the pacemakers have a set rate between 60-72, if client's pulse rate falls below the set value, the pacemaker will be initiated), utilized in both temporary and permanent pacing. The pacemaker "senses" the initiation of a beat and the following conduction. If a normal cardiac beat is initiated and conducted, the pacemaker does not initiate an impulse.

Atrioventricular - The ventricle is sensed, and the atrium is paced. If the ventricle does not depolarize, then it is also paced.

Universal atrioventricular - both the atrial and ventricular circuits sense and pace in the respective chambers. This most closely resembles the normal conduction system.

Pacemaker Failure - an ECG must be available to verify pacemaker failure. If a client with a pacemaker is experiences bradycardia below the rate set on the pacemaker, it needs to be investigated immediately.

Client Education:

1. Advise the client of the set rate of his pacemaker; teach him to take his pulse every day and record on calendar. Notify the physician if the pulse is lower than the set rate.
2. Avoid constrictive clothing that puts pressure on or irritates the site; report any signs of infection.
3. Safe environment - avoid areas of high voltage, magnetic force fields, large running motors.
4, Wear a medical alert identification, and advise all health care professionals regarding the pacemaker.
5. Avoid activity that requires vigorous movement of arms and shoulders.
6. Client's pulse rate should not drop below the preset rate; if this occurs, the pacemaker is not functioning properly and it needs to be reported.
7. Follow-up care and monitoring of pacemaker is important.

NCLEX ALERT: *Determine if client's pacemaker is functioning properly.*

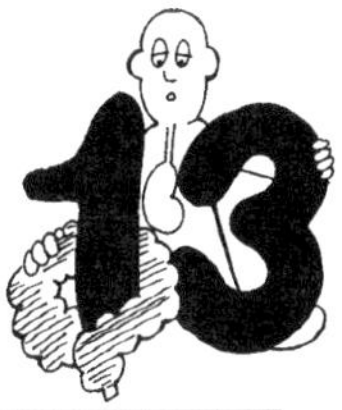

Gastrointestinal System

PHYSIOLOGY OF THE GASTROINTESTINAL (GI) SYSTEM

Organs of the Gastrointestinal System

A. Mouth, pharynx, esophagus.

B. Stomach.

1. Lies in the upper left portion of the abdominal cavity.
2. Gastroesophageal sphincter (cardiac sphincter)- opening of the esophagus into the upper portion of the stomach.

C. Small intestine.

1. Primary area of digestion and absorption of food.
2. Action.
   a. Promotes mixing of the digestive juices.
   b. Peristaltic movement maintains the forward progress of the intestinal content.
   c. Secretions of the small intestine initiates the breakdown of all three major food groups.
   d. Mucosal lining of small intestine is primary area for the absorption of nutrients.

D. Large intestine (figure 13-1).

1. Divisions.
   a. Cecum - blind pouch at the junction of the ileum and the colon; appendix arises from the cecum just below the ileocecal valve.
2. Mucus is the only secretion produced in the large intestine.
3. Action.
   a. Reabsorption of water.
   b. Peristaltic movement to propel residue toward the rectum.

E. Rectum and anus.

1. As fecal material enters the rectum, the desire for defecation is initiated.
2. If desire to defecate is ignored, it will disappear and fecal material will become hard and dry.
3. During defecation the rectum and colon contract, the individual takes a deep breath and initiates a voluntary contraction of the diaphragm and the abdominal wall with the glottis closed; this in turn increases pressure in the rectum.
   a. Valsalva maneuver is the voluntary pressure exerted against a closed glottis during defecation, straining at stool, or lifting.
   b. This activity increases intrathoracic pressure and impedes venous return to the heart.
   c. When the strain is released, there is an increase in venous return to the heart. This may precipitate problems in the cardiac client.
4. An infant has no control over external sphincter; defecation is a reflex action.

System Data Collection

A. Evaluate client's history.

1. Changes in bowel habits.
2. Changes in dietary habits.
3. Weight loss or gain.
4. Pain, location.
5. Nausea and vomiting.
   a. Associated with pain.
   b. Precipitating factors.
6. Presence or problems with flatulence.

B. Assess vital signs in client's overall status.

C. Assess for presence and characteristics of pain.

D. Assess client's mouth.

1. Overall condition of teeth.
2. Overall condition of tongue.
3. Presence of the gag reflex.

E. Evaluate the abdomen (client should be lying flat) sequence of assessment -inspection, auscultation, percussion, palpation.

1. Divide the abdomen into four quadrants and describe findings according to the quadrants.
2. Evaluate the general contour of the abdomen.
3. Evaluate for presence of surgical or trauma scars or ostomies.
4. Assess for presence of and characteristics of bowel sounds, should be audible within 2 minutes.
   a. Intensity and frequency.
   b. Sounds are usually loudest just to the right and below the umbilicus.
   c. Absence of bowel sounds over a 2 minute period should be investigated

NCLEX ALERT: *Review characteristics of client bowel sounds.*

5. Percuss for areas of distention and air.

Figure 13-1: Organs of the Gastrointestinal System
Reprinted with permission: Phipps, WJ, Sands, JK, & Marek, JF (1999). *Medical Surgical Nursing: Concepts & Clinical Practice*, 6th ed. Philadelphia: Mosby, p. 1236.

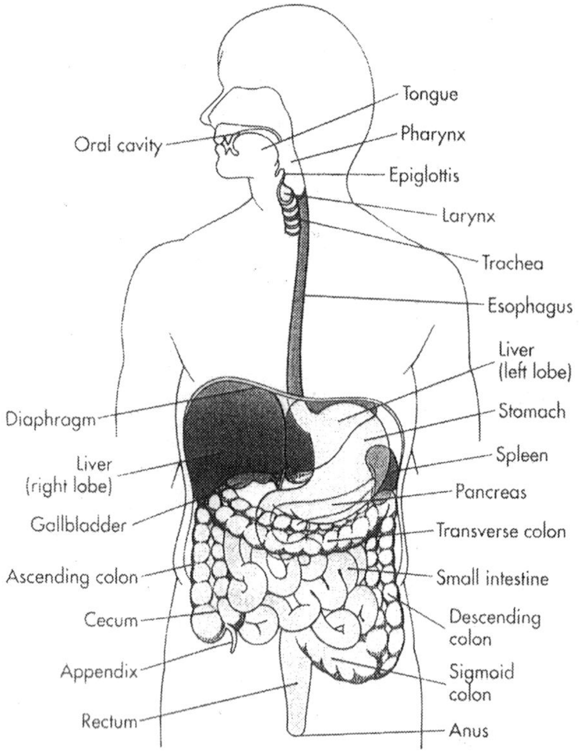

6. Palpate the abdomen. Begin with nontender areas first.
   a. Soft to palpation.
   b. Presence of distention.
   c. Presence of masses.

F. Assess rectal area.

G. Evaluate dietary pattern and fluid intake.

H. Assess stool specimen.
   1. Color.
   2. Consistency.
   3. Odor.

DISORDERS OF THE GASTROINTESTINAL SYSTEM

Nausea and Vomiting

❑ **Nausea is an unpleasant feeling that vomiting is imminent. Vomiting is an involuntary act in which the stomach contracts and forcefully expels gastric contents.**

A. Loss of fluid and electrolytes is the primary consequence of repeated vomiting; the very young and the elderly are more susceptible to complications of fluid imbalances.

B. Prolonged vomiting will precipitate a metabolic problem with acid-base balance.

Data Collection

1. Clinical manifestations.
   a. Identify precipitating cause.
      (1) Abdominal distention - especially in postoperative clients.
      (2) May be associated with medications - analgesics, NSAIDS, digitalis, and multiple other medications.
      (3) If result of food intolerance, client generally feels better after vomiting.
      (4) May be associated with virus, upper respiratory infections and postnasal drainage.
      (5) Gastritis associated with food poisoning.

NCLEX ALERT: *Determine causes of nausea and vomiting.*

   b. Assess frequency of vomiting, amount of vomiting, and contents of vomitus.
   c. Hematemesis - presence of blood in vomitus.
      (1) Bright red blood is indicative of bleeding in the stomach.
      (2) Coffee-ground material is indicative of blood retained in the stomach. The digestive process has broken down the hemoglobin.
   d. Projectile vomiting - vomiting not preceded by nausea; expelled with excessive force.
   e. Presence of fecal odor in vomitus indicates a back- flow of intestinal contents into stomach.
2. Diagnostics - clinical manifestations.

Treatment

1. Eliminate the precipitating cause.
2. Antiemetics (See Appendix 13-2).
3. Parenteral replacement of fluid if loss is excessive.

NCLEX ALERT: *Identify signs of fluid and/or electrolyte imbalance in client. Implement interventions to restore client fluid and electrolyte balance.*

Nursing Intervention

✦ *Goal: to prevent recurrence of nausea and vomiting, and ensuing complications.*

1. Prophylactic antiemetics for clients with a tendency toward vomiting (chemotherapy, postop).
2. Prompt removal of unpleasant odors, used emesis basin, used equipment, and soiled linens.

3. Good oral hygiene.
4. Position conscious client on side or in semi-Fowler's position; position unconscious client on side with head of bed slightly elevated.
5. Withhold PO food and fluid initially after vomiting; begin oral intake slowly with clear liquids.
6. Support abdominal incisions during prolonged vomiting.

✦ *Goal: to relieve nausea and vomiting.*

1. Administer antiemetics as indicated.
2. Evaluate precipitating causes; relieve if possible.
3. Gastric decompression with a nasogastric tube may be indicated.

✦ *Goal: to assess client's response to prolonged vomiting.*

1. Fluid and electrolyte status.
2. Continued presence of gastric distention.
3. Overall vital sign changes.
4. Intake and output.
5. Assess for adequate hydration.
6. Evaluate weight loss.

NURSING PRIORITY: *Any client who is experiencing vomiting it at increased risk for aspiration.*

Constipation and Diarrhea

Constipation

❑ ***Constipation* exists when the interval between bowel movements is longer than normal for the individual and the stool is dry and hard.**

Data Collection

1. Precipitating causes.
   a. Inadequate bulk in the diet.
   b. Inadequate fluid intake.
   c. Immobilization.
   d. Ignoring the urge to defecate.
   e. Diseases of the colon and rectum.
   f. Side effects of medications.
2. Clinical manifestations.
   a. Abdominal distention.
   b. Decrease in the amount of stool.
   c. Dry, hard stool.
3. Diagnostics - clinical manifestations.

NCLEX ALERT: *Identify factors that interfere with elimination.*

Box 13-1: Elderly Care Focus:
Preventing Fecal Impaction

- Increase intake of high fiber foods - raw vegetables, whole grain breads and cereals, fresh fruits.
- Increase fluid intake - water and juice.
- Maintain regular activity - daily walking in immediate area.
- Discourage use of laxatives and enemas - client becomes dependent on them.
- Encourage use of bulk- forming products to provide increased fiber -methylcellulose, psyllium.
- Encourage bowel movement at same time each day.
- Try to position client on bedside commode rather than on a bedpan.
- If client is experiencing diarrhea, check to see if stool is oozing around an impaction.

Treatment (see Appendix 13-3 and Box Text 13-1)

Nursing Intervention

✦ *Goal: to identify client at risk of developing problems and institute preventive measures.*

✦ *Goal: to implement treatment measures.*

NCLEX ALERT: *Intervene with client experiencing alteration in bowel elimination.*

Diarrhea

❑ ***Diarrhea* occurs when there is a significant increase in number of stools and stools are more liquid.**

Data Collection

1. Precipitating causes.
   a. Intestinal inflammation and infections.
   b. Food and drug intolerance.
   c. Food poisoning.
   d. Bowel disorders.
   e. Malabsorption problems.
   f. Psychological factors.
2. Clinical manifestations.
   a. Frequent, liquid bowel movements.
   b. Stools may contain undigested food, mucus, pus, or blood.
   c. Frequently foul- smelling.

d. Abdominal cramping, distention, and vomiting frequently occur with diarrhea.

e. Weight loss.

f. Hyperactive bowel sounds.

g. May precipitate dehydration, hypovolemia, hypokalemia, and shock.

h. Infants and elderly are most susceptible to complications of diarrhea.

3. Diagnostics.

a. Clinical manifestations.

b. Stool culture.

4. Complications of severe diarrhea.

a. Dehydration resulting in hypovolemia.

b. Acid-base imbalances

Treatment

1. Treat the underlying problem.
2. Decrease activity and irritation of the GI tract by decreasing intake.
3. Increase clear liquids as tolerated.
4. Parenteral replacement of fluid and electrolytes if diarrhea is severe.
5. Administer antidiarrheal medications (See Appendix 13-4).

Nursing Intervention

✦ *Goal: to decrease diarrhea and prevent complications.*

1. Identify precipitating causes and eliminate if possible.
2. Decrease food intake; more soft, nonirritating food, and increase in fluids.
3. Replace fluids as indicated, either PO or IV.
4. Maintain good hygiene in the rectal area to prevent skin excoriation.
5. Decrease activity.

✦ *Goal: to evaluate client's response to diarrhea.*

1. Evaluate changes in vital signs correlating with fluid loss.
2. Evaluate electrolyte changes and overall hydration status.
3. Intake and output, daily weight if diarrhea is progressive.
4. Assess changes in abdominal distention and cramping.
5. Ongoing evaluation of characteristics of diarrhea.

✦ *Goal: to prevent spread of diarrhea.*

1. Good hand washing techniques, contact precautions.
2. Enteric precautions if diarrhea is of infectious origin.

Rotavirus

❑ **Most common pathogen in young children hospitalized for diarrhea.**

A. Affects all age groups and is most common in cool weather.

B. Incubation period is 1-3 days.

C. Important source of nosocomial infections in hospital.

D. Is frequently associated with an upper respiratory infection.

Data Collection.

1. Clinical manifestations.

a. Abrupt onset.

b. Nausea/vomiting and abdominal pain.

c. Persistent foul smelling, explosive, diarrhea.

d. Fever last approximately 48 hours.

2. Diagnostics.

a. History regarding onset and duration.

b. Laboratory electrolytes to determine status of hydration.

Nursing Intervention.

✦ *Goal: to maintain fluid and electrolyte balance (see nursing interventions for client with diarrhea)*

1. Fluid and electrolyte replacement, initially oral rehydration therapy with solutions to replace electrolytes (oral rehydration solutions)
2. Monitor IV fluids in situations of severe diarrhea.
3. Antidiarrheal medications (Appendix 18-4).
4. Monitor stools; is at increased risk for developing a paralytic ileus.
5. Strict monitoring of hydration status.
6. May begin food as soon as child can tolerate, generally soft, easily digestible food, but does not have to be clear liquids.

✦ *Goal: to decrease infection and prevent spread.*

1. Contact precautions in hospital.
2. Instruct parents regarding importance of handwashing, and how to care for infant/child at home.
3. Maintain "clean" and "dirty" areas in the room.
4. Antibiotics are most often not indicated because of the risk of developing pseudo-membranous colitis.

NCLEX ALERT: *Identify client risk factors for infection. Identify signs and symptoms of infection.*

Oral Cancer

A. May occur in any area of the mouth; frequently curable if discovered early.

B. Sites of oral cancer.
1. Lips.
2. Tongue.
3. Salivary glands.
4. Floor of the mouth.

Data Collection

1. Risk factors/etiology.
   a. Increased incidence in males.
   b. Smoking.
   c. Continuous oral irritation due to poor dental hygiene.
   d. Chewing tobacco.
2. Clinical manifestations.
   a. Leukoplakia - whitish patch on oral mucosa or tongue.
   b. Painless oral lesions that is fixed and hard with raised edges.
   c. Advances symptoms include dysphagia, difficulty chewing or speaking, and enlarged lymph nodes.
3. Diagnostics - biopsy of suspected lesion.

Treatment

1. Surgery.
   a. Surgical resection.
   b. Reconstructive surgery.
2. Radiation.
3. Chemotherapy.

Nursing Intervention

✦ *Goal: to prepare client for surgery.*
1. General preoperative care (Chapter 3).
2. Discuss with RN the anticipated extent of surgery; reiterate and reinforce information with client.
3. Emphasis on good oral hygiene.

✦ *Goal: to maintain patent airway postoperatively.*
1. Immediate postoperative position should be supine with head turned or client positioned on side; when client is awake, elevate head of bed slightly to promote venous and lymphatic drainage.
2. *Notify RN immediately of swelling at incision site.*
3. Evaluate ability of client to handle oral secretions.
4. Respiratory assessment to identify problems of hypoxia.
5. Occasionally the client may have a tracheostomy; depends on the extent of surgery.
6. Good pulmonary hygiene.

NURSING PRIORITY: *Airway maintenance and respiratory distress are potential problems with any operative procedure that involves the face and neck.*

✦ *Goal: to maintain oral hygiene and prevent injury and infection postoperatively.*
1. Assess graft area for viability.
   a. Graft should be pale pink and warm to touch.
2. Type of oral hygiene is indicated by the extent of the procedure.
   a. Mouth irrigations.
   b. Soothing mouth rinses.
   c. If dentures are present, clean mouth well before replacing.
   d. Oral hygiene before and after PO intake.

✦ *Goal: to maintain nutrition postoperatively.*
1. Tube feedings may be indicated initially.
2. May be necessary to maintain nutrition by parenteral hyperalimentation (Appendix 13-6).
3. Oral intake - assess client's ability to swallow and control fluids.
   a. Liquid, soft, nonirritating foods.
   b. No extremes in temperature of food.
   c. Small, frequent feedings.
   d. Provide privacy and do not rush during meals.

NCLEX ALERT: *Monitor client ability to eat. Monitor client for impact of disease on nutritional status.*

Self-Care
1. Assist client to identify community resources for individual problems in rehabilitation.
   a. Speech therapist.
   b. Dietician.
   c. Counseling.
2. Stop smoking.
3. Avoid upper respiratory infections.
4. Instruct client regarding oral hygiene, dressing care, and medications.
5. Teach client symptoms of complications and to notify physician - infection, suture line bleeding

or disruption, airway problems, swallowing problems, increased pain.

Gastroesophageal Reflux Disease (GERD)

❑ **This condition is caused by backward flow of gastric contents into the esophagus, (esophageal reflux). Reflux is often associated with a *hiatal hernia;* the herniation of the upper portion of the stomach through the diaphragm into the thoracic cavity.**

Data Collection

1. Reflux esophagitis (heartburn, dyspepsia).
2. May be associated with intake of nicotine, high fat foods, and caffeine.
3. Pain after meals, may be relieved with antacids.
4. Regurgitation (effortless return of stomach contents into the mouth).
5. Discomfort occurs with increase in abdominal pressure - lifting, straining.
6. Dysphagia.
7. Diagnostics - barium swallow, esophagoscopy.

Treatment

1. Medications (Appendix 13-5).
2. Surgical correction if hiatal hernia is present.

Nursing Intervention

✦ *Goal: to decrease symptoms of esophageal reflux.*

1. Administer antacids.
2. Dietary modifications.
   a. Decrease intake of highly seasoned foods.
   b. Frequent small meals, to prevent gastric dilation.
   c. Avoid carbonated beverages.
   d. Avoid any food which precipitates discomfort (fats, caffeine, chocolate; nicotine will decrease esophageal sphincter tone).
   e. Do not lie down after eating; avoid eating before bedtime.
   f. Adequate fluid intake with meals.
3. Decrease or stop smoking.
4. Elevate head of bed on four to six inch blocks.
5. Decrease weight to decrease abdominal pressure.

✦ *Goal: Perform preoperative nursing interventions as appropriate if surgery is indicated (See Chapter 3).*

✦ *Goal: Prevent complications postoperatively.*

Peptic Ulcer Disease (PUD)

❑ ***PUD* is the ulceration of the gastric mucosa as a result of the digestive action of hydrochloric acid and pepsin. The condition may be classified as acute or chronic. Duodenal ulcer is the most common type.**

A. Characteristics

1. Factors contributing to the development.
   a. Presence of *H.pylori* bacteria in the stomach.
   b. Associated with increased acid production.
   c. Increased stress in lifestyle.
   d. Smoking and alcohol.
   e. Increase in physical stress - surgery, trauma.
   f. Associated with medications - NSAIDs and steroids.
2. Clinical manifestations.
   a. Burning, cramping, midepigastric pain.
   b. Duodenal ulcers - pain may occur 1-3 hours after eating; relieved by eating
   c. Dyspepsia syndrome occur in both types: fullness, epigastric discomfort, distention, anorexia and weight loss.

Diagnostics

1. Clinical manifestations.
2. X-ray of upper GI system.
3. Endoscopy - gastroscopy with test for *H. pylori.*

Treatment

1. Medical (See Appendix 13-5).
   a. Antacids
   b. Histamine receptor antagonist and antisecretory agents to decrease acid production.
   c. Medication regimen to treat *H. pylori.*
   d. Dietary modifications - highly individual; foods precipitating pain are to be avoided.
2. Surgical interventions - gastric resection.

Complications

1. Indications of hemorrhage.
   a. Hematemesis, melena, or both.
   b. Hypovolemic shock (Chapter 11).

> ***NURSING PRIORITY:*** *Carefully evaluate the client's blood pressure. Orthostatic hypotension (a blood pressure decrease of 10 mm Hg or more) may be indicative of hypovolemia.*

2. Perforation of ulcer into the peritoneal cavity.
   a. Sudden, severe, diffuse, upper abdominal pain.

b. Abdominal muscles contract as abdomen becomes rigid.

c. Bowel sounds absent.

d. Respirations become shallow and rapid.

e. Severity of the peritonitis is proportional to size of perforation and amount of gastric spillage.

Nursing Intervention

✦ *Goal: to promote health in clients with PUD.*

1. Assist client to understand disease process.
2. Assist client to identify factors which precipitate pain and discomfort.
3. Provide information regarding dietary implications.
4. Use acetaminophen instead of aspirin products.

***NURSING PRIORITY:** Client should not take over-the-counter medications, especially aspirin and NSAID compounds.*

✦ *Goal: to relieve pain and promote healing.*

1. Dietary modifications.
   a. Encourage small, frequent meals.
   b. Nonstimulating bland foods are generally tolerated better during healing of acute episodes.
   c. Assist client to identify specific dietary habits which accelerate or precipitate pain.
   d. Promote good nutritional habits.
2. Decrease and or change activity as indicated by discomfort.

NCLEX ALERT: *Implement interventions to manage potential client circulatory complications (hemorrhage.). Monitor client for bleeding.*

✦ *Goal: to assess for complications of hemorrhage, perforation and peritonitis, and initiate nursing actions accordingly.*

1. Assess stools and nasogastric drainage for presence of blood.
2. Assess for distention, increase in pain, and tenderness.
3. Monitor vital signs and evaluate changes.
4. Maintain client NPO.
5. Prepare client for immediate surgery.

✦ *Goal: to assist client to return to homeostasis postoperative gastric resection.*

1. General postoperative care as indicated (Chapter 3).

Table 13-1: Dumping Syndrome

✦ Condition occurs when a large bolus of food enters the intestines before it is adequately mixed with normal gastric secretions.

✦ Gastric resection for trauma, ulcer perforation, cancer, gastroplasty

✦ Symptoms typically occur 5-30 minutes after eating. meal.

✦ Symptoms include: weakness, dizziness, tachycardia, diaphoresis, palpitations, and the desire to lie down.
✧ Late symptoms (2-3 hrs after eating): epigastric fullness and distention, abdominal cramping, diarrhea, loud bowel sounds.

✦ Preventing dumping syndrome.
✧ Five to six meals daily; decrease amount of food eaten at one meal.
✧ Decrease carbohydrates, decrease salt intake, increase proteins and fats as tolerated; low roughage.
✧ No added fluid with meal or for one hour before meal or following meal; *liquids between meals only*.
✧ Position client in semi recumbent position during meals; client should lie down for 20-30 minutes after meals to delay stomach emptying.

NCLEX ALERT: *Assist with teaching client about dietary modifications.*

2. Assess for the bowel sounds that indicate return of peristalsis.
3. Maintain nasogastric suction until peristalsis returns -assess color and consistency of drainage.

NCLEX ALERT: *Monitor gastrointestinal output.*

4. After removal of nasogastric tube, assess for:
   a. Increasing abdominal distention.
   b. Nausea, vomiting.
   c. Changes in bowel sounds.
5. NPO until removal of nasogastric tube.
6. Begin PO fluids slowly - clear liquids, then progress to bland soft diet.
7. Encourage ambulation to promote peristalsis.

✦ *Goal: to identify complication of dumping syndrome and initiate preventive nursing measures postoperative gastric resection (Table 13-1: Dumping Syndrome).*

1. Assess for symptoms of condition.
2. Prevent dumping syndrome (Table 13-1).

NCLEX ALERT: *Use measures to improve a client's nutrition.*

✦ *Goal: to initiate measures to prevent the development of pernicious anemia postoperative total gastric resection: (vitamin B12 deficiency).*

✦ *Goal: to assist client to understand implications of the disease and measures necessary to maintain health postoperative total gastric resection.*

1. Modification of dietary habits.
2. Stop smoking.
3. Understand medication regimen.
4. Continue medical follow-up.
5. Identify factors in lifestyle which precipitate stress and if necessary obtain counseling to decrease stress in lifestyle.

Cancer of the Stomach

❑ **Cancer may occur in any portion of the stomach. The majority of the lesions occur in the pyloric area.**

A. Metastasis generally occurs by direct extension of the malignant growth into adjacent organs and structures (esophagus, spleen, pancreas, etc.).

B. Due to the ability of the stomach to accommodate the growing tumor, symptoms may not be evident until metastasis has occurred.

Data Collection

1. Risk factors/etiology.
   a. Chronic changes in gastric mucosa.
   b. Familial tendencies.
2. Clinical manifestations.
   a. Weight loss.
   b. Feeling of discomfort or fullness.
   c. Anemia from chronic blood loss.
   d. Presence of a palpable mass.
3. Diagnostics.
   a. Endoscopy, biopsy, cytologic washings.

Treatment

No successful treatment other than removal of tumor (gastrectomy). The gastric tumor is frequently not diagnosed until the advanced stages.

Nursing Intervention

See nursing intervention for gastric resection.

Pyloric Stenosis

❑ **This is the obstruction of the pyloric sphincter by hypertrophy and hyperplasia of the circular muscle of the pylorus.**

Table 13-2: Undiagnosed Abdominal Pain

✦ **DO NOT:**
Give anything by mouth.
Put any heat on the abdomen.
Give an enema or laxatives.
Give strong narcotics.
✦ **DO:**
Put on bed rest.
Place in position of comfort.
Assess hydration status.
Assess abdominal status: distention, bowel sounds, passage of stool or flatus, generalized or localized pain

Data Collection

1. Onset of vomiting may be gradual, or may develop forceful, projectile vomiting.
2. Vomiting occurs shortly after feeding.
3. Vomitus does not contain bile.
4. Infant is hungry and nurses well.
5. Infant does not appear to be in pain or acute distress.
6. Failure to gain weight.
7. Stools decrease in number and in size.
8. Evidence of dehydration as condition progresses.
9. Upper abdomen is distended and an "olive-shaped" mass may be palpated in the right epigastric area.

Treatment

Surgical release of the pyloric muscle (pyloromyotomy).

NCLEX ALERT: *Monitor client ability to eat and nutritional status. Position client to prevent complications. Implement measures to resort client fluid and/or electrolyte balance.*

Nursing Intervention

✦ *Goal: to restore and maintain hydration and electrolyte balance; initiate appropriate preoperative nursing activities.*

1. If infant is being fed PO:
   a. Feed slowly with infant in upright position.
   b. Frequent bubbling during feeding; to prevent gastric distention.
   c. After feeding, position infant slightly on his right side in high-Fowler's or in an infant seat.
   d. Minimal handling after feeding.
2. Monitor vital signs and correlate with problems of dehydration.
3. Assess for signs of dehydration.

4. If child is dehydrated, may be placed NPO with continuous IV infusion.
5. Accurate intake and output records - complete description of all vomitus and stools.
6. Gastric decompression and suction may be utilized preoperatively; maintain patency of tube and record drainage.
7. Preoperative teaching for parents.
8. Child should be in optimum hydration and electrolyte balance preoperatively.

✦ *Goal: to maintain adequate hydration and promote healing postoperative pyloromyotomy.*

1. Postoperative vomiting in the first 24 to 48 hours is not uncommon.
2. Assess infant's response to surgery.
3. Continue to monitor infant in the same manner as in the preoperative period.
4. Feedings are initiated early, beginning with clear liquids including glucose and electrolytes.
5. Continue feedings in the same manner as preoperatively.
6. Monitor infant's response to feedings.

✦ *Goal: to assist parents to provide appropriate home care postoperative pyloromyotomy.*

1. Generally, there are no residual problems after surgery.
2. Modifications of feedings should be continued at home.

Appendicitis

❑ ***Appendicitis* is characterized by an inflammation of the appendix and is the most common reason for abdominal surgery during childhood.**

A. Obstruction of the blind sac of the appendix precipitates inflammation, ulceration, and necrosis.
B. Problems arise when the necrotic area ruptures, spilling intestinal contents into the peritoneal cavity, causing peritonitis.

Data Collection

1. More common in older children and adolescents.
2. Child may complain of severe abdominal pain and may not be able to stand upright.
3. Pain becomes more persistent and consistent; more intense at McBurney's point (right lower quadrant).
4. Pain may be characterized as rebound pain or tenderness, may have referred pain around the perimeter of the abdomen near umbilicus.
5. Anorexia, nausea and vomiting, diarrhea.
6. Low-grade fever.
7. Client assumes a characteristic position of side-lying with the knees flexed.
8. Sudden relief from pain may be indicative of ruptured appendix.
9. Elevated WBC.
10. Complications - peritonitis.

Treatment

1. Appendectomy to remove appendix if inflammatory condition is localized.
2. More extensive abdominal surgery must be done if appendix has ruptured (abdominal laparotomy).

Nursing Intervention

✦ *Goal: to assist in evaluating child for clinical manifestations and to prepare the child for surgery as indicated.*

1. Careful nursing assessment for clinical manifestations.
2. Maintain child NPO until otherwise indicated.
3. Maintain bed rest in position of comfort.
4. Do not apply heat to the abdomen; cold applications may provide some relief or comfort.
5. Do not administer enemas.
6. Avoid unnecessary palpation of abdomen.
7. *Notify the RN immediately of any changes or sudden decrease in pain.*

✦ *Goal: to maintain homeostasis and healing postoperative appendectomy (Chapter 3).*

✦ *Goal: to prevent abdominal distention and promote bowel function postoperative abdominal laparotomy (ruptured appendix).*

1. Remain NPO.
2. Gastric decompression by nasogastric tube; maintain patency and suction.
3. Monitor abdomen for distention.
4. Assess peristaltic activity.
5. Evaluate and record character of bowel movement.
6. Encourage ambulation as soon as indicated.

✦ *Goal: to decrease infection and promote healing postoperative abdominal laparotomy.*

1. Position client in semi-Fowler's to localize infection and prevent spread of infection and development of abdominal abscess.
2. Antibiotics are usually administered via IV infusion, then as oral preparations; monitor response to antibiotics as well as status of IV infusion site.

3. Provide appropriate wound care; evaluate drainage from abdominal Penrose drains and incisional area.
4. Assess abdomen for increase in distention, tenderness, and for presence of bowel sounds.

✦ *Goal: to maintain adequate hydration and nutrition, and promote comfort postoperative abdominal laparotomy.*

1. Maintain adequate hydration via IV infusion.
2. Evaluate tolerance to PO liquids when nasogastric tube is removed.
3. Begin clear liquids PO when peristalsis returns.
4. Progress diet as tolerated.
5. Administer analgesics as indicated.

Peritonitis

❑ **Peritonitis is a generalized inflammatory process of the peritoneum.**

A. Intestinal motility is decreased and fluid accumulates as a result of the inability of the intestine to reabsorb fluid.

B. Fluid will leak into the peritoneal cavity, precipitating fluid, electrolyte and protein loss as well as fluid depletion.

NCLEX ALERT: *Identify client risk factors for infection. Identify client signs and symptoms of infection.*

Data Collection

1. Risk factors/etiology - primary source of problem is rupture of an area of the gastrointestinal tract.

NCLEX ALERT: *Monitor status of postoperative client - peritonitis is a potential complication anytime the abdomen is entered, either from trauma or from surgery.*

2. Clinical manifestations.
   a. Presence of precipitating cause.
   b. Pain over involved area; rebound tenderness.
   c. Abdominal distention
   d. Abdominal muscle rigidity ("board-like" abdomen).
   e. Fever.
   f. Anorexia, nausea, vomiting.
   g. Increased pulse, decreased blood pressure, shallow respirations.
   h. Decreased or absent bowel sounds.
   i. Dehydration.
3. Diagnostics.
   a. CBC - increased white cell count.
   b. X-ray of abdomen.
   c. Paracentesis to evaluate abdominal fluid.
   d. Clinical manifestations.

Treatment

1. Identify and treat precipitating cause (may require surgical intervention).
2. Antibiotics.
3. IV fluids.
4. Decrease abdominal distention.

Nursing Intervention

✦ *Goal: to maintain fluid and electrolyte balance and reduce gastric distention.*

1. Maintain nasogastric suction.
2. Monitor IV fluid replacement.
3. Evaluate peristalsis and return of bowel function.
4. Maintain intake and output records.
5. Assess for problems of dehydration.
6. Encourage ambulation as soon as indicated.

✦ *Goal: to reduce infectious process.*

1. Assess client's tolerance of antibiotics and status of infusion site.
2. Evaluate vital signs and correlate with progress of infectious process.
3. Maintain semi-Fowler's position to enhance respirations as well as to prevent abdominal abscess from forming.

✦ *Goal: to prevent complications associated with immobility (See Chapter 3).*

✦ *Goal: to provide postoperative care as indicated (See Chapter 3).*

NCLEX ALERT: *Identify factors that may interfere with wound healing.. Monitor client of signs and symptoms of infection. Provide emergency care for wound disruption.*

Intestinal Obstruction

❑ **Interference with normal peristalsis and impairment to forward flow of intestinal contents is known as *intestinal obstruction.***

A. Regardless of the precipitating cause, the ensuing problems are a result of the obstructive process.

B. The higher the obstruction in the intestine; the more severe the symptoms.

C. The location of the obstruction determines the extent of fluid and electrolyte imbalance and acid-base imbalance.

1. Dehydration and electrolyte imbalance do not occur rapidly if obstruction is in the large intestine.
2. If obstruction is located high in the intestine, dehydration occurs rapidly due to the inability of the intestine to reabsorb fluids.

Data Collection

1. Clinical manifestations.
   a. Vomiting (occurs early if obstruction is high).
   b. Abdominal distention.
   c. Bowel sounds initially may be hyperactive proximal to the obstruction and decreased or absent distal to the obstruction; eventually all bowel sounds will be absent.

NCLEX ALERT: *Determine characteristics of bowel sounds. This is of particular importance in the diagnosis, treatment, and nursing care of client with an obstructed bowel.*

   d. Colicky-type abdominal pain.
2. Diagnostics.
   a. X-ray of the abdomen.
   b. Evaluation of history of abdominal problems.
   c. Barium enema.
3. Complications - intestinal perforation and peritonitis.

Treatment

1. Mechanical and vascular intestinal obstructions are generally treated surgically; ileostomy or colostomy may be necessary.
2. Treatment of neurogenic obstruction (paralytic ileus) may consist of intestinal intubation and decompression (Appendix 13-7).
3. Maintain fluid, electrolyte balance, and nutrition.

Nursing Intervention

✦ *Goal: to prepare client for diagnostic evaluation and to maintain ongoing nursing assessment for pertinent data (Appendix 13-1).*

✦ *Goal: to decrease gastric distention, maintain hydration and electrolyte balance.*

1. Client maintained NPO.
2. Maintain nasogastric suction.
3. Monitor IV fluid replacement.
4. Evaluate peristalsis and return of bowel function.
5. Maintain accurate intake and output records.
6. Assess for problems of dehydration and hypovolemia.
7. Measure abdominal girth to determine if distention is increasing.
8. Encourage activities to facilitate return of bowel function.

✦ *Goal: to provide appropriate preoperative preparation when surgery is indicated (See Chapter 3).*

✦ *Goal: to maintain homeostasis and promote healing postoperative abdominal laparotomy (See Chapter 3).*

✦ *Goal: to maintain fluid and electrolyte balance and prevent gastric distention postoperative abdominal laparotomy (See Preoperative Goal above).*

✦ *Goal: to decrease infection and promote healing postoperative abdominal laparotomy.*

1. Antibiotics are usually administered via IV infusion. Monitor client's response to antibiotics as well as status of IV infusion site.
2. Monitor vital signs frequently and evaluate for presence of infectious process.
3. Provide wound care, evaluate drainage from abdominal Penrose drains as well as from abdominal incisional area.

✦ *Goal: to reestablish normal nutrition, and promote comfort postoperative abdominal laparotomy.*

1. Evaluate tolerance of liquids when nasogastric tube is removed.
2. Begin clear liquids initially and evaluate presence of peristalsis.
3. Progress diet as tolerated.
4. Administer analgesics as indicated.

Intussusception

❑ **This is the telescoping of one portion of the intestine into another.**

A. Most commonly occurs during infancy.

B. Common site is the ileocecal valve.

C. As a result, there is an intestinal obstruction.

Data Collection

1. Risk factors/etiology.
   a. Most often occurs in children between ages 3 and 5 years, or in the elderly.
   b. More common in males.
   c. Increased incidence in children with cystic fibrosis.
2. Clinical manifestations.

a. Client is healthy with sudden occurrence of acute abdominal pain.

b. Pain may be episodic characterized by periods of absence of pain.

c. Vomiting occurs initially.

d. May pass one normal stool then as condition deteriorates stool may be described as "currant jelly" with a mixture of blood and mucus.

e. Abdominal tenderness and distention.

f. A "sausage shaped" mass may be palpated in the abdomen.

3. Diagnostics.

a. Clinical manifestations.

b. Water soluble contrast with air pressure to identify and to reduce intussusception.

Treatment

1. Initial treatment may consist of hydrostatic reduction by water soluble contrast and air pressure; correction of problem may be carried out the same time as diagnostic evaluation.

2. If hydrostatic pressure does not resolve problem, then surgical intervention is necessary.

Nursing Intervention

✦ *Goal: to assist in diagnostic evaluation and maintain ongoing nursing assessment for pertinent data.*

1. Careful assessment of client's physical and behavioral symptoms.

2. Assess for colicky pain associated with vomiting.

3. If condition is reduced by hydrostatic pressure:

a. Continue to monitor all stools for passage of normal brown stool. *Notify RN if there is passage of stool*

b. Assess how well the child is tolerating oral fluids and food.

c. Continue to evaluate for symptoms of obstruction.

✦ *Goal: to provide appropriate preoperative preparation if surgery is indicated (See Chapter 3).*

✦ *Goal: to maintain homeostasis and promote healing postoperative surgery (See Chapter 3).*

Diverticular Disease

❑ **The condition in which an individual has multiple diverticulum is known as diverticulosis.**

A. Diverticula - dilatation or out pouching of a weakened area in the intestinal wall.

B. Diverticulitis - a process by which circulation to the diverticulum is compromised, allowing for bacterial invasion and inflammatory reaction.

Data Collection

1. Risk factors/etiology.

a. Increased incidence in clients over 45 years old.

b. Low-fiber diet and chronic constipation.

c. Most frequently occurs in the sigmoid colon.

2. Clinical manifestations.

a. Diverticulum is usually asymptomatic; symptoms vary with degree of inflammation.

b. Intermittent left quadrant tenderness, abdominal cramping.

c. Constipation or alternating constipation and diarrhea.

d. Occult blood and or mucus in the stool.

e. Inflammatory changes may precipitate perforation or abscess formation.

f. Diverticulitis.

(1) Fever.

(2) Left lower quadrant pain, usually accompanied by nausea and vomiting.

(3) Abdominal distention.

(4) Frequently constipated.

(5) May progress to intestinal obstruction, abscess or perforation.

3. Diagnostics.

a. Stool examination.

b. Barium enema.

c. Sigmoidoscopy.

Treatment

1. Medical management of uncomplicated diverticulum.

a. High fiber diet (restrict indigestible fiber such as corn, popcorn, and tomatoes).

b. Prevent chronic constipation - bulk laxatives and stool softeners.

2. Treatment for acute diverticulitis.

a. Antibiotics.

b. May be NPO or on a low residue diet.

c. IV fluids.

d. Possible surgery and colon resection if obstruction or perforation occur.

Nursing Intervention

✦ *Goal: to assist client to understand dietary implications and maintain prescribed therapy to prevent exacerbations.*

1. Understand high-fiber diet.
2. Avoid indigestible roughage such as nuts, popcorn, raw celery.
3. Maintain high-fluid intake.
4. Avoid large meals.
5. Avoid alcohol.

NCLEX ALERT: *Use measures to improve client's nutrition - clients with diverticulosis need specific instructions regarding dietary modifications.*

6. Weight reduction if indicated.
7. Avoid activities which increase intraabdominal pressure (straining at stool, bending, lifting, tight restrictive clothing).

Hernias

❑ **A hernia is a protrusion of the intestine through an abnormal opening or weakened area of the abdominal wall.**

A. Types.

1. Inguinal - a weakness where the spermatic cord in men and the round ligament in women passes through the abdominal wall in the groin area; more common in men.
2. Femoral - protrusion of the intestine through the femoral ring; more common in women.
3. Umbilical - occurs most often in children where the umbilical opening fails to close adequately; occurs in adults where the abdominal muscle is weak.
4. Incisional - weakness in the abdominal wall due to a previous incision.
5. Classification.
    a. Reducible - hernia may be replaced into the abdominal cavity by manual manipulation.
    b. Incarcerated - hernia may not be replaced back into the abdominal cavity.
    c. Strangulated - blood supply and intestinal flow in the herniated area are obstructed; strangulated hernia leads to intestinal obstruction.

Data Collection

1. Clinical manifestations.
    a. Hernia protrudes over the involved area when the client stands or strains.
    b. Severe pain occurs if hernia becomes strangulated.
    c. Strangulated hernia occurs with symptoms of intestinal obstruction.
2. Diagnostics.
    a. History.
    b. Clinical manifestations.

Treatment

1. General elective surgery to prevent complications of strangulation (herniorrhaphy).
2. Strangulated hernia involves resection of the involved bowel.

Nursing Intervention

✦ *Goal: to prepare client for surgery if indicated (See Chapter 3).*

✦ *Goal: to maintain homeostasis and promote healing postoperative herniorrhaphy.*

1. General postoperative nursing care (See Chapter 3).
2. Assess male clients for development of scrotal edema (inguinal hernia).
3. Discourage coughing, but encourage deep breathing and turning.
4. When coughing occurs, teach client how to splint the incision.
5. Generally restrain from heavy lifting for approximately 6 to 8 weeks postoperatively.

Inflammatory Bowel Disease

❑ ***Crohn's disease*** **is a chronic, nonspecific, inflammatory disease that extends through all layers of the bowel wall. Most commonly occurs in the distal ileum and colon.**

❑ ***Ulcerative colitis*** **is inflammation and ulceration of the mucosal layer of the colon and rectum; area of inflammation is diffuse involving mucosa and submucosa of the intestinal wall. It frequently begins in the rectum, and spreads in a continuous manner up the colon; seldom is the small intestine involved.**

Data Collection

1. Risk factors/etiology.
    a. May begin in adolescence; peak incidence occurs between ages 20 and 30 years.
    b. Clients with long-standing ulcerative colitis have significant increase in cancer of the colon.
    c. Clients with ulcerative colitis may have history of difficulty in handling stress.
2. Clinical manifestations.
    a. Abdominal pain.
    b. Diarrhea, more severe in colitis clients.

c. Steatorrhea due to poorly absorbed fats.
d. Nausea and vomiting.
e. Abdominal pain and tenderness.
f. Stool may contain occult blood or bright red blood.

3. Diagnostics.
a. Stool analysis to rule out bacterial or parasitic infection.
b. Barium enema (generally the pretest procedures are modified for this client, always check with the physician).
c. Proctosigmoidoscopy and colonoscopy.

Treatment

1. Dietary modifications - low residue and ,fiber diet; increased calorie intake; increased protein and increased vitamin and iron supplements.
2. Medications.
a. Corticosteroids to reduce the inflammation (Appendix 5-7).
b. Antidiarrheal medications (Appendix 13-4).
c. Antibiotics.
d. Aminosalicylates.
3. Surgical intervention (ileostomy) if fistulas, perforation, bleeding, or intestinal obstruction occur.

Nursing Intervention

✦ *Goal (acute): to monitor inflammatory response and promote healing.*

1. Observe number and character of stool.
2. Evaluate fluid status, daily intake and output and weights.
3. Good skin hygiene around anal area to prevent excoriation due to diarrhea.
4. Evaluate character of bowel sounds.
5. Monitor lab values for anemia and electrolyte imbalance.

NCLEX ALERT: *Monitor client nutritional status. Use measurers to improve nutritional intake. Identify signs and symptoms of fluid and/or electrolyte imbalance.*

Self-Care

1. Dietary modifications - low residue, bland foods that are high in calories and protein. Diet may progress as inflammation subsides.
2. Medication regimen.
3. Symptoms of reoccurrence of the problem; when to call the physician.
a. Bleeding from the colon, or vomiting blood.
b. Significant increase in abdominal pain.
c. Increase in stools with decrease in weight.
4. Identify appropriate measures to decrease stress in lifestyle.
5. Avoid smoking and alcohol.

NCLEX ALERT: *Reinforce client and family teaching about managing problems.*

Gastritis

❑ **This is an inflammatory process involving the mucosa of the stomach.**

Data Collection

1. Risk factors:
a. Ingestion of contaminated food (Salmonella and Staphylococcal bacteria).
b. Alcohol
c. NSAID's, aspirin
d. Radiation therapy
2. Clinical manifestations.
a. Abdominal cramping.
b. Nausea, vomiting, and diarrhea.
3. Diagnostics - identify precipitating cause.

Treatment

Appropriate medication for causative agents.

Nursing Management

✦ *Goal: to evaluate and maintain hydration and electrolyte balance, and to prevent spread of disease.*

NURSING PRIORITY: *Problem is usually self-limiting; fluid imbalance is of increased concern in the elderly and in the infant.*

1. NPO until vomiting ceases.
2. Begin clear liquids gradually after vomiting ceases.
3. Enteric precautions until organism is identified, then precautions as indicated.

✦ *Goal: to provide symptomatic nursing care for diarrhea, nausea, and vomiting (See general intestinal disorders).*

Hirschsprung's Disease (Congenital Aganglionic Megacolon)

❑ **This disease is characterized by congenital absence of innervation in a segment of the colon wall.**

A. Precipitates a neurogenic bowel obstruction.

B. Most common site is the rectosigmoid colon; colon proximal to the area dilates (i.e., megacolon).

Data Collection

1. Clinical manifestations.
   a. Varies according to age and amount of colon involved.
   b. Newborn (first 24-48 hours).
      (1) Failure to pass meconium.
      (2) Bile-stained vomitus.
      (3) Abdominal distention.
   c. Older infant.
      (1) Failure to thrive.
      (2) Abdominal distention.
      (3) Constipation and overflow diarrhea.
2. Diagnostics.
   a. Rectal biopsy for aganglionic cells.
   b. Barium enema.

Treatment

1. Surgery - usually done in two stages, first a temporary colostomy, than later more complete repair.

Nursing Intervention

✦ *Goal: to promote normal attachment and prepare infant and parents for surgery:*

1. Allow parents to ventilate feelings regarding congenital defect of infant.
2. Foster infant-parent attachment.
3. Bowel preparation - NPO, isotonic enemas, antibiotics.
4. Careful explanation of colostomy to parents.

✦ *Goal: to assist parents to understand and provide appropriate home care for the child postoperative colostomy.*

1. Colostomy is generally temporary.
2. Parents should be actively involved in colostomy care prior to discharge. (Appendix 13- 8)

Cancer of the Colon and Rectum

❑ **Second most frequent cause of cancer in the United States.**

Data Collection

1. Risk factors/etiology.
   a. Most common in older adults, highest incidence in clients over 85years.
   b. May be associated with ulcerative colitis.
   c. Family history of colon cancer.
   d. Adenomatous polyps.
   e. Majority of malignant tumors are found in the rectal area.
2. Clinical manifestations.
   a. Symptoms are vague early in disease state.
   b. Change in bowel habits.
   c. Passage of bright blood or melena stools
   d. Change in shape of stool (pencil- or ribbon-shaped due to sigmoid or rectal cancer).
   e. Weakness and fatigue, weight loss.
   f. Anemia
   g. Constipation and distention, abdominal cramping.
   h. Tenesmus - ineffective, painful straining at stool.
   i. Pain is a late symptom.
3. Diagnostics.
   a. Sigmoidoscopy/colonoscopy.
   b. Rectal examination.
   c. Fecal occult stool test.

Treatment

1. Surgical resection of tumor - a temporary or permanent colostomy may be done.
2. Radiation therapy.
3. Chemotherapy.

> ***Geriatric Priority:*** *Abdominal pain, obstruction, tenesmus, and rectal bleeding are most common symptom in elderly, they are also at increase risk for complications.*

Nursing Intervention

✦ *Goal: to provide preoperative care as indicated for abdominal laparotomy and colostomy (Appendix 13-8).*

1. Usually undergo extensive preoperative bowel preparation.
2. If colostomy is going to be done, discuss with client placement on abdomen.

✦ *Goal: to provide appropriate wound care postoperative abdominal- perineal resection.*

1. For rectal cancer, client will frequently have three incisional areas:
   a. Abdominal incision.
   b. Left abdominal incision for colostomy.
   c. Perineal incision.
2. Perineal wound may be closed with a Penrose drain inserted, or may be left open to heal by secondary intention.

a. Generally irrigate the perineal wound with saline.
b. Warm sitz bath to promote debridement and increase circulation to the perineal area.

3. Abdominal wound may need frequent dressing changes due to profuse serosanguineous drainage immediately postoperative.

NCLEX ALERT: *Promote the progress of wound healing. Monitor for signs and symptoms of infection*

✦ *Goal: to prevent complications of immobility postoperative abdominal-perineal resection (See Chapter 3).*

✦ *Goal: to maintain homeostasis and promote healing postoperative abdominal-perineal resection (See Chapter 3).*

Self-Care

1. Due to age of most clients, recovery period is long; assist client and family to identify community resources.
2. Assist client and family to perform colostomy care (Appendix 13-8).
3. Return for frequent medical checkups.
4. Understand symptoms to report to physician.
   a. Increased pain.
   b. Change in stool or bleeding.
   c. Weight loss.
   d. Sustained vomiting and diarrhea.

Hemorrhoids

❑ **Dilated varicose veins of the anus and rectum are called *hemorrhoids*.**

Data Collection

1. Risk factors/etiology.
   a. By age 50, approximately 50% of people have them.
   b. May appear periodically depending on amount of anorectal pressure.
   c. Caused by conditions which increase anorectal pressure.
      (1) Pregnancy.
      (2) Prolonged constipation.
      (3) Prolonged standing or sitting.
      (4) Heavy lifting.
      (5) Portal hypertension.
2. Clinical manifestations.
   a. External hemorrhoids appear as reddish protrusions at the anus.
   b. Internal hemorrhoids become constricted, are painful and will bleed during defecation.
3. Diagnostics - rectal examination.

Treatment

1. Ointments to shrink mucous membranes.
2. Stool softeners.
3. Sitz bath.
4. Removal of the hemorrhoid - ligation of internal hemorrhoids; cryosurgery and laser surgery are also used.

Nursing Intervention

✦ *Goal: to provide appropriate information to assist client to manage problem at home.*

1. Avoid prolonged standing or sitting.
2. Sitz bath to decrease discomfort.
3. Over-the-counter ointments to decrease discomfort.
4. Ice pack followed by a hot sitz bath if severe discomfort occurs.
5. Avoid constipation and straining at stool.
6. Dietary modifications to prevent constipation; take bulk laxatives.

✦ *Goal: to maintain homeostasis and promote healing postoperative hemorrhoidectomy.*

1. Rectal pain may be quite severe
2. Assess for urinary retention.
3. Sitz bath 2-3 times a day, beginning 12 hours after surgery - promotes cleanliness, decreases pain, and increases healing.
4. Promote passage of normal stool.
   a. Stool softeners.
   b. Teach client not to resist urge to defecate.
   c. Encourage activity to promote peristalsis.

Study Questions—Gastrointestinal

1. A client has had extensive oral surgery for cancer of the mouth. What is an important nursing measure when providing oral care for this client?

① irrigate the mouth with normal saline after every meal.
② using a bulb syringe, irrigate the mouth with peroxide.
③ frequent oral care with a bactericidal mouthwash.
④ offer only cold foods that are non irritating.

2. A client is placed on NPO status due to a bowel obstruction. A nasogastric tube is inserted. What is the purpose of this tube?

① decrease gastric distention.
② eliminate nausea and vomiting.
③ reduce pain postoperatively.
④ provide a route for a tube feeding.

3. What type of stool can the nurse expect from a client who has a colostomy of the lower descending colon?

① liquid.
② bloody.
③ black.
④ formed.

4. A client has just had his nasogastric tube removed. What would be the best immediate nursing intervention?

① Check for presence of bowel sounds.
② Assist client with oral hygiene.
③ Offer the client some ice cream.
④ Palpate the abdomen for distention.

5. A nurse is changing the ileostomy bag the day after surgery. What is a normal finding around the base of the stoma?

① pitting edema.
② dusky gray color.
③ small amount of capillary bleeding.
④ tissue sloughing in the area.

6. What is important for the nurse to assess and document in clients who have digestive tract problems?

① peripheral edema and urinary output.
② changes in bowel activity and weight fluctuation.
③ decrease in eating and blood sugar of 110.
④ alteration in appetite with a change in ADLs.

7. When attempting to auscultate bowel sounds that are decreased or not audible, how long should the nurse listen to each quadrant?

① 2 minutes.
② 6 minutes.
③ 30 seconds.
④ 15 seconds.

8. While preparing a client for radiography, the client complains of excessive fatigue and says he does not want this procedure done. What is the best nursing management?

① wait five minutes, then return to prepare the client.
② explain to the client how important the procedure is.
③ stop the preparation and call the physician.
④ call the nurse's station and ask for assistance.

9. The nurse is caring for a client who is being prepared for surgery for appendicitis. What is the preoperative preparation?

① ambulate to decrease problems with distention.
② administer meperidine (**Demerol**) for pain.
③ allow position of comfort, maintain NPO.
④ put a warm pad on abdomen, offer clear liquids.

10. The client returns to his room after a gastrectomy. What are important nursing measures regarding the care of the nasogastric tube?

① irrigate gently with normal saline every hour.
② clamp tube for 30 minutes every 4 hours.
③ measure gastric output every hour.
④ do not reposition tube if drainage decreases.

11. A client is receiving tube feedings via his nasogastric tube three days after surgery. What method of administration of the tube feeding would cause the client to experience the most problems with tolerance and absorption of the feeding?

① dilute formula given intermittently via drip method.
② concentrated formula given at 50cc/hour via continuous drip.
③ 250cc of dilute formula given as a bolus via gravity.
④ bolus feeding of 300 cc full strength via gravity.

12. What would be appropriate teaching for a client who is experiencing gastroesophageal reflux (GERD)?

① take an antacid after eating.
② lay down on your right side after eating.
③ do not drink fluids with meals.
④ avoid eating within three hours of bedtime.

13. A client with nausea and vomiting would be placed in what position to prevent aspiration?

① supine with head turned to the right.
② prone with head of bed at 45 degrees.
③ side lying.
④ Trendelenburg.

14. What is the desired action of ranitidine (Zantac) in the treatment of the gastric ulcer client?

① increase gastric acid production.
② increase production of bile.
③ neutralize hydrochloric acid production.
④ decrease production of hydrochloric acid.

15. The nurse notes the vomitus in a client's emesis basin appears to be of a coffee ground nature. What is the nurse's interpretation of this emesis?

① it contains mucus.
② it represents old blood.
③ the client is actively bleeding.
④ there is excessive bile present.

16. A client who is postoperative gastrectomy surgery is at risk for what type of vitamin deficiency?

① vitamin B12.
② vitamin C.
③ vitamin D.
④ vitamin B6.

17. The peptic ulcer client should be taught to avoid what type of drug?

① H2 blocker.
② aspirin.
③ antacid.
④ antiemetic.

18. What is the common medication classification of psyllium husk (Metamucil), ducosate calcium (Surfak), and ducosate sodium (Colace)?

① antidiuretics.
② antidiarrheal.
③ stool softener.
④ antiemetic.

19. The nurse is admitting a client with an intestinal obstruction. What will be the nurse include in the initial plan of treatment?

① nasogastric tube for GI decompression.
② soap suds enema to evacuate the bowel.
③ clear liquid diet to decrease production of stool.
④ ambulation to increase peristaltic activity.

20. In performing a nursing assessment on a client with inflammatory bowel disease, what finding would be of most concern?

① dehydration.
② bloody stool.
③ distended abdomen.
④ hyperglycemia.

Appendix 13-1: GASTROINTESTINAL SYSTEM DIAGNOSTICS

X-RAY:

- ***Upper Gastrointestinal Series or Barium Swallow:*** X-ray examination utilizing barium as a contrast material; used to diagnose structural abnormalities and problems of the esophagus and stomach.
  Nursing Implications:
  1. Explain procedure to client.
  2. Maintain client NPO at least 6 hours prior to procedure.
  3. After examination, administer laxative to promote elimination of barium to prevent impaction.

- ***Barium Enema:*** X-ray examination of the colon using barium as a contrast medium; barium is administered rectally.
  Nursing Implications:
  1. Liquid or clear liquids for 24 hours prior to examination, NPO 6-8 hours prior to examination.
  2. Colon must be free of stool; laxatives and enemas are administered the evening prior to surgery; enemas may also be given the morning of the procedure.
  3. Explain to client that he/she may experience cramping and feel urge to defecate during the procedure.
  4. After the procedure, increase fluids and administer a laxative to assist in expelling the barium.

ENDOSCOPY:

- ***Esophagoscopy, Gastroscopy, Duodenoscopy:*** The direct visualization of the esophagus, stomach, and duodenum via a lighted scope; inflammation, ulcerations, tumors, and esophageal varices may be observed.
  Nursing Implications prior to procedure:
  1. Maintain client NPO for 6 to 8 hours prior to procedure.
  2. May give preoperative medication for relaxation and to decrease oral secretions.
  3. Explain to client that local anesthesia will be utilized to anesthetize the throat prior to insertion of the scope.
  4. Assess client's mouth for dentures and removable bridges.
  Nursing Implications after the procedure:
  1. Maintain client NPO until the gag and cough reflexes returns.
  2. Use throat lozenges or warm saline gargles for relief of sore throat.
  3. Observe for signs of perforation - bleeding, fever, dysphagia, substernal or epigastric pain.

- ***Proctosigmoidoscopy and Colonoscopy:*** Direct visualization of the colon.
  Nursing Implications prior to procedure:
  1. Clear liquid diet 24 hours before examination; osmotic laxative the day before, enemas the evening, and possibly the morning, of the procedure.
  2. Sigmoidoscopy - knee-chest position or left lateral Sim's for elderly clients. Explain the need to take a deep breath during the insertion of the scope; client will feel urge to defecate as scope is passed.
  3. Sedatives may be administered prior to test.
  4. Colonoscopy - conscious sedation, client is generally placed on left side during procedure.
  Nursing Implications after the procedure:
  1. Observe for signs of perforation - bleeding, pain, fever.
  2. Assist client to upright position - observe for orthostatic hypotension.
  3. Client may take a sitz bath for relief of anal discomfort.

ANALYSIS OF SECRETIONS:

- ***Gastric Analysis:*** Utilized to determine the amount of hydrochloric acid and pepsin. Assists in the diagnosis of gastric carcinoma, pernicious anemia, and to determine the presence of *H. pylori* bacteria.
  Nursing Implications:
  1. NPO for 8 to 12 hours prior to examination.
  2. Explain to client the insertion of the nasogastric tube.
  3. Withhold medications affecting gastric secretions.
  4. No smoking prior to the examination.
  5. Specimens of gastric secretions will be obtained via a nasogastric tube at specific intervals.
- Geriatric Priority: Geriatric clients may have difficulty with bowel preparation prior to colon and intestinal diagnostic procedures, they may need assistance in understanding and complying with the guidelines..

Appendix 13-1: GASTROINTESTINAL SYSTEM DIAGNOSTICS

- ***Paracentesis:***

Purpose: To determine intraabdominal bleeding, to determine presence of ascites.

Procedure: Catheter or trocar is inserted into the peritoneal cavity, most often just below the umbilicus. A liter of solution (normal saline, or Ringers lactate) is rapidly infused into the peritoneal cavity. The fluid may be aspirated or allowed to drain by gravity. Normal fluid return should be clear with a slight yellow cast. If a positive tap is obtained, the client is most often prepared for abdominal exploratory surgery.

Nursing Implications:

1. Nasogastric tube may be inserted to maintain gastric decompression during the procedure.
2. Have the client void or insert a Foley prior to the procedure.
3. Maintain sterile field for the puncture, drainage, and place sterile dressing over the puncture site when finished.
4. Observe client for development of complications.

Complications:

1. Peritonitis from bacteria introduced via the puncture, or from puncture of the bowel on insertion of the trocar.
2. Free air in the peritoneal cavity. Client will complain of referred shoulder pain from air under the diaphragm.
3. If the client had a full bladder at the time of insertion of the trocar, there is the possibility the bladder will be perforated.

NCLEX ALERT: *Prepare client for procedure. Monitor client diagnostic test results.*

Appendix 13-2: ANTIEMETICS

MEDICATIONS	SIDE EFFECTS	NURSING IMPLICATIONS
PHENOTHIAZINE DERIVATIVES: Depresses the chemoreceptor trigger zone and vomiting center.		
Chlorpromazine hydrochloride (**Thorazine**): *PO, suppository, IM* Promethazine (**Phenergan**): *PO, IM, suppository* Prochlorperazine (**Compazine**): *PO, suppository, IM* Thiethylperazine maleate (**Torecan**): *PO, suppository, IM*	Central nervous system depression, drowsiness, photosensitivity	1. Sub-q injection may cause tissue irritation and necrosis. 2. Use with caution in pediatrics; do not administer **Thorazine** to infants under six months, **Compazine** to children under 20 pounds or under two years old, or **Torecan** to children under 12. 3. **Thorazine** should be used only in situations of severe nausea or vomiting.
ANTIHISTAMINES: Depresses the chemoreceptor trigger zone.		
Hydroxyzine (**Atarax, Vistaril**): *PO, IM* Dimenhydrinate (**Dramamine**) *PO, suppository, IM*	Sedation; anticholinergic affects - blurred vision, dry mouth, difficulty in urination and constipation; paradoxical excitation may occur in children	1. Caution client regarding sedation - should avoid activities that require mental alertness. 2. Administer early in order to prevent vomiting. 3. Use with caution in clients with glaucoma and asthma. 4. Sub-q injection may cause tissue irritation and necrosis.
GI STIMULANT: Stimulates motility of upper GI tract.		
Metoclopramide (**Reglan**): PO, IM, IV)	Restlessness, drowsiness, fatigue	1. Used to decrease problems with esophageal reflux. 2. Use with caution when increase in GI mobility may be dangerous (intestinal perforation, obstruction.)

Appendix 13-3: LAXATIVES

MEDICATIONS	SIDE EFFECTS	NURSING IMPLICATIONS

❖ GENERAL NURSING IMPLICATIONS ❖

— Laxatives should be avoided in clients who have nausea, vomiting and/or undiagnosed abdominal pain and cramping, or any indications of appendicitis.
— Dietary fiber should be taken for prevention of and in first line of treatment for constipation.
— Daily intake of fluids should be increased.
— Constipation is determined by stool firmness and frequency.
— Increasing activity will increase peristalsis and decrease constipation.
— Narcotic analgesics and anticholinergics will cause constipation.
— A laxative should be used only briefly and in the smallest amount necessary.
— Use with caution during pregnancy.

NCLEX ALERT: *Intervene with client experiencing alteration in bowel elimination.*

MEDICATIONS	SIDE EFFECTS	NURSING IMPLICATIONS
BULK LAXATIVES: Stimulates peristalsis and passage of soft stool.		
Methylcellulose (**Citrocel**) Psyllium (**Metamucil, Perdiem**) Fibercon Bran	Esophageal irritation, impaction, abdominal fullness, flatulence.	1. Not immediately effective; 12 to 24 hours before effects are apparent. 2. Use with caution in clients with difficulty swallowing. 3. Administer with full glass of fluid to prevent problems with irritation and impaction. 4. Fibercon is a tablet form, others are powder form to be mixed with fluids.
STOOL SOFTENERS OR SURFACTANTS: Decreases surface tension allowing water to penetrate feces		
Ducusate Potassium (**Colace**) *Combination with stimulant:* Ducosate Calcium (**Doxidan**) Ducusate sodium (**Dialose Plus**)	Occasional mild abdominal cramping	1. Do not use concurrently with mineral oil. 2. Not recommended for children under 6 years old.
STIMULANT OR CONTACT LAXATIVES: Stimulates and irritates the large intestine to promote peristalsis and defecation.		
Bisacodyl (**Dulcolax**): suppository, PO Phenolphthalein (**Modane, Ex-lax**): PO Senna concentrate (**Senokot**): PO, suppository	Diarrhea, abdominal cramping	1. Do not crush or chew tablets. 2. Not recommended for long term use.
BOWEL EVACUANTS: Nonabsorbable osmotic agent that pulls fluid into the bowel.		
Polyethylene glycol (**Golytely, Nulytely**) Magnesium Citrate		1. Primary use is in preparing the bowel for examination 2. Client should fast 4-5 hours prior to administration. 3. Food (except clear liquids) is contraindicated within 2 hours of medication. 4. Polyethylene glycol involves large amount of fluid for client to drink (3-4L), provide 8-10 ounces chilled at a time to increase client consumption and taste, best if consumed over 3-4 hours.

Appendix 13-4: ANTIDIARRHEAL AGENTS

MEDICATIONS	SIDE EFFECTS	NURSING IMPLICATIONS
OPIOIDS: Suppress peristalsis, facilitating water and electrolyte reabsorption.		
Paregoric: PO Diphenoxylate HCL + Atropine (**Lomotil**): PO Loperamide (**Imodium**): PO	Nausea, vomiting, paralytic ileus, abdominal cramping.	1. Interacts with MAO inhibitors. 2. Not recommended during pregnancy 3. Not recommended for children under 2 years old.
ABSORBENTS AND EMULSANTS: Soothing effects and absorbs toxic substances.		
Attapulgite (**Donnagel**):	May precipitate an impaction	1. May interfere with absorption of PO medications. 2. Should not be given to clients with high fever.

Appendix 13-5: ANTI-ULCER

MEDICATIONS	SIDE EFFECTS	NURSING IMPLICATIONS
ANTACIDS: An alkaline substance that will neutralize gastric acid secretions, non systemic.		
Aluminum Hydroxide (**Amphojel**): PO	Constipation Phosphorus depletion with chronic utilization	1. Avoid administration within 1 to 2 hours of other oral medications. Medications should be taken frequently, before and after meals and at bedtime. 2. Instruct clients to take medication even if they do not experience discomfort.
Aluminum hydroxide and magnesium salt combinations (**Gelusil, Maalox, Di-gel**, and **Gaviscon**)	Constipation or diarrhea Hypercalcemia Renal calculi	3. Clients on low sodium diets should evaluate sodium content of various antacids 4.Administer with caution to the cardiac client as GI symptoms may be indicative of cardiac problems.
Sodium preparation: Sodium bicarbonate, (**Rolaids, Tums**): PO	Rebound acid production Alkalosis	1. Discourage use of sodium bicarbonate due to occurrence of metabolic alkalosis. 2. Tums maybe used for daily calcium supplement.
HISTAMINE H_2 RECEPTOR ANTAGONISTS: Reduces volume and concentration of gastric acid secretion and prevents stress-induced ulcers.		
Cimetidine (**Tagamet**): PO, IV, IM	Rash, confusion, lethargy, diarrhea, arrhythmias	1. Take with or after meals. 2. May be used prophylactically or for treatment of PUD. 3. Do not take with PO antacids.
Ranitidine (**Zantac**): PO, IM, IV	Headache, GI discomfort, jaundice, hepatitis	1. Use with caution in clients with liver and renal disorders. 2. Do not take with aspirin products. 3. Wait 1 hour after administration of antacids.
Niaztidine (**Axid**): PO	Anemia, dizziness	
Famotidine (**Pepsid**) PO, IV	Headache, dizziness, constipation, diarrhea	1. Used with caution in clients with renal or hepatic problems. 2. Dosing may be done with meals or without regard to meal time. 3. Caution clients to avoid aspirin and other NSAIDs.
ACID PUMP INHIBITORS: Inhibits the enzyme that produces gastric acid.		
Omeprazole (**Prilosec**): PO Lansoprazole (**Prevacid**): PO	Headache, diarrhea, dizziness	1. Administer before meals. 2. Do not crush, chew or open capsules 3. Sprinkle granules of **Prevacid** over food, do not chew granules.
CYTOPROCTECTANT: Binds to diseased tissue provides a protective barrier to acid.		
Sucralfate (**Carafate**): PO	Constipation, GI discomfort	1. Avoid antacids. 2. Use: prevention and treatment of duodenal ulcers. 3. May impede the absorption of medications that require an acid medium.
PROSTAGLANDIN ANALOGUE: Suppresses gastric acid secretion, increases protective mucus and mucosal blood flow.		
Misoprostol (**Cytotec**)	GI problems, headache.	1. Contraindicated in pregnancy. 2. Indicated for prevention of NSAID induced ulcers.
ANTICHOLINERGICS: Inhibit secretion of gastric acids.		

Appendix 13-5:
ANTI-ULCER

MEDICATIONS	SIDE EFFECTS	NURSING IMPLICATIONS
Dicyclomine hydrochloride (**Bentyl**): PO Propantheline (**Pro-banthine**): PO, IM	Drowsiness, dry mouth, urinary retention	1. Use with caution in clients with glaucoma. 2. Evaluate for anticholinergic side effects. 3. Do not administer at same time as antacids

Appendix 13-6:
NURSING PROCEDURE ■ **Total Parenteral Nutrition (TPN)** ■

❑ **Definition: A method for providing nutrients that support healing as well as maintaining body systems.**

Indications for TPN are:
1. Inadequate protein intake to support tissue healing.
2. Conditions that interfere with nutrition — ingestion, digestion, absorption.

Routes of Administration:
1. Central parenteral line is inserted via the jugular or subclavian vein and threaded into the vena cava.
2. Utilized for long term nutritional support.
3. Peripheral hyperalimentation may be utilized. Solution is not as strong and is utilized for shorter period of time.

✦ *Goal: to maintain client in positive nitrogen balance and promote healing.*

✓ Key Points: Nursing Implications
- Solution should be at room temperature before administering.
- Infusion pump is utilized to maintain constant flow rate; no "catching up."
- Do not mix any other medications (IVPB) or blood components with parenteral solutions.
- Antiseptic occlusive dressing should be utilized at the central catheter site. It should be changed at least every 48 to 72 hours (depending on hospital policy) utilizing sterile technique.
- Infusion is initiated and discontinued on a gradual basis to allow for the pancreas to compensate for increased glucose intake.
- Maintain record of daily weight, as well as intake and output.
- Monitor blood sugar every 6 hours, or as hospital policy requires.
- Depending on blood sugar, check for orders regarding insulin coverage for hyperglycemia.
- Closely monitor temperature for indication of possible infection.
- Assess client for weight gain and for tissue healing.

NCLEX ALERT: *Monitor TPN administration. Monitor nutritional state. Weigh client correctly.*

Appendix 13-7:
NURSING PROCEDURE ■ Nasogastric And Intestinal Tubes ■

NASOGASTRIC TUBES:

Types:
Nasogastric tube (Levine tube, gastric sump tube) (Figure 13-2).
1. Maintain gastric decompression.
2. Short-term use.
3. Not recommended for long-term or for feedings.

Nasoduodenal tube (Dubhoff)
1. Short-term feedings.
2. Less problems with aspiration because lumen is in the duodenum.

✓ **Key Points: Placement of nasogastric tubes.**
- Discuss the procedure with the client.
- Measure from the bridge of the nose to the ear lobe to the xiphoid process to determine length of tube.
- Have client drink small amount of water to moisten mouth and throat.
- Lubricate the tube with water-soluble lubricant.
- Gently pass the catheter into the nasopharynx, asking the client to swallow as tube is passed.
- If there is any sudden change in client's respiratory status, withdraw tube.
- When length of tube is inserted, check for placement.
- Connect tube to suction and observe for gastric contents.
- Secure tube to nostril and excess tubing to client's gown.

NCLEX ALERT: *Implement measures to prevent aspiration, review NG tube placement. Manage patency of client tubes to prevent complications. Monitor client for NG tube placement and to reduce potential risks. Maintaining nasogastric tubes is a common task for practical nurses.*

✓ **Key Points:** ***Verifying placement of nasogastric tube.***
- Aspirate gastric contents with a syringe.
- Place the stethoscope over the gastric area and inject a small amount of air through the nasogastric tube. Characteristic sound of air entering the stomach from the tube should be heard.

✓ **Key Points:** ***Verifying placement of a nasoenteric tube.***
- X-Ray is the only method to determine the exact placement of the tube. Air instillation can be used but will not differentiate placement in the stomach or duodenum.

NURSING PRIORITY: *ALWAYS check the placement of a gastric tube prior to infusing medications, feedings, or irrigating. Placement should be checked each shift if there is a continuous feeding infusing. Document placement in the nurse's notes.*

INTESTINAL TUBES:

✦ *Goal: to provide intestinal decompression proximal to a bowel obstruction. Prevent/decrease intestinal distention.*

Types:

Cantor and Miller-Abbott tubes
1. Approximately 6 to 10 feet long.
2. Tube is weighted on the end with a bag containing mercury.
3. Gastric/intestinal suctioning is maintained while the tube is in place.

✓ **Key Points: Nursing Implications**
- Maintain client NPO.
- Evaluate the type of gastric secretions being aspirated.
- Do not tape or secure the tube until it has reached the desired position.
- Tubes may be left in place for several days.
- Monitor client's response, (i.e., increase or decrease in abdominal distention).
- Removal of the tube depends on the relief of the intestinal obstruction.

Appendix 13-8:
NURSING PROCEDURE ■ Care of the Client with an Ostomy ■

TYPE of OSTOMY

1. **Colostomy** - opening of the colon through the abdominal wall; stool is generally semisoft and bowel control may be achieved.

2. **Ileostomy** - opening of the ileum through the abdominal wall; stool drainage is liquid and excoriating; drainage is frequently continuous, therefore difficult to establish bowel control. Fluid and electrolyte imbalance is a common complication.

Preoperative Care:
1. Preoperative education: actively involve family and client; encourage questions concerning the procedure.
2. Client frequently on a low-residue diet prior to surgery to decrease intestinal contents.

✓ Key Points: Postoperative Nursing Implications - Initial Care

- Assess the stoma postoperatively; should be moist, red, and not painful. If the stoma appears dark or dusky, notify the doctor.
- Pouch should fit around the stoma without exposed skin; however, make sure the pouch is not too tight around the stoma and impairing circulation.
- The stoma will shrink postoperatively which necessitates changing the size of the appliance.
- Prevent contamination of surgical wound when emptying the pouch.
- Observe the quantity and characteristics of the stool from the ostomy.
- Changing the stoma pouch or bag.
  1. The pouch seal is changed when the skin seal is broken; the pouch is emptied when there is drainage.
  2. Cleanse the skin around the stoma with warm water and mild soap; dry thoroughly.
  3. Carefully assess the skin around the stoma; it should not be irritated or broken.
  4. There are multiple types of skin barriers to use on the skin to provide a moisture-proof seal; this is done prior to the replacement of the pouch.

✓ Key Points: Irrigation

- Do not irrigate an ileostomy, or maintain regular irrigations in child with colostomy.
- Irrigate the colostomy at the same time each day; this will establish an elimination pattern. After the irrigation and return of fluid, the client may have very little stool for the rest of the day.
- Assist the client to control odors; foods to encourage - green leafy vegetables (especially parsley), yogurt, buttermilk.
- Generally irrigate with 500 to 1,500 cc warm tap water.

NURSING PRIORITY: *Do not:*
(1) force catheter into the stoma.
(2) insert the catheter over three inches.
(3) use more than 1,500 cc of irrigation fluid.
(4) irrigate more than once a day.
(5) irrigate in the presence of diarrhea.

- Place the client in a sitting position for irrigation, preferably in the bathroom with the irrigation sleeve in the toilet.
- Elevate the solution container approximately 12 to 18 inches or to the shoulder height of the client in a sitting position and allow solution to flow in gently. If cramping occurs, lower fluid or clamp the tubing.
- Allow 25 to 45 minutes for return flow. Client may want to walk around before the return starts.
- Encourage client to participate in care of his or her own colostomy. Have client perform return demonstration of colostomy irrigation prior to leaving the hospital.

Clinical Tips for Problem Solving

If water does not flow easily into colostomy stoma, then —

- ❑ Change angle or position of catheter slightly.
- ❑ Check for kinks in tubing from container.
- ❑ Check height of irrigating container.
- ❑ Encourage client to relax and take a few deep breaths.

If client experiences cramping, nausea, or dizziness during irrigation, then —

- ❑ Stop flow of water, leaving catheter in place.
- ❑ Do not resume until cramping has passed.
- ❑ Check water temperature and height of water bag; if water is too hot or flows too rapidly, it can cause dizziness.

If client has no return of stool or water from irrigation, then —

- ❑ Be sure to apply drainable pouch that will accommodate amount of irrigation fluid.
- ❑ Have client increase fluid intake.
- ❑ Gently massage the abdomen, or close the pouch and have the client ambulate.

If diarrhea occurs, then —

- ❑ Do not irrigate colostomy.
- ❑ Check client's medications as sometimes they may cause diarrhea.
- ❑ If diarrhea is excessive and/or prolonged, *notify RN or physician.*

NCLEX ALERT: *Provide ostomy care.*

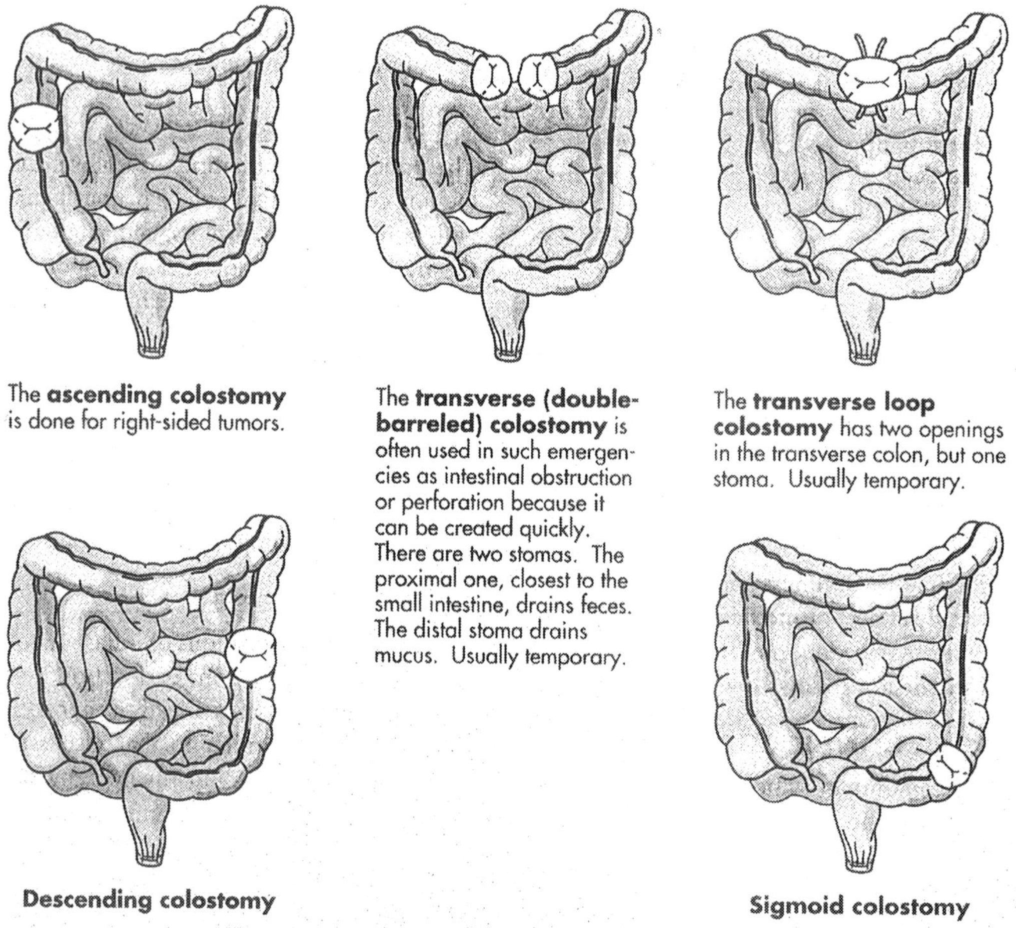

Figure 13-3: Types of Ostomies

Reprinted with permission: Phipps, WJ, Sands, JK, & Marek, JF (1999). *Medical Surgical Nursing: Concepts & Clinical Practice*, 6th ed. Philadelphia: Mosby, p. 1336.

Appendix 13-9:
NURSING PROCEDURE ■ Enemas ■

TYPES OF ENEMAS

Cleansing: Stimulate peristalsis through irritation of colon and rectum and by distention. Most common solution are tap water and normal saline. Normal saline should be used when several enemas are required for cleansing. Soap is not recommended because of the extreme irritation of the colon.

Prepackaged disposable enema (Fleets, mini enemas): Approximately 125 cc; hypertonic solution which is an irritant that causes increased peristalsis and draws fluid into the bowel. Should not be used on clients who are dehydrated. Client should retain enema for at least 20 minutes. Causes less abdominal distention and discomfort than other enemas.

✓ Key Points: Administering an Enema

- Fill water container with 500 to 1000 cc of lukewarm solution, (500 cc or less for children, 250 cc for an infant), 105° to 115°F. Solutions that are too hot or too cold or solutions that are instilled too quickly can cause cramping and damage to rectal tissues.
- Allow solution to run through the tubing so that air is removed.
- Place client on left side in a Sims' position.
- Lubricate the tip of the tubing with water-soluble lubricant.
- Gently insert tubing into client's rectum (3 to 4 inches for adult, 1 inch for infants, 2 to 3 inches for children), past the external and internal sphincters.
- Raise the water container no more than 12 inches for a small volume or 18 inches for a large volume.
- Allow solution to flow slowly. If the flow is slow, the client will experience fewer cramps. The client will also be able to tolerate and retain a greater volume of solution.
- After you have instilled the solution, instruct client to hold solution for as long as he can.
- Enemas till clear refers to return of enema solution without any fecal material.

Clinical Tips for Problem Solving

If client expels solution prematurely, then —

- ❑ Place the client in Sim's position
- ❑ Temporarily stop the flow of solution, have client take a deep breath, turn or move to facilitate the flow of fluid from the rectum into the colon, then continue the instillation of fluid.

If enema returns are not clear prior diagnostic testing, then —

- ❑ Repeat enema. If, after three enemas, returns still contain fecal material, notify physician.

If client complains of abdominal cramping during instillation of fluid, then —

- ❑ Slow the infusion rate by lowering the fluid bag.
- ❑ If cramping does not subside, discontinue the enema.

NCLEX ALERT: *Administer an enema.*

Appendix 13-10:
NURSING PROCEDURE ■ **Tube Feeding** ■

LONG-TERM TYPES

1. Percutaneous Endoscopic Gastroscopy (PEG): A tube is inserted percutaneously into the stomach; local anesthesia and sedation is used for tube placement.

2. Percutaneous Endoscopic Jejunostomy (PEJ): A tube is inserted percutaneously into the jejunum.

3. Gastrostomy: A surgical opening is made into the stomach and a gastrostomy tube is positioned with sutures.

✓ Key Point: Methods of administering a tube feeding

- Continuous—controlled with a feeding pump. Decreases nausea and diarrhea.
- Intermittent—prescribed amount of fluid instills over specific time. For example 350 cc is given over 30 minutes.
- Bolus—a prescribed amount of feeding is drawn into a syringe or poured through a funnel and allowed to instill by gravity flow; this is the least preferred method.
- Cyclic—involves feeding via a pump for a part of a day, usually 12 to 16 hours. This method may be used for weaning from feedings.

Clinical Tips for Problem Solving

- Position client on right side in high-Fowler's position for intermittent or bolus feeding.
- Aspirate contents of stomach to determine residual. If residual is over 100 cc, or more than 10-20% of an hourly amount, it may be necessary to withhold feeding and reassess the client in an hour or until residual diminishes.
- Return aspirated contents to stomach to prevent electrolyte imbalance.
- When administering bolus, hold tube feeding container no more than 18 inches above client's abdomen for short-term feeding.
- Do not force solution through the tube with pressure or a syringe.
- Following tube feeding, medications, or every 4 hours for continuous feeding, flush the tube with 30 to 50 cc of water.
- When the PEG or PEJ tubes are placed, note the length of tube protruding from the abdomen. This tube should be routinely checked to determine if the tube is migrating from the original insertion point.
- For continuous feeding (intermittent or bolus), change or clean feeding reservoir every day.
- Amount of feeding formula should not exceed the amount to infuse over 4 hours.

Avoid diarrhea:

- Slow rate of infusion.
- Keep equipment clean to avoid bacterial contamination.
- Check for fecal impaction; diarrhea may be flowing around impaction.
- Identify clients with medical conditions that would precipitate diarrhea.

NCLEX ALERT: *Administer a tube feeding. Initiate, maintain, monitor, and discontinue tube feedings according to orders. Use measures to improve nutritional intake of client.*

Appendix 13-11:
NURSING PROCEDURE ■ Stool Specimen ■

TYPES OF STOOL:

- Narrow, ribbon-like stool ➔ spastic, irritable bowel, or obstruction.
- Diarrhea ➔ spastic bowel, viral infection.
- Blood and mucus, soft stool ➔ bacterial infection.
- Mixed blood or pus ➔ colitis.
- Yellow or green stool ➔ severe, prolonged diarrhea.
- Black stool ➔ GI bleeding or intake of iron supplements.
- Tan, clay-colored, or white stool ➔ liver or gallbladder problems.
- Red stool ➔ colon or rectal bleeding; some medications and foods can may also cause a red coloration.
- Fatty stool, pasty or greasy ➔ intestinal malabsorption, pancreatic disease.

✓ Key Point: Collecting the Specimen

- Always wear gloves during procedure.
- Use clean bedpan or bedside commode to collect stool; do not use stool that has been in contact with toilet bowl water or urine.
- Collect stool specimen in a clean, dry container; use a tongue blade to obtain a small portion of the formed stool from several areas of the stool and place in the container.
- The client collecting a stool specimen for occult blood needs to follow directions regarding diet restrictions (no red meat, beets, or foods that may cause the stool to turn red or lead to a false positive).
- Do not keep specimen on the unit; take it to the lab when it is collected.
- If client has diarrhea, check to see if all of stool is required for the test.
- When checking stool for parasites, take samples of the stool from several different areas.
- Maintain standard precautions when collecting and transporting the specimen.

NCLEX ALERT: *Collect client specimens according to policies.*

Notes

Hepatic and Biliary System

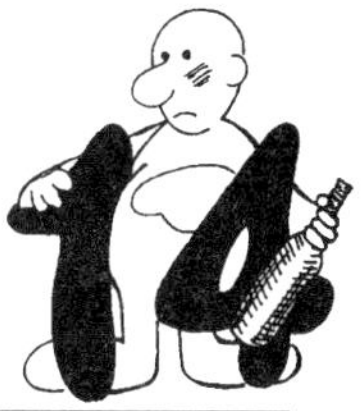

PHYSIOLOGY OF THE HEPATIC AND BILIARY SYSTEM

Organs of the Hepatic and Biliary System

A. Liver.
   1. Located in the upper right portion of the abdominal cavity just under the diaphragm; vascular organ; protected by the rib cage.
   2. Blood flow into the liver is from two sources.
      a. Portal vein carries venous blood from the stomach, intestines, pancreas, and spleen into the liver. The venous blood is rich in nutrients absorbed from the GI system.
      b. The hepatic artery provides oxygenated blood to the liver.
   3. Due to pressure differences in the hepatic and portal veins, the liver may normally store 200 to 400 cc of blood.
   4. The liver produces approximately 600 to 1200 cc of bile daily which drains from the liver via the common bile duct.
   5. The liver is susceptible to many pathologic processes. It can sustain 90 percent damage with loss of tissue and still remain functional.

B. Gallbladder.
   1. The primary function of the gallbladder is concentration and storage of bile.
   2. Gallbladder is capable of storing 20 to 50 cc of bile.

Functions of the Liver

A. Synthesis of absorbed nutrients.
   1. Serum glucose regulation.
   2. Lipid (fat) metabolism.
   3. Protein metabolism.

B. Synthesis of prothrombin for normal clotting mechanisms. Vitamin K is necessary for adequate prothrombin production.

C. Vitamin and mineral storage.

D. Drug metabolism - barbiturates, amphetamines, and alcohol are metabolized by the liver.

E. Production of bile and bile salts.

System Data Collection

A. History.
   1. History of liver, gallbladder, or jaundice problems.
   2. History of bleeding problems.
   3. History of reproductive problems.
   4. Medication intake.
   5. Recent association with anyone with jaundice.
   6. Alcohol consumption.

B. Physical data collection.
   1. Inspection.
      a. Skin.
         (1) Presence of vascular angiomas, skin lesions, or petechiae.
         (2) Hydration status.
         (3) Color of the skin (jaundiced).
         (4) Presence of peripheral edema.
      b. Abdomen.
         (1) Evidence of jaundice.
         (2) Contour of the abdomen.
         (3) Presence of visual abdominal wall veins.
   2. Palpation of the abdomen
      a. Pain, tenderness.
      b. Presence of distention.
      c. Hepatomegaly.
      d. Splenomegaly.

C. Nutritional data collection.
   1. Weight gain or loss.
   2. Dietary intake.
   3. Problems of anorexia, nausea, and vomiting.

DISORDERS OF THE LIVER

Jaundice

A. Jaundice may begin so gradually that it is not noticed immediately.

B. The increased levels of bilirubin cause a yellowish discoloration of the skin. It may be first observed as a yellow color in the sclera of the eye.

C. Types of jaundice.
   1. Prehepatic (hemolytic jaundice).
      a. Occurs with an increase in the breakdown of red blood cells, which produce an increase in the amount of unconjugated bilirubin in the blood.
      b. Causes of hemolytic jaundice.
         (1) Blood transfusion reactions.
         (2) Sickle cell crisis.
         (3) Hemolytic anemias.
         (4) Hemolytic disease of the newborn.

2. Posthepatic (obstructive jaundice).
   a. Results from an obstruction to bile flow through the liver and the biliary system.
   b. The obstruction may be within the liver, or it may be outside the liver.
   c. Causes of obstructive jaundice.
      (1) Hepatitis.
      (2) Liver tumors.
      (3) Cirrhosis.
      (4) Obstruction of the common bile duct by a stone.
3. Hepatocellular jaundice
   a. Liver dysfunction related to the uptake, conjugation and transport of bilirubin.
      (1) Hepatitis
      (2) Liver tumors
      (3) Cirrhosis

Viral Hepatitis

❑ **Widespread inflammation of the liver tissue is called *hepatitis*.**

A. Types of hepatitis (Table 14-1).
1. Hepatitis A (HAV, infectious hepatitis).
   a. Mode of transmission.
      (1) Carriers are most contagious just prior to onset of symptoms (jaundice).
      (2) The route of infection is predominately fecal-oral.
      (3) Virus is present in feces and serum during the incubation period.
   b. Administration of immune serum globulin (IgG) to exposed individuals may decrease the severity of the illness.
2. Hepatitis B (HBV, serum hepatitis).
   a. Mode of transmission.
      (1) Percutaneous inoculation with contaminated needles or instruments.
      (2) Non-percutaneous transmission-contact with body fluids containing hepatitis B surface antigen (sexual contact).
      (3) Infants of mothers with HBV may contract the disease in utero, at birth, or postnatal.
      (4) Infected asymptomatic carrier.
   b. Identification of the hepatitis B surface antigen (HB_sAg, Australian antigen).
      (1) Identification of antigen in potential blood donors has significantly decreased transmission via blood transfusions.
      (2) Antigen is present in vaginal secretions, menstrual fluid, semen, saliva, and respiratory secretions.
3. Hepatitis C (non-A non- B) - transmission and precautions are essentially the same as for HBV, multiple causative agents - per cutaneous inoculation (IV drug abuse), blood transfusions, and increased incidence in crowded living conditions.

B. The inflammatory process causes hepatic cell destruction and necrosis. Hepatitis A is generally self limiting, with liver regeneration and complete recovery. Hepatitis B and C are more serious and can progress to total destruction of the liver.

Data Collection

(Regardless of the type, the clinical picture is similar.)

NCLEX ALERT: *Identify client risk for infection. Identify signs and symptoms of infection. Apply principles of infection control.*

1. Hepatitis A.
   a. Primarily occurs in young children and young adults.
   b. Increased incidence in crowded living conditions and areas of poor hygiene.
   c. Infected food handlers may be the source of infection.
   d. May be transmitted from contaminated water, milk products or shellfish from contaminated waters.
   e. Primary route of transmission is fecal-oral.
2. Hepatitis B.
   a. Percutaneous inoculation, IV drug abuse.
   b. Blood transfusions.
   c. Affects all ages.
   d. Onset of hepatitis B is more insidious; symptoms are more severe.
3. Clinical manifestations.
   a. Anorexia, nausea.
   b. Upper right quadrant discomfort.
   c. Pruritus.
   d. Malaise, headache.
   e. Jaundice (may not occur in children).
   f. Low-grade fever.
   g. Bleeding tendencies.
   h. Dark urine.
   i. Light and clay colored stools.

Table 14-1: Hepatitis

HEPATITIS A (HAV)	HEPATITIS B (HBV)	HEPATITIS C (HCV)
Transmission modes:		
Poor personal hygiene Oral-anal sexual practices Contaminated food, water, and shellfish (commonly spread by infected food handlers)	Blood and blood products Skin or mucous membrane break by inoculation (needle sticks, cuts, ear piercing, tattooing, or contaminated drug paraphernalia) Sexual contact	Blood and blood products Sexual contact Close contact, IV drug use Closely associate with HBV
Incubation period:		
2 to 6 weeks (average: 4 weeks); also the most contagious period	6 weeks to 6 months (average: 12 weeks) Contagious as long as serum marker (surface antigen) appears	Variable
High-Risk Individuals:		
Household contacts Sexual contacts Institutions, day care centers, schools	Household contacts Sexual contacts Dental, laboratory, and medical personnel Multiple blood transfusion recipients IV drug users	Multiple blood transfusion recipients Sexual contacts IV drug users
Isolation precaution: Isolation is the same for all forms of hepatitis. Private room - necessary only for client with poor hygiene Gown - for direct contact with blood or body fluid Gloves - for direct contact with blood or body fluid Needles and syringes - dispose of in properly labeled, puncture-resistant container Dressings and tissues - double bag and dispose of in hospital's designated area Linen - double bag in isolation bags if contaminated with blood or body fluid Specimens - properly labeled specimens "Blood and body fluid precautions"		

NCLEX ALERT: *Apply principles of infection control*

4. Diagnostics
   a. Specific serologic markers for each type of hepatitis.
   b. Presence of specific antibodies in serum.
   c. Serum aminotransferases are elevated initially.
   d. Serum bilirubin is increased.

Treatment

1. No specific medications.
2. Dietary modifications - increased calories, increased carbohydrates, protein as tolerated, low fat.
3. Decreased activity.

Nursing Intervention

✦ *Goal: to control and prevent hepatitis.*

1. Understand characteristics of transmission and preventive measures for hepatitis A.
   a. Good personal hygiene, especially handwashing.
   b. Identification of individuals at an increased risk of exposure; includes household, intimate sexual, and institutional contacts with the active disease.
   c. Administer immune serum globulin (IgG) within two weeks of exposure.
   d. Enteric/standard precautions.
2. Understand characteristics of transmission and preventive measures for hepatitis B.
   a. Identification of individuals at increased risk of exposure; IV drug users, or sexual contact.
   b. Administration of hepatitis B vaccine, administration of hepatitis B immune globulin (HBIG) to individuals with one-time exposure.
3. Maintain standard precautions in hospitalized client with questionable diagnosis of hepatitis (Table 14-1).

***Geriatric Priority:** Elderly clients are at a higher risk for liver damage and for complications.*

✦ *Goal: to promote healing and regeneration of liver tissue.*

1. Activity restrictions based on level of fatigue; avoid excessive activity that causes undue fatigue.
2. Promote psychological and emotional rest.
   a. Bedrest may increase anxiety; generally activities as tolerated.
   b. Frequently, young adults are very concerned about body image; encourage verbalization and emphasize temporary nature of symptoms.
   c. Maintain communication and frequent contact if client is on isolation precautions.

NCLEX ALERT: *Initiate measures to improve nutritional status.*

3. Promote nutritional intake.
   a. Anorexia and decreased taste for food potentiate the problem.
   b. Anorexia may be decreased in the morning.
   c. Small, frequent feedings of favorite foods, good oral hygiene, and food served in a pleasant atmosphere.
4. Promote adequate fluid intake.

Self-Care

1. There will be a continued need for adequate rest and nutrition until liver functions are normal.
2. If possible, client should have his own bathroom.
3. Stress to client and family the importance of handwashing and personal hygiene.
4. Avoid alcohol and OTC medications especially those containing acetamnophen and phenothiazine.
5. Clients with hepatitis B should avoid intimate and sexual contact until HBsAg is negative and serum enzyme levels are normal.
6. Continue regular medical follow-ups for at least one year.
7. Client should not donate blood.
8. Educate client to recognize symptoms of recurrence.

NCLEX ALERT: *Review client teaching about health risks and health promotion.*

Hepatic Cirrhosis

❑ **Hepatic cirrhosis is a chronic, progressive disease of the liver characterized by degeneration and destruction of liver cells.**

Data Collection

1. Clinical manifestations.
   a. Early.
      (1) GI disturbances - anorexia, indigestion, change in bowel habits.
      (2) Malaise.
      (3) Right upper quadrant discomfort, due to enlarging liver.
   b. Later.
      (1) Jaundice.
      (2) Spider angiomas on the face, neck and shoulders.
      (3) Palmar erythema - reddened areas in the palm that blanche with pressure.
      (4) Anemia.
      (5) Increased risk of infection due to leukopenia.
      (6) Coagulation disorders, thrombocytopenia.
      (7) Changes in sexual characteristics: gynecomastia, impotence in males; amenorrhea, vaginal bleeding in females.
      (8) Peripheral neuropathy - probably due to inadequate intake of vitamin B complex.
      (9) Hepatomegaly, splenomegaly.
   c. Portal hypertension.
      (1) Esophageal varices which bleed easily.
      (2) Hemorrhoids.
      (3) Veins visible on abdominal wall.
      (4) Development of edema and ascites.
   d. Peripheral edema and ascites.
      (1) Edema generally occurs in feet, ankles, and presacral area.
      (2) Severe abdominal distention and weight gain with ascites.
   e. Hepatic encephalopathy (coma) — secondary to ↑ serum ammonia.
      (1) Changes in mental responsiveness.
      (2) Memory problems.
      (3) Asterixis (liver flap).

Treatment

1. Cirrhosis.

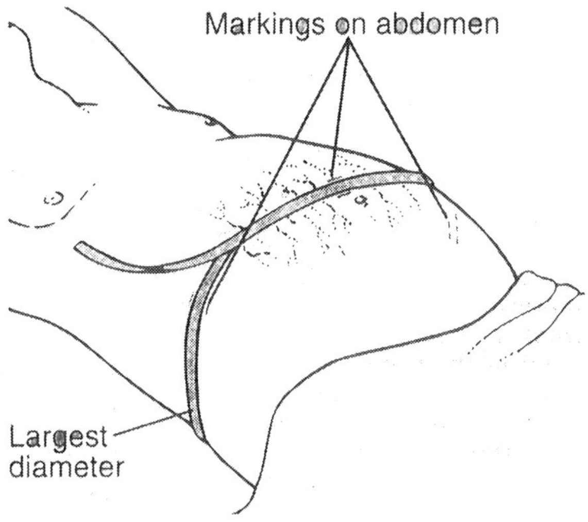

Figure 14-1: Measuring Abdominal Girth
With the client supine, the nurse brings the tape measure around the client and takes a measurement at the largest diameter of the abdomen. Before removing the tape, the nurse marks the client's abdomen along the sides of the tape on the client's flanks (sides) and midline to ensure that later measurements are taken in a consistent manner.
Reprinted with permission: Ignatavicius, D., Workman, L., Mishler, M. (1995). *Medical Surgical Nursing: A Nursing Process Approach,*Philadelphia: W.B. Saunders, p. 1671.

a. Rest.
b. Dietary modification - increase calories and carbohydrates; protein and fat as tolerated.
c. Vitamin supplement, especially vitamin B complex.
d. Abstinence from alcohol.
e. Corticosteriods.

2. Portal hypertension -surgical creation of a portacaval shunt decreases the pressure by shunting the blood from the portal system to an adjacent vein in the systemic system.
3. Ascites.
   a. Sodium restriction in dietary intake.
   b. Fluid restriction in severe ascites.
   c. Diuretics.
   d. Paracentesis.
   e. Peritoneal venous shunt (LeVeen shunt) - a surgical procedure for reinfusion of ascitic fluid.
   f. Measure abdominal girth (Figure 14-1).
4. Esophageal varices (generally not treated unless bleeding).
   a. Surgical procedures to decrease portal hypertension by shunting portal blood flow.
   b. Blood transfusions to restore volume from bleeding varices, preferably fresh whole blood.
   c. Administration of vitamin K and vasopressin to control bleeding.
5. Hepatic encephalopathy coma (treatment is directed toward decreasing ammonia formation).
   a. Restriction of dietary protein intake.
   b. Sterilization of the intestine by neomycin to reduce bacterial activity on protein.
   c. Lactulose - produces an acidic environment in the intestine and thereby decreases bacterial activity.

Nursing Intervention

✦ *Goal: to promote health in the cirrhotic client.*

1. Proper diet.
2. Adequate rest.
3. Avoid potential hepatotoxic over-the-counter drugs.
4. Abstain from alcohol and avoid aspirin.
5. Daily weight with intake and output records.
6. Attention and care should be given to the alcoholic client without being judgmental or moralizing.
7. Client should understand symptoms indicative of complications and when to seek medical advice.
8. Regular medical checkups.

✦ *Goal: to maintain homeostasis and promote liver function in the hospitalized client.*

1. Rest and activity schedule based on clinical manifestations and lab data.
2. Measures to prevent complications of immobility (See Chapter 3).
3. Assist client to maintain self-esteem.
   a. Maintain positive, accepting atmosphere in the delivery of care.
   b. Encourage ventilation of feelings regarding disease.
   c. Be a supportive listener.
4. Assist in ADL as necessary to prevent undue fatigue.
5. Promote nutritional intake.
   a. Good oral hygiene.
   b. Between-meal nourishment.
   c. Provide food preferences when possible.
   d. Antiemetic prior to meals if necessary.
   e. Iron and vitamin supplements, especially vitamin B complex.

f. Nasogastric or parenteral feeding if unable to maintain adequate intake.

6. Decrease discomfort of pruritus secondary to jaundice.
7. Good skin care to prevent breakdown.
8. Monitor temperature closely due to increased susceptibility to infection.
9. Assess for bleeding tendencies and prevent trauma to the mucous membrane.

✦ *Goal: To assess for and decrease bleeding tendencies if esophageal varices are present.*

1. Soft, nonirritating foods; discourage coffee.
2. Discourage straining at stool.
3. Decrease esophageal reflux.
4. No salicylate compounds (aspirin).
5. Evaluate for active bleeding.
   a. Monitor vital signs.
   b. Assess for melena.
   c. Assess for hematemesis.
6. *Notify RN immediately of any bright red vomiting (bleeding) or significant changes in vital signs.*

✦ *Goal: to assess for and prevent complications associated with ascites.*

1. Decrease sodium intake.
2. Diuretics, potassium supplements.
3. Daily measurements of abdominal girth. (Fig 14-1)
4. Maintain semi Fowler's position to decrease pressure on the diaphragm.
5. Evaluate daily weight for fluid loss or gain.

✦ *Goal: to assess for and prevent complications of hepatic encephalopathy (coma).*

1. Frequent assessment of responsiveness.
2. Decrease production of ammonia.
   a. Decrease protein diet.
   b. Increase carbohydrates and fluids.
   c. Decrease activity since ammonia is by-product of metabolism.
   d. GI bleeding will increase ammonia levels, due to breakdown of red blood cells.
3. Prompt treatment of hypokalemia.

✦ *Goal: to provide appropriate pre-and postoperative care if surgical procedure is indicated (See Chapter 3).*

a. Portacaval shunt requires general postoperative care (Chapter 3).
b. Peritoneal - venous shunt (LaVeen) to provide for continuous reinfusion of ascitic fluid into the venous system.
c. Client at increased risk for operative procedures.
d. Postoperative care is similar to that for any abdominal surgery; postoperative complications include:
   (1) Hemorrhage.
   (2) Electrolyte imbalance.
   (3) Seizures.
   (4) Delirium tremens.
e. Surgical procedures do not alter course of progressive hepatic disease.

Cancer of the Liver

❑ **Primary cancer of the liver is rare. Metastatic cancer is more common.**

A. Liver is common site for metastases, due to increased rate of blood flow and capillary network.
B. Metastases are found in liver in approximately one-half of all late-stage cancer victims.
C. Prognosis is poor.

Data Collection

1. Anorexia, weight loss.
2. Fatigue.
3. Anemia.
4. Abdominal pain with rapid liver enlargement.
5. Ascites and jaundice may occur.
6. Diagnostics — liver scan and biopsy (Appendix 14-2).

Treatment

Primarily palliative.

1. Surgical excision of tumor if it is localized.
2. Chemotherapy.
3. Pain control.

Nursing Intervention

Focused on maintaining comfort; nursing care is very similar to care required for the advanced cirrhotic client.

DISORDERS OF THE BILIARY TRACT

Cholelithiasis and Cholecystitis

❑ **Cholelithiasis is the presence of stones in the gallbladder; this is the most common form of biliary disease.**

❑ **Cholecystitis is an inflammation of the gallbladder which is frequently associated with stones; this condition may be acute or chronic.**

Data Collection

1. Cholelithiasis — presence of gallstones.
   a. Increased incidence in females, especially during pregnancy.
   b. Obesity
   c. Pain in upper midline area, radiating to the back.
   d. Epigastric distress, feeling of fullness.
   e. Nausea and vomiting.
2. Cholecystitis — inflammation of the gallbladder.
   a. Associated with stones.
   b. Abdominal guarding and rigidity with rebound tenderness.
   c. Fever.
   d. Pain radiating to back and aggravated by deep breathing.
   e. May present suddenly with severe pain or pain occurs after eating.
3. Obstruction of cystic duct by stones, precipitating biliary colic.
   a. Severe abdominal pain radiating to the back and shoulder.
   b. Nausea, vomiting, tachycardia, diaphoresis.
   c. Jaundice may occur.
   d. Urine may become very dark and stools clay colored.
   e. Sometimes fatty foods will precipitate the attack.

Treatment

1. Cholelithiasis - surgical removal of the stones.
2. Cholecystitis.
   a. Anticholinergics to decrease secretions and promote relaxation of the gallbladder.
   b. Analgesics - usually meperidine (**Demerol**). Morphine may cause a spasm in the sphincter of Oddi, causing increase in pain.
   c. Antibiotics.
   d. Decrease dietary fat intake.
3. Surgery

✦ *Goal: to decrease attack of pain and inflammatory response.*

1. Low-fat liquid diet during acute attack.
2. Low-fat solids added as tolerated.
3. IV fluids and gastric decompression if nausea and vomiting are severe.

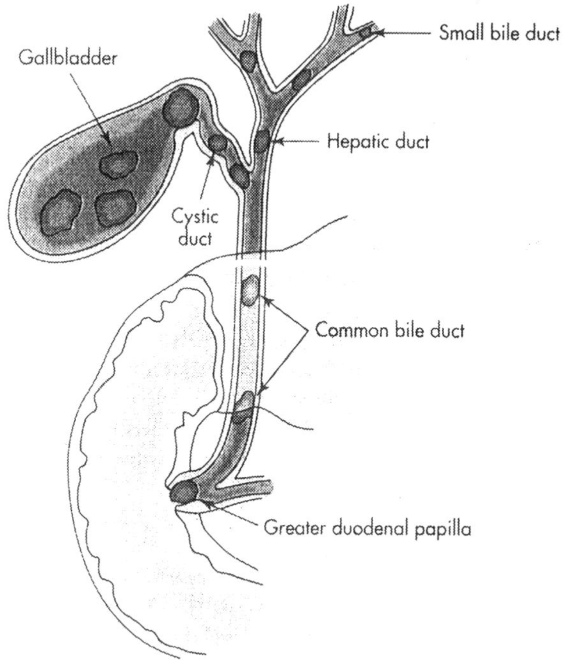

Figure 14-2: Gallstones
Reprinted with permission: Ignatavicius, D., Workman, L., Mishler, M. (1999): *Medical-Surgical Nursing : A Nursing Process Approach*, Philadelphia: W.B. Saunders, p. 1708.

4. Antibiotics and analgesics.

✦ *Goal: to provide appropriate preoperative nursing care if surgery is indicated. (See Chapter 3).*

✦ *Goal: to maintain homeostasis and prevent complications postoperative cholecystectomy.*

1. General postoperative care for clients having surgery (See Chapter 3).
2. Evaluate tolerance to diet and progress diet gradually to low-fat solids.
3. T-tube may be utilized to maintain patency of bile duct and bile drainage if common bile duct was opened during surgery.

> ***NURSING PRIORITY:*** *Maintain T-tube to gravity drainage; do not irrigate. Observe amount and color of bile drainage.*

   a. Do not irrigate or clamp tube.
   b. Observe for bile drainage around the tube.
   c. Observe and record drainage.
   d. As edema in the common duct subsides, the drainage will decrease.
   e. Drainage usually around 500 cc per day for several days postoperative; gradually; drainage will decrease and the doctor will usually remove the tube after 5 to 7 days.
4. Monitor urine and stool for changes in color.
5. Post laparoscopy
   a. 3 small incisions.

b. Decreased risk to client.
c. One day admit or out patient.
d. Early ambulation and decreased pain.

Self-Care

1. Dietary teaching regarding low-fat diet.
2. Weight reduction if appropriate.
3. Avoid heavy lifting.
4. Postoperative care of the incision and signs of infection.

Study Questions—Hepatic & Biliary

1. Which client would be considered at an increased risk for developing hepatitis A?

① elderly man with daily alcohol consumption.
② young woman who had to have multiple blood transfusions.
③ male client who regularly donates blood.
④ older woman who regularly eats raw oysters.

2. Which nursing activity would put the nurse at increased risk for exposure to Hepatitis B virus?

① cleansing the client's anal area without wearing gloves.
② recapping syringes and needles.
③ hand contact with client's blood.
④ spraying of blood into nurses eyes.

3. What is important to teach a client who is being discharged after treatment for hepatitis B regarding over the counter medications?

① do not take acetaminophen products.
② increase your intake of Vitamin A.
③ do not take decongestive products.
④ use cough medications with caution.

4. What are critical vaccinations for a person who is working in the health care field?

① hepatitis B.
② hepatitis A.
③ human immunodeficiency virus (HIV).
④ varicella.

5. What is another name for hepatitis A?

① serum hepatitis.
② noninfectious hepatitis.
③ hepatitis C.
④ infectious hepatitis.

6. Why is it important for a client with end-stage liver failure to be very cautious when taking any form of medication?

① the liver metabolizes many medications for utilization and excretion from the body.
② the liver inactivates most medications
③ a diseased liver will increase the action of medications.
④ the client usually has to take a larger dose to get the actual therapeutic value.

7. What physiological characteristics would the nurse find while checking the skin of a client with cirrhosis of the liver?

① spider angiomas on the chest, yellow tinted skin color, bruises.
② cyanosis, red to pink colored extremities, glassy eyes.
③ dusky blue color, fruity breath, yellow tinted skin color.
④ yellow tinted skin color, varicose veins, glassy eyes.

8. While taking vital signs, the nurse notices that the client has yellow tinted sclera. What term best describes this condition?

① conjunctivitis.
② sclerosis.
③ exophthalmos.
④ jaundice.

9. A client being treated for ascites is placed on a strict low-sodium diet. Considering his diet, what would be an appropriate food to select?

① pasta and milk.
② whole wheat bread.
③ four slices of apple.
④ peanut butter on crackers.

10. A client with advanced liver disease would present with which symptoms?

① hypotension.
② nocturia.
③ melena.
④ ascites.

11. The client is returning to his room after a cholecystectomy. What is the best position for this client?

① side lying to decrease pain.
② semi-Fowler's to promote breathing.
③ prone to decrease problems of aspiration.
④ supine to decrease stress on suture line.

12. A charge nurse tells her staff nurse that the client with advanced liver disease has a high level of

blood ammonia. What would the nurse expect to find with this client?

① increased problems breathing.

② altered level of consciousness.

③ fragile skin and easy bruising.

④ yellowish skin discoloration.

13. The nurse understands that preoperative pain medication for cholelithiasis will most likely be meperidine (Demerol), as opposed to morphine. What is the rationale for this drug for pain control?

① **Demerol** can be given SQ, if needed.

② morphine has a lesser effect than **Demerol**.

③ **Demerol** is less expensive for long-term use.

④ morphine may cause bile duct spasms.

14. A client with chronic liver problems is to receive Vitamin K prior to surgery. What is the purpose of this medication?

① decreases bleeding tendencies.

② increases healing after surgery.

③ assists to maintain fluid balance.

④ prevents nausea and vomiting.

Appendix 14-1: DIAGNOSTICS OF THE HEPATIC AND BILIARY SYSTEM -LABORATORY TESTS

LABORATORY TESTS	CLINICAL / NURSING IMPLICATIONS
SERUM STUDIES:	
• Bilirubin	A rise in the serum level of bilirubin will occur if there is excessive destruction of red blood cells or if the liver is unable to excrete normal amounts of bilirubin.
• Total serum protein	Proteins are responsible for maintaining the colloid oncotic pressure in the serum. Synthesis of protein and normal serum protein levels are affected by various liver impairments.
• Prothrombin time	Prothrombin time may be prolonged in liver disease. Evaluates vitamin K deficiency. (See Chapter 11 for specific values and detailed nursing interventions.)
• Serum blood ammonia	Increasing blood ammonia is indicative of the inability of the liver to convert ammonia to urea.
TRANSAMINASE STUDIES:	
• Lactic dehydrogenase (LDH) • Aspartate aminogransferase (AST) formerly serum glutaminic oxaloacetic transaminase (SGOT) • Alanine aminotransferase (ALT) formerly serum glutaminic pyruvic transaminase (SGPT)	ALT (SGPT) is primarily found in liver tissue and is a sensitive index of hepatic injury. (AST) SGOT and LDH are also elevated in liver damage, but are not specific to liver tissue.

Appendix 14-2:
DIAGNOSTICS OF THE HEPATIC AND BILIARY SYSTEM -INVASIVE PROCEDURES

PROCEDURE	NURSING IMPLICATIONS
LIVER BIOPSY:	
Needle aspiration of liver tissue.	1. Client NPO 6 hours prior to biopsy. 2. Blood coagulation studies should be available on the chart prior to biopsy procedure. 3. Immediately prior to needle insertion, have client take a deep breath, exhale completely and hold his/her breath. This immobilizes the chest wall and decreases the risk of penetration of the diaphragm with the needle. ***NURSING PRIORITY:*** *After the biopsy, position the client on his/her right side with a pillow under the costal margin to facilitate compression of the liver.* 4. Client generally on bedrest for 24 hours. 5. Assess for complications of pneumothorax, and hemorrhage immediately after biopsy, observe for development of bile peritonitis, and assess for right upper abdominal pain or right referred shoulder pain. 6. Vital signs should be evaluated hourly for 8 - 12 hours. 7. Purpose is to obtain tissue samples for diagnosis of liver diseases.
CHOLANGIOGRAPHY:	
IV injection of radiopaque dye to visualize the common bile duct.	1. Evaluate client for history of allergy to iodine or seafood. 2. Client may be in X-Ray for several hours; dye is injected at intervals. 3. Assess for iodine reaction - dyspnea, tachycardia, nausea and vomiting, chills. 4. Increase fluids after test to increase excretion of dye. 5. Purpose is to visualize passage of dye into bile ducts to determine patency. 6. Observe for allergic reaction. 7. May have discomfort on urination due to the iodine dye.
ORAL CHOLECYSTOGRAM (GALLBLADDER SERIES):	
X-ray visualization of the gallbladder to determine the gallbladder's ability to concentrate and store the dye ingested and the patency of the biliary duct system.	1. Evaluate client for history of sensitivity to iodine. 2. Administer radiopaque dye PO evening prior to examination: six tablets, one given every 5 minutes. Client is NPO after dye ingestion. 3. Evaluate for side effects of the dye. 4. Client may be given a fatty meal before or during the x-ray procedure. This depends on the type of diet, type of radiopague contrast media being used and what particular function is being assessed (i.e., emptying of gallbladder, contraction of gallbladder, etc.). 5. Increase fluids after test to increase excretion of the dye. 6. Purpose is to visualize gallbladder to determine disease or obstruction. 7. *Notify RN if nausea and vomiting occur. The tablets may not be absorbed.*
CHOLECYSTOSONOGRAPHY & ABDOMINAL ULTRASONOGRAPHY	
Use of sound waves to visualize gall bladder and abdominal organs.	1. No preparation required. 2. Non invasive. 3. No specific preparation pre or post test.

NCLEX ALERT: *Determine if client is prepared for procedure Monitor client diagnostic test results.*

Notes

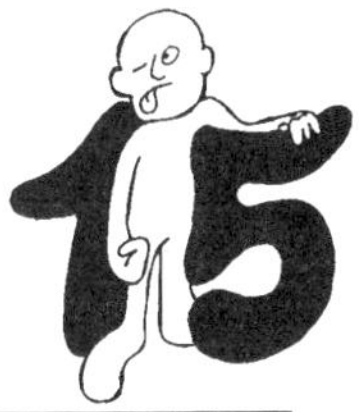

❑ The neurologic or nervous system is composed of two primary areas: the central nervous system, which includes the brain and the spinal cord, and the peripheral nervous system, which includes all of the network of nerves extending from the central system.

PHYSIOLOGY OF THE NEUROLOGIC SYSTEM

Central Nervous System

The brain and the spinal cord within the vertebral column make up the *central nervous system.*

A. The brain and the spinal column are protected by the rigid bony structure of the skull and the vertebral column.

B. Meninges - the protective membranes that cover the brain and are continuous with those of the spinal cord.

1. Pia mater - covers the surfaces of the brain and the spinal column.

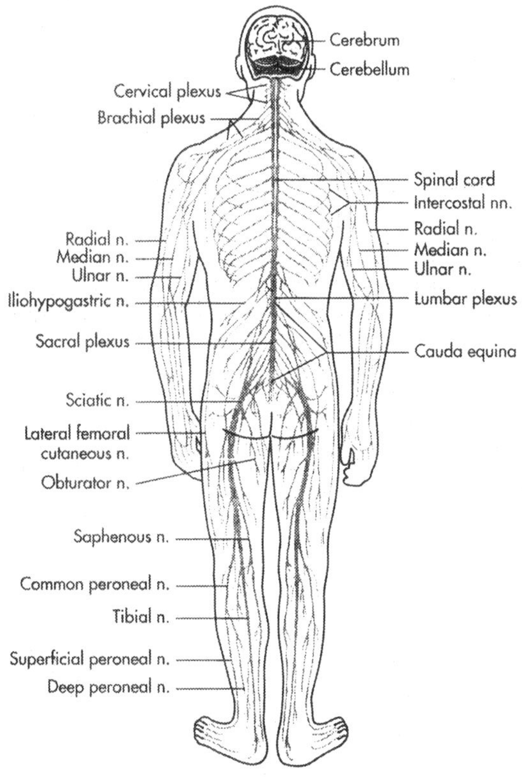

Figure 15-1:The central and peripheral divisions of the nervous system. CNS consists of the brain and spinal cord. Reprinted with permission: Phipps, WJ, Sands, JK, & Marek, JF, (1999). *Medical Surgical Nursing: Concepts & Clinical Practice*, 6th ed. Philadelphia: Mosby, p. 1673.

2. Arachnoid - waterproof membrane that encases the entire CNS; the subarachnoid space contains the cerebrospinal fluid.
3. Dura mater - a tough membrane that provides protection to the brain and spinal cord.

C. Cerebrospinal fluid (CSF).

1. Serves to cushion and protect the brain and spinal cord; brain literally floats in CSF.
2. CSF is clear, colorless, watery fluid; approximately 100 to 200 cc total volume, with a normal fluid pressure of 70 to 150 cm of water (average - 125 cm water pressure).
3. Formation and circulation of CSF - since CSF is formed continuously, it is reabsorbed by the arachnoid villi in the ventricles at the same rate it is formed.

D. Brain.

1. Cerebrum - the largest portion of the brain is separated into hemispheres; the cerebral cortex is the surface layer of each hemisphere.
2. Motor areas of the cerebral cortex - primary function is to coordinate and control skeletal muscle activity.
3. Brain stem - consists of the pons and the medulla.
   a. Pons - is responsible for alertness.
   b. Medulla oblongata - a continuation of the spinal cord as it enters into the cranial vault in the brain.
      (1) Respiratory center for changes in rate and depth of breathing.
      (2) Controls cardiac rate.
      (3) Vomiting reflex center.
      (4) Swallowing reflex center.
   c. Hypothalamus — area of body temperature regulation.

E. Spinal cord.

1. The spinal cord is continuous with the medulla and extends down the vertebral columns to the level of the first and second lumbar vertebra.
2. Each column is divided into functional groups of nerve fibers - ascending tracts (sensory pathways)and descending tracts (motor pathways)
3. Structure.
   a. Vertebrae provide protection for the spinal cord and nerve roots.
   b. Intervertebral discs lie between each vertebra to provide flexibility to the spinal column.

c. Nucleus pulposus is a gelatin substance in the vertebral disc.

4. Upper motor neurons - originate in the brain; transmit impulses from the brain to the lower motor neuron.

5. Lower motor neurons - originate in the spinal cord; transmit impulses to the muscles and organs. These neurons form the reflex arc.

Peripheral Nervous System (PNS)

The cranial and spinal nerves which connect the CNS with the body parts constitute the PNS. The peripheral nervous system is further divided into subdivisions based on the destination of the nerves. The autonomic nervous system is part of the subdivision.

A. Cranial nerves.

1. Twelve pairs of cranial nerves.
2. Originate from under the surface of the brain.

B. Spinal nerves — each pair of nerves is numbered according to the level of the spinal cord from which it originates.

C. Autonomic nervous system - regulates involuntary activity (cardiovascular, respiratory, metabolic, body temperature, etc.) (Table 15-1).

1. Parasympathetic division - maintains normal body functions.
2. Sympathetic division - prepares the body to meet a challenge or an emergency.
3. Most of the organs of the body receive innervation from both the parasympathetic and the sympathetic divisions.

System Data Collection

A. History.

1. Neurologic history

> ***Geriatric Priority:*** *mental status must be assessed before assuming the history data from the client is accurate.*

2. Medical history.
   a. Chronic, concurrent medical problems.
   b. Medications (especially tranquilizers, sedatives, narcotics, etc.).
   c. If client is an infant or young child, a pregnancy and delivery history of the mother is obtained..
   d. Sequence of growth and development.
3. Family history - presence of hereditary or congenital problems.
4. Personal history - activities of daily living; any change in routine.
5. History and symptoms of current problem.

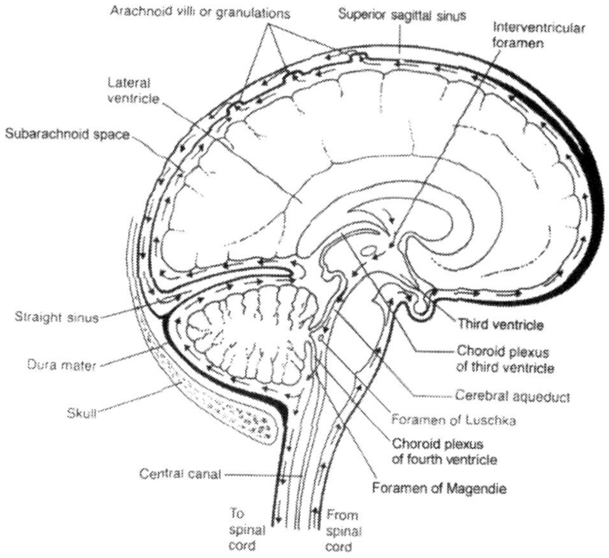

Figure 15-2: Circulation of cerebrospinal fluid.
Reprinted with permission: Ignatavicius, D., Workman,L., Mishler, M., (1995). *Medical Surgical Nursing: A Nursing Process Approach,* Philadelphia: W.B. Saunders, p. 1098.

   a. Paralysis or paresthesia.
   b. Syncope, dizziness.
   c. Headache.
   d. Speech problems.
   e. Visual problems.
   f. Changes in personality.
   g. Memory loss.
   h Nausea, vomiting.

B. Physical assessment.

> **NCLEX ALERT:** *Review changes in client neurological status.*

1. General observation of client.
   a. Posture, gait.
   b. Position of rest for the infant or young child.
   c. Personal hygiene, grooming.
   d. Evaluate speech and ability to communicate.
      (1) Pace of speech - rapid, slow, halting.
      (2) Clarity - slurred or distinct.
      (3) Tone - high pitched, rough.
      (4) Vocabulary - appropriate choice of words.
   e. Facial features may suggest specific syndromes in children.
2. Mental status (must take into consideration the client's culture and educational background).

a. General appearance and behavior.

b. Level of consciousness.

(1) Oriented to time, person, place.

(2) Appropriate response to verbal and tactile stimuli.

(3) Memory, problem-solving abilities.

> ***Geriatric Priority:*** *Judgement and problem solving abilities are critical for the safety of the elderly client.*

c. Mood.

d. Thought content and intellectual capacity.

e. Judgment and abstract thinking.

f. Perceptual distortion.

> ***NURSING PRIORITY:*** *Level of consciousness is a very sensitive indicator of change in the client with neurological problems.*

3. Assess pupillary status and eye movements.

a. Size of pupils should be equal.

b. Reaction of pupils.

(1) Direct light reflex - constriction of pupil when light is shown directly into eye.

(2) Accommodation - pupillary constriction to accommodate near visions.

c. Evaluate eye movements.

(1) Note nystagmus - fine, jerking eye movement.

(2) Ability of eyes to move together.

(3) Resting position should be at mid- position of the eye socket.

d. PERRLA - indicates that pupils are equal, round, reactive to light and accommodation is present.

4. Evaluate motor function.

a. Assess face and upper extremities for equality of movement, sensation, and evaluate swallow reflex.

b. Evaluate appropriateness of motor movement, spontaneous and on command.

Box 15-1: Elderly Care Focus

Causes of Confusion in Elderly Client

Decreased cardiac output
- Myocardial infarction
- Dysrythmias
- CHF

Hypoxia/respiratory acidosis
- Pneumonia
- Infection
- Hypoventilation

Neurological
- Vascular insufficiency
- Infections
- Cerebral edema

Metabolic
- Electrolyte imbalance
- Hypo/hyperglycemia
- Dehydration

Environmental
- Strange surroundings
- Hypo/Hyperthermia
- Sensory overload/deprivation

> **NCLEX ALERT:** *Provide care to meet special needs of the older adult client. Plan interventions to manage confusion.*

c. Movement of extremities should always be evaluated bilaterally, comparing tone, strength, and muscle movement of each side.

d. Presence of inappropriate, non-purposeful movement, (i.e., posturing).

(1) Decerebrate - extension and adduction of the arms, hyperextension of the leg.

(2) Decorticate - flexion, internal rotation of the arms, extension of the leg.

Table 15-1: AUTONOMIC NERVOUS SYSTEM

AREA AFFECTED	SYMPATHETIC	PARASYMPATHETIC
Pupil	Dilates	Constricts
Bronchi	Dilates	Constricts
Heart	Increases rate	Decreases rate
Gastrointestinal	Inhibits peristalsis Decreases secretions	Stimulates peristalsis Increases secretions
Bladder	Relaxes bladder muscle Constricts sphincter	Contracts bladder muscle Relaxes sphincter
Peripheral vessels	Constricts	Generally no effect

(3) Presence of non-purposeful involuntary movements such as tremors, jerking, twitching.

(4) Opisthotonos position - rigid arching of the back

e. Ability of an infant to suck and to swallow.

f. Asymmetrical contraction of facial muscles.

5. Evaluate reflexes.

a. Gag or cough reflex.

b. Swallow reflex.

c. Babinski reflex - normal sign is negative in adults and children over one year; positive sign is dorsal flexion of the foot and large toe with fanning of the other toes.

6. Assess vital signs and correlate with other data; changes often occur slowly, and the overall trend needs to be evaluated.

a. Blood pressure and pulse - intracranial problems precipitate changes: blood pressure may increase and pulse rate may decrease.

b. Respirations - rate, depth, and rhythm are sensitive indicators of intracranial problems.

c. Temperature - evaluate changes in temperature as related to a neurological control versus infection.

NCLEX ALERT: *Assess changes in a client's neuro status. Implement interventions to prevent potential neurological complications.*

Table 15-2: GLASCOW COMA SCALE

Eye opening	
Spontaneous	4
To sound	3
To pain	2
Never	1
Motor response	
Obeys commands	6
Localizes pain	5
Normal flexion (withdrawal)	4
Abnormal flexion posturing	3
Extension posturing	2
None	1
Verbal response	
Oriented	5
Confused conversation	4
Inappropriate words	3
Incomprehensible sounds	2
None	1

A score of 7 or less indicates coma.

The highest possible score is 15.

C. Bedside neuro checks — parameters for frequent nursing evaluation of neurological symptoms.

1. Assess level of consciousness (LOC).

a. Verbal and motor response to command.

b. Appropriate conversation and speech.

c. Appropriate behavior in infants and young children.

d. Be explicit in describing LOC; may utilize a specific coma scale (Table 15-2).

2. Respiratory patterns - evaluate current respiratory pattern and assess for changes in pattern.

3. Pupillary response.

a. Equality of pupils.

b. Presence of direct and accommodation reflexes.

c. Position of pupils at rest.

4. Motor function.

a. Ability to move all extremities with equal strength.

b. Presence of posturing.

c. Babinski reflex.

d. Presence of seizure activity.

e. Presence of gag and cough reflexes.

5. Vital signs.

a. Correlate blood pressure and pulse changes.

b. Assess respiratory pattern.

c. Assess temperature in regard to overall condition.

6. Assess for presence of pain, headache.

7. Presence of projectile vomiting not associated with nausea.

8. Infants - assess fontanel and suture lines.

a. Size of fontanel for growth and development level.

b. Fontanel should be soft to touch, with slight pulsations.

c. Normal approximation of cranial suture lines.

DISORDERS OF THE NEUROLOGICAL SYSTEM

Concept of Increased Intracranial Pressure (IICP)

❑ **An increase in intracranial pressure occurs any time there is an increase in the size of the intracranial contents.**

A. The cranial vault is rigid, and there is minimal area for expansion of the intracranial components - brain tissue, blood, cerebrospinal fluid.

B. An increase in any one of the components necessitates a reciprocal change in other cranial contents; this frequently results in ischemia of brain tissue. An increase in ICP results from one of the following:
  1. Structural lesions that put pressure on the brain (brain tumors, cerebral hemorrhage, trauma, congenital defects.)
  2. Metabolic disorders that impair brain functions (hypoxia, increased blood ammonia levels, cerebral edema).

C. Regardless of the cause, increased intracranial pressure will result in a reduction of cerebral blood flow, and tissue ischemia. Specific deficiencies are determined by the area of compression and ischemia of brain tissue.

D. In infants where the cranial suture lines are open, increased ICP will cause further separation of the suture lines and increased the circumference of the head.

Data Collection

1. Risk factors/etiology.
   a. Cerebral edema secondary to the initial damage.
   b. Brain tumors.
   c. Intracranial hemorrhage due to closed head injuries and or ruptured vessels.
   d. Cerebral embolism
   e. Cerebral thrombosis
   f. Hydrocephalus.
   g. Reye's syndrome.
      (1) Hepatic dysfunction resulting in increased levels of ammonia.
      (2) Characterized by neurological changes secondary to the high ammonia levels.
      (3) Problem associated with aspirin intake in children with viral infections.
2. Clinical manifestations.

NCLEX ALERT: *Plan and implement interventions to prevent client complications of neurologic system. Provide care for a client experiencing increased intracranial pressure.*

   a. Assess for changes in level of consciousness.

NURSING PRIORITY: *The first sign of a change in the level of intracranial pressure is alteration in level of consciousness.*

      (1) Increased irritability, restlessness, or lethargy in the infant and young child.
      (2) As the client loses consciousness, hearing is the last sense to be lost.
   b. Changes in vital signs.
      (1) Decreased pulse rate with increasing systolic blood pressure.
      (2) Widening of the pulse pressure.
      (3) Alteration in respiratory pattern (Cheyne-Stokes, hyperventilation).
      (4) Temperature usually increases.
   c. Pupillary changes.
      (1) Pupillary response to light may be from slow, sluggish reaction to fixed, dilated with no response.
      (2) Unilateral dilatation of pupil.
   d. Decrease in motor and sensory function.
      (1) Weakness.
      (2) Hemiplegia.
      (3) Failure to withdraw from painful stimuli.
      (4) Posturing.
   e. Headache.
      (1) Constant with increasing intensity.
      (2) Aggravated by movement.
   f. Vomiting - projectile vomiting with no preceding nausea.
3. Infant may have persistent, irritable crying.
   a. Infants.
      (1) Tense, bulging fontanel.
      (2) Separated cranial sutures.
      (3) Increasing frontal- occipital circumference.
      (4) High-pitched cry.
      (5) Increased restlessness
4. Diagnostics (Appendix 15-1).
   a. CT scan.
   b. MRI
   c. Cerebral angiogram.
   d. Electroencephalogram (EEG).

Treatment

1. Treatment of the underlying cause of increasing pressure.
2. Fluid balance.
3. Medications.
   a. Osmotic diuretics.
   b. Corticosteroids.
   c. Anticonvulsants.
4. Maintain good ventilation -prevent respiratory acidosis which dilates cerebral vessels.

Complications

1. Herniation - the shifting of the intracranial contents from one compartment to another.
   a. Brain compression occurs.
   b. Obstruction of the cerebrospinal fluid.
   c. Irreversible brain damage and death.

Nursing Intervention

✦ *Goal: to identify and decrease problem of IICP.*

1. Neuro checks as indicated by client status.
2. Maintain semi-Fowler's position to promote venous drainage and respiratory function.
3. Change client's position slowly and gently; avoid jerky movements.
4. Monitor fluid intake carefully.
5. Evaluate intake and output.
   a. In response to diuretics.
   b. As correlated with changes in daily weight.
6. Maintain intake evenly over twenty-four hour time period.
7. Avoid use of sedatives or narcotics.
   a. Depress respiration.
   b. May mask symptoms indicating increasing ICP.
8. Client should avoid strenuous coughing, the valsalva maneuver, and isometric muscle exercises.
9. In infants, measure frontal-occipital circumference to evaluate increase in size of the head.
10. Control hyperthermia as indicated.

✦ *Goal: to maintain respiratory function.*

NURSING PRIORITY: *Airway is one of the most common problems in the unconscious client; position him to maintain patent airway, or use airway adjuncts.*

1. Prevent respiratory problems of immobility.
2. Evaluate patency of airway frequently; as level of consciousness decreases, client is at an increased risk for respiratory obstruction by the tongue and accumulating secretions.
3. Suction as necessary, but in short duration with rest periods.
4. Do not suction the nasopharyngeal area of a client with a head injury or basilar skull fracture.

✦ *Goal: to protect from injury.*

1. Maintain seizure precautions (Appendix 15-5).
2. Restrain client only if absolutely necessary to maintain safety; struggling against restraints will increase ICP.

NCLEX ALERT: *Identify and use least restrictive restraint. Document use and monitor client response.*

3. Do not clean the ears or nasal passages of a head injury or neurosurgery client.
   a. Bleeding or drainage occurs from these areas may be cerebrospinal fluid.
   b. Check fluid for a halo sign - separation of CSF products on the dressing.
4. Aspiration is a major problem in the unconscious client.
   a. Carefully assess the swallow reflex in clients who are not fully conscious.
   b. Position the client in semi-Fowler's for tube feeding.

NCLEX ALERT: *Identify potential for aspiration.*

5. Maintain quiet, nonstimulating environment if condition is unstable.
6. Inspect eyes and prevent corneal ulceration.
   a. If protective patches are used to prevent corneal drying, frequent assessment is necessary to prevent patch from coming in contact with cornea and causing an abrasion.
   b. Normal saline irrigation or methylcellulose drops q2h to maintain moisture.

✦ *Goal: to maintain psychological equilibrium.*

1. Neuro checks are a continuous reminder of potential problem.
2. Encourage verbalization of fears regarding condition.
3. Give simple explanation of procedures to client and family.
4. Altered states of consciousness will cause increased anxiety and confusion; maintain reality orientation.
5. If client is unconscious, continue to talk to him/her; describe procedures and treatments; always assume that client can hear.
6. Assist parents and family to work through feelings of guilt and anger.

✦ *Goal: to prevent complications of immobility (Chapter 3).*

✦ *Goal: to maintain elimination.*

1. Urinary incontinence - may use condom catheter or indwelling bladder catheter may be necessary due to retention or to measure hourly urine output.
2. Keep perineal area free from excoriation.
3. Monitor bowel function; evaluate for fecal impaction.

Brain Tumors

❑ **Brain tumors may be benign, malignant, or metastatic. Regardless of the origin, site, or presence of malignancy, problems of increased intracranial pressure occur because of the limited area in the brain to accommodate an increase in the intracranial contents.**

Data Collection

1. Clinical manifestations (due to the local destructive effect of the tumor or to an increase in ICP).
   a. Behavioral and mental status changes.
   b. Seizures.
   c. Dizziness and vertigo.
   d. Localized symptoms.
      (1) Focal weakness.
      (2) Sensory disturbances.
      (3) Language disturbances.
      (4) Coordination disturbances.
      (5) Visual disturbances (diplopia).
2. Diagnostics (Appendix 15-1).
   a. Clinical manifestations exhibited in the neurological exam.
   b. EEG.
   c. CAT scan.
   d. Brain scan.

Treatment

1. Medical.
   a. Dexamethasone (Appendix 5-7).
   b. Anticonvulsants (Appendix 15-2).
   c. Radiation and chemotherapy if malignant.
2. Surgical excision - craniotomy.

Complications

Meningitis, respiratory aspiration, brain stem herniation, diabetes insipidus.

Nursing Intervention

Preoperative management - see nursing goals for increased intracranial pressure.

✦ *Goal: to provide appropriate preoperative nursing intervention.*

1. General preoperative care (Chapter 3) with exceptions as noted.
2. If there is increased ICP, generally do not administer an enema.
3. Prepare client, family, and parents for appearance of the client postoperatively.
4. Encourage verbalization regarding concerns of surgery.

✦ *Goal: to maintain homeostasis and monitor changes in increased intracranial pressure postoperative craniotomy.*

1. Neuro checks as necessary.
2. Maintain pulmonary function and hygiene.
   a. Patent airway.
   b. Prevent aspiration.
   c. Increase respiratory excursion by deep breathing.
   d. Antiemetics to decrease vomiting and possibility of aspiration.
   e. Discourage vigorous coughing.
3. Careful evaluation of the level of consciousness; regression to more lethargic or irritable state may be indicative of increasing ICP.
4. Evaluate dressing.
   a. Location and amount of drainage.
   b. Evaluate for CSF leak through the incision, nose and ears.
   c. Do not change dressing initially, but reinforce it.
5. Position in semi-Fowler's if there is a spinal fluid leak from ears or nose.
6. Maintain fluid regulation.
   a. Begin clear liquids PO after swallow and gag reflexes return and client is awake.
   b. Maintain IV fluid until client tolerates fluids.
   c. Closely monitor intake and output.
7. Evaluate neuro status in response to fluid balance and diuretics.
8. Provide appropriate pain relief.
   a. Narcotic analgesics are used with caution; may mask signs of increased intracranial pressure.
   b. Maintain quiet, dim atmosphere.
   c. Avoid sudden movements.
9. Prevent complications of immobility (Chapter 3).
10. Maintain seizure precautions (Appendix 15-5).

Head Injury

❑ **Trauma to the cranium and its contents.**

A. Children and infants are more capable of absorbing direct impact, due to pliability of the skull.

B. Injury to the brain occurs by compression, tearing, and shearing stresses on vessels and nerves.

C. Although brain volume remains unchanged, cerebral edema occurs in response to the injury and frequently precipitates an increase in intracranial pressure.

D. Types of head injuries.

1. Concussion.
   a. Immediate brief period of unconsciousness, but no structural damage.
   b. Generally followed by amnesia from the moment of injury impact and short period afterward.
2. Intracranial hemorrhage.
   a. Epidural (extradural) hematoma - a large vessel (generally an artery) in the dura mater is damaged; a hematoma rapidly forms between the dura and the skull, precipitating an increase in intracranial pressure.
   b. Subdural hematoma - bleeding between the dura and arachnoid area, usually due to the rupture of veins in the subdural space; leads to increase in ICP. A chronic subdural bleed may not be identified for weeks to months after the incident.

***Geriatric Priority:** a seemingly minor impact may cause the development of a chronic subdural hematoma in the elderly client.*

Data Collection

1. Clinical manifestations - symptoms of increasing intracranial pressure, history of head impact or fall..
2. Diagnostics.
   a. Neurologic history.
   b. Skull X-ray.
   c. MRI.
   d. CT scan.

Complications

Increased intracranial pressure, meningitis, permanent brain damage.

Treatment

***NURSING PRIORITY:** The initial treatment of the head injury client is to maintain adequate respiratory function, to prevent hypoxia and respiratory acidosis.*

1. Majority of clients who experience concussion are treated at home.
2. A period of unconsciousness or presence of seizures increases concern regarding neurological damage.
3. Surgical intervention - surgical evacuation of the hematoma.

Nursing Intervention

See Nursing Diagnosis for Increased Intracranial Pressure.

Self-Care

1. Problems frequently do not occur until twenty-four hours or more after the initial injury.
2. Teach family/caretaker to observe the client for increased periods of sleep; if client is asleep, awaken every two to three hours to see if he can be aroused normally.
3. Client/family should maintain contact with health care professionals for re-evaluation if complications occur.
4. Family/caretaker should immediately return the client to the health care facility for:
   a. Any changes in LOC (increased drowsiness, confusion).
   b. Unable to arouse client.
   c. Seizures occur.
   d. Bleeding or watery drainage from the ears or nose.
   e. Loss of feeling or sensation in any extremity.
   f. Blurred vision.
   g. Slurring speech.
   h. Vomiting.

***NURSING PRIORITY:** Instructions should be given to the client and the family in writing. Frequently, clients and family do not remember verbal directions, especially from the ER.*

✦ *Goal: to maintain homeostasis; monitor and identify early symptoms of increased intracranial pressure in the hospitalized client.*

1. Generally on bed rest and clear liquids initially.
2. Frequent neuro checks for increased ICP.
   a. Decreased level of consciousness frequently the first indication.

TABLE 15-3: Risk Factors Associated With Cerebral Vascular Accident

Reversible:
* Smoking
* Obesity
* Increased salt intake
* Sedentary life style
* Increased stress
* Oral contraceptives

Partially Reversible:
* Hypertension
* Cardiac valve disease
* Dysrhythmias
* Diabetes mellitus
* Hypercholesterolemia

Non reversible:
* Age - increased incidence after be 75
* Increased incidence in black population
* Family history

b. Seizures are common in children.

c. Instruct head injury client not to cough, sneeze or blow his/her nose.

3. Evaluate drainage from nose, ears and mouth.

a. *Notify the RN immediately of any drainage from the ears or nose.*

b. Check continuous clear drainage from the nose with a Dextrosstix; if glucose is present, it is indicative of CSF.

c. Do not suction a client with a cerebrospinal fluid leak.

4. Seizure precautions (Appendix 15-5).

5. Maintain adequate fluid intake via IV or PO.

✦ *Goal: to provide appropriate nursing intervention for the client experiencing an increase in intracranial pressure (see nursing goals for IICP).*

Hydrocephalus

❑ **A condition caused by an imbalance in the production and absorption of CSF in the ventricles of the brain.**

Data Collection

1. Risk factors/etiology.

a. Neonate — congenital malformations.

b. Older child, adult — space-occupying lesion.

2. Clinical manifestations - infant.

a. Head enlargement, increasing circumference.

b. Separation of cranial suture lines.

c. Fontanel becomes tense and bulging.

d. Opisthotonos positioning.

e. Increasing irritability and lethargy.

3. Clinical manifestations - older child, adult.

a. Symptoms of increasing ICP.

b. Specific manifestations related to site of the lesion.

4. Diagnostics.

a. MRI, CT scan

b. Increasing head circumference is diagnostic in infants.

Treatment

1. Obstructive - removal of the obstruction (cyst, hematoma, tumor).

Nursing Intervention

✦ *Goal: to monitor for the development of increasing ICP.*

1. Daily measurement of the frontal-occipital circumference of the head in infants.
2. Assess for symptoms of increasing ICP.
3. Infant is often difficult to feed; administer small feedings at frequent intervals.
4. Evaluate for increasing restlessness and lethargy; this is frequently the first symptom of increasing ICP in the infant.

✦ *Goal: to maintain patency of the shunt and monitor intracranial pressure post shunt procedure.*

1. Position on the unoperative side to prevent pressure on the shunt valve.
2. Keep head of the bed flat to decrease risk of rapid reduction of intracranial fluid.
3. Monitor for increasing ICP and compare data with previous data.
4. Monitor for infection (a common problem from shortly after surgery to 1-2 months later).

Self-Care

1. Teach parents symptoms of increasing ICP.
2. Have parents participate in care of the shunt prior to client's discharge.
3. Encourage parents and family to ventilate feelings regarding client's condition.
4. Refer client to appropriate community agencies.

Cerebral Vascular Accident (CVA)

❑ **Also known as a stroke or brain attack, CVA is the disruption of the blood supply to an area of the brain resulting in tissue necrosis and sudden loss of brain function.**

A. Ischemia.

1. Thrombosis — often occurs from atherosclerosis and endothelial damage to the vascular wall.

a. Common internal carotid problem.

Figure 15-3: Transfer to wheelchair
Client education guide for transfer from bed to wheelchair by a hemiplegic. (Shading on right side of client indicates the affected side.) Lock the wheelchair for safety and keep it placed beside the bed on your nonaffected side. Use your nonaffected arm and leg (A and B) to move your affected arm and leg. As your legs drop over the edge of the bed, swing your torso up to a sitting position (C). Push yourself up to a standing position (D) by using your nonaffected arm and leg. Reach across the wheelchair (E) to grasp the far arm of the chair, and turn to seat yourself.
(Reprinted with permission: Black, J. and Matassarin-Jacobs, E (1999). *Luckmann and Sorensen's Medical-Surgical Nursing: A Psychophysiologic Approach*, 5th Ed., Philadelphia: W.B. Saunders, p.719).

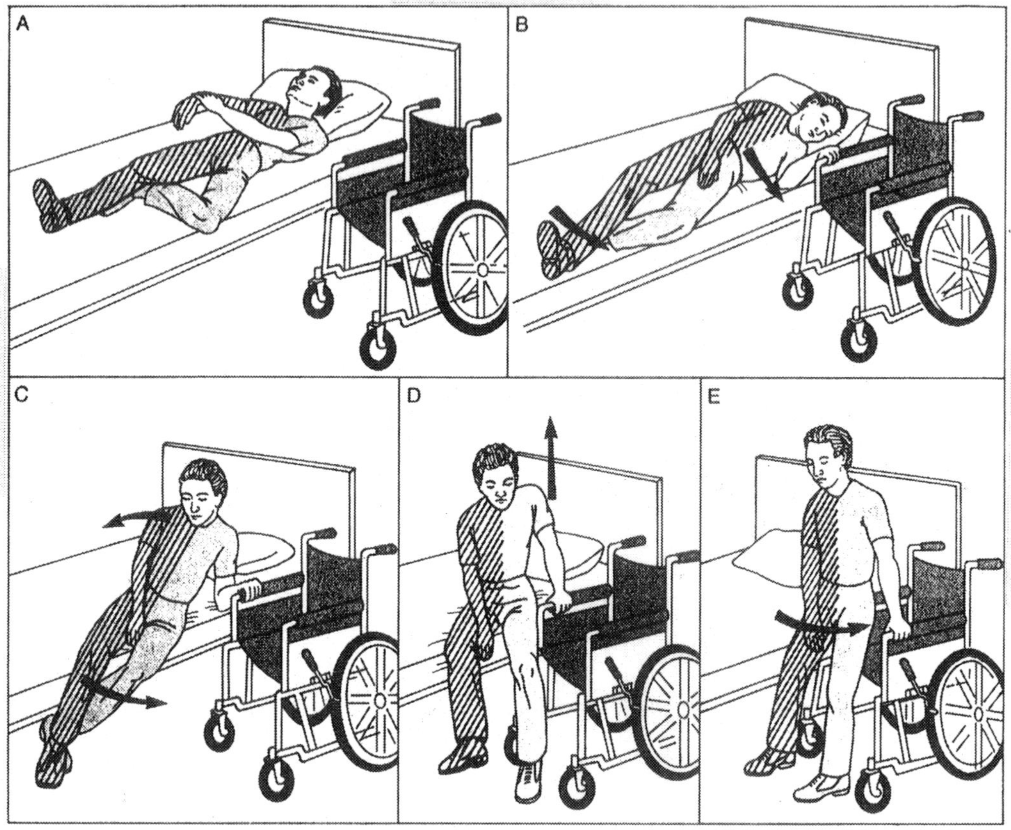

b. Most common stroke caused by diabetes.

2. Embolism — occurs as the result of an emboli, most common cause is plaque.
   a. Occurs in cardiac valve replacements.
   b. Atrial fibrillation.
   c. Endocarditis.

B. Hemorrhage
1. Intracerebral hemorrhage — occurs from rupture of a cerebral vessel which causes bleeding into the brain tissue.
2. Aneurysm rupture.

C. The area of edema resulting from tissue damage may precipitate more damage than the vascular damage itself.

D. Transient ischemic attack (TIA).
1. Brief episode of neurological dysfunction.
2. Should be considered a warning symptom of an impending CVA.
3. Neurologic dysfunction is present for minutes to hours, but no permanent neurological deficit remains.

E. Neuromuscular deficits.
1. Damage to one side of the brain will result in paralysis of opposite side of the body.
2. Damage to the left side of the brain will result in paralysis of the right side of the body (hemiplegia - paralysis of one side of the body).
3. Both upper and lower extremities of the involved side are involved.

> ***Geriatric Priority:*** *The problem of CVA is frequently complicated by presence of other chronic diseases.*

Data Collection

1. Risk factors/etiology (See Table 15-3).
2. Clinical manifestations.
   a. TIA.

(1) Temporary loss of vision in one eye.
(2) Transient hemiparesis.
(3) Tinnitus.
(4) Vertigo.
(5) Confusion.
(6) Aphasia

b. Completed CVA (occurs suddenly with an embolism, more gradually in hemorrhage or thrombosis).

(1) Loss of voluntary movement on affected side.
(2) Problem of neuromuscular control of respiration.
(3) Swallowing and cough reflex may be affected.
(4) Initially may be incontinent.
(5) Communication problems - aphasia (Appendix 15-6).
(6) Change in mental status, emotional lability.
(7) Impairment of judgment and memory.
(8) Hypotonia (flaccidity) for days to weeks, followed by hypertonia (spasticity).
(9) Visual disturbances.

3. Diagnostics (Appendix 15-1).

a. Clinical manifestations.

Treatment

1. Preventive — control diabetes, hypertension and cholesterol levels.(Table 15-3)
2. Medical.

a. Medications to decrease cerebral edema.

(1) Osmotic diuretics.
(2) Corticosteroids (dexamethasone).

b. Antihypertensive therapy.

c. Thrombolytic therapy - needs to be administered within about 3 hours after stroke occurs (Appendix 12-2).

3. Surgical - carotid endarterectomy. Done most often in clients who have experienced a TIA.

Nursing Intervention

✦ *Goal: to maintain patent airway and adequate cerebral oxygenation.*

1. *Report to RN immediately any changes in respiratory status.*
2. Position side-lying with head elevated and neck straight.
3. Assess for symptoms of hypoxia, provide oxygen (Chapter 10).
4. Maintain patent airway; use oropharyngeal airway to prevent airway obstruction by the tongue.
5. Client is prone to obstructed airway and pulmonary infection; have him/her cough and deep breathe as indicated.
6. Control of high blood pressure.

✦ *Goal: to assess for and implement measures to decrease intracranial pressure (see nursing goals for IICP).*

✦ *Goal: to maintain adequate nutritional intake.*

NCLEX ALERT: *Monitor client ability to eat. Monitor client nutritional status. Provide nutritional supplements. Identify potential and prevent aspiration.*

1. Administer PO feedings with caution; check presence of gag reflex and swallowing reflex before feeding.
2. Place food on the unaffected side of the mouth.
3. Select foods that are easy to control in the mouth and swallow (gelatin); use "thicket" to thicken liquids so client is better able to control them.
4. Maintain high Fowler's position for feeding.
5. Maintain privacy and unrushed atmosphere.
6. If client is unable to tolerate PO intake, tube feedings may be initiated (Appendix 13-10).

NCLEX ALERT: *Identify client complications of immobility. Monitor client responses to immobility*

✦ *Goal: to preserve function of the musculoskeletal system to prevent joint contraction and muscle atrophy.*

1. Passive ROM on affected side.
2. Active ROM on unaffected side.
3. Passive ROM and sitting client up with his feet on the floor, to prevent foot drop.
4. Legs should be maintained in a neutral position; prevent external rotation of affected hip by placing a trochanter roll or sandbag at the thigh.
5. Position every two hours but limit the period of time spent on the affected side.
6. Assess for adduction and internal rotation of the affected arm; maintain arm in a neutral (slightly flexed) position with each joint slightly higher than the preceding one.
7. Client may be placed in prone position for 30-45 minutes several times a day to prevent knee and hip flexion contractures and to prevent decubitus ulcer formation.

8. Assist client to move from bed to chair, promote independence in learning how to transfer alone.(Figure 15-4)

✦ *Goal: to maintain homeostasis through continued nursing assessment and appropriate nursing intervention.*

NCLEX ALERT: *Be familiar with basic nursing care required to maintain homeostasis in the CVA client - nutrition, immobility, oxygenation, psychosocial needs.*

1. Evaluate adequacy of cardiac output.
2. Monitor hydration status - prevent fluid overload.
   a. Carefully evaluate intake, encourage fluids unless contraindicated.
   b. Evaluate response to diuretics.
   c. Assess for the development of peripheral edema.
   d. Assess respiratory parameters indicative of fluid overload (rales, dyspnea, etc.).
3. Maintain and promote normal elimination.
   a. Avoid urinary catheter if possible; if catheter is necessary, remove as soon as possible.
   b. Offer bedpan or urinal every two hours; help establish a schedule.
   c. Prevent constipation - increase bulk in the diet, stool softeners, adequate fluid intake, etc.
4. Prevent problems of skin breakdown through change of position q2h and proper positioning with good skin hygiene.
5. Maintain psychological homeostasis.
   a. Client is very anxious due to the lack of understanding of what has happened to him/her and the inability to communicate.
   b. Speak slowly, clearly, and explain what has happened.

✦ *Goal: to assist client to become independent in activities of daily living as rehabilitation phase progresses.*

1. Encourage independence and participation in activities of daily living.
2. Provide clothing easy to get in and out of.
3. Active participation in ROM; do his/her own ROM on affected side using unaffected extremities.
4. When in the sitting position, assist client to maintain sense of balance; client will frequently fall to the affected side.
5. Continue with bowel and urinary schedule.
6. Encourage social interaction.
   a. Allow client plenty of time to respond.
   b. Speak slowly and clearly; do not give too many directions at one time.
   c. Do not "talk down to" or treat as a child.
   d. Mental status may be normal; do not assume it is impaired.

Intracranial Aneurysm

❑ **An intracranial or cerebral aneurysm is the dilation of the wall of a cerebral artery (berry aneurysm). Aneurysms most often arises from an arterial junction.**

A. Rupture of the aneurysm produces sudden severe headache, and often loss of consciousness.

B. Symptoms occur when aneurysm enlarges and exerts pressure on the brain tissue, or when it ruptures.

Data Collection

1. Clinical manifestations.
   a. Rupture may be preceded by:
      (1) Severe headache.
      (2) Intermittent nausea.
   b. Rupture frequently occurs without warning.
      (1) Severe headache.
      (2) Seizures.
      (3) Stiff neck.
      (4) Hemiparesis.
      (5) Loss of consciousness.
      (6) Overall symptoms of increasing intracranial pressure.
   c. Severity of symptoms depends on the site and amount of bleeding.
2. Diagnostics.
   a. Lumbar puncture, reveals blood in the spinal fluid.
   b. Cerebral angiogram.
   c. CT scan.

Treatment

1. Osmotic diuretics.
2. Antihypertensive medications.
3. Corticosteroid medications.
4. Surgical intervention - ligation or "clipping" of the aneurysm, strengthening of arterial wall.

Nursing Intervention

✦ *Goal: to prevent further increase in intracranial pressure and possible rupture.*

1. Immediate, strict bed rest.

2. Prevent the Valsalva maneuver.
3. Client should avoid straining, sneezing, pulling up in bed, acute flexion of the neck and cigarette smoking.
4. Elevate head of the bed 30° to 40°.
5. Quiet, dim, nonstimulating environment.
6. Constant monitoring of condition to identify occurrence of bleeding as evidenced by symptoms of increasing intracranial pressure.

NURSING PRIORITY: *If the client survives the rupture of the aneurysm, it is most likely to re-bleed within the next 24 to 48 hours.*

✦ *Goal: to assess for and implement nursing measures to decrease intracranial pressure (see nursing goals for increased intracranial pressure).*

✦ *Goal: to provide appropriate preoperative nursing intervention (see nursing goals for brain tumor).*

✦ *Goal: to maintain homeostasis and monitor changes in intracranial pressure postoperative craniotomy (see nursing goals for craniotomy).*

Meningitis/Encephalitis

❑ **Meningitis is an inflammatory condition of the meningeal tissue covering the brain. Inflammatory process results in the development of cerebral edema.**

❑ **Encephalitis is an inflammatory process of the CNS. Cerebral edema may develop. Condition is usually less severe than meningitis.**

NURSING PRIORITY: *When admitting a client with CNS irritation, clarify with physician what type of isolation, if any, may be required.*

Data Collection

1. Risk factors/etiology.
   a. Meningitis.
      (1) Bacteria may gain entry from an infection elsewhere in the body.
      (2) Meningococcal meningitis is contagious via droplet infection from the nasopharyngeal secretions, the only form readily contagious.
      (3) Occurs primarily in young children.
   b. Encephalitis.
      (1) Transmitted by vectors (mosquitoes and ticks).
      (2) May occur as a complication following a viral infection, especially herpes simplex.
2. Clinical manifestations - older child, adult.
   a. Stiff neck.
   b. Fever.
   c. Headache, photophobia.
   d. Increasing irritability, changes in LOC.
   e. Difficulty chewing and swallowing.
   f. Anorexia.
   g. Generalized seizures.
   h. Altered mental status.
   i. Opisthotonos positioning - a stiffening of the back with the legs extended.
3. Clinical manifestations - neonate and infant.
   a. Fever.
   b. Apneic episodes.
   c. Bulging fontanel (neonate).
   d. Seizures.
   e. High-pitched cry.
   f. Changes in sleep pattern, increasing irritability.
   g. Poor sucking, may refuse feedings.
   h. Poor muscle tone, diminished movement.
4. Diagnostics.
   a. Blood culture identification of causative organism.

NCLEX ALERT: *Identify signs and symptoms of infection. Identify changes in neurological status.*

Treatment

1. Isolation until positive organism is identified.
2. IV antibiotics (Appendix 5-10).
3. Optimum hydration.
4. Anticonvulsant medications (Appendix 15-2).
5. Maintain ventilation.

Complications

1. Increasing ICP, resulting in permanent brain damage.
2. Meningococcal sepsis
3. Respiratory complications.
4. Damage to hearing and vision.

Nursing Intervention

✦ *Goal: to identify the organism, control spread, and initiate therapy.*

1. Maintain isolation as indicated.
2. Begin IV antibiotics after lumbar puncture and fluid sample are obtained.
3. Monitor IV infusion as indicated.

✦ *Goal: to monitor course of infection and prevent complications.*

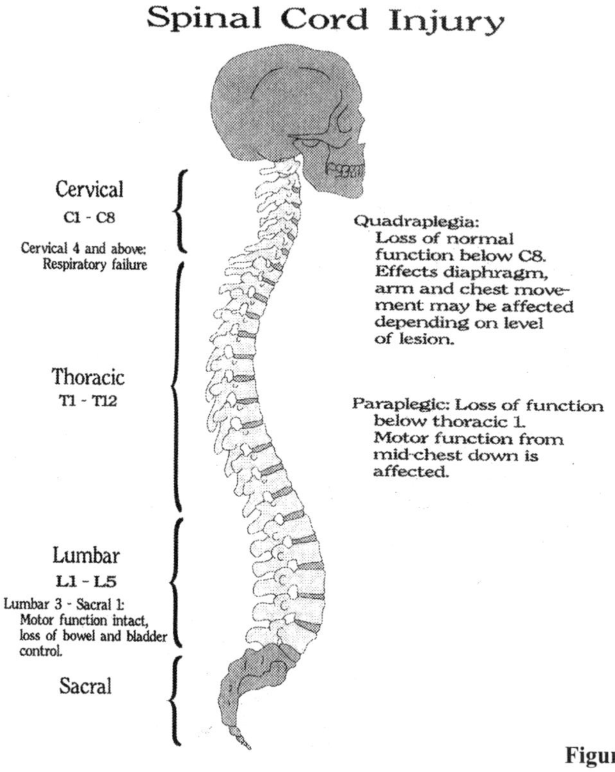

Figure 15-4: Spinal Cord Injury.

1. Frequent nursing assessment for increased ICP.
2. Maintain hydration.
3. Monitor infusion site for complications of IVPB antibiotics.
4. Decrease stimuli in environment - dim lights, quiet environment, no loud noises.
5. Avoid movement or positioning that increases discomfort; client generally assumes a side-lying position.
6. Seizure precautions.
7. Prevent complications of immobility.
8. Good respiratory hygiene.
9. Measures to decrease fever.
10. Assess for increased ICP.

Spinal Cord Injury

❑ **Generally occurs as a result of direct trauma to the vertebrae in the spinal column.**

A. Initially after the injury, the nerve fibers swell and circulation to the spinal cord is decreased; this decrease in blood to the area of injury will cause further deterioration of the area of injury.

***NURSING PRIORITY:** Within twenty-four hours of the injury, edema secondary to the inflammatory process results in compression of the cord; the edema extends above and below the area of injury and increases the area of ischemic damage.*

B. Consequences of cord injury depend on the extent of damage as well as the level of cord injury (Fig. 15-3).
   1. The higher the lesion, the more severe the injury.
   2. Complete transection (complete cord dissolution, complete lesion) - paralysis below the level of injury; minimum, if any, return of function.

C. Spinal cord shock (areflexia) - occurs predominantly in complete cord lesions. The muscles below the level of injury will become flaccid ,with loss of all functional control.
   1. Condition may persist for several weeks and reverse spontaneously.
   2. When spinal cord shock is resolved, the muscles become spastic.

D. Bladder dysfunction will occur as a result of the injury. Normal bladder control is dependent on intact sensory and motor pathways.

E. Long-term rehabilitation potential depends on the amount of damage done to the cord, which may not be evident for several weeks after the injury.

Data Collection

1. Clinical manifestations - depend on level of cord injury.
   a. Frequently associated with other injuries.
   b. Flaccid paralysis and sensory loss below the level of injury.
   c. Spinal shock - a total disruption of spinal cord function below the level of injury.
      (1) Generally occurs within one to two hours and may last for several weeks.
      (2) Flaccid paralysis.
      (3) Loss of sensation and absence of reflexes.
      (4) Loss of bowel and bladder control.
      (5) Hypotension and bradycardia.
      (6) Absence of temperature control and pain below level of injury.
      (7) No perspiration evident below level of injury.
   d. After spinal shock, reflexes and autonomic activity return as evidenced by development of spasticity.
2. Diagnostics.
   a. History of accident.
   b. Clinical manifestations.
   c. CT scan, x-rays to determine level of damage.

Treatment

1. High doses of corticosteroids within the first 8 hours may significantly reduce the inflammation and significantly improve the prognosis.
2. Maintain high levels of arterial PO2 to prevent worsening of the neurological defect.
3. Surgical intervention to decrease cord compression, and to stabilize the area of injury.
4. Traction and immobilization to prevent further injury.
   a. Halo vest.
   b. Cervical traction
   c. Rigid collars.
   d. Special beds to provide cord stabilization - stryker frames, kinetic beds, etc.

Nursing Intervention

✦ *Goal: to maintain stability of the vertebral column and prevent further cord damage.*

1. Emergency care and treatment.
   a. Suspect spinal cord injury if there is any evidence of direct trauma to the head or neck area (contact sports, diving accidents, MVA).
   b. Immobilize and place on spinal board with the head and neck in a neutral position; do not allow the neck to flex or rotate.

> ***NURSING PRIORITY:*** *Do not hyperextend the neck in the client with a suspected cervical injury. Airway should be opened by the jaw lift method. Improper handling of the client at the scene of the accident often results in extension of the damaged area.*

   c. Maintain in extended position with no twisting or turning; do not remove from the spinal board until area of injury is identified.
   d. Maintain patent airway during transportation.
2. Maintain stability of the vertebral column as indicated by the level of injury (hospitalized client).
   a. Bed rest on firm mattress with supportive devices (sandbags, skin traction, etc.); maintain alignment in the supine position; logroll without any flexion or twisting.
   b. Maintain cervical traction - halo vest, or tongs inserted into the skull, with traction and weights applied; do not remove weights.
   c. Maintain extremities in neutral, functional position.
3. Maintain immobilization via halo vest with cranial pins.
   a. Keep wrench taped to the brace for quick removal in case of emergency.
   b. Do not use the rods on the vest to assist the client to move.
   c. Perform pin care to pin sites at least daily.
   d. Client's center of gravity is off and he is at high risk for falling.

✦ *Goal: to maintain ongoing assessment to identify level of damage and changes in neurological status.*

1. Motor and sensory evaluation.
   a. Ability to move all extremities; strength of extremities.
   b. Sensory examination, including touch and pain.
2. Ongoing assessment and status of:
   a. Bladder function.
   b. Gastric function.
   c. Respiratory and cardiovascular systems.

> **NCLEX ALERT:** *Identify progressive changes sin respiratory status. Intervene to improve client respiratory status.*

✦ *Goal: to maintain respiratory function.*

1. Frequent assessment of respiratory function during first forty-eight hours.
   a. Evaluate for changes in breathing pattern.
   b. Evaluate client's complaints of increasing difficulty in breathing.
   c. Evaluate for presence of increasing hypoxia.
2. Maintain adequate respiratory function.
   a. Chest physiotherapy.
   b. Incentive spirometry.
   c. Changing position within limits of injury.
   d. Assess for complications of atelectasis and pneumonia.
   e. Nasopharyngeal or endotracheal suctioning.

✦ *Goal: to maintain cardiovascular stability.*

1. Evaluate cardiovascular responses when turning or suctioning.
2. Anti-embolism stockings, elastic wraps, pneumatic compression devices to the legs to facilitate venous return. A decrease in venous return secondary to the injury puts the client at increased risk for the development of deep vein thrombosis.
3. Evaluate cardiovascular response to changes in client's neurological status.

✦ *Goal: to maintain adequate fluid and nutritional status.*

1. During the first forty-eight hours, evaluate GI function frequently; decrease in function may necessitate utilization of a nasogastric tube to decrease distention.
2. Prevent complications of nausea and vomiting.
3. Evaluate bowel sounds and client's ability to tolerate PO fluids.
4. Increase protein in diet; may need to decrease calcium intake.
5. Evaluate for development of paralytic ileus.
6. Increase roughage in diet to promote bowel function.

✦ *Goal: to prevent complications of immobility (Chapter 3).*

✦ *Goal: to promote bowel and bladder function.*

1. Urine is retained due to the loss of control of the bladder.
   a. Intermittent catheterization or indwelling catheter initially, to prevent bladder distention.
   b. Nursing intervention to prevent urinary tract infection.
   c. If voiding, evaluate for residual.
2. Assess client's awareness of bladder function.
3. Initiate measures to institute bladder control.
   a. Establish a schedule for voiding; have client attempt voiding every two hours.
   b. May be necessary to teach client self-catheterization.
   c. Record output and evaluate for residual urine.
4. Evaluate for development of paralytic ileus.
   a. Incontinence and paralytic ileus frequently occur with spinal shock.
   b. Incontinence and impaction are common later.
5. Initiate measures to promote bowel control
   a. Identify client's bowel habits prior to injury.
   b. Maintain sufficient fluid intake and adequate bulk in the diet.
   c. Establish specific time each day for bowel evacuation.
   d. Assess client's awareness of need to defecate.
   e. Induce defecation by digital stimulation, suppository, or as a last resort, enema.

✦ *Goal: to maintain psychological equilibrium.*

1. Simple explanation of all procedures.
2. Anticipate outburst of anger and hostility as client begins to work through the grieving process and adjustments in body image.
3. Anticipate and accept periods of depression in client.
4. Encourage independence whenever possible; allow client to participate in decisions regarding care and to gain control over environment.
5. Encourage family involvement in identifying appropriate diversional activities.
6. Avoid sympathy and emphasize client's potential.

Myasthenia Gravis

❑ **Myasthenia gravis is a neuromuscular disease characterized by a decrease in chemicals at the junction of the nerve and muscle. This produces a disturbance in the transmission of nerve impulses.**

Data Collection

1. Risk factors/etiology.
   a. More common in women.
   b. Peak incidence between ages 20 and 30.
2. Clinical manifestations.
   a. Primary problem is skeletal muscle fatigue; symptoms are predominantly bilateral.
      (1) Muscular fatigue increases with activity.
      (2) Ptosis (drooping of the eyelids) and diplopia (double vision) are frequently the first symptoms.

(3) Impairment of facial mobility and expression.

(4) Impairment of chewing and swallowing.

(5) Speech impairment (dysarthria).

b. Course is variable.

(1) May be progressive.

(2) May stabilize.

(3) May be characterized by short remissions and exacerbations.

c. Myasthenic crisis - an acute exacerbation of symptoms of the condition characterized by weakness of the muscles controlling swallowing and breathing (dysphagia, dysarthria, dyspnea). Occurs as a result of insufficient acetylcholine (anticholinesterase) or exacerbation of disease state.

(1) Difficulty breathing, swallowing, chewing, or speaking.

(2) Increased secretions (saliva, bronchial).

(3) Restlessness and apprehension.

3. Diagnostics.

a. Clinical manifestations.

b. Electromyography - shows a decreasing response of muscles to stimuli.

c. Tensilon test.

Treatment

1. Anticholinesterase medications (Appendix 15-3).
2. Steroids (Appendix 5-7).

Nursing Intervention

(Client generally hospitalized for acute myasthenic crisis or for respiratory infection).

✦ *Goal: to maintain respiratory function.*

1. Assess for increasing problems of difficult breathing.
2. Determine client's medication schedule; when was medication last taken?
3. Assess ability to swallow; prevent problems of aspiration.

NURSING PRIORITY: *Do not give the client in myasthenic crisis anything to eat or drink as there is significant increased risk for aspirating during this time.*

4. Evaluate effectiveness of cough reflex.
5. Have emergency tracheotomy set available.

Self-Care

1. Importance of taking medication on a regular basis; peak effect of the medication should coincide with mealtimes.
2. If ptosis becomes severe, client may need to wear an eye patch to protect cornea (alternate eye patches if problem is bilateral).
3. Emotional upset, severe fatigue, infections, and exposure to extreme temperatures may precipitate myasthenic crisis.

Multiple Sclerosis

❑ **Multiple sclerosis is a disease which is characterized by multiple areas of damage to the neurons in the brain and spinal cord (CNS).**

A. The progression of the disease results in total destruction of the nerve.

B. The condition is chronic, with unpredictable remissions and exacerbations; with repeated exacerbations, there is a progressive nerve scarring and deterioration of the neurological function.

Data Collection

1. Risk factors/etiology.

a. Autoimmune disorder.

b. Increased incidence in women.

c. Considered a disease of young adults; onset generally between ages 20 and 40.

2. Clinical manifestations (vary from person to person as well as within the same individual, depending on the area of involvement).

a. Two major courses of disease

(1) Exacerbating, remitting - episodes of dysfunction, may recover or have increased problems with each exacerbation.

(2) Chronic progressive - Steady decline in neurological function over several years.

b. Sensory problems.

(1) Diplopia.

(2) Blurred vision.

(3) Vertigo, ataxia.

(4) Decreased hearing.

c. Motor problems.

(1) Weakness.

(2) Spasticity in muscles of involved extremities.

(3) Dysphagia (difficulty swallowing).

d. Bowel and bladder problems.

NCLEX ALERT: *Monitor client elimination pattern. Use alternative methods to promote client voiding.*

(1) Urinary retention.

(2) Spastic bladder.

(3) Constipation.

e. Psychosocial.
(1) Intellectual functioning remains intact.
(2) Emotional lability - increased excitability and inappropriate euphoria.

3. Diagnostics.
a. No definitive diagnostics, MRI, and electrophoresis of spinal fluid are helpful.
b. Diagnostics based on history and clinical manifestations.

Treatment

1. No cure; medical treatment is directed toward delaying of disease process and treatment of the symptoms.
2. Medications to decrease edema and inflammation of the nerve site.
a. Anti-inflammatory (Appendix 5-7).
b. Antispasmodic.
c. Immunosuppressive.
d. Interferon.

Nursing Intervention

(Client hospitalized generally for diagnostic work up or for acute exacerbation and complications).

✦ *Goal: to maintain homeostasis and prevent complications in an acute exacerbation of disease symptoms.*

1. Maintain adequate respiratory function.
a. Prevent respiratory infection.
b. Good pulmonary hygiene.
c. Prevent aspiration; sitting position for eating.
d. Evaluate adequacy of cough reflex.
2. Maintain urinary tract function.
a. Prevent urinary tract infection.
b. Increase fluid intake.
c. Evaluate voiding - assess for retention and incontinence.
d. Provide good perineal care.
3. Maintain nutrition.
a. Evaluate coughing and swallowing reflexes.
b. Provide food that is easy to chew.
c. If client is experiencing difficulty swallowing, observe closely with fluid intake.
4. Assess for activity intolerance
a. Avoid excessive temperature - heat or cold.
b. Strengthening exercises for muscle weakness.

✦ *Goal: to prevent complications of immobility (Chapter 3).*

Guillain-Barré Syndrome (*Polyradiculitis*)

❑ **Condition involves segmental demyelination of nerve roots in the spinal cord and medulla. This causes decreased nerve conduction and rapidly ascending paralysis. Both sensory and motor impairment.**

Data Collection

1. Clinical manifestations.
a. Begins in the lower extremities and ascends bilaterally.
(1) Weakness.
(2) Ataxia.
(3) Bilateral paresthesia progressing to complete paralysis.
2. Diagnostics - based primarily on the clinical manifestations.

Treatment

(Supportive).

1. Corticosteroids (Appendix 5-4).
2. Maintain respiratory function; may require mechanical ventilation.

Nursing Intervention

✦ *Goal: to evaluate progress of paralysis and initiate actions to prevent complications.*

1. Evaluate rate of progress of paralysis; careful assessment of changes in respiratory pattern.
2. Frequent evaluation of cough and swallow reflexes
3. Prevent complications of immobility during period of paralysis (Chapter 3).

✦ *Goal: to prevent complications of hypoxia if respiratory muscles become involved (Chapter 10).*

Muscular Dystrophy

❑ **The term *pseudohypertrophy* describes the characteristic muscle enlargement due to fatty infiltration that occurs with muscular dystrophy.**

A. Muscular dystrophy is the most significant group of childhood diseases of the muscles.
B. Duchenne's is the most common type and is also the most severe.
C. Condition is characterized by gradual degeneration of muscle fibers and progressive symmetrical weakness and wasting of skeletal muscle.

Data Collection

1. Risk factors/etiology.

a. Genetic - sex-linked disorder primarily affecting males.
b. Onset generally between 1 to 5 years.

2. Clinical manifestations.
   a. Difficulty ambulating - child has difficulty keeping up with their friends.
   b. Abnormal waddling gait.
      (1) Falls frequently and develops characteristic manner of rising.
      (2) Gower's sign - from sitting or squatting position, the child assumes a kneeling position and pushes his/her torso up by walking his/her hands up the thighs.
   c. Ultimately destroys essential muscles of respiration; death occurs from respiratory infection or cardiac failure.
3. Diagnostics.
   a. Electromyography (EMG).
   b. Muscle biopsy.
   c. Serum enzymes.

Treatment

No definitive therapy.

Nursing Intervention

(Child is frequently cared for at home; hospitalized only for complications).

✦ *Goal: to maintain function as long as possible.*

1. Maintain child's independence in ADL and maintain social contact with peers as long as possible.
2. Assist parents to identify resources for assistance with physical therapy and exercise program at home.
3. Assist family to identify resources to adapt to physiological barriers within the home and to promote mobility of the child in a wheelchair.
4. Assist family to identify methods of preventing respiratory infection and to assess for increasing respiratory problems.

Cerebral Palsy (CP)

❑ **A non-progressive abnormality resulting in impairment of muscle control. May be classified according to the specific area of brain involvement and to the resulting clinical manifestations.**

Data Collection

1. Risk factors/etiology - associated with cerebral anoxia during pregnancy or perinatal period.
2. Clinical manifestations.
   a. Poor motor development, delayed achievement of developmental milestones.
   b. Spasticity of extremities.
   c. Abnormal posture; tend to walk on their toes.
   d. Strabismus and speech difficulties.
3. Diagnostics.
   a. Neurological examination and contributing history.
   b. Diagnostic tests to rule out other neurological dysfunction.
   c. Frequently difficult to diagnose in early months; condition may not be evident until child attempts to walk.

Treatment

(Generally supportive).

1. Maintain and promote mobility with orthopedic devices and physical therapy.
2. Skeletal muscle relaxants.

Nursing Intervention

(Child is frequently cared for at home and on an outpatient basis unless complications occur).

✦ *Goal: to assist child to become as independent and self-sufficient as possible.*

1. Physical therapy program designed to assist individual child to gain maximum function.
2. Assist child to progress according to developmental level and functional abilities; encourage crawling, sitting, and balancing appropriate to developmental level.
3. Assist child to carry out activities of daily living as age and capacities permit (feeding, dressing, and personal hygiene).
4. Encourage play appropriate for age.

Parkinson's Disease

❑ **A progressive neurological disorder causing destruction and degeneration of nerve cells in the brain. Damage to the nerves causes difficulty in control and regulation of movement.**

> ***Geriatric Priority:*** *Develops most often after age 60; client frequently has other chronic conditions.*

Data Collection

1. Tremor.
   a. Generally affects the arms and hands bilaterally - often the first sign.
   b. Tremors usually decrease with movement.
   c. Described as "pill-rolling" tremor.
   d. Aggravated by emotional stress and increased concentration.

2. Muscle rigidity.
   a. Increased resistance to passive movement.
   b. Movement may be described as "cog wheel rigidity" due to jerky movement of extremities.
   c. Precipitates slowness of movement -bradykinesia.
3. Significant decrease or loss of muscle tone and movement.
   a. Decreased blinking of the eyelids.
   b. Loss of ability to swallow saliva.
   c. Loss of tone of facial muscles, expression is blank or "masklike."
   d. Loss of normal arm swing while walking.
   e. Difficulty initiating movement.
4. Stooped posture.
5. Shuffling propulsive gait.
6. Onset usually gradual.

Treatment

1. Medication to enhance CNS function (Appendix 15-4).

Nursing Intervention

✦ *Goal: to maintain homeostasis.*

1. Encourage independence in ADL, utilizing self-help devices.
2. Maintain nutrition.
   a. Increase calories, protein, and easily chewed foods.
   b. Frequent small meals.
   c. Allow ample time for eating.
   d. Monitor weight loss.
   e. Provide pleasant atmosphere at mealtime; client frequently prefers to eat alone due to difficulty swallowing and inability to control saliva.
   f. Increase fluid intake with increased bulk in the diet to decrease problem with constipation.
3. Maintain muscle function.
   a. Full range of motion to extremities to prevent contracture.
   b. Decrease effects of tremors.
   c. Encourage activity - stationary bicycle, swimming, walking.
   d. Physical therapy as indicated.

✦ *Goal: to promote a positive self-image.*

1. Encourage diversional activities.
2. Assist client to set realistic goals.
3. Assist client in gaining control of environment.
4. Assist client to identify and avoid activities that increase frustration levels.
5. Encourage good personal hygiene.

Trigeminal Neuralgia (Tic Douloureux)

❑ **A disorder of the nerve that controls sensory and motor function of the face (trigeminal nerve , or cranial nerve V).**

> ***Geriatric Priority:*** *Commonly occurs between 50-70 years; majority of clients are female.*

Data Collection

1. Abrupt onset of paroxysmal pain in the lower and upper jaw, cheek, and lips.
   a. Tearing of the eyes and frequent blinking.
   b. Facial twitching and grimacing.
   c. Pain usually brief; ends as abruptly as it begins.
2. Recurrence of pain is unpredictable.
3. Pain is initiated by stimulation of the affected nerve area.
   a. Chewing.
   b. Washing the face.
   c. Extremes of temperature - either on the face or in food.
   d. Brushing teeth.

Treatment

1. Medical management of pain.
2. Surgical intervention.
   a. Local nerve block.
   b. Surgical intervention to interrupt nerve impulse transmission.

Nursing Intervention

✦ *Goal: to control pain.*

1. Assess the nature of a painful attack.
2. Identify triggering factors; adjust environment to decrease factors.
   a. Keep room at an even, comfortable temperature.
   b. Avoid touching client.
   c. Avoid jarring the bed.
   d. Allow client to carry out own ADL as necessary.

✦ *Goal: to maintain nutrition.*

1. Frequently, client does not eat due to reluctance to stimulate the pain.
2. Provide lukewarm food which is easily chewed.
3. Increase protein and calories.

Bell's Palsy (Peripheral Facial Paralysis)

❑ **A nerve disorder affecting the facial nerve characterized by a disruption of the motor branches on one side of the face. The disruption of the motor branches results in muscle flaccidity of the affected side of the face.**

Data Collection

1. Clinical manifestations.
   a. Lag or inability to close eyelid on affected side.
   b. Drooping of the mouth.
   c. Decreased taste sensation.
   d. May experience pain behind the ear of the affected side.
2. Diagnostics - no specific diagnostic test.

Treatment

1. Corticosteroids.
2. Vasodilators.

Nursing Intervention

✦ *Goal: to assess nerve function and prevent complications.*

1. Analgesics to decrease pain.
2. Evaluate ability of client to eat.
3. Meticulous oral hygiene.
4. Prevent drying of the cornea on the affected side.
   a. Instill moisture drops in the eyes frequently during the day.
   b. Ophthalmic ointment and eye patches may be required at night.

Study Questions—Neurological

1. An elderly client has been placed on levodopa (L-Dopa). What nursing observations would indicate the medication is working?

① decrease in tremors in upper extremities.
② blood pressure goes from 180/90 to 140/80.
③ urine output increases to 60cc per hour.
④ increased strength on affected side.

2. The nurse is planning to assist a client with right sided paralysis out of bed into the wheel chair. What is an important safety principle for this transfer?

① position the client close to the edge of the bed.
② position the wheel chair on the non affected side.
③ assist the client to stand and pivot to the wheelchair.
④ assist the client to sit, with two people move him to the chair.

3. Hypoxia, premature birth, or trauma at birth is said to be related to what neurological disease?

① cerebral palsy.
② poliomyelitis.
③ Parkinson's disease.
④ bell's palsy.

4. What complication is associated with clients who have had a craniotomy?

① transient ischemic attack.
② seizures.
③ complete heart block.
④ acute renal failure.

5. A client with multiple sclerosis experiences difficulties in mobility. Why does this client have a significance decrease in mobility?

① peripheral neuropathy has occurred in the extremities.
② there is an increase in pressure in the spinal column.
③ impaired conduction of the nerve impulses from the spine.
④ damage has occurred in the central nervous system.

6. After a lumbar puncture, the client's post-treatment care plan states to keep him in a flat position for 6 hours. What is the purpose of this position?

① to decrease effects of hypertension.
② to increase the rate of replacement of spinal fluid.
③ increase ventilation and lung expansion.
④ to prevent a headache due to withdrawing the spinal fluid.

7. A client experiencing problems with their hypothalamus would have a loss of control of what function?

① temperature.
② blood pressure.
③ pulse.
④ respiration.

8. A client is placed on his side, with his knees drawn up to his chest. This is the position for what procedure?

① electrocardiogram.
② electroencephalogram.
③ magnetic resonance imaging.
④ lumbar puncture.

9. What nursing assessment data would be indicative of a neurological problem in the postoperative craniotomy client?

① bradycardia.
② hypotension.
③ hypoglycemia.
④ dyspnea.

10. How can the nurse reliably assess the mental status of a client?

① determine sensory function.
② assess level of consciousness.
③ evaluate vital signs.
④ perform reality checks every 2 hours.

11. A client is experiencing increased intracranial pressure. Which response would be a characteristic change in the client's pupils?

① reactive to light and pinpoint.
② dilated and reactive to light.
③ dilated and fixed.
④ fixed and pinpoint.

12. Why are clients who experience a brain accident more prone to the development of constipation?

① IV therapy.
② immobility.
③ hemiparalysis.
④ infection.

13. What is a common complication of clients who experience a brain accident?

① increased bleeding tendencies, jaundice. liver failure.
② decreased cardiac output, with left ventricular failure.
③ BUN increases with a decrease in urinary output.
④ increased pooling of secretions in the lung causing pneumonia.

14. What would be a significant finding in a client admitted with a diagnosis of meningitis?

① elevated temperature.
② increased lethargy.
③ purple appearing skin rash.
④ tachycardia.

15. In order to prevent tongue obstruction and/or aspiration in the airway of a CVA client, what position would the nurse place the client?

① side-lying.
② prone.
③ full-Fowler's.
④ semi-Fowler's.

16. What is the focus of nursing care immediately after a client has experienced a brain accident.

① elimination.
② airway.
③ range of motion.
④ skin breakdown.

17. Mannitol (Osmitrol) is administered to a client who is experiencing problems with increased intracranial pressure. What nursing measures are taken when this medication has been administered?

① measure intake and output.
② suction to maintain airway.
③ assess for bradycardia.
④ active range of motion.

18. An adult client with a history of grand mal seizures is admitted to the hospital because of recurrent seizures. What is a common factor that contributes to this problem?

① increased stress in lifestyle.
② not taking medications as directed.
③ mixture of drug and alcohol abuse.
④ complications of neurological problems.

19. A client is described as being quadriplegic. What is the best description of this condition?

① one side of the body is paralyzed.
② the client is paralyzed with no sensation from his waist down.
③ there is no sensation to pain below the waist.
④ there is minimal, if any movement, from the arms down.

20. Strict bed rest and immobility of spinal cord injuries places the client at a high risk for what complication?

① bradycardia.
② hypoglycemia.
③ pedal edema.
④ skin breakdown.

Appendix 15-1: NEUROLOGIC SYSTEM DIAGNOSTICS

- **SKULL AND SPINE X-RAYS** - Simple X-rays to determine fractures, calcifications, etc.

Nursing Implications: Explain procedure to client.

- **ELECTROENCEPHALOGRAPHY (EEG)** - a recording of the electrical activity of the brain to physiologically assess cerebral activity; useful for diagnosing seizure disorders; used as a screening procedure for coma; also serves as an indicator for brain death. Electrodes are attached to various areas of the skull. Procedure may be done in the client's room or in a diagnostic area.

Nursing Implications:

1. Explain to client that procedure is painless and there is no danger of electrical shock.
2. Consult with RN for any medications that should be withheld prior to test (especially tranquilizers and sedatives).
3. Frequently, coffee, tea, and cola are not allowed for several hours prior to examination.
4. Client's hair should be clean prior to the examination; after the exam, assist client to wash electrode paste out of hair.

- **MAGNETIC RESONANCE IMAGING (MRI)** - Cell nuclei have magnetic properties; the MRI records the signals from the cells in a manner that provides information to evaluate soft tissue structures (tumors, blood vessels). May be used to diagnose problems throughout the body.

Nursing Implications:

1. Procedure will take approximately 1 ½ hours and is painless.
2. All metal objects should be removed from the client (hearing aids, hair clips, jewelry, buckles, etc.).
3. The client will be placed in a long magnetic tunnel for the procedure. Explain to client that he/she will not be left alone while in the "tunnel."
4. Contraindications.
   a. Clients with pacemakers (the magnetic field interferes with the function of the pacemaker, and interferes with the test as well).
   b. Clients with implanted insulin pumps.
   c. Pregnant clients and very obese clients.
   d. Any client who requires life support equipment (the equipment will malfunction in a magnetic field).

- **LUMBAR PUNCTURE** - a needle is inserted into the lumbar area at L4 - L5 level, spinal fluid is withdrawn, and spinal fluid pressure is measured; contraindicated in presence of increased intracranial pressure. Spinal fluid is evaluated for presence of blood, bacteria, protein, and glucose.

Nursing Implications:

Pretest:

1. Have client empty bladder.
2. Explain position to client (lateral recumbent with knees flexed).

Posttest:

1. Keep client flat for 3 to 6 hours after the procedure.
2. Encourage high fluid intake.
3. Observe for spinal fluid leak from puncture site; if leakage occurs it may cause a severe headache.
4. Label CSF specimens as they are withdrawn -#1, #2, #3.
5. *Notify RN of spinal fluid leak.*

NCLEX ALERT: *Determine if client is prepared for procedure. Document client response to procedure.*

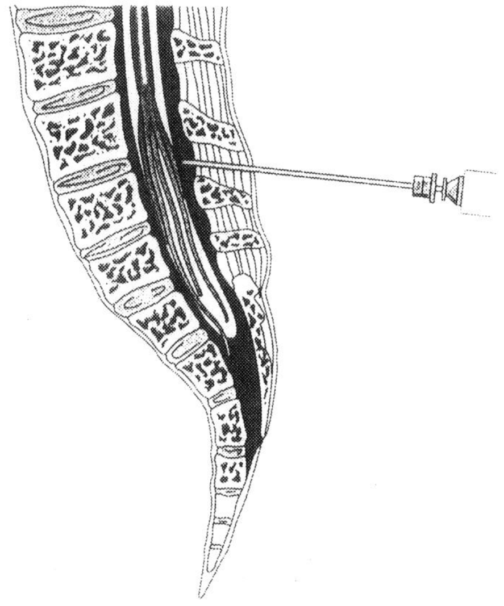

Figure 15-5: Lumbar puncture technique
Reprinted with permission: Phipps, WJ, Sands, JK, & Marek, JF, (1999). *Medical Surgical Nursing: Concepts & Clinical Practice*, 6th ed. Philadelphia: Mosby, p.1688.

Appendix 15-1: NEUROLOGIC SYSTEM DIAGNOSTICS

- **COMPUTERIZED AXIAL TOMOGRAPHY (CAT or CT SCAN)** - computer-assisted X-ray of thin cross sections of the brain to identify hemorrhage, tumor, edema, infarctions, and hydrocephalus. Frequently used to diagnose problems throughout the body. May be used with or without contrast material, depending or organ or area of concern.

Nursing Implications:

1. Explain appearance of scanner to client and explain importance of remaining absolutely still during the procedure.
2. Dye will be injected via venipuncture; advise the client he may experience a flushing or warm sensation when the dye is injected.
3. If a dye is used, it is most often iodine-based. Determine if client is allergic to iodine or shellfish.
4. Closely observe client for reaction to iodine -especially difficulty breathing.
5. Remove any objects from the hair and head.

- **BRAIN SCAN** - A scanner traces the uptake of the radioactive dye in the brain tissue. The dye is concentrated in the damaged tissue.

Nursing Implications:

1. *Consult with RN or physician for any medications that need to be withheld prior to procedure.*
2. Client will be asked to change positions during the test in order to visualize the brain from different angles.
3. The client should not experience any pain.

- **MYELOGRAM** -injection of dye into the subarachnoid space and utilization of X-rays of the spinal cord and vertebral column to identify spinal lesions.

Nursing Implications:

Pretest:

1. Same as for lumbar puncture.
2. Check if client has any allergies to dye.
3. *Check with RN regarding any medications that should not be given.*
4. Increase fluid intake 12 hours prior to procedure.

Post test:

1. *Consult with RN regarding client position.*
2. Check with physician regarding position after myelogram; most often head is elevated 15-30 degrees.
3. Generally on bed rest for 6-8 hours, then normal activity.
4. Need to increase fluid intake

- **CEREBRAL ANGIOGRAM** -injection of contrast material into the cerebral circulation; series of X-rays taken to study the cerebral blood flow; a catheter is inserted into the femoral artery and guided into the area of the carotid vertebral arteries, then dye is injected.

Nursing Implications:

Pretest:

1. Client should be well-hydrated and void prior to procedure.
2. Inform client he/she should remain very still during the procedure.
3. A feeling of warmth in the face and mouth and a metallic taste in the mouth common when dye is injected.
4. Document client's neurological status for comparison after the test.
5. Iodine dye may be used; assess for history of allergy to iodine or seafood.

Posttest:

1. Evaluate client's neurological status; complications involve spasm of cerebral arteries.
2. Observe injection site for hematoma formation and circulation distal to puncture.
3. May be on bed-rest initially after test, possibly as long as 12 hours.

- **ELECTROMYOGRAPHY (EMG)** - measures the electrical currents produced by skeletal muscles. Small needle electrodes are inserted into the muscle and measurements of electrical potentials are recorded.

Nursing Implications:

1. Explain to the client that the procedure will not be painful; he may feel some of the electrical stimulation, but it will be mild.
2. Avoid stimulants, depressants, or sedatives for 24 hours prior to test.
3. The client needs to be cooperative and follow directions during the test.

- **POSITRON EMISSION TOMOGRAPHY (PET)** - allows visualization of physiologic functions in body areas; can differentiate diseased tissue from normal tissue. Radioactive tracers are injected and concentration of the tracers are picked up by the scanner. Single positron emission computed tomography (SPECT) is a type of PET scanning that requires a less precise but more stable and available isotope.

Nursing Implications:

1. Client should eat a meal 3-4 hours prior to test, then nothing after the meal prior to the test.
2. Scanner is very quiet, no noise is made, client may be placed in a reclining chair.
3. Alcohol, tobacco and caffeine should not be taken for 24 hours prior to test.
4. Test may take 1-1½ hours and requires client cooperation.

Appendix 15-2: ANTICONVULSANTS

MEDICATIONS	SIDE EFFECTS	NURSING IMPLICATIONS
ANTICONVULSANTS: Reduce and prevent seizure activity.		
Phenobarbital (**Sodium Luminal**): IM, PO, rectal, IV Primidone (**Mysoline**): PO	Drowsiness, ataxia, excitation in children and in the elderly	1. Client should avoid potential hazardous activities requiring mental alertness. 2. Sudden withdrawal may precipitate symptoms. 3. Close observation of response in children and elderly. 4. Used to treat grand mal and focal seizures. 5. See Appendix 15-5 for care of client with seizures.
Phenytoin (**Dilantin**): PO, IV	Gingival hyperplasia, skin rash, hypoglycemia Visual changes: nystagmus, diplopia, blurred vision dysrhythmias	1. Administer PO preparations with meals or milk to decrease gastric irritation. 2. Frequently used with phenobarbital for control of grand mal seizures. 3. IM injection not recommended. 4. Do not mix with any other medications when administering IV solution. 5. Promote good oral hygiene. 6. See Appendix 15-5 for care of client with seizures.
Valproic acid (**Depakene**): PO	Transient nausea, hepatotoxic	

NCLEX ALERT: *Maintain care of client with seizures. Observe for effects of medications.*

Appendix 15-3: CHOLINERGIC (ANTI-CHOLINESTERASE) MEDICATIONS

MEDICATIONS	SIDE EFFECTS	NURSING IMPLICATIONS
CHOLINERGENIC MEDICATIONS: Intensify transmission of impulses throughout the CNS, where acetylcholine is necessary for transmission.		
Neostigmine bromide (**Prostigmin**): PO, SQ, IM Pyridostigmine bromide (**Mestinon**): PO, IM, IV Edrophonium chloride (**Tensilon**): IV, IM	Excessive salivation, increased GI motility, urinary urgency, bradycardia, visual problems	1. Primary group of medications used for treatment of myasthenia gravis. 2. Atropine is the antidote for treatment of overdose. 3. In treatment of myasthenia gravis, medication is frequently administered 30 to 45 minutes prior to meals. 4. **Mestinon** is given for maintenance of the myasthenia client. 5. **Tensilon** is utilized for diagnostic purposes; not recommended for maintenance therapy. 6. Teach client symptoms of side effects and advise them to call the doctor if present.

Appendix 15-4:
ANTI-PARKINSONISM AGENTS

MEDICATIONS	SIDE EFFECTS	NURSING IMPLICATIONS
ANTI-CHOLINERGIC: Decreases synaptic transmissions in the CNS.		
Benztropine mesylate (**Cogentin**): PO, IM, IV Trihexyphenidyl hydrochloride (**Artane**): PO, IM, IV Procyclidine (**Kemadrin**): PO	Paralytic ileus, urinary retention, cardiac palpitations, blurred vision, nausea and vomiting, sedation, dizziness	1. Administer PO preparations with meals to decrease gastric irritation. 2. Medication should not be abruptly discontinued. 3. Are generally used in younger clients, increased risk of CNS problems with geriatric clients. 4. Monitor client carefully for bowel and bladder problems.
DOPAMINERGIC: Assists to restore normal transmission of nerve impulses.		
Levodopa (**L-dopa, Larodopa**): PO	***Early:*** anorexia, nausea and vomiting, abdominal discomfort, postural hypotension ***Long term:*** abnormal, involuntary movements, especially involving the face, mouth and neck; behavioral disturbances involving confusion, agitation, and euphoria	1. Administer PO preparations with meals to decrease GI distress. 2. Almost all clients will experience some side effects which are dose related; dosage gradually increased according to client's tolerance and response. 3. Onset of action is slow; therapeutic response may require several weeks to months. 4. Vitamin B6 (pyridoxine) is antagonistic to the effects of the medication; decrease client's intake of multiple vitamins and fortified cereals.
Carbidopa/levodopa (**Sinemet**): PO	(Same as for levodopa)	1. Same as for levodopa. 2. Utilization of carbidopa significantly decreases the amount of levodopa required for therapy. 3. Prevents the inhibitory effects of levodopa on vitamin B6.
Amantadine hydrochloride (**Symmetrel**): PO	Orthostatic hypotension, dyspnea, dizziness, drowsiness, blurred vision, constipation, urinary retention (side effects are dose-related)	1. Less effective than levodopa; produces a more rapid clinical response.
Pramipexole (**Mirapex**) PO	Nausea, vomiting, weakness Constipation	1. Food will reduce the absorption. 2. Frequently combined with levodopa/carbidopa 3. Dosage usually started slow than increase.

Appendix 15-5: SEIZURE DISORDERS

❑ **DEFINITION:** Interruption of normal brain functioning by uncontrolled paroxysmal discharge of electrical stimuli from the neurons.

CLASSIFICATIONS OF SEIZURES:

Partial Seizures:

1. **Focal seizures (motor)** - confined to a specific area (hand, arm, leg).
2. **Jacksonian seizures (motor)** - activity begins slowly and progresses. May start with slow clonic movement in the hand and progress up the arm and over the side of the body. May be several minutes in duration.
3. **Complex partial** -characteristically produces automatisms (lip smacking, grimacing, repetitive hand movements). Client may become violent; period may be followed by amnesia and confusion.

Generalized Seizures:

1. **Absence (petit mal)** - characterized by a short period of time when the client is in an altered level of consciousness. Staring, blinking period (followed by resumption of normal activity) is characteristic. May occur over 100 times per day, may go unnoticed; generally, onset in children between ages of 4 and 12.
2. **Tonic-clonic seizures** - may experience an aura prior to the development of the seizure (auditory, visual, sensory, olfactory disturbances). Full recovery may take several hours; client may be confused, amnesic, and irritable during this recovery period.

Tonic phase -client may lose consciousness and fall, followed by muscle spasms. Apnea and cyanosis are common during this period; generally last for about one minute.

Clonic phase -hyperventilation, with rapid jerking movements. Tongue biting, incontinence, heavy salivation may occur during this period.

SEIZURE ETIOLOGY:

Acute Disorders:

1. Increased intracranial pressure.
2. Metabolic alterations.
3. Febrile episodes in children (generally between 6 mos and 3 yrs).
4. Infections.

Chronic (recurrent):

1. Brain injury at birth.
2. Trauma.
3. Vascular disease.
4. Brain tumors.
5. Idiopathic.

Nursing Assessment:

1. Identify any activities that occurred immediately prior to the seizure.
2. Was the client aware a seizure was going to occur? If so, how did he know?
3. Describe type of movements that occurred and the body area affected - jaw clenched, tongue biting.
4. Presence of incontinence.
6. Period of apnea and cyanosis.
7. Presence of automatisms (lip smacking, grimacing, chewing).
8. Duration of seizure.
9. Changes in level of consciousness.
10. Condition of client post-seizure: oriented, what level of activity, any residual paralysis or muscle weakness.

> **NCLEX ALERT:** *Determine changes in client's neurologic status. Maintain care of client with seizures.*

Nursing Management:

1. Remain with the client who is in seizure activity, note the time the seizure began and how long it lasted.
2. Do not attempt to force anything into the client's mouth if the jaws are clenched shut.
3. If the jaws are not clenched, place an airway in the client's mouth. This protects the tongue and also provides a method of suctioning the airway should the client vomit.
4. Protect the client from injuring himself by falling out of bed or by striking himself on bedrails, etc.
5. Loosen any constrictive clothing.
6. Do not restrain client during seizure activity; allow seizure movements to occur, but protect client from injury.
7. Evaluate respiratory status, if vomiting occurs; be prepared to suction the client to clear the airway and prevent aspiration.
8. Maintain calm atmosphere and provide for privacy after the seizure activity.
9. Re-orient client.

Client Education:

1. Identify activities/events that precipitate the seizure activity.
2. Avoid alcohol.
3. Take medications as directed.
4. Counseling for the family and for the client to assist them in maintaining positive coping mechanisms.

> ***NURSING PRIORITY:** Artificial ventilation cannot be performed on a client in a tonic-clonic seizure. After the seizure is over, evaluate the airway and initiate ventilations if necessary.*

Appendix 15-6: APHASIA

❑ **Aphasia is a defect in the ability of the client use and interpret the symbols of language. The most common cause of aphasia is a vascular problem (CVA). Aphasic clients are often frustrated and irritable. Emotional lability is common, accept the behavior in a manner that prevents embarrassment for the client.**

TYPES OF APHASIA:	*Nursing Implications:*
Sensory Aphasia (receptive) - Cannot understand oral or written communication. Client cannot interpret the incoming speech or read. ***Motor Aphasia (expressive, Broca's aphasia)*** - Inability to speak or to write; however, the client can comprehend incoming speech and can read. ***Mixed*** - Most aphasia involves both the sensory and the motor aspect of speech. Rarely is aphasia only sensory or only motor.	1. Stand in front of the client, speak clearly and slowly. 2. Do not shout or speak loudly, the client can hear. 3. Be patient, give the client time to respond, do not press him for immediate answers. 4. Use nonverbal communications - touch, smile, show objects. 5. Assist the client with motor aphasia to practice repeating simple words - yes, no, please. 6. Listen carefully, try to understand, try to communicate; this conveys to the client that you care. 7. Provide directions as simply as possible. 8. Involve the family in practice and assist them to identify ways they can support the client.

NCLEX ALERT: *Use alternative methods to communicate with a client.*

1866 4365701
1866 436 57 02

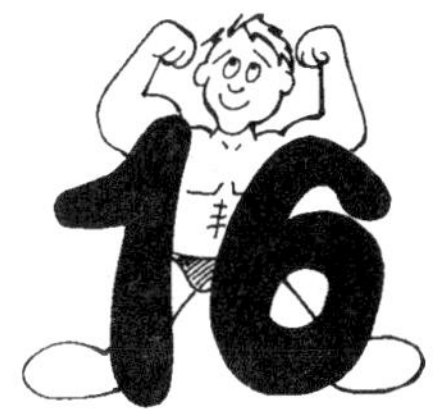

16 Musculoskeletal and Connective Tissue System

PHYSIOLOGY OF THE MUSCULOSKELETAL AND CONNECTIVE TISSUE

Skeletal System

A. Bone structure.
   1. Periosteum - dense fibrous membrane covering the bone; periosteal vessels supply bone tissue.
   2. Epiphysis - a cartilage area in children which provides for longitudinal growth of the bone.
   3. Red bone marrow - primary function is production of red blood cells.

B. Bone maintenance and healing.
   1. Regulatory factors determining both formation and resorption.
      a. Weight-bearing stress stimulates local bone resorption and formation; therefore, in states of immobility where weight bearing is prevented, calcium is lost from the bone.
      b. Vitamin D promotes absorption of calcium from the GI tract and accelerates mobilization of calcium from the bone to increase or maintain serum calcium.

Connective Tissue - Joints and Cartilage

A. Joints.
   1. The action of joints permits bones to change position and facilitate body movement.
   2. The synovial joint is the most common type of joint in the body.

B. Cartilage is rigid connective tissue.

C. Ligaments and tendons are tough fibrous connective tissue providing stability while continuing to permit movement.

Skeletal Muscle

A. Muscles are attached to tendons, bones, and connective tissue.

B. Lower motor neurons control the activity of the skeletal muscle.

C. Energy is consumed when skeletal muscles contract in response to a stimulus.

D. Muscle contraction.
   1. Muscles accomplish movement only by contraction.
      a. Flexion - bending at a joint.
      b. Extension - straightening of a joint.
      c. Abduction - action moving away from the body.
      d. Adduction - action moving toward the body.

> ***NURSING PRIORITY:*** *In caring for orthopedic clients, it is essential to know the terms used in referring to movement of joints.*

   2. Hypertrophy, or increased muscle mass, will occur if muscle is exercised repeatedly.
   3. Atrophy, or decreased muscle mass, will occur with muscle disuse.

System Data Collection

A. History.
   1. History of musculoskeletal injuries, neuromuscular disabilities, inflammatory and metabolic conditions directly or indirectly affecting the musculoskeletal system.
   2. Familial predisposition to orthopedic problems.
   3. Level of normal activity.
      a. Occupation.
      b. Exercise, recreation.
   4. Existence of other chronic health problems.

B. Physical assessment.
   1. Initial inspection for gross deformities, asymmetry, swelling, and edema.
   2. Nutritional status - appropriateness of client's weight and body frame.
   3. Joints.
      a. Movement - active and passive; examine active movement first; compare movement and range of motion to opposite side.
      b. Inflammation and tenderness - with or without movement.
      c. Presence of joint deformities or dislocations.
   4. Evaluate client's spinal alignment, posture, and gait.
   5. Evaluate skeletal muscle.
      a. Muscle strength bilaterally.
      b. Coordination of movement.
      c. Presence of atrophy or hypertrophy.
      d. Presence of involuntary muscle movement.
   6. Assess peripheral pulses and peripheral circulation, capillary refill should take about 2-3 seconds in normal circulation.

Box 16-1: Elderly Care Focus

Musculoskeletal Changes

- Decreased bone density leads to more frequent fractures.
- Decrease in subcutaneous tissue results in less soft tissue over bony prominences.
- Degenerative changes in the spine alter posture and gait.
- Degenerative changes in cartilage result in decreased movement of joints.
- Decreased range of motion of extremities; may need increased assistance with ADLs.

7. Assess for presence of and characteristics of pain.
   a. Most musculoskeletal pain is relieved by rest.
   b. Identify precipitating activities and/or precipitating factors.
   c. Type of pain and location.

***NURSING PRIORITY:** Orthopedic situations frequently contain questions that are based on the concepts of immobility, nursing assessment of an extremity for compromised circulation, and general operative care. Pay close attention to the direction of the question.*

MUSCULOSKELETAL DISORDERS

Developmental Dysplasia of the Hip

❑ **Malformations of the hip as a result of imperfect development of the femoral head, the acetabulum, or both.**

Data Collection

1. Ortolani's sign - infant supine, knees flexed, hips fully abducted; a click is heard or felt as the hip is reduced by abduction.
2. Asymmetrical gluteal and thigh folds.
3. Shortening of the leg on the affected side
4. Limited abduction.

Treatment

1. Treatment should be initiated prior to 2 months of age.
2. The dislocated hip is securely held in a full abduction position to keep the femur in the acetabulum and stabilize the area. (Pavlik Harness).
3. Successful reduction becomes increasingly difficult after age 4.

Nursing Intervention

✦ *Goal: to identify problem in the newborn prior to discharge.*

✦ *Goal: to assist parents to understand mechanism to maintain reduction.*

1. Double diapering - may be done until more definitive appliance is available.
2. Cast and braces - observe for areas of irritation, a evaluate peripheral circulation and maintain cleanliness.

✦ *Goal: to facilitate developmental progress and adapt nurturing activities to meet infant and parent needs.*

1. Provide appropriate stimuli and activity for developmental level.
2. Encourage parents to hold and cuddle child.
3. Maintain normal home routine.

Herniated Intervertebral Disk

❑ **The intervertebral disk forms a cushion between the vertebral bodies of the spinal column. As stress on an injured or degenerated disk occurs, the cartilage material of the disk (nucleus pulposa) herniates inward toward the spinal column, causing compression or tension on the spinal nerve root.**

Data Collection

1. The problem generally occurs in the lumbar sacral area.
2. Clinical manifestations.
   a. Low back pain radiating down the posterior thigh (sciatica pain).
   b. Coughing, straining, sneezing, bending, and lifting aggravate the pain.
   c. Lying supine and raising the leg in an extended position will precipitate the pain.
3. Diagnostics: myelogram, MRI.
4. Treatment - medical
   a. Analgesics, muscle relaxants, anti-inflammatory medications.
   b. Weight reduction if appropriate.
   c. Heat treatments and physical therapy.
   d. Bed rest with good body alignment for up to 4 days.
5. Surgical.
   a. Laminectomy - removal of the herniated portion of the disk.
   b. Micro-laminectomy - removal of the herniated disk utilizing a microscope. There is less trauma in the disk area, improved hemostasis, minimal nerve root involvement, and quicker recovery.

Nursing Intervention

✦ *Goal: to relieve pain via conservative measures and prevent recurrence of problem.*

1. Decrease muscle spasm with bed rest and medications.
2. Begin ambulation slowly and avoid having client bend, stoop, sit, or lift.
3. Instruct the client regarding the principles of body mechanics.
4. The client may need to utilize a bed board if the mattress at home is not firm; avoid sleeping in the prone position.
5. Encourage correct posture; avoid prolonged standing.
6. Sit in straight-backed chairs.

✦ *Goal: to prepare client for laminectomy.*

1. General preoperative nursing intervention as appropriate.
2. Have client practice logrolling preoperatively.
3. Have client practice voiding from supine position.
4. Explain to client that postoperative pain is very similar to preoperative pain, due to the temporary inflammation and edema of the area around the spinal cord.
5. Evaluate bowel and bladder function.
6. Identify specific characteristics of pain for data base postoperatively.

✦ *Goal: to maintain spinal alignment postoperative laminectomy.*

1. Keep the bed in flat position.
2. Logroll client when turning.
3. Keep pillows between the legs when positioned on the side; do not place pillow under the knees.
4. Elastic stockings or pneumatic compression stockings to increase venous return.
5. Good pulmonary hygiene - fluids, coughing, deep breathing, and spirometry
6. The client with micro-disk surgery will have less limitations on his mobility. Generally he may assume a position of comfort.

✦ *Goal: to maintain homeostasis and assess for complications postoperative laminectomy.*

1. Evaluate incision area for possible leakage of spinal fluid and bleeding.

NCLEX ALERT: *Identify changes in neurologic system. A hematoma in the incisional area may be manifested by swelling around the incision site or by neurological deficits in the lower extremities.*

2. Evaluate pain; pay particular attention to areas of pain radiation.
3. Evaluate sensation of extremities.
4. Evaluate ability to move feet and toes.
5. Evaluate circulatory status of legs and feet.
6. Assess for urinary retention and loss of sphincter control. *Need to notify RN or physician immediately, it may be an indication of cord compression.*

NURSING PRIORITY: *The laminectomy client frequently experiences difficulty voiding due to edema in the area of surgery that may interfere with normal bladder sensation.*

7. Ambulate as soon as indicated (frequently on first postoperative day if no fusion was done).
8. Analgesics as indicated.
9. The client with the micro-laminectomy generally experiences less pain, is frequently out of bed the day of surgery, and has fewer complications.

Scoliosis

❑ **Adolescent idiopathic scoliosis is a lateral curvature of the spine. Without treatment, it will severely affect the shape of the thoracic cavity and impair ventilation.**

Data Collection

1. Decreased spinal flexibility.
2. Visible curvature of the spinal column; head and hips are not in alignment.
3. When client bends forward from the waist, there is visible difference in the level of the shoulders. The ribs and shoulder are more prominent on one side.
4. Waistline is uneven.
5. One hip is more prominent.
6. Defect is progressive.

Treatment

1. Brace if spinal curvature progresses, general initial treatment (i.e., Cotrel's traction - early correction, Milwaukee brace).
2. Surgery - spinal fusion and placement of a rod or instrument to maintain alignment of the fused seg-

ment. The rod may be left in place permanently unless it becomes displaced.

Nursing Intervention

✦ *Goal: to identify defects early and promote effective conservative therapy.*

1. Promote health programs in school to identify condition.
2. Assist client and parents to properly utilize braces.
   a. Make sure brace is properly fitted and does not inadvertently rub bony prominences.
   b. May put light T-shirt under brace for comfort.
   c. Initially, the brace is worn 20 to 23 hours per day.
   d. Brace is regularly adjusted to promote correction.
   e. If progress is good, child is weaned from the brace during the daytime and wears it only at night.
   f. Supplemental exercises.

✦ *Goal: to maintain spinal alignment postoperative correction (See postoperative laminectomy goal above).*

✦ *Goal: to maintain homeostasis and assess for complications postoperative correction (See postoperative laminectomy goal above).*

Fractures

❑ **A disruption or break in the continuity of the bone, which generally occurs from a traumatic injury.**

A. Pathological fractures occur secondary to a disease process.

B. Classification of fractures.

1. Type.
   a. Comminuted - fractures with multiple bone fragments; more common in the adult.
   b. Greenstick - an incomplete fracture with bending and splintering of the bone; more common in children.
2. Classified according to location on the bone - proximal, middle, or distal.
3. Simple, closed fracture - does not produce a break in the skin.
4. Complex, open, or compound - fracture involves an open wound through which the bone has protruded.

Data Collection

1. Clinical manifestations.
   a. Edema, swelling of soft tissue around the injured site.
   b. Pain.
   c. Abnormal positioning of extremity; deformity.
   d. Loss of function due to disruption of bone integrity.
   e. False movement; movement occurs at the fracture site.
   f. Crepitation - palpable or audible crunching as the ends of the bones rub together.
   g. Discoloration of the skin around the affected area.
   h. Sensation may be impaired if there is nerve damage.
2. Diagnostics.
   a. Clinical manifestations and history.
   b. X-ray of involved area.

Treatment

1. Immediate immobilization of suspected fracture area.
2. Fracture reduction.
   a. Closed reduction - manual realignment of the bones; injured extremity is usually placed in a cast for continued immobilization until healing occurs.
   b. Open reduction internal fixation (ORIF)- surgical correction of alignment with steel plates and screws to reinforce area of fracture. Allows for earlier weight bearing.
3. Traction (Figure 16-1).
   a. Purposes.
      (1) Immobilization of fractures until surgical correction is done; immobilization or alignment of fracture until sufficient healing occurs to permit casting.
      (2) Decrease, prevent, or correct deformities associated with muscle diseases and bone injury.
      (3) Decrease muscle spasm by fatiguing involved muscles.
   b. Types.
      (1) Skeletal - wire or metal pin is inserted into or through the bone (Kirschner wires, or Steinmann pins).
      (2) Skin - force of pull is applied directly to the skin and indirectly to the bone.
4. Cast application to maintain immobility of affected area above and below the injured area.
5. External fixation - rigid external device consisting of pins placed through the bone and held in place by a metal frame.
   a. May be used to treat open comminuted fractures.

b. A cast may also be applied until healing is complete.

Complications

1. Infection - especially in injuries resulting in open fracture and soft tissue injury.
2. Compartmental syndrome - there are compartments in the extremities that are lined by fascia. This fascia does not expand in response to an increase in the contents of the compartment.
   a. Any increase in the size of the compartment due to bleeding or swelling will put pressure on the structures within that compartment.
   b. May cause permanent damage if not relieved within 4 to 6 hours.
   c. Earliest sign is paresthesia; pulselessness is a late sign. Clients may complain of pain unrelieved by analgesics.
   d. Evidence of decreased circulation distal to the involved area.
   e. Treatment is directed toward immediate release of pressure. If the client has a cast, the cast may be "bivalved." The cast is split in half, the halves are secured around the extremity by a wrap such as an elastic bandage.
   f. Volkmann's contracture - compartmental syndrome that compromises arterial and venous circulation, resulting in prolonged ischemia. Commonly occurs with fractures to the elbow and forearm; results in crippling contracture of the hand.
3. Impaired blood flow - most common in casted extremities.
   a. Decreased to absent pulse distal to cast or injury.
   b. Pain and swelling
   c. Paresthesia
   d. Motor paralysis
4. Venous stasis and thrombus formation related to immobility.
5. Fat embolism.
   a. Often associated with fractures of long bones; primarily occurs in adults.
   b. Clinical manifestations generally occur within 24-48 hours of injury.
   c. Fat globule is transported to the lungs, producing symptoms of acute respiratory distress and hypoxia.
   d. Disuse syndrome while in cast.

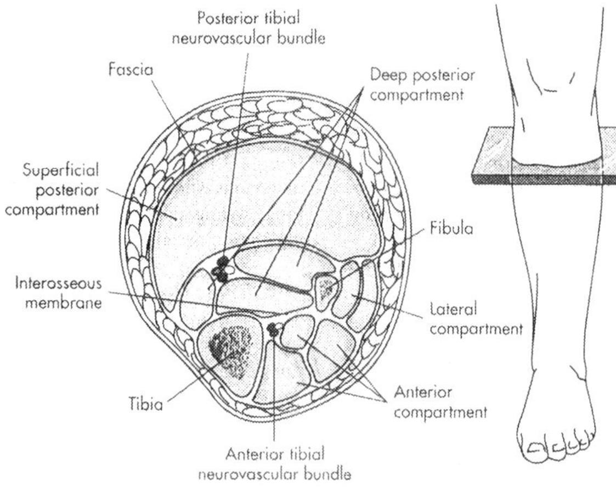

Figure 16-1: Compartmental Syndrome
Compartments of the proximal third of the lower leg - anterior, lateral, deep posterior, superficial posterior. As the compartment swells, pressure is exerted on vessels and nerves within the compartment.
Reprinted with permission: Phipps, WJ, Sands, JK, & Marek, JF (1999). *Medical Surgical Nursing: Concepts & Clinical Practice*, 6th ed. Philadelphia: Mosby, p. 1936.

NCLEX ALERT: *Immediately report pain that is unrelieved by analgesics in order to avoid paralysis and necrosis.*

Nursing Intervention

✦ *Goal: to provide immobility and emergency care prior to transporting victim.*

1. Evaluate circulation distal to injury.
2. Splint and immobilize extremity prior to transfer.
3. Elevate the affected extremity, if possible, to decrease edema.

✦ *Goal: to identify complications early; frequent peripheral nerve and vascular assessment distal to the area of injury (prior to treatment and ongoing after immobilization of injury).*

Figure 16-2: Traction

Reprinted with permission: Wong, D., et. Al., (1999). *Whaley & Wong's Nursing Care of Infants and Children*, St. Louis: Mosby, p. 1921.

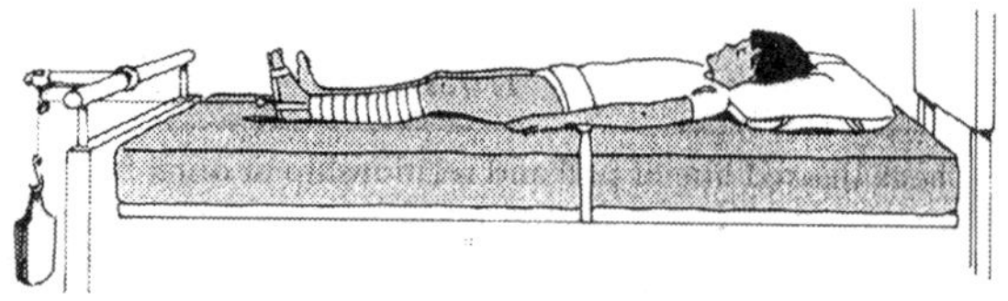

Buck extension traction.

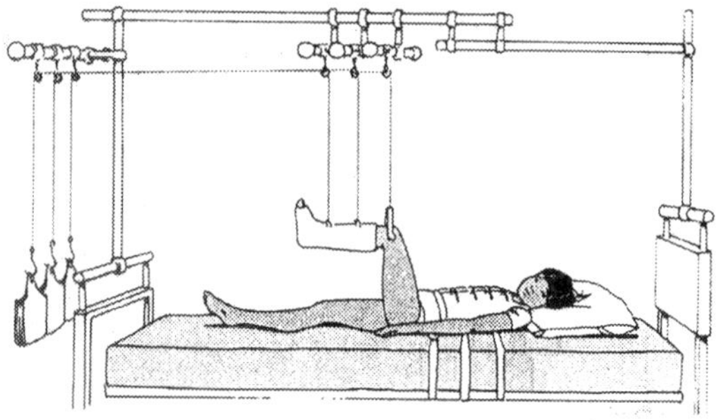

"90-90" traction.

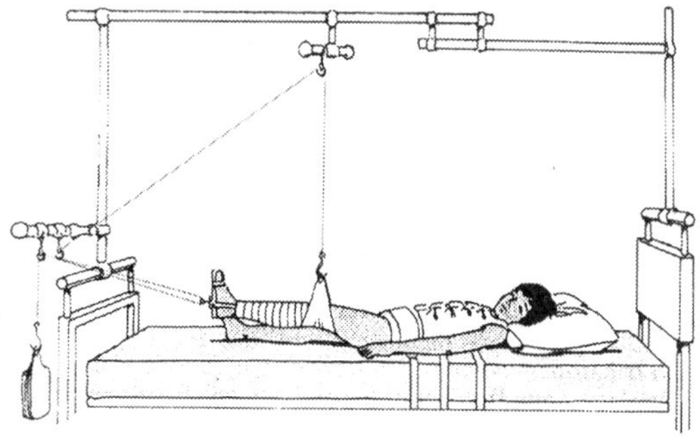

Russell traction.

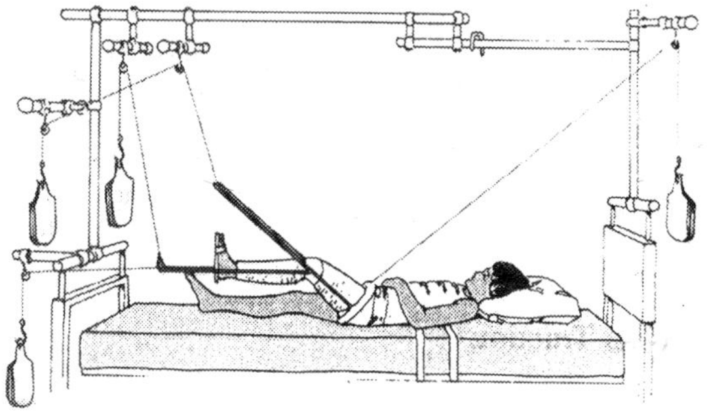

Balance suspension with Thomas ring splint and Pearson attachment.

5 P's of Circulatory Assessment

1. **P**ain.
   a. Location.
   b. Increasing or decreasing, throbbing, response to analgesics.
   c. Precipitating factors.
2. Presence of peripheral **P**ulses.
3. **P**allor of skin.
   a. Skin pale and cool to touch.
   b. Nail beds - capillary refill within 2-3 seconds.
4. **P**aresthesia.
   a. Decreased sensation.
   b. Numbness, tingling.
5. **P**aralysis.

NCLEX ALERT: *Implement measure to prevent neurological complications (e.g., foot drop, numbness, tingling.)Recognize client with conditions resulting in insufficient vascular perfusion.*

NURSING PRIORITY: *It is critical for the nurse to assess for signs and symptoms of compartmental syndrome and decreased arterial circulation. The RN or physician should be notified immediately.*

✦ *Goal: to maintain immobilization via traction (see Fig. 16-1).*

NCLEX ALERT: *Maintain client traction devices. Implement measures to promote client venous return. Recognize client with conditions resulting in insufficient vascular perfusion.*

1. Assume that traction is continuous unless the doctor orders otherwise.
2. Carefully assess for skin breakdown, especially under the client.
3. Do not change or remove traction weight on a client with continuous traction.
4. The traction ropes and weights should hang free from any obstructions.

5. Traction applied in one direction requires an equal counter traction to be effective.
   a. Do not let the client's feet touch the end of the bed; it will cause the counter traction to be lost.
   b. Do not allow the traction weights to rest on anything at the end of the bed; this negates the pull of the traction.
6. Carefully assess the pin sites in clients with skeletal traction. Osteomyelitis is a serious complication of skeletal traction.

✦ **Goal: to maintain immobilization via cast.**

1. Allow plaster cast to dry adequately before handling or moving the client.
   a. Do not cover the cast with a blanket.
   b. Encourage cast to dry by utilizing fans and maintaining adequate circulation.
   c. Synthetic casts dry in about 20 minutes; cast will feel warm during the drying process.
   d. Plaster casts take several hours to dry completely; the cast will also feel warm during drying.
   e. Avoid handling wet cast to prevent indentions which may cause pressure areas inside the cast.
   f. Position client to allow drying on all cast surfaces.

NURSING PRIORITY: *Do not apply any type of heat to a cast to enhance drying.*

2. Continue to assess for compartmental syndrome.
3. Body jacket cast and hip spica cast.
   a. Evaluate for abdominal discomfort due to cast compression of mesenteric artery against duodenum.
   b. Relief of pressure via nasogastric tube and suction, or cast removal and reapplication.
   c. Evaluate for pressure areas over iliac crest.
4. Do not allow cast to become excessively damp or to get wet.
5. Elevate casted extremity, especially during the first 24 hours after application.
6. Apply ice packs directly over the area of injury during the first 24 hours.
7. Assess the cast surface for drainage.

✦ *Goal: to provide care to client with external fixation device.*

1. Assess for neurovascular complications.
2. Inspect exposed skin and pins for infection.
3. Do not use frame to pull or lift client.
4. Frame will be removed when fracture has healed.
5. Do not adjust the clamps on the external fixator frame.

NCLEX ALERT: *Recognize client with conditions resulting in insufficient vascular perfusion.*

✦ *Goal: to prevent complications of immobility (Chapter 3).*

NURSING PRIORITY: *Check for complications due to a cast, traction, or other immobilizing equipment.*

Self-Care

1. Client should not:
   a. Bear weight on the cast until instructed to do so.
   b. Allow the plaster cast to get wet; discuss alternatives in bathing.
   c. Insert anything under or in the cast.
2. Client should report any symptoms associated with swelling or increase in pain.
3. Maintain follow-up care.

Specific Fractures

A. ***Colle's fracture.***

1. Fracture of the distal radius.
2. Primary complication is compartmental syndrome.

B. ***Fractured pelvis.***

1. Frequently occurs in elderly and is associated with falls.
2. May cause serious intra-abdominal injuries and urinary tract injury.
3. Bed rest is utilized for stable fractures.
4. Combination of external fixation, open reduction and internal fixation may be utilized in complex fractures.
5. Turn client only on specific orders.

C. ***Fractured hip.***

1. Common in elderly women over 60 years old with osteoporosis.
2. Clinical manifestations.
   a. External rotation and adduction of the affected extremity.
   b. Shortening of the length of the affected extremity.
   c. Severe pain and tenderness.
3. Treatment.

Box 16-2: Elderly Care Focus

Musculoskeletal Nursing Implications

- Difficulty maintaining immobility after fractures, therefore, they are frequently repaired with surgical, intervention (ORIF).
- Heal more slowly, so use of extremity and weight bearing are frequently delayed.
- Complications of immobility occur more frequently; mobilize hospitalized clients as early as possible.
- Do not rely on fever as the primary indication of infection; decreasing mental status is more common.
- Contractions are more common.
- More frequent use of assistive devices - canes and walkers.

a. Initially, Buck's or Russell's traction with sandbags and trochanter to immobilize fracture, decrease muscle spasms, and control external rotation (Fig. 16-1).

b. Surgical repair when client's condition allows (permits earlier mobility and prevents complications of immobility).

4. Nursing intervention postoperative.

a. Circulatory and neurologic checks distal to area of injury.

b. Position to prevent flexion, adduction and internal rotation, which cause dislocation of the prosthesis.

(1) Do not adduct the affected leg past the neutral position.

(2) Maintain the affected leg in an abducted position.

(3) It is important to maintain neutral rotation and abduction.

(4) Prevent external rotation by utilizing sandbags, pillows, and trochanter rolls at the thigh.

(5) Maintain abduction with an A-frame pillow or by keeping pillows between the knees.

(6) Avoid acute flexion of the hip.

NURSING PRIORITY: *Watch positioning on the fractured hip client*

c. Check physician's order regarding positioning and turning.

d. Evaluate blood loss.

(1) Check under the client for hemorrhage.

(2) Measure the diameter of the thigh to evaluate the presence of internal bleeding.

e. The client is prone to complications of immobility - thigh-high antiembolic stockings, pneumatic compression devices on legs; encourage foot flexion, prophylactic low dose Heparin.

Joint Replacement

1. Hip replacement may be done due to a pathological fracture or due to a disease process such as rheumatoid arthritis.

2. Preoperative Care.

a. Encourage client to practice using either crutches or a walker, whichever is anticipated to be used postoperatively. (See Appendix 16-4)

b. Encourage client to practice moving from the bed to the chair in the same manner he will postoperatively.

3. Postoperative care. (Chp 2)

a. Client may be out of bed to stand at the bedside on the first postoperative day.

b. Encourage postoperative exercises.

c. Do not allow the hip to flex greater than 90 degrees, therefore do not elevate the bed greater than 60 degrees.

d. Maintain abduction and prevent external rotation of extremity.

e. When sitting, keep client's knees below level of hip.

f. Frequent assessment of circulatory status.

g. Pain control is frequently difficult secondary to age, respiratory status, and need to mobilize client.

h. Monitor wound drainage, frequently will have a portable wound suction device.

Total knee Replacement

A. Most often done due to joint complications of arthritis.

B. Postoperative care.

1. Usually returns from surgery with a compression dressing, monitor neurovascular status of extremity,

2. Cold packs to incision site to decrease edema and bleeding.

3. Portable wound suction - monitor drainage.

4. Continuous passive motion - promotes haling by increasing circulation and movement of joint, check device to make sure amount extension and flexion are maintained.

5. When client is out of bed, apply the knee immobilizing device and elevate the extremity.

6. Weight bearing limits postoperative, gradually increase with healing.

NCLEX ALERT: *Provide assistance with prescribed exercises. Monitor client mobility gait and strength.*

Osteoporosis

❑ **A metabolic bone disease that involves an imbalance between new bone formation and bone resorption.**

A. Primary osteoporosis is most common type — occurs most often in women after menopause, greatest prevalence is in women over 80 years old.

B. Bone loss occurs predominantly in the vertebral bodies of the spine and the femoral neck in the hip. The bone mass declines, leaving the bone brittle and weak.

Geriatric Priority: *Aging is the major risk factor. Problem occurs predominantly in women between ages of 55-65 years due to decrease in estrogen.*

Data Collection

1. Clinical manifestations.
   a. May be asymptomatic until X-rays demonstrate skeletal weakening. Bone loss of 25% to 40% occurs before osteoporosis can be identified on standard X-rays.
   b. Spinal deformity and "dowager's hump."
      (1) May be diagnosed after a fracture or a vertebral compression frame.
      (2) Gradual loss of height.
      (3) Increase in spinal curvature (kyphosis).
   c. Vertebral fractures may occur spontaneously, or as a result of minimal trauma.
   d. Chronic low thoracic and midline back pain.
   e. Height loss may precipitate thoracic problems, decrease in abdominal volume and exercise tolerance.
2. Diagnostics.
   a. Serum lab values of calcium, phosphorus, and alkaline phosphatase are usually normal.
   b. Computed tomography to evaluate bone loss.
   c. Bone scan to identify bone density.

Treatment

1. Dietary - increased protein, calcium and vitamin D.
2. Calcium supplements- (Appendix 16-2).
3. Vitamin D supplements to enhance utilization of calcium.
4. Estrogen replacement therapy as indicated.
5. Exercise - activities that put moderate stress on bones by working them against gravity (walking, racquet sports, jogging). This type of exercise is believed to decrease the development of osteoporosis and possibly increase new bone formation.
6. Compression fractures of the vertebra usually heal without surgical intervention.

Complications

Bone fracture occurring in the vertebral bodies, distal radius, or the hip.

Nursing Intervention

✦ *Goal: to decrease pain and promote activities to diminish progress of disease.*

1. Pain relief.
   a. Bed rest initially.
   b. Firm mattress.
   c. Analgesics.
2. Assess bowel and bladder function; client prone to constipation and paralytic ileus if vertebra are involved.
3. Regular daily weight-bearing exercise; encourage outdoor exercises, increases utilization of Vitamin D.
4. Discourage use of caffeine and alcohol.

Self-Care

1. Decrease falls and injury by maintaining safe home environment; use assistive devices.
2. Understand need to continue medications, even if they do not make the client feel better. Important for client to understand that the calcium supplements are to prevent further damage.
3. Do not exercise if pain occurs.
4. Avoid heavy lifting, stooping, and bending. Review and demonstrate good body mechanics with the client.

Osteomyelitis

❑ **An infection of the bone. The most common organism is *Staphylococcus*.**

Data Collection

1. Tenderness, swelling, and warmth of affected area.
2. Drainage from infected site.
3. Fever, chills.
4. Constant pain of affected area.
5. Remission and exacerbation of problem.
6. Diagnostics.

a. Wound culture.
b. Blood culture.
c. MRI, bone scans

Treatment - prevention is primary goal

1. Intensive IV antibiotics.
2. Immobilization of affected area.

Nursing Intervention

✦ *Goal: to decrease pain, promote comfort, and decrease spread of infection.*

NCLEX ALERT: *Monitor client wounds for infection, Identify signs and symptoms of infection.*

1. Maintain correct body alignment.
   a. Move affected extremity gently and with support.
   b. Prevent contractures, especially of affected extremity.
   c. Warm moist soaks to increase circulation and healing.
2. If there is an open wound, maintain wound contact precautions (Chapter 5).
3. Client is usually discharged with antibiotics and should maintain close follow-up care.
4. Condition may become chronic with reoccurrence after primary infection.

Malignant Bone Tumors

A. The most common primary bone cancer is osteogenic sarcoma; it advances very rapidly with metastasis to the lungs via the blood. (See Chapter 2).
   1. Most commonly affects the long bones, especially the distal end of the femur.
   2. Occurs predominantly in males aged 10-30 years.

B. Metastatic bone cancer occurs when there is a malignancy in another part of the body that has metastasized to the bone (breast and prostate).

Data Collection

1. Clinical manifestations- generally nonspecific.
   a. Localized pain and swelling
   b. Tender, palpable bony mass.
2. Diagnostics.
   a. Computerized tomography to determine the extent of the lesion.
   b. Radioisotope scans to evaluate the metastasis.
   c. Bone biopsy
   d. X-ray will reveal the tumor location, and assist in determining an appropriate biopsy site.

Treatment

1. Primary site - extensive resection of area around tumor; amputation may be necessary.
2. Metastatic site - identify primary site, chemotherapy and radiation.

Nursing Intervention

✦ *Goal: to assist the client and family to cope with the diagnosis and build basis for rehabilitation.*

1. Honest, straightforward information to client and family regarding the situation.
2. Allow opportunity to express their concerns and fears.
3. Anticipate sense of loss of control and anger over changes in body.
4. Encourage normal growth and developmental activities as appropriate; allow client to be as independent as possible.

✦ *Goal: to assist the client and the family to cope with the side effects of chemotherapy and radiation. (See Chapter 2).*

NCLEX ALERT: *Provide support to client with changes in body image.*

Rheumatoid Arthritis

❑ **A systemic disease that produces a chronic inflammatory process, most often involving synovial joints.**

A. Exacerbations and remissions occur. Condition tends to be progressive with each exacerbation. Seldom does the client return to the previous level of functioning prior to the exacerbation.

B. Early diagnosis may prevent or delay permanent damage.

Data Collection

1. Clinical manifestations.
   a. Gradual onset.
   b. Joint involvement (hands and feet).
      (1) Warm, tender, red, painful joints.
      (2) Decrease in range of motion.
      (3) Decrease in strength.
      (4) Stiffness and pain worse in the morning.
      (5) Joint involvement is bilateral and symmetrical.
   c. Subcutaneous nodules on the fingers.

d. Systemic effects.
   (1) Low fever.
   (2) Malaise and weakness.
   (3) Anorexia and weight loss.
   (4) Depression.
   (5) Fatigued by afternoon.

e. Chronic deformities develop most often in the hands and feet.

f. Exacerbation of symptoms may be associated with physical or emotional stress.

2. Diagnostics.
   a. Positive serum rheumatoid factor.
   b. Increased erythrocyte sedimentation rate (ESR).
   c. Antinuclear antibody titer.
   d. Aspiration of synovial joint fluid.

Treatment

1. Nonsteroidal anti-inflammatory drugs (NSAIDs).
2. Corticosteroids.
3. Heat and/or cold applications.
4. Physical and rehabilitative therapy.
5. Surgery - joint replacements.

Nursing Intervention

✦ *Goal: to relieve pain and preserve joint mobility and muscle strength.*

1. Use warm, moist compresses to relieve pain and stiffness of muscle spasms associated with chronic stiffness.
2. If acute inflammation is present, cold compresses may be used.
3. Inflamed joints may be immobilized in a device that maintains a functional position.
4. Position client to maintain correct body alignment and prevent contractures, especially flexion contractures.
5. Exercises to maintain joint mobility and to decrease pain.
6. Anti-inflammatory medications should be taken with meals or food, to decrease gastric upset.
7. If client is on steroids, an identification tag should be worn.

NURSING PRIORITY: *Nursing care of the client with rheumatoid arthritis is directed toward decreasing pain and maintaining joint function.*

✦ *Goal: to assist client to understand implications of the disease process and measures to maintain health.*

1. Regularly scheduled rest periods to relieve fatigue and pain; amount of rest varies with the individual and the disease process.
2. Protect small joints.
   a. Maintain joint alignment; avoid positions which precipitate joint contraction (do not use pillow under the knees; encourage activities which involve pressing down the fingers).
   b. Change position frequently; maintain good body alignment.
   c. Use large muscle groups instead of smaller ones; avoid repetitive movements in small joints.
   d. Modify home routine to decrease or avoid stress on joints - dressing activities, ADL.
3. If joint becomes painful during exercise, and the pain persists for 2 hours after the exercise, the activity should be evaluated.
4. Discuss with client importance of identifying false advertising regarding claims of cure and relief of chronic pain.
5. Encourage client to be independent in ADL as long as possible.

NCLEX ALERT: *Maintain correct body alignment. Monitor client response to interventions for preventing complications. Implement measures to maintain range of motion.*

Osteoarthritis

❑ **It is a progressive degenerative joint disease that primarily affects the joints in long bones.**

Data Collection

1. Clinical manifestations.
   a. Joints involved
      (1) Primarily involves weight-bearing joints; may occur as a result of mechanical stress.
      (2) May be unilateral and involve a single joint.
   b. Pain, swelling and tenderness, stiffness of the joint.
   c. Pain occurs on motion and with weight bearing.
   d. Pain increases in severity with activity.
2. Diagnostics.
   a. X-ray to determine structural joint change.
   b. No specific diagnostic test.

Treatment

1. NSAIDS may be effective in pain relief.
2. Methotrexate to decrease swelling and pain.
3. Activity balanced with adequate rest.

4. Joint injection with corticosteriods
5. Physical therapy and exercise.
6. Surgical intervention with joint replacement.

Nursing Intervention

✦ *Goal: to relieve pain, prevent further stress on the joint, and maintain function.*

1. Maintain functional joint alignment; desired position may not be position of comfort.
2. Plan ADL to prevent stress on involved joints and provide adequate rest periods.
3. Warm compresses and hot showers to reduce stiffness and pain.
4. Cold compresses may be used if the joint is acutely inflamed.
5. Local rest of an affected joint - splint or brace.

✦ *Goal: to assist client to understand implications of the disease process and measures to maintain health.*

1. Identify activities requiring increased stress on involved joints.
2. Maintain regular exercise program to preserve muscle strength and joint mobility.
3. Encourage independence in ADL as indicated.

✦ *Goal: to maintain psychological equilibrium and promote positive self-esteem (see rheumatoid arthritis goal).*

Gout

❑ **An arthritic condition resulting from the defect in the metabolism of uric acid (hyperuricemia).**

Data Collection

1. Clinical manifestations.
   a. Characterized by remissions and exacerbations of acute joint pain.
   b. Onset is generally rapid.
   c. Rapidly swelling, painful joint.
   d. Great toe is frequently the joint involved; may also involve ankles and knees, wrists and elbows.
2. Diagnostics.
   a. Urate crystals present in synovial fluid.
   b. High serum uric acid levels.

Treatment

1. Medications for acute attack (see Appendix 16-2)
2. Medications to prevent attack.
3. Low purine diet. (Chapter 3).
4. Avoid aspirin, alcohol, and diuretics, as they precipitate an attack.

Nursing Intervention

✦ *Goal: to prevent acute attack, promote comfort, and maintain joint mobility.*

1. Medications should be given early in the attack to decrease the severity .
2. Protect affected joint.
   a. Immobilize.
   b. Elevate the joint.
   c. No weight-bearing.
3. Cold packs may decrease pain.
4. Provide client with information regarding a low purine diet.
5. Encourage high fluid intake to increase excretion of uric acid and to prevent the development of uric acid kidney stones.

NCLEX ALERT: *Check client discomfort and pain levels. Check client response to medications.*

Study Questions—Musculoskeletal

1. What is the main contributing factor to hip and knee contractures in an elderly client?

① prolonged sitting.
② passive range of motion.
③ active range of motion.
④ use of a wedge pillow.

2. What nursing observations would the nurse be most concerned about on a client three days following a below the knee amputation?

① warmth at the end of the stump.
② serosanguineous drainage on the dressing.
③ bright red blood on the dressing.
④ bilateral femoral pulses of 80 and 78.

3. A client is admitted with a fractured hip, prior to surgery the client is placed in Buck's traction. What are important nursing interventions for this client?

① remove the traction boot every 4 hours to check circulation.
② check the pin sites for infection and cleanse three times a day.
③ check for adequate circulation at the fracture site.
④ make sure the client's feet are not touching the end of the bed.

4. The nurse is checking a client for capillary refill. What is the normal time for the nail bed to return to its pink color?

① 1 minute.
② 2-3 seconds.
③ 10 seconds.
④ 15 seconds.

5. The client tells the nurse that he is feeling pain in the area where his leg has been removed. What is the best nursing response?

① because there was severe pain previously, this is a subconscious pain.
② the pain is referred from another area that is injured.
③ the injured nerve endings do not accurately reflect the area of the pain.
④ this is pain that is really occurring at the stump.

6. A client is being treated with a long leg cast for his leg fracture. What are important nursing measures while the cast is still wet?

① the fingertips should be used when handling the cast.
② support the cast on a pillow with a plastic cover.
③ apply a heat lamp and a fan to increase the drying time.
④ do not reposition client until cast is dry.

7. A client had a Steinman pin inserted for repair of a fractured leg. This client is at increased risk for what postoperative complication?

① osteomyelitis.
② poor bone realignment.
③ hip flexion contraction.
④ compartmental syndrome.

8. An elderly client had a fractured hip repaired. The client returns to the unit with a wound drainage system that is connected to low suction. Over the next four hours the client has 75cc of bright bloody drainage. What is the best nursing action?

① notify the doctor of the abnormal amount of bleeding in the container.
② empty the drainage container, record the amount, and continue to observe.
③ apply pressure at the incisional area and evaluate for increase in drainage.
④ check the operative record for the placement of the drain.

9. The nurse is checking a child in a left hip spica cast and suspects an infection. What findings would validate the nurse's conclusion?

① increased complaints of pain and a hot spot found over the incision area.
② complaints of itching and discomfort inside the cast.
③ dusky colored toes with weak pedal pulses.
④ tingling of the leg with a three second capillary refill.

10. A client has a compound fracture and has required increased amount of pain medication, but without therapeutic results. What complication should the nurse assess for in this client?

① infection.
② compartmental syndrome.
③ deep vein thrombosis.
④ muscle cramping.

11. A client complains that the cast on his leg is rubbing his skin raw. What is the best nursing action?

① call the physician to have the cast cut back.
② apply aloe vera lotion to the irritated area.
③ petal the edges of the cast.
④ increase the client's pain medication.

12. What is the major reason pathological hip fractures occur?

① advancing age.
② vitamin deficiency.
③ osteoporosis.
④ calcium deposits at the fracture site.

13. The nurse is caring for a client with an acute problem resulting from an exacerbation of her rheumatoid arthritis. Her hands and fingers are painful, swollen, and inflamed. What is an important nursing measure for this client?

① assist with active range of motion in affected extremity.
② place hand in position of comfort and apply cold packs.
③ apply warm packs to increase circulation to the area.
④ explain the importance of therapeutic joint exercises to increase mobility.

14. A child with a femoral fracture is to be scheduled for a open reduction and internal fixation. Prior to surgery, the nurse would anticipate what nursing measure for this client?

① check for circulation under the temporary hip spica cast.
② evaluate the counterbalance and appropriate amount of weight on the Buck's traction.
③ position the client in a pressure traction bed to decrease skin breakdown.
④ assist with the evaluation and alignment of the Bryant's traction.

15. What modifications would be important to make in the diet of a client in skeletal traction?

① increased carbohydrates.
② increased calcium.
③ decreased vitamin C.
④ increased protein.

16. The nurse is caring for a client in the immediate postoperative period following a lumbar laminectomy? What nursing observations would cause the nurse the most concern?

① complaints of pain when moving either leg.
② pain radiating down the hip and thigh.
③ bilaterally delayed capillary refill on lower extremities.
④ complaints of numbness and tingling in his right foot.

17. What is the nursing management for a client in balanced suspension traction?

① check under the boot for skin irritation and circulation.
② remove the weights to help the client reposition himself.
③ adjust the weights every eight hours to increase circulation.
④ check the weights to make sure they are hanging freely in place.

18. A client is learning to use crutches. What is important for the nurse to teach the client?

① when going up stairs, advance the affected leg first.
② the axillary bar on the crutches should be firmly in the axillary area for full weight bearing.
③ always keep arms and elbows straight when walking.
④ the axillary bar on the crutches should be two fingers below the axillary area.

19. A client is complaining of pain due to a bone fracture. The nurse would expect the client to describe the pain as:

① sharp and piercing.
② dull and spreading.
③ aching like a muscle cramp.
④ burning and dull.

20. What will assist the elderly female client to prevent the development of osteoarthritis?

① vitamin B supplements.
② non-weight bearing exercises.
③ low calcium diet.
④ progesterone replacement therapy.

Appendix 16-1: DIAGNOSTIC STUDIES

SERUM DIAGNOSTICS

Rheumatoid Factor)—Used to determine presence of autoantibodies (rheumatoid factor) seen in clients with connective tissue disease; if antibody is present, it is suggestive of rheumatoid arthritis; the higher the antibody titer the greater the degree of inflammation.

Antinuclear antibody (ANA)—Measures the presence of antibodies that destroy the nucleus of body tissue cells, (i.e., those seen in connective tissue diseases; a positive test is associated with systemic lupus erythematosus).

INVASIVE DIAGNOSTICS

Arthroscopy—Involves the utilization of an arthroscope inserted into a joint for visualization of the joint structure; procedure is conducted preferably in the operating room with strict asepsis; performed under either local or general anesthesia; frequently utilized to diagnose structural abnormalities of the knee.

Nursing Implications:

1. Preoperative nursing intervention as appropriate with the level of anesthesia to be used.
2. After procedure, wound is covered with a sterile dressing.
3. A compression bandage may be applied for 24 hours posttest; teach client symptoms of vascular compromise.
4. Weight bearing is limited.
5. Teach the client signs of infection (increased temperature, local inflammation at site).

Arthrocentesis—Incision of a joint capsule to obtain samples of synovial fluid; local anesthesia and aseptic preparation utilized prior to fluid aspiration. Synovial fluid is examined for infection, bleeding into the joint, and to confirm specific types of arthritis.

Nursing Implications:

1. Explain procedure to client.
2. May be done at bedside or in an examination room.
3. Compression dressing usually applied and joint rested for several hours posttest.
4. Observe dressing for leakage of blood or fluid.

Arthrography—Used to visualize soft tissue structures. Contrast medium is injected into the joint for visualization on X-ray.

Myelogram—Used to determine status of vertebral disk. See Appendix 15-1.

Bone Biopsy—May be performed in client's room or in a treatment room. After satisfactory local anesthetic, a long needle is inserted into the bone or a small incision is made to obtain bone tissue.

Nursing Implications:

1. Plan for analgesic to be administered prior to procedure.
2. If an incision was made, maintain a pressure dressing over the site.
3. Extremity is usually immobilized for several hours post biopsy.
4. Assess the puncture or incision for evidence of infection.

NON-INVASIVE DIAGNOSTICS

X-Rays—The most common diagnostic procedure to determine musculoskeletal problems.

1. Identify musculoskeletal problems.
2. Determine progress of disease or condition.
3. Evaluate effectiveness of treatment.

Bone Scan—Radioisotopes are injected intravenously and bone is scanned to determine where the isotopes are "taken up". May be used to determine malignancies, arthritis, and osteoporosis.

Nursing Implications:

1. Explain procedure to client: procedure is not painful and will take about an hour to complete.
2. Have client void prior to procedure.
3. Increase fluids after procedure.

Computerized Axial Tomography—(computerized tomography, CT, CAT scan) See Appendix 15-1.

Magnetic Resonance Imaging (MRI)—See Appendix 15-1.

NCLEX ALERT: *Determine if client is prepared for procedure. Monitor client diagnostic test results.*

Appendix 16-2: MEDICATIONS

MEDICATIONS	SIDE EFFECTS	NURSING IMPLICATIONS
ANTIGOUT: Decreases the plasma uric acid levels by either inhibiting the synthesis of uric acid or by increasing the excretion of uric acid.		
Colchicine: PO, IV	Nausea Vomiting Diarrhea	1. Take medication at earliest indication of impending gout attack. 2. Take medication with food. 3. Promote high fluid intake to promote uric acid excretion. 4. In acute attack, administer one tablet every hour until symptoms subside, or until GI problems occur, or a total of 8mg has been taken.
Allopurinol (**Zyloprim**): PO	Rash GI distress Fever Headache	1. Administer with food to decrease gastric upset. 2. Discontinue medication if rash occurs. 3. Use with caution in clients with renal insufficiency. 4. May be used to decrease serum uric acid levels in clients on chemotherapy.
Probenecid (**Benemid**): PO Probenecid + Colchicine (**Colbenemid**) PO	GI disturbances, Headache, Skin rash, Fever	1. Urate tophi deposits should decrease in size with therapy. 2. Lifelong therapy is usually required.
SKELETAL MUSCLE RELAXANTS: Relaxes skeletal muscle by depressing synaptic pathways in the spinal cord.		
Methocarbamol (**Robaxin**): PO, IM, IV Cyclobenzaprine (**Flexeril**): PO Baclofen (**Lioresal**): PO	Drowsiness, dizziness, GI upset, rash, blurred vision Drowsiness, dizziness, headache, GI upset, orthostatic hypotension Drowsiness, weakness, fatigue, confusion	1. Use: muscle spasm associated with MS, and spinal cord injury. 2. Caution clients to avoid activities that require mental alertness for safety (driving, power tools, etc) 3. Evaluate client for postural hypotension. 4. Advise client to avoid CNS depressants (alcohol, opioids, antihistamines)
Dantrolene (**Dantrium**): PO, IV	Hepatotoxcity, muscle weakness, drowsiness	1. Teach clients symptoms of liver dysfunction. 2. Acts directly to relax skeletal muscle.
CALCIUM MEDICATIONS: Hormones that prevent the reabsorption of bone, and decrease serum calcium.		
Calcitonin-salmon (**Calcimar**): SQ, IM	GI upset, local inflammation at injection site, flushing	1. Monitor levels of serum calcium. 2. Only given parenterally.
Aminobisphosphonate (**Fosamax**) PO (**Miacalcin**) nasal spray	GI upset, nasal ulceration with spray, flushing, rash	1. Have client swallow tablet whole, do not chew. 2. Take in AM with large glass of water and wait at least 30 minutes before eating or lying down. 3. Make sure client has adequate intake of Vitamin D. 4. Use: prevention of postmenopausal osteoporosis.
CORTICOSTEROIDS: (See Appendix 5-7)		

Nonsteroid anti-inflammatory: See Appendix 5-8.

Appendix 16-3:
AMPUTATIONS

❑ Definition: Removal of all or part of an extremity.

POSTOPERATIVE CARE:

NURSING PRIORITY: *Be familiar with the nursing management of a client with an amputated extremity, especially regarding positioning to prevent contractures.*

Stump Wound Care:

1. The stump may be elevated for approximately 24 hours; after that time, keep the joint immediately above the stump in an extended position. Flexion contracture hinders prosthetic utilization.

2. Discuss the phenomenon of phantom limb pain; it does not help for the nurse to point out to the client that the extremity is gone.

3. Administer analgesics; phantom limb pain is very real to the client.

4. Evaluate stump for good tissue perfusion and healing.

5. A rigid compression dressing (plaster molded over stump dressing) may be applied to prevent injury and to decrease swelling. Controlling the edema will enhance healing and promote comfort.

6. If the client is not fitted with a rigid compression dressing, the stump will be shaped with a compression bandage. Ace bandage elastic wrap is often used.

7. Discourage semi-Fowler's position in the client with above-the- knee amputation; position encourages flexion contraction at the hip.

8. Compression wrap is done from the distal to proximal.

Stump Care After Wound Has Healed:

1. Continually assess for skin breakdown; visually inspect the stump.

2. The stump should be washed , carefully rinsed and dried daily. Soap and moisture contribute to skin breakdown.

3. Do not apply anything to the stump (alcohol increases skin dryness and skin cracking; lotions keep skin soft and hinder prosthetic use).

4. Client should put the prosthesis on when he gets up and should wear it all day. The stump tends to swell if the prosthesis is not applied. The more the person wears the prosthesis, the less the swelling.

NCLEX ALERT: *Provide support to client with changes in body image. Maintain correct body alignment of client. Monitor client mobility, gait and strength.*

Appendix 16-4:
ASSISTIVE DEVICES FOR MOBILITY

CRUTCHES

Measuring a client

- With the client standing with his shoes on, measure the distance from the axillary fold to a point six inches lateral to the heel.
- Adjust hand bars so that client's elbows are slightly flexed (25° to 30°)
- Have client stand, then measure distance between client's axilla and arm pieces.
- Two fingers should fit between client's axilla and the crutch bar.
- Assist the client to stabilize on the crutches and demonstrate how to bear weight on the cross bars, not under the arms.

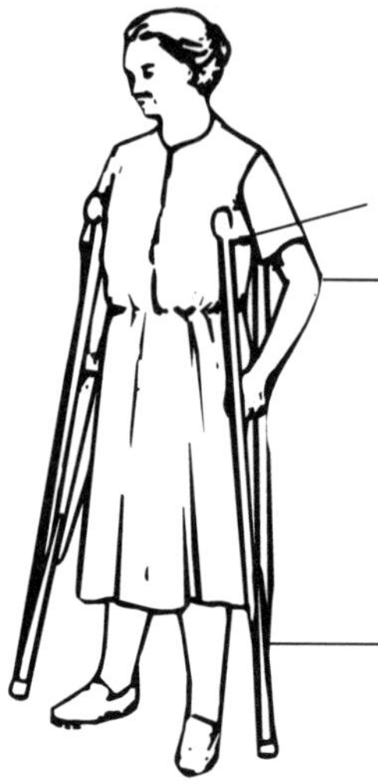

✓ Four-point Alternate Gait

- The four-point alternate gait is used by patients who can bear partial weight on both feet
- This gait provides a normal walking pattern and makes some use of the muscles of the lower extremities.

✓ **Three-point Alternate Gait**

- For the three-point alternate gait the patient must be able to bear the total body weight on one foot; the affected foot or leg is either partially or totally non-weight-bearing.
- In this gait both crutches are moved forward together with the affected leg while the weight is being borne by the patient's hands on the crutches. The unaffected leg is then advanced forward.

✓ **Going Downstairs**

- Crutches are advanced to the lower step and affected leg goes down the stairs first.
- Transfer weight to the crutches and move the good leg down.

✓ **Going Upstairs**

- Unaffected leg moves up the stair first, followed by the crutches and affected leg.

CANES

- The cane is used on the side opposite the affected leg.
- The cane and the affected leg move together.

WALKERS

- The arms should be bent about 30° degrees when the client is standing in front of the walker.
- Lift the walker and place it approximately two feet in front, provides equal weight bearing.
- Gain balance before moving walker forward again.

NCLEX ALERT: *Monitor client for presence/appropriate use of assistive devices(e .g., walkers, canes, crutches). Review changes in client neurological status.*

Reproductive System

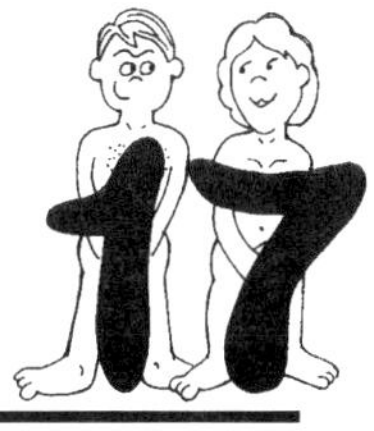

PHYSIOLOGY OF THE REPRODUCTIVE SYSTEM

Male Reproductive System

A. External genitalia

1. Penis - serves both a reproductive and urinary function.
2. Scrotum - a wrinkled, double sac of skin divided by an internal septum; functions as protection of the testes and sperm by maintaining a temperature lower than that of the body.

B. Internal genitalia.

1. Testes (gonads) - a pair of oval glandular organs normally contained in the scrotum. Function is sperm formation and production of testosterone.
2. Excretory duct system.
   a. Epididymis - produces some semen.
   b. Vas deferens - two short tubular structures extending from the epididymis up through the inguinal canal to the ejaculatory ducts;
   c. Ejaculatory ducts - a passage for semen and seminal vesicle fluid.

C. Semen.

1. Sterility: sperm count less than 20 million per milliliter; (normal sperm count 100 million per milliliter.)
2. Storage of sperm: varies from a period of several hours to 40 days, depending primarily on the frequency of ejaculation.

Female Reproductive System

A. External genitalia (vulva).

1. Mons pubis (mons veneris) - soft, rounded, pad of fat covering the interior portion of the synthesis pubis.
2. Labia majora - two longitudinal folds of skin extending from the mons pubis around the external vaginal opening or the introitus, to the perineum; smaller inner folds of tissue called labia minora .
3. Perineal body (perineum) - an area of fibromuscular tissue located between the vagina and the anal opening.

B. Internal genitalia.

1. Vagina.
2. Cervix (neck of the womb).
   a. Cervical mucosa functions to provide lubrication.
   b. Provides an alkaline environment to shelter sperm from the acidic vagina.
   c. Cervical mucus pH increases (alkaline) and becomes clear and more viscous at ovulation.
3. Uterus - a hollow, pear-shaped muscular pelvic organ; located between the bladder and the rectum.
4. Fallopian tubes - two small tubular structures; attached to the upper, outer section of the uterus.
5. Ovaries - two almond-shaped organs located behind and below the fallopian tubes. Produce ovum, estrogen, and progesterone.

C. Breasts

1. Function to provide nourishment through the lactation process.
2. Nipples - sensitive, erectile tissue which becomes more rigid and prominent during the menstrual cycle, sexual excitement, pregnancy and lactation.
3. Areola - a heavily pigmented area surrounding the nipple.

D. Menstrual cycle.

1. The cyclical hormonal changes occurring from menarche to menopause.
2. Phases.
   a. Menstrual phase - shedding of the superficial two-thirds of the endometrium; initiated by periodic vasoconstriction of the spiral arteries.
   b. Proliferative phase - a period of rapid growth; extends from day five to ovulation.
   c. Secretory phase - follows ovulation; large amounts of progesterone are produced; uterine lining is prepared to receive and nourish a fertilized ovum if one is available.
3. Fertilization - generally occurs in the outer third of the fallopian tube; a single ejaculation deposits 2.5 to 4.0 cc of semen, containing approximately 200 to 400 million spermatozoa.
4. Implantation - the zygote (fertilized ovum) is propelled by ciliary action of the fallopian tube into the uterine cavity; implants into the endometrium about seven to ten days after fertilization.

Data Collection

A. External assessment.

1. Inspect penis, scrotum, and vulva for normal hair distribution.

2. Assess vulvar area for discharge, erythema, or growths.
3. Assess penis for growths, masses, discharge, ulcers, or vesicles.
4. Inspect breasts for inversion, retraction, secretions, nodules, lumps, or masses.
5. Determine if there is any abdominal pain or tenderness upon palpation.

B. History.

1. Menstrual history.
   a. Age of onset.
   b. Last menstrual period.
   c. Duration of cycle, amount of flow, and use of birth control methods.
2. Obstetric history.
3. Urinary system.
   a. Pattern of voiding - dysuria, urgency, nocturia, frequency.
   b. Difficulty starting stream, stopping stream, changing the force of stream, or a feeling of incomplete emptying of bladder.
4. Change in sexual function.
   a. Ability to achieve erection and ejaculation.
   b. Problems with intercourse.
   c. Bleeding after intercourse.
   d. Contact with sexually transmitted diseases.

DISORDERS OF THE MALE REPRODUCTIVE SYSTEM

Prostate Disorders

❑ **Benign prostatic hyperplasia (BPH) - enlargement and increase in size of prostate gland tissue.**

❑ **Cancer of the prostate - a malignancy of the prostate gland.**

> ***NURSING PRIORITY:*** *Prostate problems occur in the majority of men over 60 years old. Questions may be asked regarding assessment, care after surgery, and teaching.*

Data Collection

1. Common to both disorders.
   a. Urinary hesitancy, frequency, urgency, and dribbling.
   b. Nocturia, urinary retention, and a sensation of incomplete emptying of the bladder.
2. BPH.
   a. Prostatic enlargement noted primarily in the median and lateral lobes of the prostate.
   b. Often first symptom is nocturia.
3. Prostatic cancer.
   a. Unilateral prostatic enlargement - "stony hard" and fixed.
   b. Pain in the lumbosacral area radiating down into the hips or legs.
   c. Weight loss and anorexia.
   d. Urinary tract symptoms occur late in a malignancy.
4. Diagnostics.
   a. BPH.
      (1) Digital rectal examination.
      (2) Prostate biopsy.
      (3) Urinalysis
   b. Prostatic cancer.
      (1) Elevated serum acid phosphatase.
      (2) In advanced stages, bone scan will show metastatic areas in the bone.
      (3) Prostatic specific antigen (PSA) serum test; value should be below 4ng/dl.
      (4) Sexual dysfunction

> ***NURSING PRIORITY:*** *Carefully assess the client with BPH in regard to anticholinergic medications that cause urinary retention as a side effect. A common medication causing problems is atropine, which may be included in preoperative medications.*

Treatment

1. Surgical
   a. Transurethral resection of the prostate (TURP) - removal of prostatic tissue via a resectoscope which is passed through the urethra; primary treatment for BPH.
   b. Suprapubic prostatectomy - removal of the prostate through a lower midline abdominal incision, through the bladder, into the anterior aspect of the prostate.
   c. Retropubic prostatectomy - a low abdominal incision is made into the prostate gland without entering the bladder.
   d. Perineal prostatectomy - incision is made between the scrotum and the anus; most often used for cancer of the prostate; often results in impotence and urinary incontinence.
2. Medical
   a. Medications (See Appendix 17-1)
   b. Transurethral probe, balloon dilation

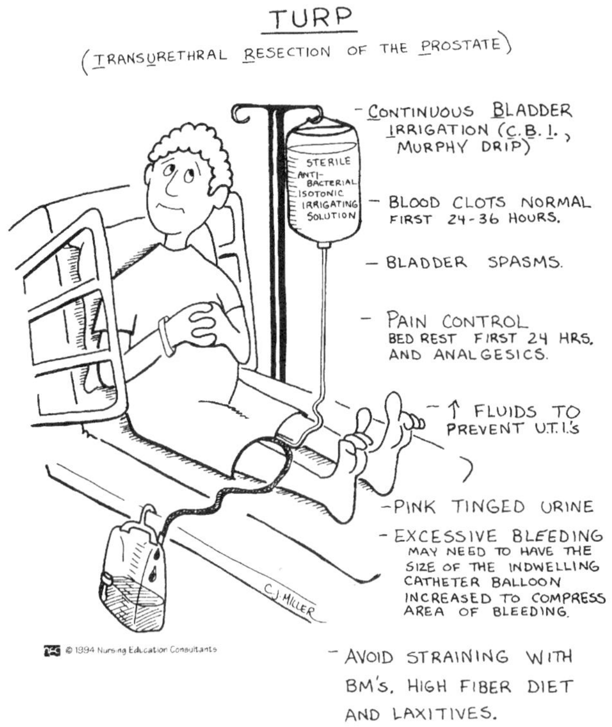

Figure 17-1: Transurethral Resection of the Prostate
Zerwekh, J. & Claborn, J. (2000). *Memory Notebook of Nursing*, Vol. 1, Dallas, TX: Nursing Education Consultants, Inc.

Complications

1. BPH.
   a. Preoperative.
      (1) Urinary tract infection.
      (2) Renal calculi.
      (3) Rupture of overstretched blood vessels in the bladder - hematuria.
      (4) Hydroureter and hydronephrosis, causing increased pressure on the kidney.
      (5) Dribbling and incontinence of urine
   b. Postoperative.
      (1) Hemorrhage.
      (2) Urethral stricture.
      (3) Bladder spasms.
      (4) Retrograde ejaculation - semen passed into the bladder rather than out through the penis.
      (5) Epididymitis.
2. Prostatic cancer.
   a. Preoperative.
      (1) Complications are similar to BPH.
      (2) Cancer may spread via the perineal lymphatic system to the regional lymph nodes; from the veins of the prostate it spreads to the pelvic bones, bladder, lungs and liver.
   b. Postoperative - same as BPH, but most often does experience sexual dysfunction.

Nursing Intervention

✦ *Goal: to promote elimination, treat urinary tract infection, and provide client education related to surgery and sexual functioning.*

1. Assess for adequate bladder emptying.
2. Assess for symptoms of urinary tract infection; promote adequate fluid intake
3. Determine client's ability to discuss concerns related to sexual functioning and implications for surgery.

NCLEX ALERT: *Monitor client elimination status.*

✦ *Goal: to provide postoperative care by assessing and preventing complications (hemorrhage, bladder spasms, and infection), restoring normal urinary control, and providing opportunity to discuss sexual concerns.*

1. Continuous bladder irrigation (CBI) with sterile isotonic irrigating solution.
   a. Continuous bladder irrigation is usually accomplished with a triple lumen catheter: one lumen for inflating the balloon, one for maintaining outflow of urine, one for the instillation of the continuous irrigating solution.
   b. Provides continuous irrigation to prevent infection and rid the bladder of tissue and clots following TURP.
   c. Frequent assessment of urinary drainage to determine patency of catheter and presence of bleeding or clots.
2. Blood clots are normal for first 24 to 36 hours.
3. If client has excessive bleeding, the physician may increase the size of the balloon on the indwelling catheter and put traction on the catheter to compress the area of bleeding.

***NURSING PRIORITY:** Prevent over distention of the bladder. If client complains of pain, check the urinary drainage system first and make sure it is patent. Obstruction most commonly occurs in the first 24 hours, due to clots in the bladder. Over distention of the bladder precipitates hemorrhage as well as bladder spasms.*

4. Bladder spasms can occur -often spasms occur due to presence of clots in the catheter.

5. Decrease pain with bed rest and analgesics; after client is ambulatory, encourage walking rather than sitting for prolonged periods.
6. Evaluate ability to empty bladder completely and presence of dribbling prior to discharge.

NCLEX ALERT: *Monitor effective funtioning of therapeutic devices prescribed for client.*

Self-Care

1. Teach client exercises to control urinary stream and maintain continence.
   a. Contract perineal muscle by squeezing buttocks together.
   b. Practice starting and stopping the stream several times during voiding.
2. Prevent straining during bowel movement by eating a diet high in fiber and taking stool softeners.
3. Encourage high fluid intake to prevent bladder infections.

Inflammatory Disorders

❑ **Prostatitis - inflammation of the prostate; usually caused by bacteria or by a sudden decrease in sexual activity.**

❑ **Epididymitis - inflammation of epididymis usually secondary to prostatitis or a urinary tract infection; often develops as a complication of gonorrhea; in men under age 35 major cause is Chlamydia trachomatis.**

Data Collection

1. Prostatitis.
   a. Perineal, rectal, or back pain.
   b. Burning, frequency, urgency, and dysuria.
   c. Prostate is enlarged, firm, and tender when palpated.
2. Epididymitis.
   a. Pain and tenderness in the inguinal canal.
   b. Swelling in the scrotum and groin.
   c. Temperature and chills.
   d. Pyuria and bacteriuria.

Treatment

1. Prostatitis - analgesics, stool softeners, and sitz baths.
2. Epididymitis.
   a. Bed rest with elevation of the scrotum (scrotal support or scrotal bridge).

Box 17-1: Elderly Care Focus

Benign Prostatic Hypertrophy (BPH)

General

All men over 60 years of age should be assessed for urinary retention and adequacy of bladder emptying.

Increased problem with urinary stasis; increased straining to urinate; increased incidence of infections.

Postoperatively

Closely evaluate for presence of infection, especially UTI, respiratory.

Assess fluid balance; confusion and agitation may be symptoms of fluid overload.

Assist the client to ambulate as soon as possible - increased risk for pooling of blood in pelvic cavity and pulmonary emboli from immobility.

Increased risk for falls.

Determine psychological response to physical stress (confusion, disorientation); orient to surroundings frequently.

   b. Treatment of client's sexual partners (chlamydial infection).

Complications

1. Chronic prostatitis can lead to recurrent urinary tract infection and epididymitis.
2. May have chronic recurring incapacitating infections.

Nursing Intervention

✦ *Goal: to assist client to understand the implications of the disease and measures to maintain health.*

1. Encourage early treatment to prevent complications.
2. In chronic prostatitis encourage activities that drain the prostate such as intercourse, masturbation, and prostatic massage.
3. Client should avoid straining (lifting) and sexual excitement until acute infection is under control.
4. Encourage treatment of sexual partners when epididymitis is of chlamydial origin.

Undescended Testes (Cryptorchidism)

❑ **This condition is the failure of one or both testes to descend into the scrotal sac. If testis remains undescended it will cause problems of sperm production and increased risk of testicular cancer.**

Data Collection

1. Inability to palpate the testes in the scrotal sac.
2. Inguinal hernia most often present also.

Treatment

1. Surgical intervention - (orchidpexy).
   a. Usually done around 2 years of age or before.
   b. Generally done on an outpatient basis.
   c. Testis is brought through the inguinal canal and anchored in the scrotum.

NCLEX ALERT: *Review teaching with cliet about health promotion - testicular sefl-exams.*

Nursing Intervention

Self-Care

1. Keep the scrotal area clean of urine and stool.
2. Long- term follow-up regarding fertility.
3. Teach parents to instruct the child of the importance of self examination when he is old enough.

Tumors of the Testes

❑ **These tumors are often malignant and tend to metastasize quickly; condition is most often unilateral.**

Data Collection

1. Most common cancer in men age 15 to 35.
2. More common in clients who have had cryptorchidism and infections.
3. A mass is palpated in the scrotum; the client may or may not complain of pain; most men experience a heaviness in the scrotum.
4. Backache, pain in the abdomen, loss of weight may occur in a malignancy.

Treatment

1. Surgical intervention - orchiectomy (removal of the testis) and/or a radical retroperitoneal lymph node resection.
2. Medical.
   a. Radiation.
   b. Chemotherapy.

Nursing Intervention

✦ *Goal: to detect any abnormality of the testes through client's self-examination.*

1. Teach client, especially those between ages 15 and 35, to self-examine monthly while showering or bathing, to detect any abnormal mass or change of contents of the scrotum.
2. Emphasize importance of follow-up of client with a history of undescended testis or a previous testicular tumor.

✦ *Goal: to assist the client to understand the implications of surgery.*

DISORDERS OF THE FEMALE REPRODUCTIVE SYSTEM

Common Gynecological Problems

Vaginal Inflammatory Conditions

Common predisposing factors

1. Excessive douching.
2. Oral contraceptives.
3. Antibiotics - especially broad-spectrum, which wipe out normal vaginal flora.
4. Steroids.
5. Stressful situations.
6. Improper cleaning after voiding and defecating.
7. Diabetics or prediabetics are more predisposed to the development of chronic vaginal problems.

Bacterial Vaginitis

1. Causative organism - *Gardnerella vaginalis*.
2. Malodorous vaginal discharge (fishy smell).
3. Sexual partner usually is not treated.

Candidiasis

1. Organism - *Candida albicans* (fungus or yeast infection).
2. Internal itching, beefy red irritation, inflammation of vaginal epithelium.
3. White, cheese-like discharge which clings to the vaginal mucosa.

Trichomoniasis

1. Organism - *Trichomonas vaginalis* (protozoan).
2. Itching, burning, painful intercourse.
3. Frothy, yellowish white or yellowish-brown, malodorous vaginal discharge.
4. Sexual partner needs to be treated because of cross infection. Men are usually asymptomatic.

Postmenopausal Vaginitis (Atrophic Vaginitis)

1. Due to lack of estrogen.
2. Itching and burning.
3. Dyspareunia.

Nursing Intervention

✦ *Goal: client education regarding personal hygiene to prevent infection and promote comfort.*

1. Appropriate cleansing from front of vulva to back of perineal area.
2. Frequently infection is worse around the menstrual period. Teach client to change tampons 3 to 4 times a day.
3. Do not douche. The normal protective bacteria are washed out and other bacteria are introduced.
4. If infection is chronic, it may be necessary to have sexual partner tested; he may be reinfecting the woman.

✦ *Goal: to assist the woman to decrease the inflammation.*

1. Sitz baths may decrease inflammation and promote healing and comfort.
2. Nylon underware, wet bathing suits encourage excessive moisture and heat which interferes with the healing process and comfort.
   a. Avoid tight clothing and panty hose.
   b. Encourage the client to wear cotton-lined undergarments.
3. Avoid use of feminine hygiene sprays.

✦ *Goal: to educate the woman regarding correct utilization of medications .*

1. Vaginal suppositories, ointments, and creams are often utilized (Appendix 17-1).
   a. Teach client importance of hand washing before and after insertion of suppository or application of cream.
   b. Advise client to remain recumbent for 30 minutes after application to promote absorption and prevent loss of the medication from the vaginal area.
   c. Encourage client to wear a perineal pad to prevent soiling of clothing with vaginal drainage.

Abnormal Uterine Bleeding

Amenorrhea -

1. Absence of menses - primary, (no menstruation has occurred), or secondary, (previously had menses).
2. May be indicative of menopause,
3. May be first indication of pregnancy.
4. Occurs when woman has lost a critical fat percentage(athletes, anorexia).

Menorrhagia

1. Excessive vaginal bleeding.
2. Single episode of heavy bleeding may indicate a spontaneous abortion.
3. May be associated with IUD.
4. Hypothyroidism.

Metrorrhagia

1. Vaginal bleeding between periods.
2. May be normal menopause.
3. Ectopic pregnancy.
4. Breakthrough bleeding from oral contraceptives.
5. Cervical polyps.

***NURSING PRIORITY:** Vaginal bleeding after menopause or surgical hysterectomy is a symptom of problems and needs to be evaluated.*

Nursing Intervention

1. Assist to determine most likely cause of problem.
2. Next period may not occur, or may not be on schedule.
3. Report excessive bleeding, abdominal pain, fever.

Pelvic Inflammatory Disease (PID)

❑ **PID is an infectious condition of the pelvic cavity that involves the fallopian tubes, the ovaries, or the peritoneum.**

Data Collection

1. Risk factors/etiology.
   a. Frequent complication of gonorrhea or staphylococcal infections.
   b. Can occur following abortion, pelvic surgery and childbirth.
   c. Intrauterine devices (IUD) are correlated with increased incidence of PID.
2. Clinical manifestations.
   a. General malaise, fever, nausea, and vomiting.
   b. Leukocytosis.
   c. Bilateral lower abdominal pain.
   d. Vaginal discharge which is heavy and purulent.
   e. Chronic PID - persistent pelvic pain, secondary dysmenorrhea, dysfunctional uterine bleeding, and periodic episodes of acute symptoms.
3. Complications.
   a. Sterility.
   b. Ectopic pregnancy.

Treatment

1. Medical.
   a. Antibiotics.
   b. Analgesics.
2. Surgical.
   a. Incision and drainage of abscesses with or without a laparotomy.

Nursing Intervention

✦ *Goal: to prevent the spread and extension of the infection.*

1. Semi-Fowler's position may decrease spread of infection by gravity.
2. Frequent change of pad and tampons during menses.
3. Good hand washing before and after voiding or changing pads or tampon.
4. Provide frequent perineal care.
5. Encourage oral fluids and adequate nutrition.
6. Client should avoid sexual activities until advised by health care provider.

✦ *Goal: to provide psychological support.*

1. Encourage expression of feelings related to guilt and possibility of sterility.

Endometriosis

❑ **Endometriosis is the presence of endometrial tissue outside of the uterus. The tissue responds to hormonal stimulation by bleeding into areas within the pelvis, causing pain and adhesions.**

Data Collection

1. Dysmenorrhea; deep-seated aching pain in the lower abdomen, vagina, posterior pelvis, and back occurring one to two days before menses.
2. Abnormal excessive uterine bleeding and painful intercourse.
3. Painful or difficulty in defecation.
4. Diagnosed by a culdoscopy and laparoscopy.

Treatment

1. Medications - oral contraceptives or hormones to decrease proliferation of tissue.
2. Surgical intervention.
   a. Excision of endometrial tissue in the extrauterine sites.
   b. Panhysterectomy (may be done for women close to the menopause).

Nursing Intervention

✦ *Goal: to assist client to understand the implications of the disease process and postoperative care.*

1. Reproductive ability and menses will be lost.
2. Provide reassurance that sexual activity will be normal after the surgery.
3. Determine from the physician if the client will be on hormone replacement after the surgery - discuss hormone replacement with her.
4. Avoid activities that increase pelvic congestion - sitting or prolonged standing.
5. Provide opportunity for her to share her feelings regarding change in her body.

Cervical Cancer

Data Collection

1. Risk factors/etiology.
   a. Early sex life including several partners.
   b. Smoking and use of oral contraceptives.
   c. Daughters of women who took diethylstilbestrol (DES) during their pregnancies.
2. Clinical manifestation.
   a. May be asymptomatic.
   b. Leukorrhea (a yellow or whitish vaginal discharge).
   c. Painless vaginal discharge between periods.
   d. Thin and watery drainage which later becomes dark and foul- smelling as the disease progresses.
3. Diagnostics - Papanicolaou smear (Pap Smear)
   a. Annual PAP smear should begin at 18 years old, or when woman becomes sexually active.
   b. PAP smears are continued after menopause and hysterectomy.
   c. Client should not douche or use vaginal medications 24 hours prior to smear.
   d. Classification of Pap smears.
      (1) Normal result - no malignant cells.
      (2) Significant inflammation - no malignant cells.
   e. International classification of cervical cancer.
      (1) Stage 0 - preinvsive, carcinoma in situ.
      (2) Stage 1 - cancer strictly confined to cervix.
      (3) Stage 2 - Cancer extends beyond the cervix, but not the pelvic wall.
      (4) Stage 3 - cancer extends to one or both pelvic walls.
      (5) Stage 4 - extension of cancer beyond pelvis.

> ***NURSING PRIORITY:** If cancer of the cervix is identified prior to becoming invasive, there is virtually a 100% cure rate.*

   f. Biopsy and conization of the cervix.
      (1) Avoid strenuous activity for 24 hours.
      (2) Remove vaginal packing as directed.
      (3) Abstain from sexual intercourse for approximately 24 hours.
      (4) Avoid using tampons and douching.

Treatment

(Surgical intervention)

1. Conization - used for microinvasive cervical cancer.
2. For invasive cervical cancer, the following procedures may be done:
   a. Vaginal hysterectomy - removal of the uterus; fallopian tubes and ovaries remain intact.
   b. Total abdominal hysterectomy - bilateral salpingo-oophorectomy (TAH-BSO) - total hysterectomy includes removal of fallopian tubes and ovaries.
   c. Pelvic exoneration - radical hysterectomy plus total vaginectomy, removal of bladder with urinary diversion, bowel resection, and colostomy.
3. Radiation therapy either intracavitary implants (radium implant) or external.

Nursing Intervention

✦ *Goal: to provide pre-and postoperative teaching in preparation for a total abdominal hysterectomy.*

1. General preoperative care.
2. Postoperatively assess for complications involving urinary output
   a. Foley catheter - evaluate urinary output.
   b. Assess for difficulty urinating after catheter is removed.
   c. Assess for urinary tract infection.
3. Early ambulation is encouraged.
4. Prevent postoperative thrombophlebitis.

Self-Care

1. Sexual activity when physician advises.
2. Avoid straining abdominal muscles.
3. Report any bleeding or discharge.
4. Continue with annual physical and PAP smear.
5. Client who has had a pelvic exoneration will have many concerns regarding sexual function, as the vagina will be lost, surgical menopause will occur, and there will be a urinary or bowel diversion to the abdominal wall (an ileoconduit or colostomy).

Cystocele and Rectocele

Data Collection

1. Cystocele - outward displacement of the bladder into the vagina.
   a. Stress incontinence - during coughing, lifting, or sneezing.
   b. Frequency and urgency.
2. Rectocele - herniation of the bowel into the vagina.
   a. Constipation.
   b. Incontinence of gas or liquid feces.
3. Common complications.
   a. Infection.
   b. Hemorrhoids.
   c. Cystitis.

Treatment

1. Surgical intervention.
   a. Cystocele - repaired by a procedure called an anterior colporrhaphy.
   b. Rectocele - repaired by a posterior colporrhaphy.
   c. Procedure is usually called A and P repair.

Nursing Intervention

✦ *Goal: to assist client to understand the implications of and be prepared for surgery.*

1. Preoperative teaching.
2. Postoperative period.
   a. Prevent wound infection.
   b. Prevent pressure on suture line in the vagina.
   c. Perineal care usually BID and after each voiding or defecation.

Self-Care

1. Encourage the use of mild laxatives to prevent straining at stool.
2. Discuss a low-residue diet.
3. Activities that are restricted include heavy lifting, prolonged standing, walking, sitting, and intercourse until area has healed.

Breast Carcinoma

Data Collection

1. Risk factors/etiology.
   a. Increased incidence in women over 50 years old.
   b. Family history of breast cancer.
   c. Nulliparous women or those whose first pregnancy occurred after age 30.
   d. Early menses, late menopause. Removal of the ovaries prior to age 40 significantly decreases the risk of breast cancer.
   e. The incidence of recurrence of breast cancer is significant. Almost 25% of women who have a malignancy will develop recurrences even with surgical intervention and negative lymph nodes. The incidence of recurrence, increases dramati-

cally in those women who have positive detection of malignant cells in the lymph nodes.

2. Clinical manifestations.
   a. Asymmetry of the breast.
   b. Skin dimpling, flattening, or nipple retraction.
   c. Skin coloring and thickening, large pores, sometimes called peau d'orange (orange peel appearance).
   d. Changes in the nipple, discharge from the nipple.
   e. Painless, nontender, and irregular mass
3. Diagnostics.
   a. Mammography.
   b. Breast biopsy.
4. Complications - Metastases via the lymphatic system to the bone, lung, brain, and liver.

Treatment

1. Surgical.
   a. Lumpectomy - Removal of the mass along with some normal tissue.
   b. Axillary node dissection - may be done to stage the malignancy and determine appropriate chemotherapy/radiation therapy.
   c. Mastectomy - removal of all of the breast tissue, axillary nodes, and overlying skin. Extent of surgery depends on invasiveness of malignancy.
2. Radiation - may be used in combination with lumpectomy and axillary node resection for early stage treatment.
3. Hormonal therapy
4. Chemotherapy

Nursing Intervention

✦ *Goal: to promote early detection of breast cancer through public education and self breast examination.*

NCLEX ALERT: *Review teaching with client about health promotion - self breast exam.s*

1. Risk factors; educate women regarding who is at an increased risk.
2. Perform self breast examinations (SBE) on a regular basis in order to determine abnormalities (Table 17-1).
3. Women over 40 should have a mammogram every 1 to 2 years; women over 50 should have a mammogram every year.

Table 17-1: Self-Breast Examination

✦ **Step 1:** Inspect your breasts before a mirror to determine asymmetry or changes in size, breast should be evaluated from three positions: with the arms relaxed at the side; with the arms high over the head; with the hands on the hips, pressing down firmly to flex chest muscle.

✦ **Step 2:** Lie down; flatten the right breast by placing a pillow under the right shoulder and extending the right arm with fingers flat, using the sensitive pads of the middle three fingers of your left hand, press firmly enough to feel the different breast tissue. Systematically examine all of the breast from the collarbone to the base of your bra and the axillary area. Gently squeeze the nipple of each breast to determine presence of any discharge.

✦ **Step 3**: Examine your breasts in the shower or during a bath - this allows the hand to glide over the skin more smoothly. With your fingers flat, systematically and gently move over every part of each breast.

***NURSING PRIORITY:** When teaching a woman, SBE should be done about a week after menses or for postmenopausal women, at same time each month.*

4. The American Cancer Society provides extensive information for women regarding early detection of breast cancer and rehabilitation after a mastectomy.

✦ *Goal: to prepare the client physiologically and psychologically for surgery (normal pre-and postoperative care, Chapter 3).*

1. Assist woman to decrease emotional stress and anxiety; encourage spiritual and social resources.
2. Anticipate concerns related to sexuality and fear of rejection by husband or sex partner after the mastectomy.

✦ *Goal: to recognize and prevent postoperative complications (modified radical mastectomy).*

1. There may be one or more portable suction drains in the incisional area.
2. Elevate the bed about 30 degrees and keep the affected arm elevated, to promote lymphatic drainage.
3. Do not take blood pressure or perform any injections or venipuncture on the arm of the affected side.

NCLEX ALERT: *Provide support to client with changes in bdoy image.*

NURSING PRIORITY: The arm on the affected side will be at increased risk for developing problems of edema and infection due to the removal of the axillary lymph node tissue, causing altered lymph drainage. Any procedure that hampers circulation or causes any loss of skin integrity should be avoided. This must be discussed with the woman and the arm protected throughout the rehabilitation and during activities of daily living for an indefinite period of time.

4. Arm exercises are usually started 24 hours after surgery.
   a. Assist/teach the woman to perform flexion and extension exercises with the wrist and elbow frequently throughout the day. Squeezing a ball is good exercise at this period.
   b. The affected arm should not be abducted, or externally rotated in initial exercises. Encourage gentle use of the arm in activities of daily living (brushing her hair, eating, washing her face).
5. Active exercises are begun after wound healing is well-established. Exercises may still be done from the supine position, but more complete range of motion is encouraged, with some abduction and external rotation of the upper arm.
6. Approximately two to three weeks after surgery and with good wound healing, more active exercises are begun.
   a. Pendulum arm swings.
   b. Pulley-type rope exercise to promote forward and lateral movement of the arms.
   c. "Wall climbing" with the fingers.

✦ *Goal: to promote client's return to homeostasis and understand implications of modified lifestyle; identify measures to maintain health.*

1. Discuss symptoms of recurrence and importance of maintaining regular visits to the physician to monitor recovery and to detect changes.
2. Promote a positive self-image and reintegration with family.
3. Discuss obtaining breast prosthesis about 6 to 8 weeks after surgery.
4. Encourage the woman to participate in the Reach for Recovery Program through the American Cancer Association. Check with the physician to see if representatives may visit with the client prior to the surgery.

SEXUALLY TRANSMITTED DISEASES

A. Characteristics of sexually transmitted diseases (STD).
   1. Are transmitted by sexual activity; including oral and rectal activities and between people of the same and opposite sex.
   2. One person can have more than one STD at a time.
   3. All sexual partners need to be evaluated.

B. Nursing role to recognize and provide factual information.
   1. Mode of transmission.
   2. Prevention of transmission.
   3. Importance of contacts being identified and treated.
   4. Information provided in accepting, non-judgmental manner.

NURSING PRIORITY: Consider all oral, genital, and rectal lesions on a client to contain pathologic organisms until documented otherwise.

Syphilis

❑ **A sexually transmitted disease caused by the spirochete *Treponema pallidum*.**

Data Collection

1. Incubation period: 10 to 90 days, average is 20 to 30 days.
2. Transmission: direct contact with primary chancre lesion, body secretions (saliva, blood, vaginal discharge, semen), and transplacentally to the fetus.
3. Communicability: highly infectious during the primary stage; blood contains spirochete during the secondary stage; during the latent stage usually noninfectious after 1 year, and late (tertiary) stage is noninfectious.
4. Primary stage.
   a. Chancre - painless lesion found on the penis, vulva, lips, vagina, or rectum.
   b. Usually heals spontaneously within 2 to 3 weeks, with or without treatment.
   c. Regional lymphadenopathy.
5. Secondary stage.
   a. Client may be asymptomatic for a period of time; secondary stage usually begins anywhere

from 2 weeks to 6 months after the chancre has healed.

b. Maculopapular rash on the palms of the hands and on the soles of the feet.

c. Generalized lymphadenopathy, gray mucous patches in the mouth.

d. Condylomata lata- flat lesions that may appear in moist areas, are highly infectious (not to be confused with venereal warts).

e. Symptoms will disappear within 2 to 6 weeks.

6. Latent stage.

a. Absence of clinical symptoms.

b. Serologic tests for syphilis remain positive.

c. Transmission through blood contact can occur.

d. The majority of clients remain in this stage without further symptoms.

7. Late syphilis - severe irreversible complications; is not contagious. (CNS, cardiovascular, bone and joint involvement).

8. Congenital syphilis.

a. Maculopapular rash over face, genital region, palms and soles.

b. Snuffles - a mucopurulent nasal discharge.

c. Nephrotic syndrome may develop.

9. Diagnostics.

a. Serologic screening tests - Venereal Disease Research Laboratories (VDRL)

b. Rapid plasma reagin (RPR).

c. Fluorescent Treponema Antibody Absorption (FTA-ABS) test.

d. The VDRL and FTA-ABS are based on presence of antibodies and are not positive until about 4 weeks after the appearance of the chancre.

Treatment

1. Antibiotics.

Nursing Intervention

✦ *Goal: to promote early detection and treatment.*

1. Public education of sexually transmitted diseases.

2. Education regarding hand washing and hygienic measures.

3. Encourage clients to seek serologic testing after 1, 3, 9 and 12 months of therapy.

4. Prenatal screening on first visit; early treatment of syphilis in pregnancy reduces incidence of congenital anomalies.

✦ *Goal: to report all cases to local public health authorities.*

Gonorrhea

❑ **Most common STD; an infection of the genitourinary tract; however, may affect the rectum, pharynx, and the eyes; caused by the bacteria *Neisseria gonorrhoeae*.**

Data Collection

1. Incubation period: 2 to 7 days.

2. Transmission: direct contact with exudate via sexual contact.

3. Communicability: contagious as long as organism is present.

4. Men.

a. Urethritis, dysuria, and purulent urethral discharge.

b. Increased evidence of asymptomatic disease or a chronic carrier state in males.

5. Women.

a. May be asymptomatic or have minor symptoms.

b. Vaginal discharge, dysuria, urinary frequency.

c. If untreated, may result in pelvic inflammatory disease (PID).

6. Neonate - ophthalmia neonatorum.

7. Diagnostics.

a. Antigen detection test for *C. trachomatis.*

b. Positive culture.

8. Complications.

a. Men: prostatitis, epidymititis, urethral strictures, urethritis, and sterility.

b. Women: PID, Bartholin abscess, ectopic pregnancy, infertility, and gonococcal arthritis.

Treatment

1. Antibiotics.

Nursing Intervention

1. Antibiotics - necessary to take the full course of treatment, doses are larger then average.

2. Prophylactic treatment for gonorrhea eye infection in the neonate - ophthalmia neonatorum.

3. Encourage follow-up cultures 7 to 14 days after treatment, and again at 6 months.

✦ *Goal: to reduce infectious process.*

1. Teach importance of abstinence from sexual intercourse until diagnostics are negative.

2. Urge client to inform sexual partner so that he or she may be treated for infection.

Genitalis Herpes (HVH Type II)

❑ **A highly contagious infection caused by the herpes virus hominis (HVH) Type II, which is characterized by painful vesicles surrounded by an erythematous area.**

Data Collection

1. Lesions characteristically occur below the waist, generally in the genital area. It is possible for the Type II lesions to cause oral lesions.
2. Initial sensation of tingling and itching prior to the appearance of the lesion.
3. Painful genital lesions that ulcerate.
4. Virus enters a latent phase and is harbored by the individual - recurrences of the infection occur when the virus is activated, usually by stress, sunburn, sexual activity, or fever.
5. Incubation period: unknown.
6. Transmission: by direct contact with the vesicles.
7. Lesions in pregnant women or a positive viral tissue culture confirming the diagnosis are a concern. Considerations will be made regarding the method of delivery.

Treatment

1. Antiviral medication (see Appendix 5-12).

Nursing Intervention

✦ *Goal: to assist client to understand implications of STD and measures to maintain health.*

1. Teach importance of genital hygiene and avoidance of sexual contact while lesions are present.
2. Teach good hygiene practices. If the lesions break open, the fluid contains the virus. The virus can be spread by contact and cause a lesion in any area of the body where it comes in contact with area of broken skin.

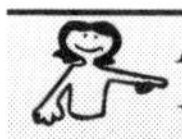

NURSING PRIORITY: *Always wear gloves when cleaning the perineal area of clients, to prevent herpetic whitlow, which is a herpes lesion around the nail bed. Nurses and other medical personnel are at risk for developing this because of local contact of the HVH virus on broken skin areas around the nail.*

✦ *Goal: to teach importance of genital hygiene and avoidance of sexual contact while lesions are present.*

1. If acyclovir is started at the earliest sign of a lesion, the course of the lesion may be decreased
2. Symptomatic treatment; sitz baths, wet compresses, and analgesics for relief of pain.

Chlamydia Infection, Non-gonococcal Urethritis (NGU)

Characteristics

❑ **An sexually transmitted disease caused by the *Chlamydia trachomatis.***

Data Collection

1. Males.
   a. Urethritis, epididymitis, prostatitis.
   b. Primary reservoir is the male urethra.
2. Females.
   a. Cervicitis, dysuria, pelvic pain, abnormal bleeding, purulent vaginal discharge.
   b. Primary reservoir is the cervix.
3. Effect of maternal infection on newborn: inclusion conjunctivitis and pneumonia.
4. Need to treat sexual partner.
5. Diagnostics: isolation of the organism in a tissue culture or serologic testing.
6. Incubation period: 7 to 21 days.

Nursing Intervention

✦ *Goal: to reduce spread of organism and provide measures to reduce infection.*

1. Urge client to have sexual partner treated.
2. Complete antibiotic treatment as prescribed.

Genital Warts (condyloma acuminata)

❑ **A common sexual transmitted disease characterized by clusters of warts caused by the human papillomavirus - HPV**

Data Collection

1. Female - cluster of warts on the vulva, vagina, cervix.
2. Male - clusters of warts on the glans penis or in the urethra
3. Diagnostics - observation and biopsy of the lesions

Treatment

1. Cryotherapy.

Nursing Intervention

✦ *Goal: Client education and health maintenance.*

1. Education regarding transmission and increased risk of genital malignancy .
2. Female- continue to follow up with annual PAP smears.
3. Transmitted by direct contact.

Study Questions—Reproductive

1. A client is one day postoperative from a suprapubic prostatectomy. The nurse notices pink-tinged urine in the client's urine bag. What is the best nursing interpretation of this finding?

① this is a normal occurrence at this time after this type of surgery.
② there is increased bleeding and the client should be kept on bed rest.
③ this is probably due to an infection, a urinalysis needs to be collected.
④ the continuous bladder irrigation should be increased to flush the bladder.

2. The nurse is evaluating her teaching with a client who has herpes genitalia (HVH II). How would she know her teaching was effective?

① client understands that after blisters break, she is no longer contagious.
② client understands the importance of washing her hands after touching her perineal area.
③ client understands the need to take **Zovirax** for the rest of her life to prevent additional outbreaks.
④ client understands that after initial outbreak she will be immune and have no further lesions.

3. Why are all sexually transmitted diseases (STDs) reported to the public health department?

① to slow transmission by informing all who may have had contact with the client
② to help the bureau of statistics study characteristics and decrease the incidence.
③ so the public health department will know who to treat.
④ to develop educational programs for the infected client and their sexual partners.

4. What tests are most often ordered for the routine screening of sexually transmitted diseases (STDs)?

① hematocrit, hemoglobin, and electrolytes.
② Western blot, urinalysis, and Chlamydia culture.
③ VDRL, urinalysis, GC culture.
④ VDRL, ELIZA, vaginal/urethral cultures.

5. A client has a painless lesion on the side of his penis. What is the nurses best interpretation of this finding?

① the presence of chancre lesion is characteristic of syphilis.
② lesion is characteristic in clients with long term gonorrhea.
③ the lesion may indicate the outbreak of herpes simplex virus.
④ area should be cultured for presence of papillomavirus.

6. The nurse is preparing a client for a pelvic examination. What is important for the nurse to do prior to the examination?

① make sure the client had a bowel prep and cleansing enema.
② carefully document the menstrual cycle, client should not be in last third of cycle.
③ question the client regarding her last period and possibility of pregnancy.
④ make sure the client voids prior to the procedure beginning.

7. The nurse is caring for a client the first postoperative day after a left side mastectomy. What observations would cause the nurse the most concern?

① temperature of 100.6° F, pulse at 110.
② moderate amount serosanguineous drainage on dressing.
③ left forearm and hand swollen, palpable radial pulse.
④ urine output at 40cc hour, slight increase in blood sugar.

8. An elderly client complains of vaginal itching and burning. What would be the best nursing management?

① douche daily with a weak vinegar solution.
② apply estrogen vaginal creme .
③ wash the perineal area well with soap and water.
④ encourage the use of petroleum jelly during intercourse.

9. The nursing assessment of a client with prostatic hypertrophy would identify which symptom?

① pain when voiding.
② urinary frequency.
③ distended bladder.
④ scrotal edema.

10. What equipment will be needed by the physician to check a client's prostate?

① straight catheter tray.
② urethral stints and gloves.
③ a lubricant and gloves.
④ stethoscope and rectal tube.

11. A client is post transurethral resection of the prostate (TURP) and is receiving a continuous bladder irrigation. The nurse notices that the fluid is not draining into the urinary catheter bag. The nurse attempts to irrigate in an attempt to clear the catheter line, but is unsuccessful. What would be the nurse's next action be?

① call the physician.
② irrigate again, increasing the pressure.
③ observe for 30 minutes before irrigating again.
④ replace the current catheter.

12.What is important to include in a teaching plan on testicular cancer?

① typical symptoms are frequency and urgency.
② it is usually a painless lesion that appears on the scrotum.
③ the tumor is slow growing tumor with a good prognosis.
④ it occurs primarily in the young adult male.

13. What is a common screening laboratory test to rule out prostate cancer?

① prostate specific antigen.
② prostatic fluid culture.
③ serum alkaline phosphatase.
④ urine specific gravity.

14. A 15 year old boy is being seen for orchitis. What would be important for the nurse to ask the boy's mother?

① has he had a recent urinary tract infection?
② has a severe sore throat or tonsillitis been a recent problem?
③ did her son have his routine childhood vaccinations?
④ does she know if her son has become sexually active?

15. A client complains of vaginal itching and irritation. What is important to teach this client?

① avoid douches and feminine hygiene products.
② increase intake of fluids and vitamin C.
③ perform a daily douche with a weak vinegar solution.
④ she does not have a sexually transmitted disease.

16. What is the recommended time for the woman to perform a self-breast examination?

① one week prior to her menstrual period.
② at the same time every month.
③ every time she takes a shower.
④ one week after her menstrual period.

17. The nurse is positioning a client for a pelvic examination. What position will the nurse place the client for the examination?

① lithotomy.
② semi-Fowler's
③ Trendelenburg.
④ left Sim's.

18. A client is postoperative mastectomy. What is an important nursing measure to assist in preventing complications?

① keep the affected arm below the heart to increase circulation.
② keep the affected arm elevated to decrease the edema to the extremity.
③ take her scheduled diuretics to reduce fluid level in the body.
④ apply lanolin cream to the incisional area to decrease scar formation.

19. A client is about 6 hours postoperative after a trans urethral resection of the prostate (TURP) with continuous bladder irrigation in place. What observation would indicate the development of a complication?

① catheter drainage of 50 cc and increase in complaints of pain.
② 200 cc of dark bloody drainage in catheter collection bag.
③ moderate amount of bloody drainage around the catheter insertion site.
④ client complains of burning and urge to void.

20. An elderly client with BPH is started on doxazosin (Cardura). What is important to evaluate after he has started the medication?

① presence of postural hypotension.
② development of tachycardia.
③ increase in difficulty voiding.
④ gastrointestinal disturbances and rash.

Appendix 17-1:
MEDICATIONS USED IN REPRODUCTIVE SYSTEM DISORDERS

MEDICATIONS	SIDE EFFECTS	NURSING IMPLICATIONS
ALPHA -1 ADRENERGIC BLOCKER: Medications decrease the size of the prostate, therefore decreasing pressure on the urinary tract in clients with BPH.		
Doxazosin (**Cardura**): PO Terazosin (**Hytrin**): PO	dizziness, fatigue, hypotension, dyspnea	1. Advise client of possible problems of decreased blood pressure and orthostatic hypotension. 2. Prostatic cancer should be ruled out before medications are started. 3. Medication should decrease problems of urination associated with BPH.
Finasteride (**Proscar**): PO	impotence, decreased libido	1. Client should take contraceptive precautions or not have sexual intercourse with women who could potentially get pregnant.
ANTIFUNGAL/PROTOZOAL MEDICATIONS: Used to treat vaginal infections.		
Over-the-counter: Clotrimazole (**Gyne-lotrimin**): intravaginally Miconazole (**Monistat 3**): intravaginally *Prescription only:* Fluconazole (**Diflucan**): PO, IV, intravaginally Terconazole (**Terazol**): intravaginally Metronidazole (**Flagyl**): PO, IV		1. Creams are not recommended to be used with tampons or diaphragms. 2. Not recommended for use in pregnancy or lactation. 3. **Flagyl** is used to treat trichomoniasis; teach client urine may turn red-brown and *to avoid alcohol*, as it can lead to serious side effects of throbbing headaches, nausea, excessive vomiting, hyperventilation, and tachycardia. 4. Suppositories or applicators are used to place medication in vagina. 5. If client does not see improvement within 3 days, she should return to her health care provider. 6. **Diflucan** can be given as a single dose for vaginal candidiasis.

Notes

PHYSIOLOGY OF THE KIDNEY AND URINARY TRACT

A. Kidneys.
  1. Two bean-shaped structures located in the back of the abdominal cavity (retroperitoneal).
  2. Structure.
    a. Cortex - outer layer, contains blood vessels and nephrons.
    b. Medulla - inner layer, contains the collecting tubules.
    c. Renal pelvis.
      (1) Funnel-shaped sac which collects the urine.
      (2) Calix (calices) drain the urine from the collecting ducts into the renal pelvis.
  3. Blood supply.
    a. 25% of cardiac output flows to the kidneys; approximately 1,200cc per minute.
    b. Renal arteries arise from the abdominal aorta.
    c. Renal veins carry blood back into the inferior vena cava.
  4. Function.
    a. Rid the body of metabolic wastes.
    b. Regulate fluid volume; normally 125cc of fluid is filtered each minute (glomerular filtration rate), however *only* one cc is excreted as urine; average urine output is about 1,440cc per day.
    c. Regulate the composition of electrolytes.
    d. Assist in maintaining acid-base balance.
    e. Regulation of blood pressure.
    f. Regulates red blood cell production through synthesis of erythropoietin; released in response to hypoxia.
    g. Aids in calcium metabolism by activating vitamin D.

B. Nephron.
  1. The functional unit of the kidney.
  2. Kidney composed of over a million nephrons.
  3. Structure.
    a. Glomerulus - a network of capillaries encased in a thin-walled sac (Bowman's capsule).
    b. Tubular system.
      (1) Proximal convoluted tubule.
      (2) Loop of Henle.
      (3) Distal convoluted tubule.
      (4) Collecting duct.
  4. Function of nephron.
    a. Filtration - occurs in the glomerulus via a semipermeable membrane.
    b. Glomerular filtration rate (GFR) is the amount of blood filtered by the glomeruli in a given time (approximately 125cc per minute).

NURSING PRIORITY: *Clients with a decrease in urinary output should be carefully evaluated regarding blood pressure level, to maintain adequate renal circulation. The level of blood pressure to maintain renal circulation varies greatly from one client to another.*

C. Urinary tract. (Figure 18-1)
  1. The excretory system and its blood supply.
  2. Ureters - convey urine from the kidneys to the bladder.
  3. Bladder.
    a. As the bladder fills, the stretch receptors are stimulated. In the adult, the first urge to void will occur when 150 cc to 200 cc have collected,;approximately 400 cc of urine will initiate a feeling of bladder fullness.

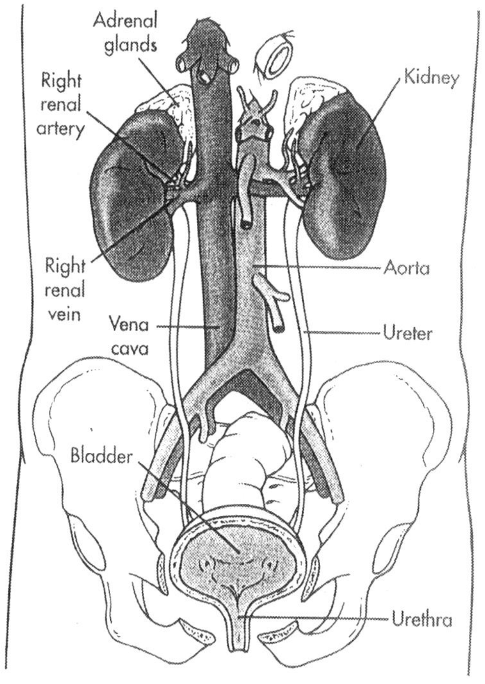

Figure 18-1: Structures of the urinary system
Reprinted with permission: Phipps, WJ, Sands, JK, & Marek, JF (1999). *Medical Surgical Nursing: Concepts & Clinical Practice*, 6th ed. Philadelphia: Mosby, p. 1396.

b. Bladder capacity varies from 1,000 to 1,800cc.

4. Urethra - a small tube which carries urine from the bladder to the exterior of the body.

5. Voiding - stimulation is sent to the sacral area of the spinal column, where the micturition reflex or voiding reflex is initiated.

System Data Collection

A. External assessment.

1. Inspect skin for changes in color, pallor, turgor, and texture (urate crystals).
2. Assess face, abdomen, and extremities for edema.
3. Determine weight gain.

B. History.

1. Presence of renal or urological congenital defect.
2. Determine if client has received antibiotics which may be nephrotoxic -aminoglycosides, amphotericin B, or sulfonamides.
3. Assess dietary intake - determine levels of calcium intake.
4. Evaluate level of activity - immobility leads to demineralization of the bones, which can predispose to infection and calculi formation.
5. Evaluate complaints of pain - dysuria, flank, or suprapubic.
6. Assess changes in pattern of urination - frequency, nocturia, urgency, or enuresis.
7. Assess changes in urine output - polyuria, oliguria, or anuria.
8. Assess changes in urine consistency - hematuria, pyuria, diluted, concentrated, or change in color.

DISORDERS OF THE URINARY TRACT

Urinary Tract Infections (UTI)

❑ **Stasis of urine in the bladder and reflux of urine back into the kidney are the primary factors in causing UTI.**

A. Upper urinary tract infection - ***pyelonephritis***, an inflammation of the renal pelvis.

B. Lower urinary tract infection.

1. ***Cystitis*** - inflammation of the bladder.
2. ***Urethritis*** - inflammation of the urethra.

C. Urinary tract infections occur in an ascending route up the urinary tract system.

Data Collection

1. Causative bacterial organisms - *E. coli* (80% to 90% of the time).
2. Factors contributing to UTI.

a. Adult female urethra is short; in close proximity to the rectum and vagina, which predisposes it to contamination from fecal material.

b. The reflux of urine from the urethra into the bladder. This causes a constant residual of urine in the bladder after voiding and precipitates UTI.

c. Instrumentation - catheterization or cystoscopic examination.

d. Stasis of urine in the bladder, leading to urinary retention for any reason (clients with prostate disease).

e. Obstruction to urinary flow - congenital anomalies, urethral strictures, ureteral stones, contracture of the bladder neck, BPH.

f. Bladder hypotonia, mechanical compression of the ureters, and hormone changes predispose the pregnant woman to increased urinary tract infections.

g. Metabolic disorders such as diabetes.

h. Sexual intercourse promotes development of UTI.

3. Clinical manifestations.

a. Cystitis.

(1) Frequency and urgency.
(2) Suprapubic pain.
(3) Voiding small amounts
(4) Hematuria.
(5) Fever, nausea, vomiting.
(6) Incomplete emptying of bladder.

b. Pyelonephritis.

(1) Fever, chills, flank pain.
(2) Painful urination (dysuria).
(3) Pain and tenderness at the costovertebral angle.
(4) Symptoms of cystitis.

4. Diagnostics.

a. Urinalysis - pus, bacteria, and RBCs found in the urine.

b. Urine test for culture and sensitivity -determines the specific bacteria and antibiotic sensitivity.

c. Acute pyelonephritis.

(1) Elevated WBC count.
(2) Cystourethrogram
(3) Intravenous pyelogram - indicates enlargement of involved kidney and abscess into renal tissue.

5. Complications.

a. A lower urinary tract infection may result in an upper urinary tract infection.

b. Chronic pyelonephritis may occur after repeated bouts of acute pyelonephritis.

Treatment

1. Medical.
   a. Sulfonamides (Appendix 5-10).
   b. Urinary antiseptics (Appendix 18-2).
   c. Urinary analgesics (Appendix 18-2).
2. Dietary.
   a. Encourage fluid intake of 3,000 cc per day.
      (1) A Dilute urine causes less irritation.
      (2) The increase in flow of urine through the urinary tract system decreases the movement of bacteria up the urinary tract.
      (3) Discourage carbonated beverages and foods or drinks containing baking powder or baking soda.
   b. A diet to increase the acidity of the urine — meats, eggs, cranberries, prunes, plums.

Nursing Intervention

✦ *Goal: to obtain relief of pain, urgency, dysuria, and fever.*

1. Antibiotics need to be taken the entire course which is usually 7 to 14 days.
2. Encourage eight to ten glasses of fluids daily.
3. Teach importance of voiding every two to three hours during the day to completely empty the bladder.
4. Sitz bath to decrease irritation of urethra.

✦ *Goal: to prevent recurrence of infection.*

1. Teach client to shower rather than bathe in tub. If client prefers to take a tub bath, she should avoid bubble bath additives.
2. Explain importance of cleansing the perineal area from front to back after each bowel movement.
3. Intercourse increases risk of infection; encourage voiding immediately after intercourse.
4. Long-term anti-microbial therapy to prevent recurrences.
5. Encourage and explain the need for follow-up care to prevent complications of chronic urinary tract infections.

NCLEX ALERT: *It is important for the nurse to initiate a toileting schedule, use methods to promote voiding, and assist the client to deal with incontinence.*

Box 18-1: Elderly Care Focus
Dealing with Incontinence

➻ *Need to determine:*

Does client have difficulty initiating urinary flow?
Is client aware of need to void?
Can client empty bladder completely or is there residual?
Is there bladder distention and overflow dribbling?
Is stress incontinence present?
What are usual voiding times?

➻ *Nursing Interventions*

Assisting the client to determine when he needs to urinate before an accident occurs.
Maintain adequate fluid intake, but limit fluids before bedtime.
Establish a voiding schedule - offer assistance and encourage voiding.
Make sure cleint has easy access to the bathroom.
Assess for presence of UTI.

Renal Calculi

❑ **Stones may form anywhere in the urinary tract;the most common location for stones is in the pelvis of the kidney. If the stones are small, they may be passed into the bladder.**

A. Stones in the bladder may increase in size if there is urinary stasis and alkaline pH.
B. Majority of stones contain calcium oxalate.

Data Collection

1. Risk factors - infection, urinary stasis, or immobility, history of previous stones.
2. Sharp, sudden, severe pain.
   a. May be described as "colic," either ureteral or renal.
   b. Nausea, diaphoresis, pallor, anxiety.
   c. Severe pain is most often precipitated by the movement of the stone into the ureter. There may be spasm in the ureter as it attempts to move the stone toward the bladder.
   d. Pain may radiate around the flank area, down into the genitalia and the bladder.
   e. Hematuria may be present from the traumatic effects of the stone on the ureter and the bladder.
   f. Pain may be intermittent.
3. Diagnostics - Intravenous pyelogram (IVP), retrograde pyelogram, and KUB x-ray (kidney, ureters, bladder).

Treatment

1. Medical.
   a. Increase fluid intake to decrease urine concentration.
   b. Insertion of ureteral catheter past the stone to maintain urine flow.
   c. Cystoscopy to manipulate stone
   d. Dietary - decrease calcium intake in client with calcium stones.
2. Surgical.
   a. Nephrolithotomy - incision into the kidney with removal of the stone.
   b. Ureterolithotomy - incision into the ureter to locate a stone and remove it.
   c. Percutaneous stone extraction - insertion of a tube through the skin into the renal collecting system; with gradual dilation the stone is extracted with forceps or by a stone basket.
3. Extracorporeal lithotripsy.
   a. Client is supported on a frame.
   b. Shock waves are directed to the stone. The force of the shock wave shatters the stone and the remains are excreted in the urine.
   c. It is essential that the client remain absolutely immobile during the procedure.
   d. Depending on the doctor and the status of the client as to the type of sedation or anesthesia. Procedure is not particularly painful; however, it is difficult for client to remain immobile for the time required.

Nursing Intervention

✦ *Goal: to relieve pain.*

1. Administer analgesics.
2. Hot baths or moist heat on flank area.
3. Encourage fluid intake.
4. Strain all urine and inspect for blood clots and passage of stone.

Self-Care

1. Client should be instructed as to importance of adhering to dietary restrictions.
2. Teach symptoms of recurring stone formation such as hematuria, flank pain, or signs of infection.
3. Encourage a 3,000 cc per day fluid intake (unless contraindicated).
4. Promote medical follow-up periodically to evaluate for symptoms of infection and recurring stone formation.

Hypospadias

❑ **Hypospadias - The urethral opening is located behind the glans penis, or along the penile shaft; fairly common problem.**

❑ **Epispadias - The urethral opening is located on the dorsal or upper side of the penis; is a rare problem.**

Data Collection

1. Visualization of defect.
2. Often, penis is crooked in appearance.
3. Stream of urine does not come out the end of the penis.
4. Often associated with undescended testes.

Treatment

1. Surgical correction of the defect; some recommend as early as 3-6 months, others 2 years.
2. Circumcison is not done on infants with hypospadias; foreskin may be used in the surgical correction of the defect.

Nursing Intervention

✦ *Goal: to provide emotional support and promote normal growth and development.*

1. Infant should not be circumcised until type of repair is determined, since foreskin may be used in repair.
2. Important not to delay repair, as child in school may be viewed differently from peers.
3. Surgical correction care.
   a. Teach parents how to care for indwelling urinary catheter.
   b. Demonstrate to parents effective methods for restraining child to prevent him from pulling on urinary catheter.
   c. Discuss with parents appropriate play activities for the child while catheter is in place.

DISORDERS OF THE KIDNEY

Nephrotic Syndrome

❑ **A problem in alteration of renal function due to glomerular injury. Cause is unknown.**

Data Collection

1. Majority of children are male and between ages of 2 and 6 years.
2. Proteinuria, hypoproteinemia, edema, and hyperlipidemia are classic signs.
3. Edema.

a. Facial edema, especially periorbital edema. May be more pronounced in the morning and subside some during the day.
b. Generalized edema of the lower extremities may increase during the day.
c. Labia and scrotum may become very edematous.
d. Edema may progress to the level of severe generalized edema (anasarca).

4. Gradual increase in weight.
5. Volume of urine is decreased and may be dark or tea-colored.
6. Irritability, fatigue, lethargy.
7. Skin is pale and is prone to break down during the edematous stage.
8. Ascites may develop.

Treatment

1. Medical.
   a. Corticosteroid.
   b. Diuretics - (frequently, child is not responsive to the diuretics; may be used when the edema is severe or the child is hypertensive).
   c. Salt-poor human albumin.
   d. Prophylactic antibiotics.
2. Dietary.
   a. Decreased sodium intake.
   b. There is usually no fluid restriction.

Nursing Intervention

✦ *Goal: to reduce edema and excess fluid retention.*

1. Support edematous organs such as scrotum.
2. Provide and encourage a salt-restrictive diet.
3. Provide meticulous skin care; change position frequently and monitor good body alignment.
4. Cleanse and powder opposing skin surfaces frequently.
5. Daily weights, accurate intake and output, measure abdominal girth.

✦ *Goal: to prevent infection.*

1. Child susceptible to infection, due to decreased immune state from steroid therapy.
2. Protect child from upper respiratory infections; good pulmonary hygiene.
3. Prevent skin excoriation and breakdown, assess carefully for indications of infection.

✦ *Goal: to promote nutrition.*

1. Encourage adequate protein intake or protein as ordered.
2. Serve small quantities of food to children.
3. Encourage input from child in selecting foods from prescribed diet.

Glomerulonephritis

❑ **An inflammatory reaction in the glomerulus as a result of an antigen-antibody response to the *group A beta-hemolytic Streptococcus.***

Data Collection

1. Acute glomerulonephritis.
   a. Disease may be mild - proteinuria.
   b. Headache and malaise.
   c. Facial edema, periorbital edema.
   d. Decrease in urine output (oliguria).
   e. Mild to severe hypertension.
   f. Tenderness over the costovertebral angle.

Treatment

1. Medical.
   a. Diuretics are usually not effective. May be utilized if the child is severely edematous.
   b. Antihypertensives.
   c. Antibiotics.
   d. Immunosuppresives.
   e. Plasmapheresis - removal of harmful blood components (antigen-antibody complex) from the plasma.
2. Dietary.
   a. Decrease sodium and potassium intake.
   b. Protein restriction if child is azotemic from prolonged decrease in urinary output. The anorexia the child experiences frequently limits the protein sufficiently.

Nursing Intervention

✦ *Goal: to maintain fluid balance.*

1. Monitor intake and output; maintain diet and fluid restrictions as ordered.
2. Monitor renal function - check characteristics and color of urine, weigh client daily, and check blood pressure every 2 to 4 hours.
3. Administer antihypertensives as ordered.
4. Frequently, the first sign of improvement is an increase in the urine output, then may progress to profuse diuresis.

✦ *Goal: to prevent complications and promote comfort.*

1. Encourage verbalization of fears.
2. Decrease anxiety by explaining treatments.

3. *Assess for complications related to hypertension, congestive heart failure, and chronic renal failure and report to RN.*

Self-Care

1. Teach client symptoms to be reported to physician - nausea, fatigue, vomiting, decrease in urinary output, or symptoms of infection.
2. Explain the need for rest, relaxation, and avoidance of people with respiratory infections.
3. Teach measures to prevent urinary tract infections.

Wilms' Tumor (Nephroblastoma)

❑ **This is one of the most common intra-abdominal tumors of childhood and is associated with congenital anomalies, especially those of the genitourinary tract. The treatment and survival rate are based on the stage of the tumor at the time it is discovered.**

Data Collection

1. Swelling or mass within the abdomen
2. Abdominal pain as tumor enlarges.
3. Hematuria, pallor, anorexia, and lethargy.
4. Hypertension.
5. Peak incidence is 2-3 years of age.

Treatment

The survival rates greatly depend on the stage of the tumor at the time of diagnosis. If the tumor is diagnosed and treated in the early stages, there is a high survival rate.

1. Surgical intervention.
   a. Surgery is scheduled as soon as the tumor is identified.
   b. Nephrectomy
2. Medical intervention.
   a. Radiation therapy pre-and post operatively.
   b. Postoperative chemotherapy

Nursing Intervention

✦ *Goal: to avoid manipulation of abdomen preoperatively to prevent spread of metastases.*

> ***NURSING PRIORITY:*** *Post a sign above the bed that reads: Do Not Palpate Abdomen.*

1. Do not palpate abdomen to determine tumor size.
2. Assist RN to prepare child and family for the surgery, including anticipation of a large incision and dressing.
3. *Assess vital signs, especially blood pressure, for indications of hypertension and report to RN.*

✦ *Goal: to assess kidney function, prevent infection, support and reassure child and parents postoperatively.*

1. Usual postoperative care for abdominal surgery.
2. Assist the child in coping with side effects related to hair loss, nausea, vomiting, etc.

Acute Renal Failure (ARF)

❑ **The loss of renal function may occur over several days or may occur over hours. Most common causes are hypotension and prerenal hypovolemia.**

Phases of Acute Renal Failure

1. Initiation phase.
   a. Begins with precipitating event (usually brings on acute tubular necrosis - ATN).
   b. Has few symptoms.
2. Maintenance phase.
   a. Begins within hours and lasts 1-2 weeks.
   b. Increase in BUN, serum creatinine, potassium, magnesium, and presence of metabolic acidosis and possible anemia.
   c. As maintenance phase ends, diuretic period begins.
   d. BUN, potassium, and phosphate remain high during diuresis.
3. Recovery phase.
   a. BUN and creatinine levels are no longer rising.
   b. Renal function may improve over 12 months.
   c. May have some type of permanent reduction occurs in glomerular filtration rate.

Data Collection

1. Risk factors/etiology.
   a. Prerenal (renal ischemia) -shock, hypovolemia.
   b. Intrarenal (kidney tissue pathology).
   c. Postrenal (obstruction to urine flow).

> ***Geriatric Priority:*** *Elderly clients are at a higher risk for developing ARF, due to their limited cardiovascular instability and decreased reserve.*

2. Clinical manifestations - see phases
3. Diagnostics.
   a. Elevated serum creatinine, BUN, and potassium.
   b. Urinalysis - proteinuria, casts, RBC, and WBC, specific gravity varies based on oliguric or diuretic period.

Treatment

1. Medical.

a. Identify and treat precipitating cause of acute renal failure (management varies according to prerenal, intrarenal, or postrenal disorder).
b. Diuretic therapy.
c. Decrease serum potassium.
2. Dietary.
a. Fluid restriction; intake may be carefully calculated with output.
b. Protein, potassium, and sodium intake is regulated according to serum levels.
c. Increased carbohydrate intake.

Nursing Intervention

✦ *Goal: to maintain client in normal homeostasis and preserve renal function while the kidneys are repairing.*
1. Accurate intake and output.
2. Daily weight.
3. Assess for hypervolemia during the oliguric phase.
4. Evaluate for postural hypotension.
5. Careful replacement of fluids to prevent overload during oliguric phase.

✦ *Goal: to prevent infection.*
1. Avoid indwelling catheter if possible.
2. Assess for development of infectious processes. Client at increased risk due to compromised immune system.

✦ *Goal: to prevent skin breakdown.*
1. Frequent turning and positioning; inspect the skin for problem areas.
2. Beds and protective devices to prevent pressure areas.
3. Frequent range of motion and activities to increase circulation.

Self-Care
1. Important to maintain follow-up to determine amount of renal damage that has occurred.
2. Teach client how to prevent UTI.

Chronic Renal Failure (CRF)

❑ **CRF is a progressive, irreversible reduction in renal function such that the kidneys are no longer able to maintain the body environment.**

Data Collection

1. Risk factors/etiology.
a. Chronic glomerulonephritis and pyelonephritis.
b. Chronic hypertension.
c. Diabetic nephropathy.
d. High serum potassium and sodium levels.
e. Metabolic acidosis.
f. Urinary system - specific gravity of urine fixed at 1.010; proteinuria; eventually oliguria leads to anuria.
g. Hematologic system - anemia and bleeding.
h. Cardiovascular system - hypertension, CHF, dysrhythmias.
i. Gastrointestinal system - anorexia, nausea, vomiting, bad odor to the breath, gastrointestinal bleeding, esophagitis, diarrhea and constipation.
j. Metabolic system - hyperglycemia, hyperlipidemia.
k. Neurologic system - central nervous system depression, seizures, impaired reasoning and judgement, peripheral neuropathy.
l. Demineralization (renal osteodystrophy) of the bones, increased serum calcium.
m. Integumentary system - sallow yellow discoloration, pruritus, and uremic frost.
n. Psychological changes - emotional lability, withdrawal, depression and psychosis.
2. Diagnostics.
a. ↑ BUN and serum creatinine level.
b. ↓ urinary creatinine clearance.
c. ↑ blood sugar and triglycerides.
d. ↑ serum potassium and sodium.
e. Anemia (↓ Hb & Hct).

Treatment

1. Medical.
a. Reduce serum potassium.
b. Antihypertensives (Appendix 11-4).
c. Diuretics (Appendix 11-5).
d. Dialysis (See next section).
2. Dietary.
a. Problems with the client losing body weight, both adipose tissue and muscle mass.
b. Restricted protein intake.
c. Water restriction - adjusted according to urinary output.
d. Sodium and potassium restriction - based upon laboratory values.
3. Surgical - kidney transplant.

Nursing Intervention

✦ *Goal: to assist the client to maintain homeostasis.*
1. Evaluate adequacy of fluid balance.
a. Daily weight.

b. Postural hypotension.

c. Level of fluid intake.

d. Discuss with the client how to monitor the fluid intake and plan for the allocated amount to be distributed over the day.

2. Encourage adequate nutritional intake within dietary guidelines.

a. Relieve GI dysfunctions prior to serving meals.

b. Plan diet according to client preferences if possible.

c. Advise client that most salt substitutes contain potassium and should not be used.

3. Prevent problems of constipation

a. Include bran in diet.

b. Stool softeners.

4. Avoid use of sedatives and hypnotics.

5. Monitor electrolyte balance, especially level of potassium.

6. Check BP and pulse; report any elevations to the RN.

7. Assess client for bleeding tendencies.

8. Evaluate client for pruritus and assist with measures to decrease the skin irritation and itching.

✦ *Goal: to maintain homeostasis for client receiving hemodialysis or peritoneal dialysis (see next section)*

✦ *Goal: to provide emotional support and promote psychological equilibrium.*

1. Encourage client to express concerns.

2. Recognize that the long-term management of a chronic disease may lead to anxiety and depression.

✦ *Goal: to provide preoperative care for kidney transplant.*

1. Maintain client's metabolic state as close to homeostasis as possible - continue with dialysis.

2. Very careful assessment regarding presence of any level of infection postoperatively.

Dialysis

❑ **The passage of particles (ions) from an area of high concentration to an area of low concentration across a semipermeable membrane.**

1. Types of dialysis (Table 18-1).

Nursing Intervention

✦ *Goal: to remove excess fluid and waste products of metabolism.*

a. Peritoneal dialysis.

Table 18-1: Types Of Dialysis

Hemodialysis
Circulation of the client's blood through a compartment that contains an artificial semipermeable membrane that is surrounded by dialysate fluid.

Peritoneal dialysis
Utilization of the peritoneal cavity and the peritoneum as the semipermeable membrane that removes excess fluid.

Continuous Ambulatory Peritoneal Dialysis (CAPD)
The dialysate is infused into the abdomen and remains there for 4 to 6 hours. The dialysate is removed by gravity drainage after the prescribed time. Most clients prefer to do the dialysis at night.

NCLEX ALERT: *Provide care for a client with vascular access for hemodialysis*

(1) Prepare client for procedure; establish baseline criteria of lab values, weight, vital signs.

(2) Complications: possible bowel perforation from catheter insertion, peritonitis, bleeding, hypoalbuminemia, and general discomfort.

b. Hemodialysis.

(1) Vascular access site must be established. Access may be temporary or permanent.

(a) External arteriovenous shunts - catheters are inserted into an artery and into a vein and may be connected together on the outside of the body in a "U" pattern.

(b) Internal arteriovenous fistulas - an artery and a vein in the arm or leg are anastomosed either directly or via a graft. Access is achieved via 2 large gauge needles inserted into the fistula site.

(c) After an internal fistula is created, it must heal prior to being used for dialysis.

(2) Do not take blood pressure or obtain blood samples from the extremity that has a vascular access site.

***NURSING PRIORITY:** Report immediately any decrease or absence of pulsations or indications of decreased blood flow through the access.*

(3) Identify dialysis disequilibrium syndrome.

(a) Occurs in the clients first few dialysis.

(b) Mental confusion, changes in level of consciousness, headache.

(c) Report problems to the dialysis nurse so adjustments can be made on next dialysis.

✦ *Goal: to provide emotional support and promote psychological equilibrium.*

1. Encourage client to express feelings of anger and depression. There is an increase in the rate of suicides in dialysis clients.

2. Encourage appropriate coping skills.

Crestor for cholesterol

3. Clients on dialysis are in limbo; they do not know if they are going to get better or not. Frequently, they have ambivalent feelings about dialysis. It maintains their life; however, it severely restricts their life style.

Renal Cancer

❑ **The majority of renal tumors are malignant; occur more frequently in men age 50 to 70 years of age. The most common areas of metastasis are the lungs and bone.**

Data Collection

1. Palpable abdominal mass.
2. Hematuria.
3. Flank pain.

Treatment

1. Medical.
   a. Radiation therapy.
   b. Chemotherapy.
2. Surgical - nephrectomy.

Nursing Intervention

✦ *Goal: to provide preoperative nursing care (See Chapter 3).*

✦ *Goal: to provide postoperative care.*

1. Urinary output is important to assess; drainage from catheters should be labeled and recorded accurately.
2. Due to the level of the incision, respiratory status is important. Encourage coughing and deep breathing, as well as incentive spirometry, every two hours while client is awake.
3. Assess for abdominal distention and paralytic ileus, which is common.

✦ *Goal: to provide supportive nursing care in relation to malignancy.*

See Chapter 2 for management of cancer client.

Study Questions—Urinary/Renal

1. A female client is diagnosed with recurrent cystitis and is asking for information about self-care. What practice would the nurse discourage?

① drink as much fluid as possible throughout the day.
② take a shower rather than bathing in a tub.
③ refrain from voiding to reduce the concentration of the urine.
④ immediately void and wash after intercourse.

2. What finding would be noted on an assessment of a client who has an acute lower urinary tract infection?

① gross painless hematuria.
② low back pain.
③ polyuria.
④ dysuria.

3. A 10am the nurse begins collection of a 24 hour urine collection. What are the guidelines for collection of this specimen?

① collect a specimen now, add it to the container and collect all urine until 10am the next day.
② ask client to void now and discard the specimen, collect all urine for 24 hours, ask client to void at 10am next day and add to specimen container.
③ collect specimen now and discard it, collect urine for 24 hours, ask client to void at 10am the following morning and discard specimen.
④ ask client to void now and discard specimen, collect all urine for next 24 hours at 2 hour intervals and save in sterile containers.

4. The nurse is caring for a group of clients in a long term care facility. What nursing measure will promote continence?

① plan schedule to facilitate assisting everyone to the bathroom every 2-3 hours.
② decrease the amount of PO fluids to increase bladder control.
③ put all clients on intake and output to evaluate adequacy of intake.
④ assess for bladder distention in clients who are increasingly restless.

5. A client has a shunt in his left arm for dialysis. How will the nurse check the patency of the shunt?

① palpate above the forearm for a rushing sound.
② check the pulse site distant to the shunt.
③ palpate the shunt site for a thrill.
④ check the shunt for warmth and color.

6. An infant is born with hypospadias. The mother asks the nurse when circumcision should be done. What is the best nursing response?

① there is no problem with circumcision, it can be done whenever the parents desire it.
② circumcision will probably be delayed until there can be further diagnostic studies of the problem.
③ circumcision is most often done when the congenital condition is repaired.
④ voiding studies will have to be completed before circumcision can be done.

7. Kidney transplant clients are on immunosuppressant drugs. What nursing measure would not be appropriate in caring for these clients?

① keep all irrigation fluids sterile.
② maintain aseptic technique.
③ give all medications by injection.
④ screen all visitors for infections.

8. The nurse is caring for a client in renal failure. What observations would indicate the development of a complication of uremia in this client?

① anorexia, nausea, and vomiting.
② pneumonia and respiratory depression.
③ tachycardia and stupor.
④ restlessness and diuresis.

9. Which client would be at the highest risk for the development of acute renal failure?

① client with placenta previa with hemorrhage controlled.
② cardiac client with frequent problems of tachycardia.
③ hypertensive client who forgets to take his medication.
④ elderly client with 20 hear history of Type II diabetes.

10. Why is it important to monitor the red blood cell count in a chronic renal failure client?

① granulocytopenia could occur which can cause infection.
② production of erythropoietin will be affected due to renal failure.
③ blood cell production could increase due to the increased production of renin.
④ an increase in waste products could cause thrombocytopenia.

11. What common medication is used to treat urinary tract infections?

① furosemide (**Lasix**).
② metoprolol (**Lopressor**).
③ nitrofurantoin (**Macrodantin**). (UTI)
④ metronidazole (**Flagyl**).

12. What is the best description of the pain that a client experiences when they begin to pass a renal calculi?

① intermittent sharp pain that radiates down the left leg.
② intermittent dull but hot pain in the upper thighs.
③ dull flank pain that only occurs with voiding.
④ sharp pain in the shoulder and chest that radiates.

13. In providing instructions to geriatric clients on the prevention of urinary tract infections, what would the nurse instruct the clients to avoid?

① take all medication ordered, regardless of symptoms.
② increase intake of fluids to 3000cc daily.
③ cleanse the perineal area from back to front.
④ increase intake of cranberry, plum, and prune juices.

14. A cystoscopy is going to be done on a client. What is important for the nurse to tell the client?

① a local anesthetic and a sedative will be given, if he is awake during the procedure he should not experience severe pain.
② a sedative will be given, but it is important for him to remain fully awake in order to cooperate with the doctor during the procedure.
③ a long black tube will be inserted through the wall of the bladder for 15 minutes to view the bladder wall and interior.
④ a three-way Foley will be inserted and dye will be injected into the urinary tract through the cystoscope.

15. What would the nurse anticipate finding when performing a skin assessment on a chronic renal failure client?

① warm, moist, pink colored skin.
② cool, clammy, dusky colored skin.
③ warm, edematous, copper-colored skin.
④ bruised, dry, yellow colored skin.

16. The nurse is caring for a client in acute renal failure. What is a complication associated with the problem of fluid volume excess in this client?

① peripheral neuropathy
② bleeding episodes.
③ congestive heart failure.
④ hyperkalemia.

17. The nurse is assessing a client in acute renal failure. What is an indication the client is progressing into the oliguric stage?

① hematuria of 600cc over 24 hours.
② increasing urine specific gravity.
③ serum potassium at 3.5meq/L.
④ urine output of 400ml/24 hours.

18. A female client is being catheterized, the nurse advances the catheter into an opening 5 to 6 inches with no urine return. What is the best interpretation of this situation?

① the catheter is too small for urine to flow without pressure.

② there must be a defect in the catheter.

③ the client was catheterized after she had voided.

④ catheter is not in the urinary meatus and is probably in the vagina.

19. What would be the best nursing action if a sterile urinary catheter has been placed in the vaginal opening in error?

① use an alcohol wipe and clean the catheter thoroughly before reinserting.

② remove the catheter and obtain a new catheter for insertion.

③ place the catheter it in a disinfectant solution and use it later.

④ discard the catheter kit and try later during the shift to catheterize the client.

Appendix 18-1: DIAGNOSTICS OF THE URINARY-RENAL SYSTEM

LABORATORY TESTS	NURSING IMPLICATIONS
• **BUN**	Common test used to diagnose renal problems; may be affected by an increase in protein intake or tissue breakdown. (Normal value: 10 - 30 mg/dL)
• **CREATININE**	End -product of protein and muscle catabolism; more accurate determination of renal function than the BUN. (Normal value: 0.5 to 1.5 mg/dL)
• **URINE SPECIFIC GRAVITY**	May be increased when the client is dehydrated. A decrease is associated with decreased tubular absorption. In chronic renal failure, it may be fixed at 1.000 - 1.010. (Normal range: 1.003 -1.030)

PROCEDURE	NURSING IMPLICATIONS
• **KIDNEYS, URETERS, AND BLADDER (KUB)** A flat plate x-ray of the abdomen and pelvis.	1. Bowel preparation may or may not be indicated.
• **IVP OR EXCRETORY UROGRAM** IV injection of radiopaque dye to visualize the urinary tract.	1. Client NPO for eight hours prior to procedure. 2. Cathartic or enema given the evening prior to procedure. 3. *Assess for sensitivity to iodine and report to RN.* 4. Instruct client that he/she will need to lie still on table while serial X-rays are taken. 5. Evaluate for iodine reaction after test and force fluids to flush out the dye.
• **RETROGRADE PYELOGRAM** An X-ray of the urinary tract which is conducted during a cystoscopic exam; ureteral catheters are inserted into the renal pelvis and dye is injected (retrograde) into the catheters.	1. Client NPO for eight hours prior to test. 2. Assess for sensitivity to iodine. 3. Explain that there may be discomfort upon insertion of the cystoscope. 4. General anesthesia may be indicated for procedure.
• **RENAL ARTERIOGRAM (ANGIOGRAM)** An IV injection of radiopaque dye into the renal artery (catheter is inserted into femoral artery) to visualize the renal blood vessels.	1. Client NPO after midnight. 2. Preoperative medication is administered. 3. Client should be assessed for sensitivity to iodine. 4. Evaluate venipuncture insertion site every 15 to 30 minutes after procedure to assess for bleeding. 5. Assess peripheral pulses to detect occluded blood flow. 6. Sandbag or pressure dressing may be applied to groin. 7. *Report to RN any indications of occlusion, bleeding or hemorrhage from puncture site.*
• **RENOGRAM** An IV injection of a radioactive nuclide (isotope) followed by a scanning device to detect radioactive emissions from the kidney; identifies renal blood flow, tubular functions, and renal excretion.	1. No specific activity or dietary restrictions. 2. Explain procedure to client.

Appendix 18-1:
DIAGNOSTICS OF THE URINARY-RENAL SYSTEM

PROCEDURE	NURSING IMPLICATIONS
• **RENAL BIOPSY** A percutaneous needle biopsy	1. Blood coagulation studies should be available on the chart prior to the biopsy procedure. 2. Type and cross-match client for two units of blood. 3. IVP or ultrasound studies report should be available prior to the biopsy. 4. Immediately after the procedure, pressure dressing is applied to biopsy site and checked frequently for bleeding. 5. *Assess urine for gross hematuria, flank pain, or a rise or fall in blood pressure and report to RN.* 6. Report any signs of backache, shoulder pain, or dysuria. 7. Encourage fluids: 3,000 cc per day. 8. Assess for complication of hemorrhage; may necessitate emergency surgical drainage or nephrectomy. 9. Contraindications: one functioning kidney, presence of infection, severe hypertension pregnancy, and bleeding disorders. 10. Procedure is preformed under local anesthesia with the client in a prone position.
• **CYSTOSCOPY** A direct method to visualize the urethra and bladder by use of a tubular lighted scope (cystoscope)	1. Force fluids or administer IV. 2. Explain lithotomy position which will be utilized. 3. Client may have general anesthesia. 4. Preoperative medication given. 5. Evaluate urine output postprocedure; check for frequency, pink-tinged color, and burning on urination (these are expected effects). 6. Evaluate for orthostatic hypotension. 7. Provide warm sitz baths and mild analgesics to alleviate urethral discomfort.
• **RENAL ULTRASOUND** A noninvasive procedure utilizing ultrasound waves which, with the aid of a computer, record images related to tissue density.	1. No specific preparation other than explanation of the procedure to the client.

Appendix 18-2: URINARY ANTISEPTICS

MEDICATION	SIDE EFFECTS	NURSING IMPLICATIONS
❖ GENERAL NURSING IMPLICATIONS ❖ —Encourage intake of 2000-3000 cc per day during treatment. —Continue medication therapy until all medication has been taken. —Most medications are better absorbed on an empty stomach; however, if GI distress occurs they may be taken with food. —Monitor intake and output, as well as symptoms of increasing renal problems. —Check drug insert package for interactions with anticoagulants.		
URINARY TRACT ANTISEPTICS: Concentrate in the urine and are active against common urinary tract pathogens. Do not affect infections in blood or tissue.		
Cinoxacin: PO Nalidixic Acid (**NegGram**): PO	GI upset is common, headache, rash, visual disturbances, photosensitivity	1. Cinoxacin and nalidixic acid, both cause photosensitivity.
Methenamine Mandelate (**Mandelamine, Mandameth**): PO	GI upset, bladder irritation, hepatotoxic	1. Requires acidic urine to be effective. 2. Should not be used with sulfonamides. 3. Used for chronic UTI, rather then acute.
Nitrofurantoin (**Furadantin, Macrodantin, Apo-nitrofurantoin, Nitrofan**): PO, IM	GI upset, blood dyscrasia, pulmonary reactions.	1. Requires adequate renal function to concentrate medication in urine. 2. Should not be administered to renal transplant clients. 3. Will turn the urine a brownish orange color.
URINARY ANALGESIC		
Phenazopyridine hydrochloride (**Azo-standard, Pyridium, Urodine, Urogesic**): PO	Headache, GI disturbances.	1. Contraindicated in renal and liver dysfunction. 2. Advise client to report any yellow discoloration to skin or eyes. 3. Urine will turn orange. 4. Administer with caution in clients with impaired renal function.

Appendix 18-3: URINARY DIVERSION

❑ A *urinary diversion* is a means of diverting urinary output from the bladder to an external device or via a new avenue.

TEMPORARY URINARY DIVERSION:

Nephrostomy Tubes (catheters) - insertion of catheters into the renal pelvis by surgical incision or percutaneous puncture, a small catheter is inserted into the renal pelvis and attached via connecting tubing to a closed system drainage.Tubes may be temporary or permanent.

Nursing Implications:

1. Catheter should *never be clamped* or *irrigated* (renal pelvis capacity is 3 to 5 cc).
2. Complications - infection and secondary renal calculi formation, erosion of the duct by the catheter.

Ureteral Catheters -small, narrow catheters placed through the ureters into the renal pelvis; draining the urinary bladder in addition to one or teo ureteral cathetersoften client has a Foley catheter. The catheter splints the ureters during healing and prevents edema from occluding ureter.

Nursing Implications:

1. Check frequently for placement of ureteral catheters; tension should be avoided.
2. Ureteral catheter *should not be clamped* or *irrigated.*
3. Maintain accurate intake and output records and label all catheters.

PERMANENT URINARY DIVERSION:

Ileal Conduit (Bricker's Procedure) the transplanting of ureters into segment of ileum which is then brought to the abdomen and a stoma is constructed.

Nursing Implications:

1. Stoma site is marked prior to surgery as a device must be worn continuously.
2. Mucus may be present in the urine postoperatively; encourage a high-fluid intake to "flush the ileal conduit."
3. Maintain meticulous skin care and changing of appliances.
4. Provide discharge instructions in regards to symptoms of obstruction, infection, and care of theostomy; client needs information relating to purchase of supplies, ostomy clubs, follow-up visits, enterstomal therapists, and the importance of not irrigating the ileal conduit.

Kock Pouch - a segment of the ileum is made into a reservoir, client is taught to use a catheter to drain the pouch and maintain continence.
Indiana Pouch - reservoir is created from an area of the ascending colon, makes a larger pouch to maintain continence.

Nursing Implications:

1. Client may still be incontinent and require continuous wearing of an appliance.
2. Obstruction and electrolyte problems occur with both types.
3. Continuous assessment of status of skin around stoma.
4. Client should understand how to care for the stoma prior to leaving the hospital.
   — types of appliances available
   — increase fluid intake to decrease infections.
   — contact physician if there are changes in the color of the stoma or urine becomes dark and foul- smelling.

Appendix 18-4:
NURSING PROCEDURE - Urine Specimen Collection

✓ ***Key Points: Random sample***

- May be collected at any time.
- May be specifically ordered to collect first voided specimen or to collect sample on second voiding.

✓ ***Key Points: Clean catch and midstream***

- Specimen is collected for culture.
- Make sure client cleans urinary meatus prior to specimen collection.
- For midstream collection, tell client to start the urinary stream and collect the specimen after the voiding has begun.

✓ ***Key Points: Catheterized specimen***

- Straight in- and -out catheterization to obtain sample for culture.
- Procedure is discouraged due to introduction of bacteria and irritation producing a UTI.

✓ ***Key Points: 12 - 24 Hour collection***

- When the collection time is started, have the client void, discard the urine, and start the collection with the next voiding.
- Mark the collection container and collect the urine over the prescribed time frame.
- When the time frame is completed, have the client void again, add it to the specimen collection, and send to lab for evaluation.

NCLEX ALERT: *Collection of urine samples is a common nursing action; be sure to know why the sample is being obtained and what type of diagnostic test it is being collected for.*

Appendix 18-5:
NURSING PROCEDURE *Urinary Catheterization*

✓ Key Points: Insertion of a Retention Catheter

- A sterile procedure.
- Lubricate catheter using sterile lubricant provided in tray.
- Cleanse the patient's meatus:
  For a female:
  a.Cleanse the patient's meatus with one downward stroke of the forceps.
  b.Repeat at least three to four times, using new sterile botton ball each time.
  c.Continue to hold the patient's labia apart until you insert the catheter.
  For a male:
  a.Hold the patient's penis upright. Hold the sides of the penis to prevent closing the urethra.
  b.Cleanse the patient's meatus with one downward stroke of the forceps.
  c.Repeat at least three to four times.
  d.Continue to hold the penis as you insert the catheter.
- Insert the catheter 2 to 3 inches beyond the point at which urine begins to flow. Inserting the catheter farther into the bladder ensures it is beyond the neck of the bladder.
- Instill sterile water into balloon after catheter is inserted.
- Tape the catheter with one-inch tape.
  a.***For a female:*** Tape catheter to the side of the leg.
  b.***For a male:*** Tape catheter to the abdomen to prevent pressure on the penoscrotal angle.
- Attach drainage bag to bed frame (not side rails), so that it hangs freely.

✓ Key Points: Providing Catheter Care

- With sterile cotton ball soaked in antiseptic solution.
- Gently pull catheter taut and cleanse with new swab or cotton ball from catheter insertion site down catheter tubing approximately 4 to 5 inches toward drainage bag.
- Place ointment around catheter at the meatus and down catheter tubing about ½ to 1 inch.

✓ Key Points: Removal of a Catheter

- Clamp catheter.
- Do not cut the catheter with a scissor. Balloon may not totally deflate if cut.
- Withdraw fluid from balloon (usually 5 to 10 cc water in balloon.)
- Pull gently on catheter to ensure balloon is deflated before attempting to remove. Damage to the urethra can occur, if balloon is not totally deflated.
- Record output on I & O bedside record.
- Wash perineum with soap and water. Dry thoroughly.
- Instruct patient to drink oral fluids as tolerated and observe for signs and symptoms of urinary tract infection (burning, frequency, urgency).
- Offer bedpan or urinal at least every 2 to 4 hours after removing catheter, until voiding occurs. Keep accurate I & O record.

Appendix 18-5:
NURSING PROCEDURE ***Urinary Catheterization***

CLINICAL TIPS FOR PROBLEM SOLVING

1. *If catheter is inserted in the vagina of female client:*
   - Leave the catheter in place so you do not reintroduce a new catheter into the vaginal area. Obtain a new catheter and new gloves.
   - If sterile field has been contaminated, obtain a whole new kit.

2. ***If unable to insert catheter into male patient:***
   - Obtain a new catheter kit.
     a. Hold penis vertical to patient's body.
     b. Insert catheter while applying slight traction by gently pulling upward on the shaft of the penis.
     c. If you encounter resistance, rotate the catheter, increase the traction, and change the angle of the penis slightly.
     d. When urine begins to flow, lower the client's penis.

3. *If pain occurs during inflation of balloon:*
   - Remove any injected water and insert the catheter farther into the bladder

4. *If urine exceeds 1000cc with catheterization*:
   - Clamp catheter for 20 to 30 minutes and then unclamp.

5. *If catheter comes out with balloon still inserted:*
   - Assess client for signs of urethral trauma, i.e., bleeding, pain.
   - Obtain a new catheter and repeat the catheterization procedure, making sure that the balloon is inflated with at least 10 cc water.
   - Monitor urine output for bleeding.

NCLEX ALERT: *Urinary catheterization is often tested, especially in relationship to maintenance of aseptic technique. Because this procedure is frequently done, be thoroughly familiar with all the information in this table.*

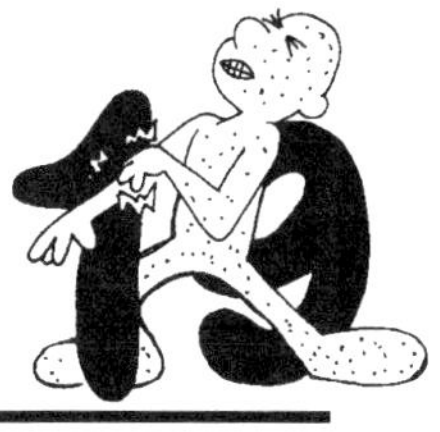

Integumentary System

PHYSIOLOGY OF THE SKIN

A. Anatomical structures.
1. Epidermis - outermost layer of the skin.
2. Dermis - layer beneath the epidermis.
3. Subcutaneous (hypodermis) - located below the dermis; anchors the muscles and bones to the skin.
4. Nail.
   a. Consists of a hard, transparent plate of keratin.
   b. Grows from the root, which lies under a thin fold of skin called the cuticle.
5. Hair.
   a. Present over the entire body except for the palms of the hands and the soles of the feet.
   b. Piloerector response - contraction of the tiny erector muscles attached to the hair follicle which lead to hair "standing on end" or "gooseflesh."
6. Sebaceous glands - secrete sebum, which is an oily secretion that is emptied into the hair shaft.

B. Functions of the skin.
1. Protection - primary function.
2. Sensory - major receptor for general sensation.
3. Water balance.
   a. 500 to 900 ml of water is lost daily through *insensible* perspiration.
   b. Forms a barrier that prevents loss of water and electrolytes from the internal environment.
4. Temperature regulation.
5. Involved in wheal and flare reaction.
   a. Wheal - swelling.
   b. Flare - diffused redness.
   c. These responses are due to local edema.

System Data Collection

A. Health history.
1. How long have you had this particular rash, lesion, problem?
2. Is there any itching, burning, or discomfort associated with the problem?
3. Have you been in contact with any irritants, sun, unusual cold or unhygienic conditions?
4. Has anyone in your family ever had this same type of problem with their skin?
5. Are you taking any medications?
6. What is your diet history? Do you have any food allergies?

B. Physical assessment.
1. Inspection.
   a. Assess the skin for color - jaundiced, cyanotic, flushed.
   b. Determine if there are areas of bruising, purpura, or petechiae (Box 19-1).
   c. Determine if skin blanches on direct pressure.
   d. Assess any lesion for type, color, size, distribution and grouping; location and consistency.
   e. Common dermatological lesions.
      (1) Macule - flat, circumscribed area of color change in the skin without surface elevation.
      (2) Papule - circumscribed, solid, and elevated lesion.
      (3) Nodule - raised, solid lesion that is larger and deeper than a papule.
      (4) Vesicle - small elevation in skin usually filled with serous fluid or blood; bulla -larger than a vesicle; pustule - vesicle or bulla filled with pus.
      (5) Wheal - elevation of the skin caused by edema of the dermis.

Box 19-1: Elderly Care Focus
Skin Concerns Of Older Adults

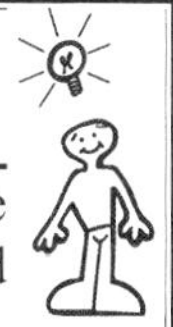

As skin ages it becomes increasingly fragile and transparent, which can lead to irritation and breakdown.

Because oil and sweat glands become less active as we age, frequent cleansing of the skin becomes unnecessary.

Encourage older clients to use oils, lotions, and creams on the skin to prevent dryness and scaliness.

Avoid use of alcohol-based lotions and creams.

Elderly clients bruise easily (causing senile purpura) due to a decrease in subcutaneous tissue and loss of skin elasticity.

Nails, especially of the feet, become dry, brittle, and thick, often needing attention and care by a nurse or podiatrist.

Development of actinic keratosis (brown spots) occur as a result of sun exposure through the years. Also, other aging changes appear, such as skin tags, lentigos ("old age spots"), and senile papillomata (yellow, brown, or black warts) making it more important to assess and monitor changes that may indicate a malignant lesion.

(6) Cyst - mass of fluid-filled tissue that extends to the subcutaneous tissue or dermis.

2. Palpation.
   a. Determine temperature and tissue turgor.
   b. Evaluate skin for moisture and texture.

DISORDERS OF THE SKIN

NCLEX ALERT: *Reinforce care of client with altered skin integrity.*

Acne Vulgaris

Acne is an inflammatory disorder of the sebaceous glands and their hair follicles.

Data Collection

1. More common in teenagers; may persist into adulthood.
2. Under hormonal influence during puberty; affected by presence of androgen; which stimulates the sebaceous glands to secrete sebum.
3. Inflammatory lesions or pustules.
4. Cysts, deep nodules that may produce scarring.

Treatment

Self-Care

1. Instruct to cleanse face twice daily - avoid over-cleansing.
2. May use a polyester sponge pad to cleanse skin.
3. Instruct to keep hands away from face and to avoid any friction or trauma to the area; avoid propping hands against face, rubbing face, etc.
4. Emphasize the importance of a nutritious diet - encourage adequate food intake and vitamin A.
5. Avoid the use of cosmetics, shaving creams, and lotion, as they may aggravate acne.
6. Counsel client that problem is not related to uncleanliness, dietary intake, masturbation or sexual activity.

Psoriasis

Psoriasis is a chronic inflammatory disorder of the skin.

Data Collection

1. Scaling, plaques on the elbow, scalp and knees.
2. If scales are scraped away, a dark red base of the lesion is seen which will procedure multiple bleeding points.
3. May improve, but often reoccurs throughout life.
4. Bilateral symmetry of symptoms is common.

Treatment

1. Coal tar preparation.
2. Corticosteroids.
   a. Photochemotherapy (PUVA therapy) - psoralen, ultraviolet A therapy.
   b. Occlusive dressing - medication applied to the skin followed by wrapping of the affected area then covering with a plastic bag.

Home Care

1. Encourage verbalization of anxiety regarding appearance.
2. Instruct client to use a soft brush to remove scales while bathing.
3. Assess client to determine factors that may trigger skin condition (i.e., emotional stress, trauma, seasonal changes).
4. Assist RN to make sure client understands treatment and implications of care related to occlusive dressings, PUVA therapy, and other treatments.

Pressure Ulcer

A *pressure ulcer* (decubitus ulcer, bedsore) is a localized area of infarcted tissue characterized by an erythematous area that does not blanche, is warm to the touch, and finally leads to a break in the skin.

Nursing Priority: *Pressure ulcers are a problem across the span of nursing. The most important aspect to remember is that the ulcer can be and should be prevented. In the prevention of the ulcer, it is important to identify those clients at increased risk for development of the ulcer and begin preventative care as soon as possible. Do not wait for the reddened area to occur before preventative measures are initiated.*

Data Collection

1. Risk factors/etiology.
   a. Prolonged pressure due to immobility.
   b. Malnutrition (overweight, underweight), hypoproteinemia, vitamin deficiency.
   c. Infection.
   d. Skin dryness, maceration, excessive skin moisture.
   e. Advancing age.
   f. Equipment such as casts, restraints, traction, etc.
2. Clinical manifestations.

a. First indication usually an erythematous area which will not blanche on pressure.

b. Four stages of ulcer formation (Table 19-1).

Treatment

1. Medical & Surgical.

a. Debridement

(1) Surgical debridement— removeal of moist, devitalized tissue, then skin grafting.

(2) Mechanical debridement—wet-to-dry dressings, hydrotherapy, wound irrigation.

(3) Enzymatic and autolytic debridement—use of enzymes or synthetic dressings that cover wound and self-digest devitalized tissue; not used if wound is infected.

b. Wound cleansing (use normal saline for most cases).

(1) Use minimal mechanical force when cleansing to avoid trauma to the wound bed.

(2) Avoid the use of antiseptics (i.e. iodine, hydrogen peroxide).

c. Dressings (should protect wound, be biocompatible, and hydrate).

(1) Film (transparent).

(2) Hydrocolloid (moisture and oxygen retaining).

***NURSING PRIORITY:** Keep the ulcer tissue moist and the surrounding intact skin dry.*

2. Dietary.

a. Increased carbohydrates and protein.

b. Increased vitamin C and zinc.

Nursing Intervention

NCLEX ALERT: *Take action to maintain skin integrity.*

✦ *Goal: to prevent or relieve pressure and stimulate circulation.*

1. Frequent change of position - turn client every 1 to 2 hours.
2. Silicone gel pads placed under the buttocks of wheelchair clients.
3. Sheepskin pads to provide a soft surface to protect the skin from abrasion.
4. Eggcrate mattress to allow circulation under the body and keep the area dry.

Table 19-1: STAGES OF PRESSURE ULCERS

Stage 1

- Skin is intact.
- Area is red and *does not blanche* with external pressure.Redness remains for 30 minutes or l onger after pressure is relieved.

Stage 2

- Skin is not intact.
- There us partial thickness skin loss of the epidermis or dermis.
- The ulcer is superficial and presents as an abrasion, blister, or shallow crater.

Stage 3

- Full thickness skin loss occurs.
- Damage or necrosis of subcutaneous tissue extends down to, but not through fascia.
- Ulcer presents as a deep crater with or without undermining of adjacent tissue.

Stage 4

- Full thickness skin loss with extensive tissue destruction, tissue necrosis or damage to muscle, bone, or supporting structures (e.g., tendon or joint capsule).
- Undermining and sinus tracts may develop.

5. Active and passive exercises to promote circulation.
6. Gentle skin massage with lotion.

✦ *Goal: to keep skin clean and healthy and prevent the occurrence of a pressure ulcer.*

1. Wash skin with mild soap and blot completely dry with soft towel.
2. Inspect skin frequently, especially over bony prominences.

***NURSING PRIORITY:** Avoid massage over bony prominences. When the side-lying position is used in bed, avoid positioning directly on the trochanter. Do not use donut-type devices. Limit the time the head of the bed is elevated. Avoid uninterrupted sitting in any chair or wheelchair.*

3. Remove any foreign material from the bed, keep sheets tightly stretched on bed to prevent wrinkles.

✦ *Goal: to promote healing of pressure ulcer.*

1. Utilize methods discussed to decrease the pressure on the area of the decubiti.
2. Keep the ulcer area dry.

a. Minimize exposure of pressure area to moisture due to incontinence, perspiration, or wound drainage.

b. Use underpads or briefs that are made of materials that absorb moisture and provide a quick-drying surface to the skin.
3. Utilize skin barriers to decrease contamination and increase healing in a non-infected ulcer.
4. Observe the ulcer for signs of infection. Infected ulcers will have to be debrided, if healing is to occur.

NCLEX ALERT: *Identify factors that interfere with wound healing.*

Atopic Dermatitis

Atopic dermatitis (also called eczema) is a superficial inflammatory disorder of genetically hypersensitive skin—condition occurs primarily during infancy, usually between 2 and 6 months of age, usually spontaneous and permanent remissions by 3 years of age.

Data Collection

1. Reddened lesions.
2. Discomfort from itching (worse at night).
3. Lesions tend to occur on the cheeks, arms, and legs.
4. As the child gets older, the lesions tend to be dry with a thickening of the skin.
5. Infants with eczema are more likely to have allergies as children and adults.

Treatment

1. Food allergies are not associated with adult atopic dermatitis; milk, eggs, wheat, and peanuts are the most common suspicious foods in children.
2. Pruritus is treated with antihistamines and topical steroids.
3. Systemic steroids, if condition is severe.

Self Care

1. Discourage exposure to sunlight (ultraviolet light).
2. Avoid perfumed soaps; generally no soap or very mild one.
3. Avoid furry, stuffed animal toys.
4. Non-irritating clothing; avoid wool or abrasive fabrics.
5. Child should avoid contact with the chicken pox virus and herpes simplex.
6. Avoid immunizations with live vaccines due to the possibility of severe reactions.

Contact Dermatitis

Contact dermatitis is an inflammatory skin reaction which results because the skin has come in contact with a specific irritant (irritant contact dermatitis that occurs immediately after injury to skin) or allergen (allergic contact dermatitis, which is usually a symptom of delayed hypersensitivity.)

Data Collection

1. Causes.
   a. Poison ivy and poison oak.
   b. Fabric - wool, polyester, etc.
   c. Cosmetics.
   d. Household products such as detergents, soap, hair dye, etc.
   e. Industrial substances - paints, dyes, insecticides, rubber compounds, etc.
2. Clinical manifestations.
   a. Pruritus and discomfort.
   b. Hive-like papules, vesicles, and plaques (more chronic).
   c. Edema.
   d. Sharply circumscribed areas (with occasional vesicle formation) that crust and ooze.

Treatment

1. Medical.
   a. Topical steroids, oral steroids for severe cases.
   b. Antihistamines and antipruritic agents.
   c. Oatmeal baths and topical soaks.
2. Skin testing to determine allergen; skin lesions usually appear within 12 to 48 hours after contact with allergen.

Self Care

1. Teach importance of washing exposed skin with cool water and soap as soon as possible after exposure (within 15 minutes is best).
2. Provide cool, tepid bath; trim fingernails, and utilize measures to control itching.
3. Teach about fallacy of blister fluid spreading the disease.

Impetigo

Impetigo* is a bacterial skin infection caused by invasion of the epidermis by pathogenic *Staphylococcus aureus and/or *group A beta-hemolytic streptococcus.*

Data Collection

1. Pustule-like lesions with moist honey-colored crusts surrounded by redness.

2. Pruritus.
3. Appears more commonly on the face, especially around the mouth.
4. Spreads to surrounding areas.

Treatment

1. Medical - topical antibiotic creams if there are only one or two lesions
2. Systemic antibiotics if there are several lesions.

Self Care

1. Teach the client and family the importance of good hand washing.
2. Encourage adherence to therapeutic regime, especially taking the full course of antibiotics.
3. Untreated impetigo may result in glomerulonephritis.

Fungal (Dermatophyte) Infections

Data Collection

1. Types.
   a. ***Tinea corporis (ringworm)*** — temporary hair loss, if scalp is affected.
   b. ***Tinea cruris ("jock itch")*** — small, red, scaly patches in the groin area.
   c. ***Tinea pedis (athlete's foot)*** — scaling, maceration, erythema, blistering, and pruritus; usually found between the toes.

Treatment

1. Topical antifungal creme.
2. Systemic therapy.
   a. Griseofulvin - used primarily for extensive cases.

Home Care

1. To prevent athlete's foot, client should be instructed to keep feet as dry as possible and use socks of absorbent cotton.
   a. Talcum powder or antifungal powder.
   b. Encourage aeration of shoes to allow them to completely dry out.
2. Ringworm of the scalp, client should maintain hygienic measures to prevent the spread of fungal diseases.
   a. Each family member should avoid using the same comb.
   b. Scarves and hats should be washed thoroughly.
   c. Examine family and household pets frequently for symptoms of the disease.
3. Client should avoid infection in affected areas
   a. Any activity that allows heat, friction, and maceration to occur may lead to skin breakdown and infection.
   b. Loose-fitting clothing and cotton underwear are to be encouraged.

Parasitic Infestations

A. ***Pediculosis.***
1. Types.
   a. *Pediculus humanus corporis* — body lice.
   b. *Phthirus pubis* — pubic lice or crabs.
2. Clinical manifestations.
   a. Intense pruritus which may lead to secondary excoriation and infection.
   b. Tiny, red, noninflammatory lesions.
   c. Eggs (nits) are often attached to the hair shaft in both head and body lice.
   d. Pubic lice are often spread by sexual contact.

B. ***Scabies (mites)*** - an infestation of the skin by itch mites.
1. Intense itching, especially at night.
2. Burrows are seen, especially between fingers, on the surface of wrists, and in axillary folds.
3. Redness, swelling, and vesicular formation may be noted.

Treatment

1. Pediculosis.
   a. Permethrin 1% (NIX) - effective with just one application.
   b. Teach parents to read the directions on the label carefully and follow them for most effective treatment.
2. Scabies.
   a. Permethrin 5% (**Elimite cream**) is considered primary treatment. Cream applied to the skin form head to soles of feet and left on for 8-14 hours, then washed off. Second application in 48 hours is recommended.
   b. Crotamiton (**Eurax**) creme.

Self Care

1. Instruct client as to the proper use of treatment medications.
2. All family members and close contacts need to be treated for parasitic disorders; nits can survive up to 3 weeks when removed from host.
3. Bedding and clothing that may have lice or nits should be washed or dry cleaned; furniture and rugs should be vacuumed or treated.

4. When shampooing hair, use a fine-tooth comb to remove remaining nits.

Viral Infections

Data Collection

1. ***Herpes virus (fever blister, cold sore)*** - herpes virus Type I.
   a. Painful, local reaction of vesicles with an erythematous base; most often occur around the mouth.
   b. Contagious by direct contact, is recurrent; there is no immunity.
   c. Not to be confused with Type II herpes virus that primarily occurs below the waist (genital herpes).
   d. It is possible for the Type I herpes to cause genital lesions, and for the Type II to cause oral lesions (See Sexually Transmitted Diseases in Chapter 17).
2. ***Herpes zoster (shingles).***
   a. Related to the chicken pox virus - varicella.
   b. Contagious to anyone who has not had chicken pox or who may be immunosuppressed.
   c. Linear patches of vesicles with an erythematous base are located along spinal and cranial nerve tracts.
   d. Often unilateral and appears on the trunk; however, may appear on the face.
   e. Pain, burning, and neuralgia occur at the site prior to outbreak of vesicles.
   f. Often precipitated by the same factors as herpes simplex.
3. ***Herpetic whitlow***
   a. Occurs on fingertips and around nail cuticle; often seen in medical personnel.

Treatment

1. Usually symptomatic - soothing moist compresses.
2. Analgesics.
3. Antiviral agents (**Acyclovir)**

Self Care

1. Alleviate pain by administering analgesics.
2. Antihistamines may be administered to control the itching.
3. Usually lesions heal without complications; herpes simplex usually heals without a scar, whereas herpes zoster may scar.
4. If hospitalized, isolate client with herpes zoster.

Cancer of the Skin

Data Collection

1. Risk factors.
   a. Overexposure to sunlight.
   b. Exposure to chemicals.
   c. Clients who have scars due to severe burns.
2. Types.
   a. ***Basal cell carcinoma*** - most common type of skin cancer.
      (1) Appears as a small, waxy nodule with a translucent pearly border.
      (2) Appears more frequently on the face, usually between the hairline and upper lip.
   b. ***Squamous cell carcinoma*** - malignant proliferation arising from the epidermis; usually on sun-damaged skin or skin that has been irradiated or excessively scarred.
      (1) May metastasize.
      (2) Appears as a firm nodule with an indistinct border; may be opaque.
   c. ***Malignant melanoma*** - has the highest mortality rate of any form of skin cancer.
      (1) Often appears in pre-existing moles in the skin.
      (2) Common sites in include back and legs.

Treatment

> Melanomas tend to have
> **A** Asymmetry
> **B** Border irregularity
> **C** Color variegation
> **D** Diameter greater than 6mm.

1. Surgical.
   a. Excisional surgery.
   b. Cryosurgery
   c. Electrodesiccation and curettage.
2. Medical.
   a. X-ray therapy.
   b. Topical and systemic chemotherapy.

Self Care

1. Teach the importance of avoiding unnecessary exposure to sunlight, apply protective sunscreen when outside.
2. Teach the warning signals of cancer.
3. Have moles treated that are in areas where there is friction or repeated irritation.

BURNS

Data Collection

A. Types of burns: chemical, electrical, thermal, and inhalation injury.
B. Fluid shift.

1. Fluid shift and edema formation occurs within 24 to 48 hours postburn; characterized by fluid loss and inflammation.
2. Fluid remobilization occurs within approximately 48 to 72 hours after the initial inflammatory response.

C. Circulatory status.
1. Tachycardia, hypotension occur early.
2. Evaluate urine output.

D. Identify when client ate last; check GI function.

E. Evaluate response to fluid therapy.

F. Evaluate circulatory status of the extremities.

NURSING PRIORITY: *The burned client is often awake, mentally alert and cooperative at first. The level of consciousness may change as respiratory status changes or the fluid shift occurs, precipitating hypovolemia. If the client is unconscious, or confused, assess him for possibility of a head injury.*

G. Identify factors contributing to severity of burn (Table 19-2).
1. Neck and face burns can lead to mechanical occlusion of the airway due to edema.
2. Circumferential burns (burns surrounding an entire extremity) can lead to impaired circulation from edema formation and lack of elasticity of the eschar.
3. Age.
   a. Infants have a immature immune system and poor body defense.
   b. Elderly clients heal slowly; more likely to have wound infection and pulmonary complications.
4. Presence of other health problems.
   a. Diabetes and peripheral vascular disease delay wound healing and ↑ risk of gangrene.
   b. Poor nutrtitional state.
   c. Presence of chronic conditions that compromise the immune system.

Treatment

1. Stabilization of the airway, breathing, and circulation.
2. Fluid resuscitation, IV fluids.
3. Nasogastric tube, NPO; paralytic ileus is common.
4. Analgesics , usually IV route; no IM or SQ meds.
5. Methods of wound care—area is cleaned and debrided of necrotic burned tissue.
   a. Open method (exposure)—burn covered with a topical antibiotic cream; no dressing applied.
   b. Closed method of dressing—fine mesh is used to cover the burned surface; may be impregnated with antibiotic ointment or ointment; may be applied prior to dressing.
   c. Escharotomy—procedure involves excision through the eschar to release pressure and to increase circulation to an extremity with circumferential burns.
   d. Wound grafting—as eschar is debrided and granular tissue begins to form; grafts are utilized to protect the wound and to promote healing.
6. Antibiotics. (Appendix 19-1 for topical).
7. Nutritional support.
   a. Diet is high in calories and protein.
   b. In clients who sustain large burned areas, supplemental gastric tube feedings or hyperalimentation may be utilized.

Nursing Intervention

✦ *Goal: to maintain patent airway and prevent hypoxia.*
1. Assess circumstances surrounding the burn.
2. As edema phase begins, evaluate respiratory status.
3. ET intubation or tracheotomy may be necessary.
4. Assess for ongoing respiratory complications.
5. *Report to RN any significant changes in respiratory status.*

✦ *Goal: to evaluate fluid status and determine where client is in fluid resuscitation.*

NCLEX ALERT: *Identify signs and symptoms of fluid imbalance.*

1. Obtain client's weight on admission.
2. Assess status of fluid resuscitation.
3. Evaluate urine output.
4. Correlate vital signs with previous readings.
5. Monitor signs indicating adequate hydration.

✦ *Goal: to prevent or decrease infection.*
1. Protective isolation - sterile linen, gloves, cap, mask, and gowns.
2. After eschar sloughs, or is removed, assess wound for infection. Infection may be difficult to identify prior to the eschar sloughing.
3. Obtain routine cultures of the wound area.

Box 19-2: Elderly Care Focus
Burns in Older Adults

Have higher mortality rate than the younger adult.

At higher risk for burn injury due to falls, decreased sensation, decreased reaction time, and immobility.

✦ *Goal: to maintain comfort and homeostasis.*

1. Maintain client's body temperature as close to normal as possible; keep room temperature warm.
2. Pressure under a dressing should be evenly distributed; elastic tubular netting may be used to maintain stability of the dressing; circulatory checks q2-3h.

✦ *Goal: to promote healing after wound is closed or grafted.*

NCLEX ALERT: *Promote progress in wound healing.*

1. Dressings are not routinely changed to prevent interruption of a new graft.
2. Graft donor site should be kept clean and dry.

✦ *Goal: to maintain nutrition and promote positive nitrogen balance for healing.*

1. Work with dietitian to maintain nutritional intake.
2. Tube feedings as indicated.
3. Monitor response to hyperalimentation.
4. Daily weight.

✦ *Goal: to prevent contractures and scarring.*

1. Assist client with mobilization and ambulation as soon as possible.
2. Passive and active range of motion should be initiated from the beginning of burn therapy and throughout therapy.
3. Position client to prevent flexion contractures; position of comfort for the client may increase contracture formation.

Table 19-2: DEPTH OF BURN

✦ ***Superficial or first-degree burn*** - area reddened and blanches with pressure; no edema present; area is generally painful to touch.

✦ ***Partial thickness or second- degree*** - Dermis and epidermis affected; formation of large, thick-walled blisters; underlying skin is erythematous.

✦ ***Full thickness or third- degree*** - All of the skin is destroyed; may be damage to the subcutaneous tissue and muscle; usually has a dry appearance, may be white or charred; will require skin grafting to cover area.

✦ ***Fourth- degree burn*** - Full thickness burn in which underlying structures (fascia, tendons, and bones) are severely damaged, usually blackened.

4. Utilize splints and exercises to prevent flexion contractures.

✦ *Goal: to promote acceptance and adaptation to alterations of body image.*

1. Utilize counselors and resource team members.
2. Maintain open communication and encourage expression of feelings.

NURSING PRIORITY: *It is important to recognize that the client's anger is not a direct attack on the care provider; it is an expression of grief and sorrow.*

3. Anticipate depression as a normal consequence of burn trauma; it should decrease as condition improves.

Self-Care

1. Physical therapy.
2. Continue high calorie, high protein diet.
3. Wound care management.

NCLEX ALERT: *Identify and provide support for client with changes in body image.*

Study Questions—Skin

1. The nurse understands that decubitus ulcers are most commonly caused by what problem?

① muscles that are not being used in passive exercises.
② poor nutrition resulting in inadequate protein intake.
③ irritation of a bony prominence that is covered by infected skin.
④ pressure cutting off blood supply to the affected area of the skin.

2. Which stage of a pressure ulcer is characteristic of nonblanching erythema?

① stage II.
② stage III.
③ stage I.
④ stage IV.

3. A client has a pressure ulcer that has necrosis in the subcutaneous level of tissue. There is undermining of the surrounding tissue. What is the stage of this ulcer?

① stage I.
② stage IV.
③ stage III.
④ stage II.

4. When turning a client, the nurse notices an area that is red and moist and the skin is broken. What is the best nursing action?

① clean with alcohol and cover with a sterile gauze dressing.
② keep the client off his left side and put a transparent film dressing over area.
③ apply skin cream to the area and carefully massage it four times a day till clear.
④ apply ice packs to the area to decrease inflammation.

5. What would the nurse teach an elderly client regarding how to care for her dry, itchy skin?

① to use a moisturizer on all dry skin areas.
② wear clothes with 80% or more of cotton fibers.
③ shower twice a day with mild soap.
④ wear protective pads on dry skin areas.

6. A child has impetigo. What is the best description of this condition?

① it is very similar to ringworms
② it is the same virus as herpes.
③ a dermatitis caused by an allergic reaction.
④ is most often a streptococcal infection.

7. What is the most common infection secondary to head lice?

① eczema.
② tinea capitis.
③ impetigo.
④ herpes zoster.

8. A elderly client has been diagnosed with herpes zoster. What is important nursing management for this client?

① daily application of an antifungal cream to affected areas.
② maintain client on standard precautions.
③ administer a herpes zoster immunization.
④ assist the client to deal with the neuralgia.

9. What would be an assessment finding of a client with basal cell carcinoma?

① a reddened area on the lip.
② small translucent nodule on the face.
③ vesicle with a clear fluid.
④ papules and plaques which slough.

10. What is the initial treatment for a client with psoriasis?

① use of topical steroids.
② debridement of dry, raised, scaly areas.
③ ice packs to the inflamed areas.
④ keep the area moist.

11. A child has scabies. What should the nurse explain to the mother?

① carefully remove nits from area and then wash with alcohol.
② spread **Elimite** cream all over body, leave on for 8 to 1-12 hours and then wash off.
③ use moist soaks of antifungal medication on burrowed skin lesions.
④ encourage exposure to sunlight to dry area.

12. What is a priority assessment finding for client who has sustained burns on the face and neck?

① spreading, large, clear vesicles.
② increased respirations.
③ difficulty with vision.
④ increased thirst.

13. When assessing a client for psoriasis, what would the nurse anticipate finding?

① pruritic vesicles.
② edema in the extremities.
③ petechiae in the lower extremities.
④ scaly, plaque-like lesions.

14. A child is diagnosed with impetigo. How would the nurse instruct the mother to take care of the child?

① apply an antibiotic cream to the dried lesion.

② wash the lesions and apply a steroid ointment.

③ administer the oral antibiotic until it is all gone.

④ keep the lesions clean and dry.

15. What is important to teach the mother regarding the management of a child with atopic dermatitis (eczema)?

① anticipate child will have chronic bronchitis.

② short time exposure to sunlight will dry lesions.

③ use ointments and oatmeal baths to keep skin moist.

④ although lesions are present, itching is not a problem.

Tolnaftate is used for ringworm

Thiabendazole is used to treat visceral roundworm, threadworm and pinworm

Permethrin (Elimite) scabies

Appendix 19-1:
TOPICAL ANTIBIOTICS FOR BURN TREATMENT

MEDICATIONS	SIDE EFFECTS	NURSING IMPLICATIONS
TOPICAL ANTIBIOTICS: Prevent and treat infection at the burn site.		
Silver sulfadiazine (**Silvadene**)	Pain, burning on application. Hypersensitivity: rash, itching, or burning sensation in unburned skin.	1. Liberal amounts are spread topically with a sterile, gloved hand or on impregnated gauze rolls over the burned surface. 2. If discoloration occurs in the **Silvadene** cream, do not use. 3. Dressings are not required, but are frequently utilized. A thin layer of cream is spread evenly over the entire burn surface. 4. Client should be bathed or tubbed daily to aid in debridement. 5. Medication does not penetrate eschar and is bactericidal. 6. On extensive burns, monitor urine output and renal function; a significant amount of sulfa may be absorbed.
Mafenide acetate **(Sulfamylon 10%)**	Pain, burning or stinging at application sites; excessive loss of body water; excoriation of new tissue; may be systemically absorbed and cause metabolic acidosis.	1. Bacteriostatic medication diffuses rapidly through burned skin and eschar and is effective against bacteria under the eschar. 2. Dressings are not required, but are frequently utilized. A thin layer of cream is spread evenly over the entire burn surface. 3. Monitor renal function, as medication is rapidly absorbed from the burn surface and eliminated via the kidney. 4. Pain on application occurs.

Appendix 19-2:
MEDICATIONS USED IN SKIN DISORDERS

MEDICATIONS	SIDE EFFECTS	NURSING IMPLICATIONS
❖ GENERAL NURSING IMPLICATIONS ❖ — Topical medications are used primarily for local effects when systemic absorption is undesirable. — For topical application: Apply after shower or bath for best absorption, as skin is hydrated. Apply small amount of medication and rub in well.		
ANTI-FUNGAL: Inhibits or damages fungal cell membrane either altering permeability or disrupting cell mitosis.		
Clotrimazole (**Lotrimin**): topical Nystatin (**Mycolog**): topical Ketoconazole (**Nizoral**): PO, topical Griseofulvin (**Fulvicin**): PO	Nausea, vomiting, abdominal pain Hypersensitivity reaction—rash, urticaria, pruritus Hepatotoxicity Gynecomastia (ketoconozole)	1. Monitor hepatic function (when on oral medication). 2. Avoid alcohol due to potential liver problems. 3. Check for local burning, irritation, or itching with topical application. 4. Prolonged therapy (weeks or months) is usually necessary, especially with griseofulvin (**Fulvicin**). 5. Take griseofulvin (**Fulvicin**) with foods high in fat, (e.g., milk, ice cream), to decrease GI upset and assist in absorption. 6. ***Uses:*** Tinea infections, fungal infections, candidiasis diaper dermatitis.
ANTIVIRAL: Reduces viral shedding, pain, and time to heal.		
Acyclovir (**Zovirax**): topical, PO, IV.	IV: phlebitis, rash, hives PO: nausea, vomiting Topical: burning, stinging, pruritus	1. Apply topically to affected area six times per day. 2. Avoid auto-inoculation; wash hands frequently; apply with gloved hand. 3. Avoid sexual intercourse for duration of genital lesions. 4. Drink adequate fluids. 5. Infuse IV preparations over 1 hour; use an infusion pump for accurate delivery. 6. ***Uses:*** *herpes infections.*
ANTI-INFLAMMATORY: Decreases the inflammatory response.		
Triamcinolone adetonide (**Aristocort**): topical	Skin thinning, superficial dilated blood vessels (teleangiectasis), acne-like eruptions, adrenal suppression.	1. Triamcinolone and hydrocortisone cremes come in various strengths and potency. Watch the percent strength. 2. Applied 2-3 times a day. 3. Use an occlusive dressing only if ordered. 4. Encourage client to use the least amount possible and for the shortest period of time.

Maternal Care 20

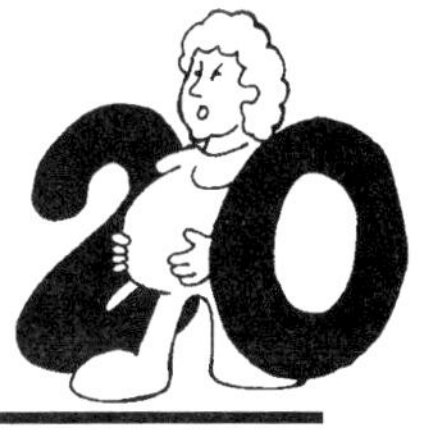

CONTRACEPTION

❑ ***Contraception* is the voluntary prevention of pregnancy. Two important factors influence the selection of the particular type of contraceptive method: acceptability and effectiveness.**

Data Collection

A. Types of Contraception.
  1. Temporary methods used to delay or avoid pregnancy.
  2. Permanent-voluntary sterilization.

B. Contraceptive methods (Appendix 20-1).

NORMAL PREGNANCY CYCLE: PHYSIOLOGIC CHANGES

Uterus

1. Increase in size as a result of the stimulating influence of estrogen and the distention caused by the growing fetus.
2. Irregular, painless uterine contractions (Braxton-Hicks) begin in the early weeks of pregnancy; contraction and relaxation assist in accommodating the growing fetus.
3. Softening of the lower uterine segment (Hegar's sign).

> ***NURSING PRIORITY:** Multigravidas tend to report a greater incidence of Braxton-Hicks contractions than primigravidas.*

4. Cervical changes.
   a. Softening of the cervix (Goodell's sign).
   b. Formation of the mucous plug to prevent bacterial contamination from the vagina.

Vagina

1. An increase in vaginal secretions.
2. A blue-purple hue of the vaginal walls is seen very early (Chadwick's sign).
3. Vaginal secretions: thickish white and acidic (pH is 3.5 to 6.0).

Breasts

1. Increase in breast size accompanied by feelings of fullness, tingling, and heaviness.
2. Superficial veins prominent; nipples erect; darkening and increase in diameter of the areola.
3. Thin, watery secretion (precursor to colostrum) can be expressed from the nipples by the end of the tenth week.

Cardiovascular System

1. Increased blood volume (30 - 50%).
2. Increase in heart rate; (ten beats per minute) by the end of the first trimester.
3. Increase in cardiac output (30 - 50%).
4. Cardiac enlargement and systolic murmurs.
5. Hematocrit (Hct) decreases by 7% - physiologic anemia.
6. BP will decrease slightly in the 2nd trimester.

Respiratory System

1. Diaphragm is elevated; change from abdominal to thoracic breathing around the twenty-fourth week.
2. Breathes deeper; only slightly increases respiratory rate.
3. Common complaints of nasal stuffiness and epistaxis due to estrogen influence on nasal mucosa.
4. Increased oxygen consumption.

Urinary/Renal Systems

1. Ureter and renal pelvis dilate (especially on the right side) as a result of the growing uterus.
2. Frequency of urination (first and last trimester).
3. Decreased bladder tone (due to effect of progesterone); bladder capacity increases: 1,300 to 1,500 cc.
4. Frequent spilling of glucose in urine (glycosuria).

Gastrointestinal System

1. Pregnancy gingivitis - gums reddened, swollen, and bleed easily.
2. Nausea and vomiting due to elevated human chorionic gonadotropin (HCG).
3. Decreased tone and motility of smooth muscles; decreased emptying time of stomach; slowed peristalsis leads to complaints of bloating, heartburn, and constipation.

Musculoskeletal System

1. Increase in the normal lumbosacral curve leads to backward tilt of the torso.

2. Center of gravity is changed ,which often leads to leg and back strain and predisposition to falling.
3. Pelvis relaxes due to the effects of the hormone relaxin; leads to the characteristic "duck waddling" gait.

Integumentary System

1. Increased skin pigmentation in various areas of the body.
   a. Facial: mask of pregnancy (chloasma).
   b. Abdomen: striae (red- purple stretch marks) and linea nigra (darkened vertical line from umbilicus to symphysis pubis).
2. Appearance of vascular spider nevi, especially on the neck, arms and legs.
3. Acne vulgaris, dermatitis, and psoriasis usually improve during pregnancy.

Placenta

1. Functions include transport of nutrients and removal of waste products from the fetus.
2. Produces human chorionic gonadotropin (HCG) and human placental lactogen (HPL).
3. Produces estrogen and progesterone after two months of gestation.
4. Production of posterior pituitary hormones: oxytocin, which promotes uterine contractility and stimulation of milk let-down reflex.

Metabolism

1. Normal weight gain: 25 to 35 lb (11.3-15.9kg).
2. Pattern of weight gain for normal weight before pregnancy.
   a. First trimester—3.5- 5 lb (1.6 - 2.3 kg).
   b. Second & third trimester—12-15 lb (5.5-6.8 kg) for each trimester or 0.97 lb (0.44kg) ***per week.***
3. There are variations of recommended weight gain based on whether the woman is overweight, underweight, or carrying twins.

NCLEX ALERT: *It is important for the nurse to be aware of the normal physiological changes during pregnancy and respond to client's questions appropriately.*

PSYCHOLOGICAL CHANGES OF THE EXPECTANT FAMILY

Changes in the Mother

A. Ambivalence.

1. If women feels comfortable in addressing ambivalent feelings, the focus is usually on changed lifestyle or the career-motherhood dilemma.
2. Indirect evidence of ambivalence:
   a. Complaints of depression or physical discomfort.
   b. Complaints of feeling ugly or unattractive.
3. Some women may consider the possibility of abortion, if pregnancy is unwanted.

B. Acceptance.

1. With an unplanned pregnancy, there is greater evidence of fear and conflict, along with more physical discomfort and depression.
2. If pregnancy is well-accepted, women experiences less discomfort and more tolerance to physical discomforts during the last trimester.

C. Introversion.

1. This "turning in on oneself" focus is normal.
2. Helps the mother plan, adjust, adapt, build, and draw strength in preparation for childbirth.

D. Mood swings.

1. Can cause difficulty in the relationship if couple doesn't realize what is occurring.
2. Husband may feel exasperated with her tears and withdraw and ignore problem when she really needs him to be affectionate and supportive.

E. Changes in body image.

1. Woman may feel negative toward body, especially during 3rd trimester.

F. Psychological tasks of the mother (Rubin, 1984).

1. Ensuring safe passage through pregnancy, labor, and birth.
2. Seeking acceptance of this child by others.
3. Seeking of commitment and acceptance of self as mother to the infant (binding-in).
4. Learning to give of one's self on behalf on one's child.

Changes in the Father

A. First trimester.

1. May feel left out of pregnancy.
2. Confused by partner's mood swings.
3. May experience "mitleiden" and develop similar symptoms of discomfort along with his partner.

B. Second and third trimesters.

1. Promote his involvement by his watching and feeling fetal movement.
2. Needs to confront and resolve his own conflicts about the fathering he received as a child.

3. Will decide on what he does and does not want to imitate from his father role figure.
4. May react differently to partner's physical body changes.

C. Developmental phases of the expectant father.
1. Announcement phase—accepts the biologic fact of pregnancy.
2. Moratorium phase—adjusts to the reality of pregnancy.
3. Focusing phase—negotiates with his partner the role he is to play in labor and to prepare for parenthood.

Changes in Siblings

A. Sibling rivalry.
1. Older child will have to share parent's time.
2. Awareness of change in family.
3. Younger children may experience separation anxiety when mother leaves for hospital.
4. Possible temporary regressive behavior demonstrated by dependency, demanding, and acting out.

B. Adequate preparation for the arrival of the new baby is important in reducing sibling rivalry.
1. Amount of parental attention focused on new baby.
2. Amount of parental attention given to the older child.
3. Parental reinforcement of regressive/aggressive behavior.

PRENATAL CARE

Data Collection

A. Initial visit.
1. Complete history and physical.
2. Obstetric history.
   a. Past pregnancies (date, course of pregnancy, labor and postpartum; information about infant and neonatal course).
   b. Present pregnancy.

B. Subsequent assessment data follow-up.
1. Vital signs.
2. Urinalysis - check for protein and sugar.
3. Monitor weight.
4. Measurement of height of uterine fundus.
5. Auscultation of fetal heart rate (FHR).

C. Definition of Common Terms (Table 20-1).

D. Signs and Symptoms of Pregnancy (Table 20-2).

E. Summary of the Antepartum Period (Table 20-3).

Diagnostics

A. Pregnancy tests.
1. Immunoassay—based on antigenic property of HCG.
   a. Hemagglutination-inhibition test or HAI (Neocept)—no clumping of cells when urine of a pregnant woman is added to the HCG-sensitized red blood cells of sheep 4 days after the first missed menstrual period.
   b. Latex agglutination tests (Gravindex and Pregnosticon slide test)—latex particle agglutination is inhibited in the presence of urine containing HCG; accurate from 4-10 days after the first missed menstrual period.
2. Radioreceptor assay — uses radioiodine.
   a. Radioreceptor Assay or RRA (Biocept-G) — uses radio-iodine labeled HCG; very sensitive test; accurate at the time of the first missed menstrual period.
   b. Beta subunit radioimmunoassay or RIA (Beta Tec, Chorio Quant)—uses radioiodinated HCG that is added to urine or serum as an antigen to specific antibodies; most reliable test as it identifies the beta subunit of HCG; accurate as early as 6 days before the first missed menstrual period.

> ***NURSING PRIORITY:** RIA is most accurate and quickest method (results in 1 hour) and it becomes positive a few days after presumed implantation, which permits earlier diagnosis.*

3. Enzyme-linked immunosorbent assay or ELISA (Pregnospia, Tandem ICON, Confidot)—uses monoclonal anti-HCG; accurate results are possible about 4 days before first missed menstrual period.
4. Home pregnancy tests (Fact, Clearblue Easy, Daisy-2)— are either HAI or ELISA type tests; best on first voided specimens; detects low levels of HCG; can be used within a few days of a missed period and give results in less than 30 minutes; false negative results should be followed up in presence of pregnancy symptoms.

B. Laboratory tests.
1. Urinalysis.
2. Complete blood count (CBC).
3. VDRL— RPR serologic screening for syphilis.
4. Vaginal cultures for gonorrhea and chlamydia in high- risk populations.

Table 20-1: DEFINITION OF COMMON TERMS

COMMON TERM	DEFINITION
✦ Gravida*	A pregnancy regardless of the duration; includes the present pregnancy.
✦ Para*	Refers to past pregnancies that continue to the period of viability (legal definition: 24 to 28 weeks gestational age amd 20 weeks, in some states i.e. texas and california).
✦ Primigravida	Woman who is pregnant for the first time.
✦ Multigravida	Woman who is pregnant for the second or subsequent time.
✦ Nullipara (para 0)	Woman who has not had children.
✦ Primipara (para 1)	Woman who has carried a pregnancy to viability; term is often used interchangeably with primigravida.
✦ Multipara (para II, para III, para IV, etc.)	Woman who has given birth to two or more children.
✦ Parturient	A woman in labor.

*The terms *gravida* and *para* refer to the number of pregnancies, not the number of fetuses. The woman who delivers twins on her first pregnancy remains a para 1, in spite of having two infants. She also is a para 1 if the fetus was stillborn or died soon after birth.

❑ **Another system used to describe reproductive status is the five-digit identification system characterized by the acronym GTPAL:**

G = total number of pregnancies
T = number of term infants (37 weeks of gestation)
P = number of preterm infants (before 37 weeks of gestation)
A = number of spontaneous or therapeutic abortions
L = number of living children

5. Antibody titers for HIV infection, rubella, and hepatitis B (HBsAg).
6. Blood type and Rh; if Rh is negative, necessary to check the father's blood group and Rh.
7. If mother is of African or Mediterrean descent, sickle cell screening.
8. Rubella titer.

C. Pelvic examination.

1. Papanicolaou smear of the cervix (PAP smear).
2. Pelvic measurements (pelvimetry).

D. Calculation of estimated date of confinement (EDC); estimated date of delivery (EDD).

1. Naegele's rule: count back three calendar months from the first day of the last menstrual period (LMP) and add seven days.
2. Examples:
   a. LMP, April 10, 1997: EDC, January 17, 1998.
   b. LMP, October 25, 1997: EDC, July 2, 1998.

Nursing Intervention

NCLEX ALERT: *The practical nurse's role in self-care education regarding common discomforts of pregnancy and general health practices is important to emphasize in your review of prenatal nursing management.*

✦ *Goal: to educate families regarding general health practices.*

1. **Hygiene:** tub baths are permitted until last trimester, when balance is altered due to change in center of gravity; no douching, no hot tubs.
2. **Clothing:** loose, comfortable clothing with good supporting brassiere; low-heeled shoes.
3. **Employment:** no severe physical straining, heavy lifting, or prolonged periods of sitting or standing.
4. **Travel:** avoid during the last month of pregnancy; when traveling by car or airplane, frequent walking and stretching is advised; use seat belts (both lap and shoulder), positioning the lap belt under the abdomen.

Table 20-2: SIGNS AND SYMPTOMS OF PREGNANCY

PRESUMPTIVE/SUBJECTIVE	PROBABLE/OBJECTIVE	POSITIVE/DIAGNOSTIC
1. Amenorrhea.	1. Positive pregnancy test (Gravidex, UCG, pregnosticon R).	1. Fetal heart tone: 10th to 12th week -Doppler. 18th to 20th week -Fetoscope.
2. Nausea and vomiting.	2. Enlarged abdomen.	2. Fetal movements.
3. Excessive fatigue.	3. Hegar's sign - softening of lower uterine segment.	3. Fetal skeleton on x-ray (not used often).
4. Urinary frequency.	4. Chadwick's sign -bluish discoloration of vagina.	4. Fetal sonography (after 16th week).
5. Breast changes - tenderness, fullness, increased pigmentation of areola, pre-colostrum discharge.	5. Goodell's sign -softening of cervical lip.	
6. Quickening - active movements of the fetus felt by the mother.	6. Ballottement - pushing on fetus (4th to 5th month) and feeling it rebound back.	
7. Increased pigmentation of skin and abdominal striae.	7. Fetal outline distinguished by palpation.	
	8. Braxton-Hicks contractions.	

NCLEX ALERT: *The signs and symptoms of pregnancy are frequently tested; be sure you are able to differentiate between presumptive, probable, and positive signs.*

5. **Rest and exercise:** adequate amounts of exercise - walking, swimming; client should stop exercising when she begins to feel tired; *moderation* is the key word.
6. **Smoking:** not advised; associated with infants who are small for gestational age (SGA).
7. **Alcohol:** recommended not to consume any alcohol; the more consumed, the greater the risk for fetal alcohol syndrome.
8. **Medications:** client advised to avoid OTC medications, especially during the first trimester. She should consult with her physician before taking any medications.

✦ *Goal: to promote relief of common discomforts through client education of self-care measures (Table 20-4).*

NCLEX ALERT: *Use measures to improve client's nutritional status.*

✦ *Goal: to promote adequate nutrition.*

1. Assess normal food intake.
2. Dietary instructions and nutrient requirements.
   a. Increase calories for pregnancy (an additional 300 calories per day) for a total of 2200 calories per day.
   b. Increase calories for lactation (an additional 500 calories per day).
   c. Increase protein to 60gm/day.
   d. Increase vitamins (generally all vitamin intake is increased, especially folic acid).
   e. Increase amount of minerals (especially iron, calcium, and phosphorous).
   f. Additional calories and protein may be recommended for the pregnant adolescent.

✦ *Goal: to educate expectant family with regard to danger signs and symptoms requiring immediate attention (Table 20-5).*

FETUS

Multiple Pregnancy

1. Fraternal twins - can be either the same sex or a different sex.
2. Identical twins - same sex, resemble each other in appearance and structure.

Placenta

1. Transfer of oxygen, nutrients, and metabolites.
2. Elimination of waste products from the fetus.
3. Production of hormones - human chorionic gonadotropin (HCG), human placental lactogen (HPL), estrogen (estriol) and progesterone.

Table 20-3: SUMMARY OF NURSING MANAGEMENT DURING THE ANTEPARTUM PERIOD

WEEKS' GESTATION	PHYSICAL SIGNS & SYMPTOMS	CHARACTERISTIC BEHAVIORS	NURSING INTERVENTIONS
0 - 16	Amenorrhea Fatigue Nausea Vomiting ↑ breast size and tenderness Urinary frequency ↑ appetite	Ambivalence with mood swings. Anxiety related to confirmation of pregnancy. Tells selected close persons of pregnancy.	1. Obtain complete history, including gynecologic and obstetric histories. Monthly followup visits. 2. Ascertain any maternal high-risk problems such as maternal age (over 35 years) heart disease, diabetes or potential high-risk neonate problems, history of congenital defects, premature births, etc. (See complete discussion in this chapter on high risk problems). 3. Identify maternal nutritional status by assessing height, weight, and frame and compare with standardized charts of normal ranges. 4. Complete a diet history and instruction. *Important to teach about necessary changes, rather than all the concepts of good nutrition.* 5. Food cravings are usually benign and may be indulged, providing a well-balanced diet is maintained. *Pica is an abnormal eating pattern and requires treatment.* 6. Encourage client to express feelings about pregnancy or ambivalence. 7. Anticipatory guidance/teaching (including family) related to: Drugs, radiation, normal signs and symptoms of pregnancy as well as reportable signs of possible complications, and the normality of her mood swings.

4. Fetal surface is shiny and slightly grayish—Schultze.
5. Maternal side is rough and beefy red—Duncan.
6. Maternal and fetal bloodstreams are in close relationship to each other, but the circulations do not mix.

Fetal Circulation

A. Fetal lungs do not participate in respiratory gas exchange.
B. There are special fetal structures to bypass blood supply to the lungs.

Monitoring of Fetal Status

A. Ultrasound—use of high frequency sound waves that detect fetal heart beat, fetal breathing activity, and fetal body movement.
   1. Purpose—identifies placental location for amniocentesis or to determine placenta previa.
   2. Procedure.
      a. Performed with a full bladder, except when ultrasound is used to localize the placenta prior to amniocentesis.
      b. Client advised to drink one quart of water two hours prior to sonogram.
      c. Requires approximately twenty to thirty minutes to perform; client must lie flat on back, which may be uncomfortable.

B. Nonstress Test (NST)
   1. Purpose—to observe the response of fetal heart rate to the stress of activity.
   2. Procedure—requires approximately thirty minutes; client in semi-Fowler's position; external monitor is applied to document fetal activity; mother activates the "mark button" on the electronic fetal monitor when she feels fetal movement.
   3. Advantages of NST.
      a. Simple; easy to perform.
      b. Does not require hospitalization.
      c. Has no contraindications.

C. Contraction Stress Test (CST)
   1. Two types.

Table 20-3: SUMMARY OF NURSING MANAGEMENT DURING THE ANTEPARTUM PERIOD

WEEKS' GESTATION	PHYSICAL SIGNS & SYMPTOMS	CHARACTERISTIC BEHAVIORS	NURSING INTERVENTIONS
16 - 30	Quickening. "Pregnant figure." Increased energy. Feeling of well-being. Round ligament pain.	Wears maternity clothes. Tells the world she's pregnant, begins to notice other pregnant women. Interested in learning about birth and babies - reads books, seeks out and questions friends and family, attends classes. Increased dependency as time goes on.	1. On-going assessment of maternal/fetal status (monthly visits up to the 5th month, then every 2-3 weeks): FHR Vital signs Fundal height Urine test for glucose (mild glycosuria is usually benign), protein, and nitrites. Finger stick for hemoglobin analysis (12-14 g/dl normal) Balanced diet 2. Prevent or minimize activity intolerance and promote adequate rest by: Encouraging 8 hours sleep each day, plus one nap Scheduling rest periods at place of employment Napping at home while other small children are sleeping Using left lateral position while resting or sleeping 3. Promote adequate exercise, (e.g., Kegel, pelvic rocking, modified sit ups), sitting tailor fashion (lotus position) 4. Anticipatory guidance/teaching (including family) related to: Libido changes, mood swings, increasing dependency, introversion, and reportable signs of possible complications.
30 - 40	Dependent edema. Pressure in lower abdomen. Frequent urination. Round ligament pain. Backache. Insomnia. Clumsiness. Fatigue.	Introversion. Increased dependency (craves attention and tenderness). Altered responsiveness and spontaneity as well as abdominal bulk and fatigue may decrease interest in genital sex uemay decrease interest in genital sex as well as abdominal bulk and fatigue. Intensifies study of labor and delivery. Increasingly feeling more vulnerable. Prepares nursery - buys baby things. Decides on feeding method for baby.	1. Ongoing continued physical assessment and every 2-3 weeks during 8th month and weekly visits from 9th month till delivery. 2. Reassure -provide emotional support related to attractiveness and self-worth. 3. Anticipatory guidance/teaching (including family) related to: Signs and symptoms of labor, environmental modification for coming infant and to provide rest for mother, teaching associated with either breast or bottle feeding, advising client concerning birthing and anesthesia options, promoting the developing parent/child attachment (encourage family to verbalize mental picture of infant and concepts of selves as parents).

Table 20-4: SUMMARY OF COMMON DISCOMFORTS AND RELIEF MEASURES

DISCOMFORT	RELIEF MEASURES
1ST TRIMESTER:	
Nausea and vomiting (morning sickness)	Frequent small meals; avoid empty stomach; between meals, eat crackers without fluid; avoid fried and spicy foods.
Urinary frequency and urgency	Practice Kegel exercises; problem may be unpreventable; use perineal pads for leakage.
Breast tenderness	Well-fitting support bra.
Increased vaginal discharge	Good hygiene; use perineal pads; no douching unless prescribed.
2ND AND 3RD TRIMESTERS:	
Heartburn	Avoid coffee, fat and fried, spicy foods; eat small, frequent meals; maintain good posture; sit upright; at night sleep with an extra pillow; swallow own saliva or chew gum.
Ankle edema	Avoid prolonged sitting or standing; support stockings applied before rising; elevate feet while sitting.
Varicose veins	Avoid prolonged periods of standing; apply support hose before rising; elevate feet while sitting; do not cross legs at knees.
Hemorrhoids	Avoid constipation, do not strain; use bulk-producing laxatives, anesthetic suppositories as prescribed.
Constipation	Increase fluid intake (6 to 8 glasses/day); eat food and fruits high in roughage; exercise moderately; use bulk-producing laxatives as prescribed.
Backache	Correct posture; low-heeled shoes; pelvic tilt exercise.
Leg cramps	Stretch affected muscle and hold till cramp subsides; warm packs; maintain adequate calcium intake.
Faintness	Sit or lie down; do not lock knees, and avoid prolonged standing.
Shortness of breath	Good posture; sleep with head elevated by several pillows.

NCLEX ALERT: *Identify signs of potential prenatal complications.*

a. Breast Self-Stimulation Test (BSST) or Nipple Stimulation Contraction Stress Test (NSCST)—stimulate breasts by rubbing nipples

b. Oxytocin Challenge Test (OCT)—administration of IV oxytocin (PITOCIN).

2. Purpose (OCT)—to observe the response of fetal heart rate to the stress of oxytocin-induced uterine contractions.

3. Procedure—OCT.

a. Client must be hospitalized and NPO.

b. Position in semi-Fowler's to avoid supine hypotension.

c. Intravenous administration of oxytocin stimulates uterine contractions - uterine activity and fetal heart rate are recorded by way of external monitoring.

D. Amniotic Fluid Analysis.

1. Purpose—analysis of the amniotic fluid obtained by the technique of amniocentesis.

2. Procedure.

a. Amniocentesis—introduction of a needle through the abdominal and uterine walls into the amniotic cavity to aspirate fluid for examination.

b. Supine position with slight elevation of the head.

c. Client should empty her bladder.

d. Abdomen is prepped: local anesthetic infiltrated subcutaneously; needle inserted and amniotic fluid aspirated and sent to laboratory for analysis.

3. Post-procedure management.

a. **Rhogam** is given post-procedure in non-sensitized Rh negative women.

b. May have mild cramping; maintain bedrest till it subsides.

E. Alpha-fetoprotein Testing.

1. Purpose—determine whether fetus has a open neural tube defect, (e.g., anencephaly or spina bifida.)

2. Procedure.

a. Between 15-18 weeks gestation, maternal blood sample can be drawn.

b. If level is above or below the normal range, ultrasound is recommended for further evaluation.

COMPLICATIONS ASSOCIATED WITH PREGNANCY

Abortion

❑ **Termination of pregnancy prior to viability (twenty to twenty-four weeks' gestation); abortions can be spontaneous (miscarriage) or induced (therapeutic or elective); approximately 75 percent to 80 percent of all spontaneous abortions occur during the second and third months of gestation.**

Data Collection

1. Risk factors.
   a. Maternal: chronic infections, fibroid tumors, structural uterine anomalies.
   b. Acute infection.
2. Clinical manifestations (types of spontaneous abortions.)
   a. Threatened abortion - slight bleeding, mild back and lower abdominal cramping, no cervical dilatation, no passage of the products of conception.
   b. Inevitable abortion—moderate amount of bleeding and cramping, internal cervical os dilates, and membranes may rupture.
   c. Incomplete abortion—only part of the products of conception are expelled.
   d. Complete abortion—all the products of conception are expelled.
   e. Missed abortion—fetus dies in utero.
   f. Habitual abortion—three or more successive, spontaneous abortions.

Treatment

(Varies according to type of abortion)

1. Threatened abortion—bedrest, sedation, and sometimes progesterone therapy (may cause congenital anomalies).
2. Inevitable and incomplete abortion.
   a. Fluid replacement: IVs, type and crossmatch for possible blood transfusion.
   b. Administration of oxytocin.
   c. Dilatation and curettage or a suction evacuation to remove products of conception.
3. Missed abortion—If abortion does not occur spontaneously after six weeks, suction evacuation or D&C will be done.
4. Habitual abortion—determination of cause, then specific therapy to correct.
5. Administration of **Rhogam** if mother is Rh negative (given within 72 hours). Given after every pregnancy.

Table 20-5: DANGER SIGNS OF PREGNANCY

- Vaginal discharge—bloody or amniotic fluid.
- Visual disturbances.
- Swelling of face or fingers.
- Fever and chills.
- Severe continuous headache.
- Pain in the abdomen
- Persistent vomiting.
- Absence of fetal movement.

Nursing Intervention

✦ *Goal: to assess or control hemorrhage.*

1. Monitoring of vital signs.
2. Accurate counting of pads to assess bleeding.
3. *Report to RN any signs of increased bleeding.*

✦ *Goal: to prevent complications.*

1. Observe for shock.
2. Prevent isoimmunization by administration of **Rhogam**.
3. Assess for elevated temperature.

✦ *Goal: to provide emotional support to the couple experiencing the loss of pregnancy.*

1. Encourage verbalization of feelings.
2. Be available and actively listen.

Self-Care

1. Report any increased bleeding.
2. Do not use tampons; peri-pads only.
3. Check temperature every 8 hours for 3 days.
4. Do not resume sexual activity until physician okays (usually after bleeding stops).

Ectopic Pregnancy

❑ **Any pregnancy that develops outside the uterus (extrauterine) is an *ectopic pregnancy.* Ninety percent of ectopic pregnancies are tubal; more common on the right side.**

Data Collection

1. If tube ruptures, sudden excruciating pain in the lower abdomen, usually over the mass.
2. Possible referred shoulder pain as the abdomen fills with blood.
3. Vaginal bleeding.
4. Shock.

Surgical treatment

1. Laparoscopy, laparotomy, salpingectomy.

Table 20-6: CLINICAL MANIFESTATIONS OF PREGNANCY-INDUCED HYPERTENSION

MILD PREECLAMPSIA	SEVERE PREECLAMPSIA	ECLAMPSIA
Elevated BP - systolic increase of 30 mm Hg. and 15 mm Hg. increase in diastolic over baseline.	Increased hypertension - systolic at 160 mm Hg; diastolic at 110 mm Hg. or more.	Elevated temperature (101°F); may precede convulsion (104°F is a grave sign).
Proteinuria - 1 gm/24 hour (1+ proteinuria).	Proteinuria - 5 gm/24 hour (3+ to 4+ proteinuria).	Tonic (15 to 20 sec) and clonic (60 sec) convulsions.
Edema -generalized, especially digital and periorbital.	Edema - excessive.	Coma (lasts from few minutes to several hours).
Weight gain - 1 lb/week in 3rd trimester.	Elevated BUN, serum creatinine, uric acid.	Hypertensive crisis or shock.
	Oliguria - less than 400 cc in 24 hours.	Renal shutdown.
	Cerebral or visual disturbances.	
	Severe headache.	
	Vomiting.	
	Epigastric pain (due to edema of liver capsule; usually indicative of impending convulsion).	

Nursing Intervention

✦ *Goal: to prevent and detect early complications.*

1. Provision of nursing care for shock as indicated.
2. Prepare for surgery (IVs, oxygen, blood, etc.).
3. Administer **Rhogam**, if indicated.

✦ *Goal: to provide emotional support (loss of pregnancy and possibly reproductive organ).*

Hyperemesis Gravidarum

❑ **This disorder is characterized by pernicious vomiting during pregnancy.**

Data Collection

1. Severe, persistent vomiting that is different from morning sickness.
2. If untreated, ketoacidosis (from loss of intestinal juices), hypovolemia, hypokalemia, jaundice, and hemorrhage.
3. Hypothrombinemia and decreased urine output.

Treatment

1. Medical - stop the vomiting, replacement of parental fluids, electrolytes, and vitamins, along with a tranquilizer or an antiemetic.
2. Dietary - NPO for first 48 hours; after condition improves, six small feedings alternated with liquid nourishment in small amounts every 1 to 2 hours; if vomiting reoccurs, NPO and IV fluids restarted.

Nursing Intervention

✦ *Goal: to assist with the medical and dietary management.*

1. Accurate recording of vomitus.
2. Daily weight checks and maintenance of intake and output.
3. Desired urine output is 1000cc in 24 hours; usually, administration of IV's at 3000cc in first 24 hours after admission to correct hypovolemia.
4. Oral hygiene measures.
5. NPO for first 48 hours, then slow diet progression.
6. Stress may contribute to condition; need to provide emotional support.

Hypertensive Disorders

❑ **Pregnancy-induced hypertension (PIH) is the term used for *hypertensive disorders* that are specifically associated with pregnancy, preeclampsia and eclampsia. Previously, the term *toxemia of pregnancy* was used.**

Data Collection

A. Risk factors.

1. Diabetes mellitus.
2. Hypertension.
3. Multiple gestations.
4. Age (less than seventeen or over thirty-five).
5. Primarily a disease of the primigravida.

Table 20-7: NURSING MANAGEMENT OF CLIENTS WITH PREGNANCY-INDUCED HYPERTENSION

✦ *Goal: Recognize the early signs of PIH and increased BP.*

1. Check BP and perform roll-over or pressor response test at weeks 28-32 in the high-risk client. Take BP in left lateral recumbent position; repeat BP after turning to supine position.

NURSING PRIORITY: *Diastolic increases of 20 mm Hg or more may be predictive of PIH.*

2. Monitor urine for proteinuria. Usually the last of the triad of symptoms to appear.
3. Monitor for nondependent pathologic edema (e.g., periorbital and hands).

✦ *Goal: Recognize progression of PIH symptoms and minimize or control their sequelae.*

1. Institute weight controls. Check for sudden increases of 2 lb/week or 6 lb/month.
2. Increase protein intake in the diet. Maintain normal sodium intake; avoid use of diuretics.
3. Institute bedrest.
4. Monitor for ominous signs of deteriorating condition: headache, visual disturbances, hyperreflexia, markedly decreased urine output, epigastric or right upper quadrant pain, dyspnea, vaginal bleeding (abruptio placentae) or any change in fetal activity.
5. Administer **Apresoline**, a vasodilator; check maternal BP, pulse, and FHR.

✦ *Goal: Prevent or control seizures.*

1. Administration of IV $MgSO_4$ by RN.
2. Have emergency items readily available, (e.g., O_2, suction, airway, sedatives, calcium gluconate).
3. Modify environment to ensure rest and quiet.
   a. Eliminate noise, bright lights, other harsh stimuli.
   b. Minimize number of personnel giving care.
   c. Initiate painful and/or intrusive procedures after sedation.
   d. Promote comfort at bed rest.

✦ *Goal: Recognize alterations in fetal well-being and promote safe delivery of the infant.*

1. Auscultate and record FHR pattern, noting presence of variability, accelerations, and report decelerations.
2. Instruct and support during amniocentesis.
3. Collect specimen for estriol determination.
4. Assist with NST and/or OCT.
5. Give instructions about induction of labor and electronic fetal heart rate monitoring.

B. Clinical manifestations of PIH (Table 20-6).

NURSING PRIORITY: *The triad of symptoms for PIH is hypertension, edema, and proteinuria.*

Treatment

A. Medical.

1. Mild preeclampsia: bedrest.
2. Severe preeclampsia: absolute bedrest, sedatives (**Valium**), antihypertensives (**Procardia, Aldomet**), anticonvulsants (magnesium sulfate) (See Appendix 20-2).
3. Eclampsia: seizure precautions (vital signs, oxygen, suction, positioning), magnesium sulfate.

B. Dietary: high-protein diet, moderate salt, and fluid intake of six to eight glasses of water per day.

Nursing Intervention

✦ *Goal: (mild preeclampsia): to initiate preventative measures.*

1. Instruction as to home care - encourage bedrest, provide dietary instruction, and regular prenatal checkups.
2. Tests to evaluate fetal status, (e.g. fetal movement record, ultrasound, NST, estriol & creatinine levels).

✦ *Goals and nursing intervention for the severely preclamptic and eclamptic client are outlined in Table 20-7.*

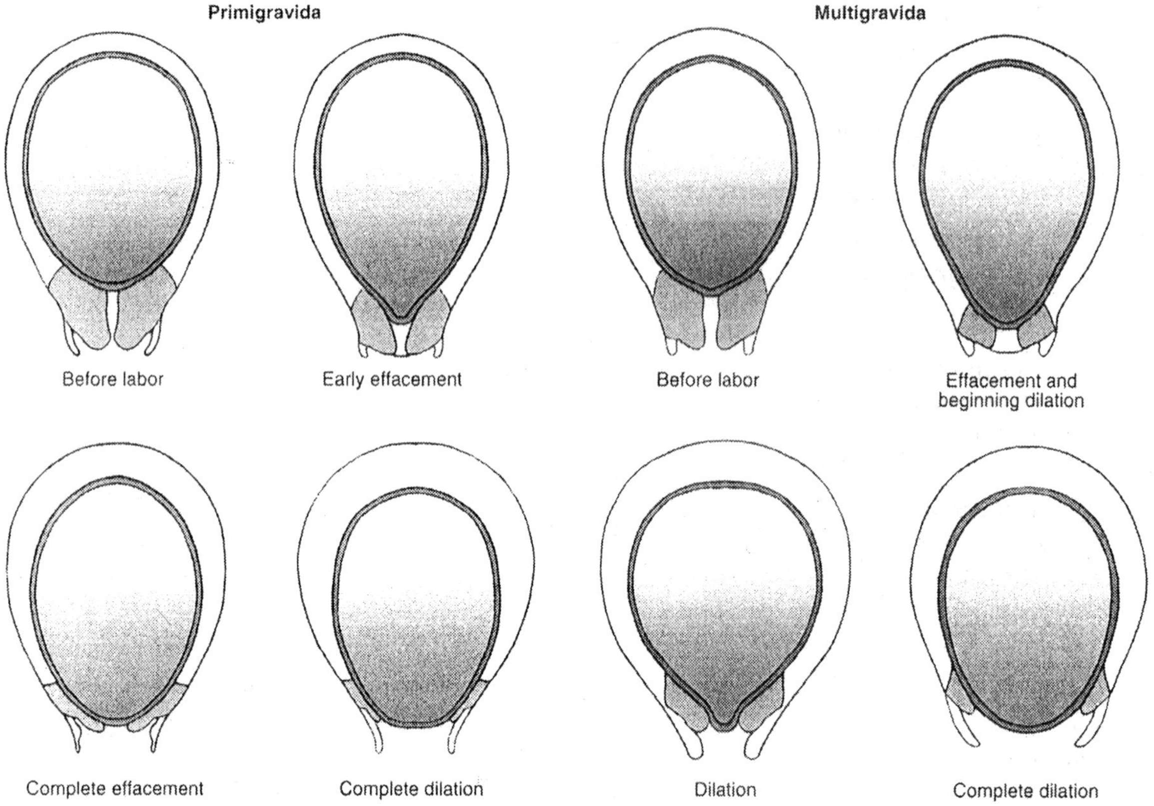

Figure 20-1: Cervical dilatation and effacement.
During labor, the multigravida's cervix remains thicker than the primigravida's.
Reprinted with permission: Gorrie, T., McKinney, E., Murray, S. (1998). *Foundations of Maternal Newborn Nursing*, 2nd ed. Philadelphia: W.B. Saunders, p. 273.

LABOR AND DELIVERY

Data Collection of the Labor Process

Maternal Data Collection

1. Signs and symptoms *prior* to true labor.
   a. Lightening - descent of the fetal head into the pelvis, experienced as "dropping" of the baby.
   b. Increased vaginal mucous discharge.
   c. Softening of the cervix.
   d. Braxton-Hicks contractions may become uncomfortable, especially at night; discomfort is usually located in the abdomen.
   e. Sudden burst of energy approximately 24 to 48 hours prior to labor.
   f. Weight loss of 1 to 3 pounds; sometimes diarrhea, indigestion, nausea and vomiting.
   g. Rupture of membranes.
      (1) If rupture occurs before onset of labor, it is called premature rupture of the membrane.
      (2) Delivery should occur within 24 hours to decrease incidence of infection.
      (3) Test with phenaphthazine (nitrazine) paper; amniotic fluid is alkaline - nitrazine paper turns blue; normal vaginal and urinary secretions are acidic.
2. Signs and symptoms of *true* labor.
   a. Cervical dilatation and effacement (Figure 20-1).

> ***NURSING PRIORITY:*** *The two most important signs indicative of true labor are cervical dilation and effacement.*

   b. Contractions occur at regular intervals and increase in duration and intensity; intensity usually increases with walking (Figure 20-2).
   c. Pain in the back which radiates around to the abdomen.
   d. Bloody show - expulsion of the mucous plug; labor begins 24 to 48 hours after bloody show or

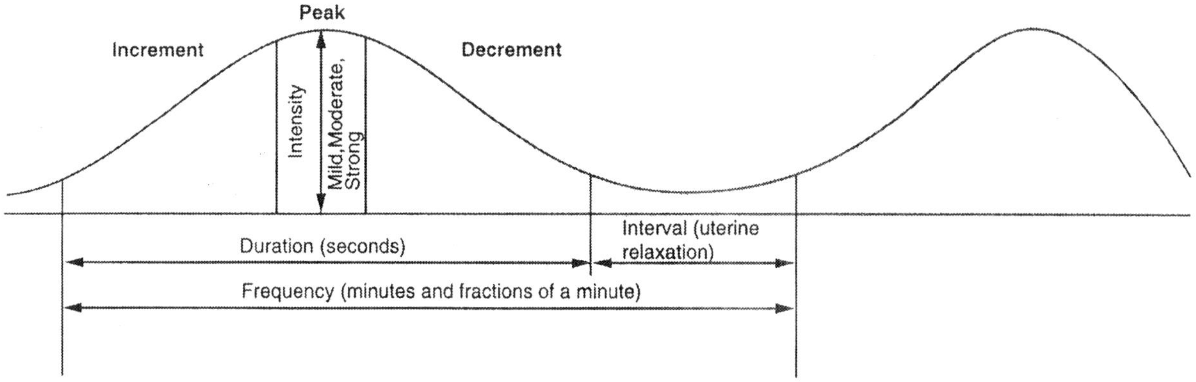

Figure 20-2: Labor contraction cycle
Reprinted with permission: Gorrie, T., McKinney, E., Murray, S. (1998). *Foundations of Maternal Newborn Nursing*, 2nd ed., Philadelphia: W.B. Saunders, p. 270.

bloody show may be observed at the onset of labor.

NCLEX-ALERT: *Monitor a client in labor.*

3. Stages of labor.
   a. First stage (stage of cervical dilation) - begins with onset of regular contractions and ends with complete cervical dilatation and effacement; divided into phases - latent, active, transition.
   b. Second stage (stage of expulsion) - begins with complete cervical dilation and ends with delivery of the fetus.
   c. Third stage (placental stage) - begins immediately after the fetus is born and ends when the placenta is delivered.
      (1) Signs of placental separation - discoid to globular shape of uterus, gush of blood, lengthening of umbilical cord, and rise of uterine fundus.
   d. Fourth stage (maternal homeostatic stabilization stage) - begins after the delivery of the placenta and continues for one to four hours after delivery.

Fetal Heart Rate Monitoring

Types of fetal heart rate monitoring.

1. *Fetoscope* - very common, inexpensive, easy-to-use method; does not give any information regarding contractions or periodic changes in FHR.
2. *Doppler* - uses ultrasound; FHR can be heard as early as 10 to 12 weeks; no information is gathered regarding contractions or periodic changes in FHR.
3. *External monitoring* - a noninvasive procedure which utilizes high-frequency sound waves to detect FHR.
4. *Internal monitoring* - also called direct fetal monitoring; invasive, however provides accurate, continuous information using a stainless steel spiral electrode inserted onto the fetal scalp.

Nursing Intervention During Labor and Delivery

Maternal

✦ *Goal: to monitor changes during each stage of labor (Table 20-8).*

✦ *Goal: to provide relief from pain and discomfort.*

1. Administer analgesic medication.
2. Do not administer analgesic medication within 2 hours of delivery. Medication may depress neonate.

Fetal

✦ *Goal: to monitor fetal status and detect early complications.*

✦ *Goal: to provide immediate care to the normal newborn.*

1. Airway: clear air passages to establish respirations.

NCLEX ALERT: *Monitor fetal heart rate.*

2. Body temperature: maintain warmth.
3. Apgar scoring: immediate appraisal of newborn's condition taken at 1 minute and again at 5 minutes (Table 20-9).

Table 20-8: SUMMARY OF OBSERVATIONS AND NURSING CARE DURING LABOR

NCLEX ALERT: *Monitor client in labor and auscultate fetal heart tones.*

PHYSICAL FINDINGS	NURSING INTERVENTION
STAGE 1: **Latent Phase**: Cervical dilatation: 0 to 3 cm Cervical effacement in primipara is usually complete before dilatation; in multipara, it occurs with dilatation Duration of latent phase: 8 to 10 hours Uterine contractions are mild, 5 to 30 minutes apart, and last 10 to 30 seconds Membranes ruptured or intact Scant brown or pink vaginal discharge or mucous plug Station: primipara - usually 0; multipara - 0 to -2 Fetal heart rates (FHR): clearest at level of or below umbilicus, dependent on fetal position	1. Orient to hospital environment and personnel. 2. Assess history and physical status. 3. Assess attitudes, past experiences, expectations. 4. Teach about labor. 5. Practice breathing and relaxation techniques. 6. Monitor physical status: Vital signs including FHR. 7. Voiding. 8. Amount and character of vaginal discharge. 9. Oral hygiene.
Active Phase: Cervical dilatation: 4 to 7 cm Duration of active phase: approximately 6 hours Uterine contractions are moderate, 3 to 5 minutes apart, and last 30 to 45 seconds Scant to moderate bloody mucus Station: 0 to +1 FHR: heard slightly below umbilicus or lower abdomen	1. Anticipate needs: Sponge face. Keep bed clean and dry. Care for dry, cracked mouth. Check bladder for fullness. 2. Stay at bedside working through each contraction with client; praise woman's efforts, point out progress. 3. Reinforce supportive efforts of the father. 4. Use touch to soothe, relax, comfort. 5. Check FHR q 15 min, B/P q 30 min. 6. Observe for hyperventilation. 7. May need analgesia to enhance coping.
Transition Phase: Cervical dilatation: 8 to 10 cm Duration of transition phase: 1 to 2 hours Uterine contractions of transition phase: strong, 2 to 3 minutes apart, and last 45 to 60 seconds Copious bloody mucus Station: +2 -+3 FHR: clearest directly about symphysis pubis	1. Continue physical and supportive care. 2. Use palpation or uterine contraction monitor to help patient define contractions and rest periods. 3. Observe perineum for bulging.

Table 20-8: SUMMARY OF OBSERVATIONS AND NURSING CARE DURING LABOR

PHYSICAL FINDINGS	NURSING INTERVENTION
STAGE 2: **Expulsion of Fetus:**	
Cervical dilatation complete at 10 cm Cervical effacement 100% Duration of Stage 2: 20 to 50 minutes Uterine contractions are strong, 2 to 3 minutes apart, and last 60 to 90 seconds; fetal bradycardia during contraction may occur Membranes may rupture Copious bloody mucus Station: fetal descent continues at a rate of 1 cm/hr in primiparas and 2 cm or more in multiparas until perineal floor is reached Urge to push begins Perineum bulges, flattens Crowning occurs Infant is born	1. Direct pushing efforts with father for each contraction. 2. Provide comfort measures and facilitate rest between contractions: Cool cloth to face. Keep perineum clean and dry. 3. Encourage efforts; point out progress. 4. Explain preparations being made for delivery. 5. Check FHR with each contraction. 6. Help with panting for delivery of head and shoulders.
STAGE 3: **Expulsion of Placenta:**	
Usually within 5 to 10 minutes of delivery Uterine shape globular, usually firmer; fundus rises Dark vaginal bleeding - gush or trickle Umbilical cord protrudes further from introitus Placenta intact: shiny presentation of fetal side of placental separation occurs from inner to outer margins (Schultze mechanism); rough presentation of maternal side of placental separation occurs from outer margins inward (Duncan mechanism).	1. Congratulate. 2. Initiate contact with infant. 3. Coach in relaxation for delivery of placenta and perineal repair. 4. Administration of oxytocics (Appendix 20-3) as needed.
STAGE 4: **Post Partum Recovery Period** *(see section on Postpartal assessment and management)*	
STAGE 4:	
Fundus firm or becomes firm when massaged, midline at level of umbilicus Moderate lochia rubra Episiotomy and laceration repair clean without ecchymosis or discharge, minimal edema; tenderness commensurate with analgesia, usually mild; edges well approximated Possible extrusion of hemorrhoids	1. Facilitation of attachment - assure parents time with newborn, mother may initiate breast feeding. 2. Ongoing assessment (q 15 min x 1 hr, then q 30 min x 2 hr) of vital signs, fundus, lochia, episiotomy and bladder function. 3. Encourage rest for both parents.

Table 20-9: APGAR SCORING SYSTEM

SIGN	0	1	2
Rate	Not detectable	Slow (below 100)	Over 100
Respiratory Effort	Absent	Slow, irregular	Good, crying
Muscle Tone	Flaccid, limp	Some flexions of extremities	Active motion
Reflex Irritability	No response	Grimace, extremities	Cough, sneeze, or cry
Color	Blue, pale	Body pink, extremities pale	Completely pink

NCLEX ALERT: *Monitor a newborn.*

4. Care of the umbilical cord: clamped after pulsation ceases; examine for number of vessels and record (one umbilical artery indicates increased incidence of congenital anomalies, especially renal and genitourinary); no dressing is applied to cord.
5. Care of the eyes: prophylaxis against ophthalmia neonatorum; ophthalmic penicillin ointment, tetracycline, erythromycin, or instillation of 1 percent silver nitrate solution.
6. Identification: wristbands fastened to both infant and mother, and appropriate footprints taken prior to leaving delivery area.

NCLEX ALERT: *Verify the identity of a client.*

7. Administration of vitamin K (**Aqua Mephyton**): 0.5 mg to 1.0 mg IM injected into the upper outer aspect of the thigh for prevention of neonatal hemorrhagic disease, due to lack of *E. coli* necessary for the synthesis of vitamin K in the intestines.
8. Inspection for gross abnormalities: clubfoot, imperforate anus, birthmarks, etc.
9. Attachment: provide contact of newborn with mother as soon as possible after birth.

OPERATIVE OBSTETRICS

Episiotomy

❑ **An episiotomy is an incision through the perineal body to facilitate delivery by enlarging the vaginal orifice.**

Types

A. Median-midline.
  1. Easy to repair; heals well.
  2. Increased chance of extension through the rectal sphincter muscle (3rd, 4th degree laceration).

B. Mediolateral - made at a 45 degree angle on either right or left side.
  1. More painful healing; increased blood loss.
  2. Less risk of extension into sphincter ani muscle.

Data Collection

A. Observe perineal site for bleeding, swelling, redness, or any discharge.

B. *Evaluate for pain and discomfort; should be minimal discomfort. Increased pain should be reported to RN.*

Nursing Intervention

✦ *Goal: to alleviate pain and swelling and promote comfort.*
  1. Ice pack (first eight hours); hot sitz baths, peri light (heat lamp treatment for 20 minutes, 3 - 4 times per day).
  2. Analgesic sprays, ointments, Tucks, as ordered.
  3. Teach importance of perineal cleansing (i.e. use of the spray bottle; direct flow from front to back).

Forceps Delivery

❑ **A *Forceps delivery* is the use of an instrument to extract the fetal head during delivery.**

Data Collection

A. Criteria for forceps delivery.
  1. Head fully engaged.
  2. Complete dilatation of the cervix.
  3. Membranes have ruptured.

B. Monitor fetal heart rate, as forceps may compress umbilical cord.

Nursing Interventions

✦ *Goal: to briefly explain procedure to couple.*

1. Monitor fetal heart rate.
2. Have client empty bowel and bladder.
3. Provide emotional support.

✦ *Goal: to detect complications for forceps application.*

1. Maternal: lacerations to birth canal and rectum.
2. Fetal: cephalhematoma, lacerations and bruising to face, facial paralysis, skull fracture, umbilical cord compression, and brain damage.

Cesarean Birth

❑ **An incision into the abdominal and uterine walls to deliver the fetus.**

Types

A. Low-segment transverse incision.

1. Preferred and most common method.
2. Decreased blood loss; less chance of uterine rupture with subsequent pregnancy as incision is made into lower uterine segment.
3. Fewer complications - peritonitis and postoperative adhesions.

B. Classic cesarean incision.

1. Used in cases of placenta previa when there are adhesions in the lower uterine segment, or in transverse fetal lie.
2. Vertical incision is made between the umbilicus and symphysis pubis.

Indications

A. Maternal.

1. Uterine dystocia.
2. Severe preeclampsia and eclampsia.
3. Previous cesarean birth or surgery on the uterus.
4. Placenta previa and abruptio placentae.

B. Fetal.

1. Fetal Distress.
2. Prolapsed cord.
3. Fetal abnormalities (e.g., hydrocephalus).

Data Collection

A. Assess for possible indication for cesarean birth.

B. "Once a section always a section"- trend is to examine the condition surrounding the previous or original section; often if original section was in lower uterine segment, a trial labor may be recommended.

C. Cesarean may be planned for a specific date or may occur as an emergency procedure; common elective reasons are previous repeat cesarean section, breech presentation, or cephalopelvic disproportion.

Nursing Intervention

✦ *Goal: to provide preoperative preparation.*

1. Preparation is similar to any abdominal surgery operation.

✦ *Goal: to provide postoperative care.*

1. Cesarean birth includes both normal abdominal postoperative care and postpartum care.

Induction of labor

Procedure

A. Aminotomy - artificial rupture of membranes (bag of water - BOW); often labor begins spontaneously.

B. Oxytocin (**Pitocin** or **Syntocinon**) is administered intravenously with physician in attendance (Appendix 20-3).

Data Collection

A. Careful assessment of uterine contractions is priority; tetanic contractions could result in uterine rupture, premature separation of placenta and fetal hypoxia.

B. Fetal heart rate (FHR) check every 15 minutes along with mother's vital signs.

Nursing Intervention

✦ *Goal: to monitor and evaluate uterine response and fetal response to induction.*

1. Frequent vital sign checks and FHR (every 15 minutes); indirect or direct fetal monitoring may be used.
2. *Report any of the following findings to the RN.*
   a. *Contractions are more frequent than every 2 minutes.*
   b. *Contraction duration exceeds 75 to 90 seconds.*
   c. *Uterus does not relax; remains contracted and tetanic.*

COMPLICATIONS ASSOCIATED WITH LABOR AND DELIVERY

Premature Labor

❑ **Premature labor is defined as labor occurring prior to thirty-eight weeks' gestation.**

Data Collection

1. Contractions occurring in increasing frequency and intensity.
2. Premature rupture of the membranes.

Treatment

A. Medications (Appendix 20-4).

1. Ritodrine (**Yutopar**).
2. Isoxsuprine (**Vasodilan**).
3. Terbutaline sulfate (**Brethine**).
4. MgSO4 (Gaining favor in treatment of premature labor, less problems with BP and pulse changes as compared to **Ritodrine** use).

Nursing Intervention

✦ *Goal: to assist in delivery if maternal complications are present.*

1. Maternal complications - diabetes, preeclampsia, hemorrhage.

✦ *Goal: to provide emotional support.*

1. Encourage expression of feelings related to anxiety and guilt.
2. Identify and support coping mechanisms for couple.

✦ *Goal: to minimize fetal complications.*

1. Promote fetal oxygenation.
   a. Avoid supine position during labor - risk of vena caval syndrome.

> ***NURSING PRIORITY:** Encourage left lateral Sim's position - promotes placental perfusion.*

   b. Avoid maternal hyperventilation which can lead to decreased oxygen to the fetus.

Dystocia

Data Collection

A. Types of uterine dysfunction.

1. Prolonged labor - labor lasting for more than twenty-four hours after onset of regular contractions.
2. Precipitous delivery - a very rapid, intense labor of two to four hours duration.
3. Hypotonic contractions - slow, infrequent, weak contractions occurring more than three minutes apart and lasting less than forty seconds.
4. Hypertonic contractions - frequent, strong, painful contractions occurring two to three minutes apart, lasting sixty seconds or more.

B. Cephalopelvic disproportion (CPD) — disproportion between the size of the fetus and that of the birth canal.

Treatment

A. Mechanical dystocia relating to CPD, or faulty presentation, is treated by a cesarean delivery.

B. Hypotonic uterine contractions or prolonged labor are treated by administration of **Pitocin** IV.

C. Hypertonic uterine contractions are treated by sedation and rest.

Nursing Intervention

✦ *Goal: to monitor level of fatigue and ability to cope with pain.*

1. Provide basic comfort measures, back rubs, change of position, clean dry linen.
2. Provide emotional support to mother and significant other.
3. Give reassurance and stay with client continually.

✦ *Goal: to assist in the medical management of dystocia.*

1. Explain procedures to rule out cause of dystocia-sonogram, x-ray studies, etc.
2. Monitor **Pitocin** if indicated for hypotonic dysfunction or prolonged labor.
3. Prepare client for cesarean delivery (indicated in CPD and faulty presentation).
4. Administer broad-spectrum antibiotics to decrease incidence of infection.
5. Maintain hydration, monitor intake and output, and administer oxygen if indicated.

✦ *Goal: to detect early complications associated with dystocia.*

1. Monitor maternal vital signs.
2. Assess mother for signs of exhaustion, dehydration, increasing temperature, and report to RN.
3. Assess fetal heart tones frequently through fetal electronic monitoring.

Supine Hypotensive Syndrome (Vena Caval Syndrome)

❑ **Shock-like symptoms seen when pregnant woman assumes a supine position. (The weight of the uterus causes partial occlusion of the vena cava, leading to decreased venous return to the heart.)**

Data Collection

1. ↓ BP, ↓ pulse.
2. Client feels faint; pale.
3. ↓ FHR.

Nursing Intervention

✦ *Goal: to decrease supine hypotensive syndrome episode.*

1. Educate mother to turn to left side; preferred position because pressure is removed from vena cava.
2. Administer oxygen if needed.
3. Assess fetal heart rates and *report any changes to RN.*

Abnormal Fetal Position

Data Collection

A. Breech presentation.

1. FHTs usually auscultated above the umbilicus.
2. Passage of meconium often occurs.
3. Increased danger of prolapsed umbilical cord.

B. Transverse lie (shoulder presentation) — dysfunctional labor patterns are seen.

Treatment

Cesarean delivery is most often performed.

Nursing Intervention

✦ *Goal: to provide reassurance and explanations of procedures as indicated.*

1. Explanation of possible cesarean delivery.
2. Assess for complications relating to prolonged labor and possible infection (temperature, fatigue).

Hemorrhage in the Pregnant Client

Nursing management of hemorrhage in the pregnant client is discussed in Table 20-10, Figure 20-3, and Figure 20-4.

Multiple Pregnancy

Data Collection

1. Increased incidence of PIH, abruptio placentae, and placenta previa, and hydraminos.
2. Auscultation of two fetal heart tones.
3. Measurement of fundal height exceeds gestational age.
4. Increased experience of more physical discomfort - shortness of breath, dyspnea on exertion, backaches, and leg edema, due to excessive size of uterus.

Treatment

A. Medical.

1. Bedrest in lateral position to treat hypertension.
2. Antiemetic for nausea and vomiting past the first trimester.

B. Dietary - increase of three hundred calories along with increased protein, iron, folic acid, and vitamin supplements.

Nursing Intervention

✦ *Goal: to provide anticipatory guidance during the antepartal period.*

1. Second trimester - prenatal visits every two weeks.
2. Third trimester - weekly visits if there are no complications.
3. Discourage travel, as labor may begin without warning.

✦ *Goal: to provide psychological support.*

1. Often, twin births are undiagnosed at the time of labor.
2. Provide assistance and advice regarding care of twins at home.
3. Since the twins are apt to be small, anticipate nursing care for a premature neonate.
4. *Assess for maternal complications,(e.g., postpartal hemorrhage) and report to RN.*
5. Ensure correct identification, Baby A and Baby B.

Prolapsed Cord

❑ **A *prolapsed cord* is the washing down of the cord in front of the presenting part.**

Data Collection

1. Commonly occurs following rupture of the membranes.
2. Cord is washed through the birth canal with a gush of amniotic fluid.
3. Visualization of the cord.
4. FHR is decreased.

Treatment

A. Medical.

1. Insert a gloved finger into the vagina and lift the fetal head off the cord to relieve the pressure.
2. Administer oxygen to the mother.
3. Positioning.
   a. Place in knee-chest position or in Trendelenburg position (head of bed or table is lowered); *administer oxygen to the mother and report to RN.*

B. Surgical.

1. If incomplete dilatation, cesarean delivery necessary.
2. Occasionally, if dilatation is complete, vaginal delivery possible.

Table 20-10: NURSING MANAGEMENT OF HEMORRHAGE IN THE PREGNANT CLIENT

NCLEX ALERT: *Implement measures to prevent circulatory complications (e.g., hemorrhage, shock).*

CAUSES AND SOURCES	SYMPTOMS	NURSING INTERVENTIONS
ANTEPARTAL PERIOD:		
Abortion	Vaginal bleeding Intermittent uterine contractions Rupture of the membranes	1. Obtain history of onset, duration, amount of bleeding, and associated symptoms. 2. Observe perineal pads for amount of bleeding (approximately 1g = 1ml blood). 3. Monitor vital signs of mother and fetus (frequency is determined by severity of clinical symptoms).
Placenta previa	Painless vaginal bleeding after the 7th month	
Abruptio placentae	Vaginal bleeding Extreme tenderness in abdomen Rigid, board-like abdomen Increase in size of the abdomen	
INTRAPARTAL PERIOD:		
Placenta previa	Bright vaginal bleeding	1. Insert IV and provide volume replacement. 2. Request type and cross-match for blood. 3. Administer fluids and blood as prescribed. 4. Monitor intake and output. 5. Minimize chances for further bleeding 6. *NO* vaginal or rectal exams. 7. Bedrest in position of comfort. 8. Anticipate delivery by Cesarean section.
Abruptio placentae	Symptoms same as above	
Uterine atony in stage III	Bright red vaginal bleeding Ineffectual contractility	
POSTPARTAL PERIOD:		
Uterine atony	Boggy uterus	1. Massage fundus of uterus and anticipate oxytocin medication for uterine atony client. 2. Reduce anxiety 3. Keep woman and family advised of treatment plan. 4. Record amount of bleeding in a specific amount of time.
Retained placental fragments	Dark vaginal bleeding Presence of clots	
Lacerations of cervix or vagina	Firm uterus Bright red blood	

Nursing Intervention

✦ *Goal: to maintain fetal oxygenation and assist with immediate delivery.*

1. Continuing assessment of FHR.
2. *Maintain woman in one of the positions described previously to alleviate compression of the cord and report to RN.*
3. Offer emotional support to the couple.

POSTPARTAL DATA COLLECTION

❑ **The puerperium is the period of time spanning the first six weeks following delivery. It is often referred to as the "fourth trimester."**

NCLEX ALERT: *Assist client with expected life transitions (e.g., attachment to newborn); monitor client's postpartum recovery.*

Physiological Changes

A. Uterus.

1. Uterine involution - process by which the uterus returns to its normal prepregnant condition.
2. Immediately after delivery, top of fundus is several finger breadths above the umbilicus.
3. Twelve hours after delivery, fundus of uterus is one finger breadth above umbilicus.
4. Fundus recedes/descends into the pelvis approximately one finger breadth per day.

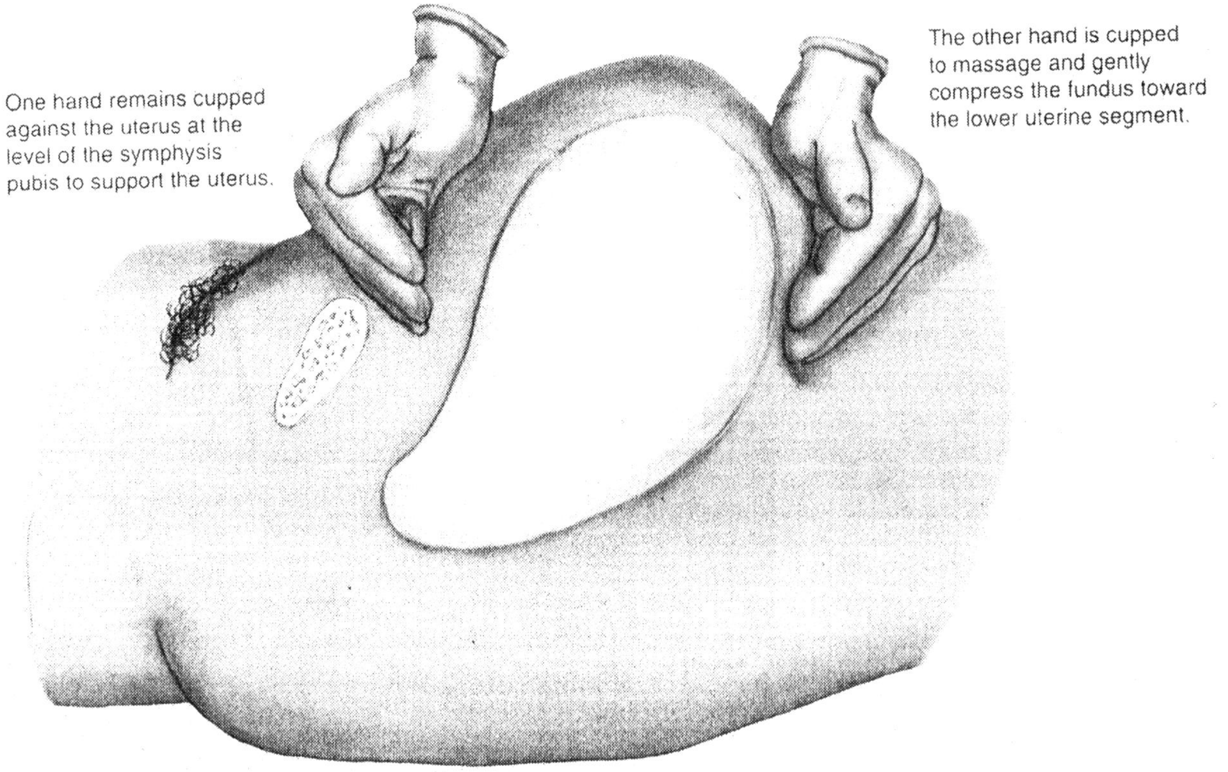

Figure 20-3: Technique for fundal massage
Reprinted with permission: Gorrie, T., McKinney, E., Murray, S. (1998). *Foundations of Maternal Newborn Nursing*, 2nd ed., Philadelphia: W.B. Saunders, p. 784.

5. By day ten fundus is below the symphysis pubis and not palpable.
6. Afterpain - alternate contraction and relaxation of the uterine muscle.
   a. Occur primarily in multiparas.
   b. May be severe, requiring analgesics.
   c. Usually subside in forty-eight hours.
7. Lochia.

NURSING PRIORITY: *The change in lochia is a common item on the examination. Always chart the amount first, followed by the character, (e.g., moderate amount lochia).*

   a. Lochia rubra - dark red discharge; occurs the first three days.
   b. Lochia serosa - pinkish, serosanguinous discharge; lasts approximately three to ten days.
   c. Lochia alba - creamy or yellowish discharge; occurs after the tenth day and may last a week or two.
   d. When lochia subsides, uterus is considered closed; postpartal infection less likely.

B. Cervix.
1. May be stretched and swollen.
2. Small lacerations may be apparent.
3. External os closes slowly; end of first week, the opening is fingertip size.

C. Vagina - labia majora and minora are more flabby.

D. Perineum.
1. May be bruised and tender.
2. Pelvic floor and ligaments are stretched.
3. Muscle tone is restored by Kegal exercises.

E. Ovulation and menstruation.
1. Non-breast-feeding women.
   a. Menstruation resumes in six weeks.
   b. Ovulation - 50 percent may ovulate during the first cycle.
2. Lactating women.
   a. Varies.

b. 45 percent resume menstruation within twelve weeks after delivery.

F. Abdomen.
1. Soft and flabby.
2. Muscle tone can be restored within two to three months with exercise.

G. Breasts.
1. Anterior pituitary releases prolactin which stimulates secretion of milk.
2. Engorgement may occur approximately thirty-six to forty-eight hours after delivery.
3. Colostrum released - thin, yellowish fluid which contains antibodies and large amounts of vitamins.

H. Gastrointestinal system.
1. Immediately after delivery, hunger is common.
2. GI tract is sluggish and hypoactive; due to decreased muscle tone and peristalsis.
3. Constipation may be a problem.

I. Urinary tract.
1. Bladder is edematous and hyperemic.
2. May be bruising and swelling due to trauma around the urinary meatus.
3. Increased bladder capacity and urinary retention.
4. Diuresis occurs during the first two days postpartum.
5. Bladder distention may displace the uterus, leading to a "boggy" uterus and increased bleeding.
6. Hematuria may occur after delivery; acetone may be present in the urine.

J. Vital signs.
1. Temperature may be slightly elevated (100.4°F) after a long labor; should return to normal within twenty-four hours.
2. Blood pressure may be slightly decreased after delivery; however, should remain stable.
3. Pulse rate slow after delivery.

K. Blood values.
1. ↑ WBC (20 to 30,000/mm).
2. Hemoglobin, hematocrit, RBC return to normal within two to six weeks.
3. Increased risk of development of thrombophlebitis and thromboembolism.

L. Weight loss.
1. Initial ten to twelve pound loss occurs due to the weight of the infant, placenta, and amniotic fluid.
2. Diuresis leads to an additional five pounds weight loss.
3. Six to eight weeks postpartum - return to prepregnant weight if an average of twenty-five to thirty pounds was gained.

Attachment—Psychosocial Response

A. Phases (Rubin, 1961).
1. Taking-in phase.
a. First few days postpartum.
b. Characterized by passiveness and dependency.
c. Preoccupied with own self-needs: food, attention, and physical comforts and care.
d. Talkative.
2. Taking-hold phase.
a. Occurs about two to three days postpartum; characterized by increase in physical well-being.
b. Emphasis on the present; woman takes hold of the task of mothering; requires reassurance.
c. Very receptive to teaching.

B. Attachment behaviors.
1. Exploration and identification pattern.
a. Touch - begins by stroking the extremities and the outline of the head with the fingertips; gradually moves toward using the entire surface of the hand; touches and observes first at arm's length, then on lap, or slightly away from the body; finally enfolds infant close to body with both arms.
b. Eye-to-eye contact - *en face position* (gazing into the eyes of the infant).

C. Postpartum blues.
1. Transient period of depression (occurring during the puerperium).
2. Complaints of anorexia, insomnia, tearfulness, and a general let-down, sad feeling.
3. Thought to be caused by fatigue, discomfort, sensory overload or deprivation, and hormonal changes.
4. Woman needs support and reassurance that it is a transient and self-limiting experience.

Nursing Intervention

✦ *Goal: to initiate routine postpartum data collection.*
1. General observations of mood, activity level, and feelings of wellness; routine vital sign data collection.
2. Inspection of breasts - check for beginning engorgement and presence of cracks in nipples, any pain or tenderness, and progress of breast-feeding.

3. Check uterine fundus - determine height of fundus in relation to umbilicus; should feel firm and globular; fundal massage if bleeding increases (Figure 20-3).
4. *Assess for bladder distention, especially during the first 24 to 48 hours and report to RN if client is distended.*
5. Perineal area.
   a. Observe episiotomy site.
   b. Apply anesthetic sprays or ointments to decrease pain.
   c. Determine presence of hemorrhoids and provide relief measures.
6. Lochia - record color, odor, and amount of discharge.
   a. *Report any significant increase in amount or foul odor of lochia to the RN.*
   b. Change peri pads frequently.
7. *Lower extremities - assess for thrombophlebitis; report positive findings to RN.*
8. Abdomen and perineum.
   a. Initiate strengthening exercises for both abdominal wall and perineum, (e.g., isometric Kegal exercises for strengthening pelvic floor), and leg raises.

✦ *Goal: to provide comfort and relief of pain.*

1. Episiotomy - ice packs, first few hours; followed by peri light, sitz baths.
2. Perineal care - use of "peri bottles" to squirt over perineum (front to back) to prevent contamination, and avoid use of toilet tissue.
3. Afterpain - use of analgesics (preferably one hour before feeding, especially for breast-feeding mothers).
4. Hemorrhoidal pain.
   a. Sitz baths, anesthetic ointments, rectal suppositories, Tucks.
   b. Encourage lying on side, and avoiding prolonged sitting.
   c. Stool softeners or laxatives may be indicated; usually normal bowel movement by 2nd or 3rd day after delivery.
5. Breast engorgement - well-fitting bra to provide support.

✦ *Goal: to promote maternal-infant attachment and facilitate integration of the newborn into the family unit.*

1. Use infant's name when talking about him or her.
2. Encourage parents to provide as much of the care to the infant while still hospitalized.
3. Accept parents' emotions and encourage expression of feelings.
4. Help parents understand sibling behavior and to plan for the arrival of the new family member.

✦ *Goal: to establish successful infant feeding patterns.*

1. Nonlactating mother.
   a. Provide supportive bra.
   b. Explain proper position for feeding.
   c. Formulas-ready-to-feed in disposable bottles often with disposable nipples.
2. Lactating mothers.
   a. Cleanse breast prior to infant nursing and afterwards.
   b. Air dry nipples at least fifteen minutes after breast-feeding; wear breast shields and change frequently when they become saturated to decrease incidence of cracking and fissuring.
   c. *Assess breasts for engorgement, nipple inversion, cracking, inflammation, or pain and report to RN.*
   d. If mother experiences uterine contractions during breast feeding, administer analgesics prior to breast feeding.

✦ *Goal: to prepare and plan for discharge.*

1. Determine if mother will need household help (especially important if birth is twins).
2. *Assist the RN to teach the following infant care skills.*
   a. Infant feeding.
      (1) Hold bottle so that air does not get into nipple.
      (2) Method of cleaning bottles and making formula.
      (3) Positioning and feeding for lactating mothers.
      (4) How to break the infant's suction on the breast.
      (5) Positioning for burping and bubbling.
   b. Diapering.
      (1) Frequent changing to prevent diaper rash.
      (2) **Vaseline** or **Desitin** ointment to prevent irritation.
      (3) Use of disposable diapers.
   c. Bathing.
      (1) Use of a mild soap.
      (2) Kitchen sink is often a good place to bathe infant.
      (3) Lotions can be applied; best advice is to avoid use of powders.
   d. Umbilical cord.

(1) Apply alcohol daily and after every diaper change.

(2) Stump usually falls off in a week to ten days.

e. Pacifiers.

(1) May be used to meet infant's sucking need.

(2) Usually discontinued around four to six months due to infant's lack of interest.

f. Sleeping.

(1) Usually sleeps through the night at around two to three months of age.

(2) Encourage mother to sleep while infant is sleeping, to avoid sleep deprivation.

g. Illness.

(1) Common behavior changes are irritability, crying, loss of appetite, and fever.

(2) Explain how to take an infant's temperature.

h. Taking the infant outside.

(1) Dress infant as you would dress yourself.

(2) Traveling - use a car seat.

i. Explain important of follow-up well-baby checkup visits with pediatrician.

COMPLICATIONS OF THE PUERPERIUM

NCLEX ALERT: *Monitor client's postpartum recovery.*

Puerperal Infection ("Childbirth Fever")

Data Collection

A. Predisposing factors.

1. Antepartal infection.
2. Premature rupture of the membranes.
3. Prolonged labor.
4. Laceration.
5. Anemia; postpartum hemorrhage.
6. Poor aseptic technique.

B. Clinical manifestations.

1. Temperature elevation 38°C (100.4°F), if taken at least four times daily on any two of the first ten postpartum days, with the exception of the first 24 hours.
2. Symptoms vary according to system involved.
3. Area of involvement characterized by five cardinal symptoms of inflammation.

Table 20-11: POSTPARTAL HIGH RISK FACTORS

✦ Preeclampsia
✦ Diabetes
✦ Cardiac disease
✦ Cesarean birth
✦ Overdistention of uterus (multiple gestation)
✦ Abruptio placentae and placenta previa
✦ Precipitous or prolonged labor
✦ Difficult delivery
✦ Extended period of time in lithotomy position (legs in stirrups)
✦ Retained placenta

4. Tachycardia, chills, abdominal tenderness common.
5. Headache, malaise, deep pelvic pain.
6. Profuse, foul-smelling lochia.

C. Area involved.

1. Uterus is most often affected - endometritis.
2. May have localized infection of the perineum, vulva, and vagina.
3. Urinary system.

a. Pyelitis.

b. Cystitis.

Treatment

A. Medications.

1. Antibiotics.
2. Antipyretics.
3. Oxytocics.

B. Dietary.

1. High-protein, high-calorie, high-vitamin diet.
2. Encourage 3,000 to 4,000 cc of fluid per 24 hours.

Nursing Intervention

✦ *Goal: to prevent puerperal infection.*

1. Maintain meticulous aseptic technique during labor and delivery.
2. Assess and treat antepartal infection.
3. *Prevent anemia - hemoglobin and hematocrit should be checked during prenatal visits and/or prior to delivery. Report any significant decrease to RN.*

✦ *Goal: to promote mother's resistance to infection.*

1. Administer antibiotic, antipyretic, and oxytocic medications.
2. Encourage good nutrition.
3. Isolate client from other maternity clients.

4. Use semi-Fowler's position to promote free drainage of lochia and prevent upward extension of infection into pelvis.

NURSING PRIORITY: The pathophysiology related to maintaining semi-Fowlers position to localize infection is important to remember, not only for obstetric clients, but others with contaminated abdominal drainage.

Mastitis

❑ ***Mastitis* is the invasion of the breast tissue by pathogenic organisms.**

Data Collection

A. Predisposing factors.
  1. Fissured nipples.
  2. Erosion of the areola.
  3. Causative agent, most frequently *Staphylococcus*, which is transmitted from the nasopharynx of the nursing infant.

B. Clinical manifestations.
  1. Occurs most often between the first and fourth weeks of the postpartal period.
  2. Chills and tachycardia.
  3. Red, swollen, painful breasts.
  4. Fever may be 39.4° C (103° F) or 40° C (104° F).

Treatment

A. Medication.
  1. Antibiotics - penicillin.
  2. Antipyretics.
  3. Analgesics.

Nursing Intervention

✦ *Goal: to prevent the complication of mastitis.*
  1. Teach mother how to cleanse breasts and nipples.
  2. Explain importance of wearing a support bra.

✦ *Goal: to promote comfort and maintain lactation if desired.*
  1. Apply ice to breasts to decrease pain.
  2. Discard milk from infected breast while temperature is elevated.
  3. Encourage good nutrition and adequate rest.
  4. Administer antibiotics as ordered.

NURSING PRIORITY: The mother can continue to nurse (providing that she is not on any antibiotics that should not be given to the infant) while infected to prevent milk stasis and engorgement; otherwise, she should pump the breast. If a breast abscess forms, she should discontinue breast feeding on that side, pump the breast and discard the milk.

Thrombophlebitis

❑ **There is an increased risk (5 times) for *thrombophlebitis* and *pulmonary* embolism during the puerperium.The reason for the increased incidence is a change in blood coagulation during pregnancy, along with engorgement of the veins of the lower extremities and pelvis, leading to pooling of blood and venous stasis. Data collection and nursing intervention are discussed in Chapter 1.**

❑ ***Cystitis* and *pyelitis* occur as a result of bladder distention and incomplete emptying of urine postpartum; three common predisposing factors are traum to the bladder mucosa, the temporary loss of bladder tone, and an increased bladder capacity (See Chapter 18).**

Parent Reaction to Premature or Malformed Infant

Data Collection

A. Period of disorganization.
  1. Grief reaction characterized by guilt, anger, and sorrow.
  2. Feelings of exhaustion, emptiness, and frequent crying.

B. Period of information seeking and resource utilization.
  1. Anxiety decreases; problem solving begins.
  2. Begins to resolve the crisis.
  3. Often information seeking leads to further anger and sorrow followed then by a period of denial or disbelief.

C. Resolution of the crisis situation.
  1. Development of new coping strategies.
  2. Acceptance and coming to terms with the situation.

Nursing Intervention

✦ *Goal: to provide emotional support to the parents.*
  1. Encourage verbalization of feelings and expression of grief.
  2. Promote parent-infant contact; point out normal characteristics.
  3. Encourage parents to visit, touch, and care for their infant as much as possible.

Study Questions—Maternal

1. How is the best way for a primigravida client to meet her increasing iron needs?

① add an extra serving of red meat to daily diet.
② include at least two eggs in her daily diet.
③ increase her daily intake of spinach.
④ take an iron supplement with orange juice.

2. During the prenatal interview, a client who is pregnant tells the nurse that she has two children. She also had a pregnancy which was terminated at seven weeks. How will the nurse document this information?

① gravida 4 para 2.
② gravida 4 para 3.
③ gravida 3 para 3.
④ gravida 3 para 2.

3. What symptom is considered a positive sign of pregnancy?

① nausea and vomiting.
② changes in breasts.
③ fetal outline on ultrasound.
④ presence of quickening.

4. A young pregnant woman comes to the clinic and complains of nausea and vomiting. What would the nurse suggest to assist in alleviating this problem?

① take 3 tablespoons of bismuth subsalicylate (Pepto-Bismol) before eating.
② increase fluids to 4000cc per day.
③ increase protein in diet.
④ eat five or more small meals a day.

5. What is important for the nurse to teach a client regarding how to prevent venous stasis and varicose veins during pregnancy?

① elevate feet and take frequent rest breaks.
② wear loose shoes and clothes to help circulation.
③ decrease salt in the diet and increase fluids.
④ wear thigh-high TED hose throughout the night.

6. What is a maternal task that usually starts during the first trimester and lasts through the neonatal period?

① seeking acceptance of this child by other family members.
② developing selflessness.
③ developing a bond with the baby.
④ establishing a support base in the event of unexpected problems.

7. The client is in her last trimester and is concerned regarding the presence of "stretch marks" on her abdomen and breast. What is the best nursing response?

① they cannot be prevented and occur in all pregnancies.
② application of cocoa butter or vitamin E oil will decrease formation of scars.
③ after delivery the reddish marks will gradually fade.
④ there is nothing that can be done to prevent them.

8. What is considered a sign of true labor?

① effacement and cervical dilatation.
② uterine contractions eight minutes apart.
③ Braxton Hicks contractions every four minutes.
④ bloody show with contraction every 30 minutes.

9. How does the nurse measure the duration of a contraction?

① from the beginning of the contraction to the end of the contraction.
② from the beginning of one contraction to the end of the next contraction.
③ from the point of maximal intensity until the contraction subsides.
④ from the beginning of one contraction to the start of the next contraction.

10. In order for a pregnant woman to fulfill her daily need for folic acid, what would the nurse suggest adding to or increasing in her diet?

① beef and chicken.
② milk, yogurt, cheese.
③ green leafy vegetables.
④ whole grain breads.

11. What would be the difference between a diet for a lactating woman and a diet during pregnancy?

① pregnant woman needs more calories.
② lactating woman needs more protein and iron.
③ pregnant woman requires less fat.
④ lactating woman needs more calories and protein.

12. Considering a woman is of normal weight, what is the average recommended weight gain during pregnancy?

① 20 to 40 pounds.
② 25 to 35 pounds.
③ 5 to 10 pounds.
④ 15 to 20 pounds.

13. What is considered the triad of symptoms of preeclampsia?

① oliguria, hypotension, proteinuria.
② hypertension, tachycardia, tachypnea.
③ edema, tachycardia, nausea.
④ hypertension, edema, proteinuria.

14. Which condition would the nurse identify as contributing to the complication of intrapartal bleeding?

① placenta previa.
② third degree laceration.
③ vena caval syndrome.
④ retained placental fragments.

15. What is the best position for a client during labor?

① position of comfort.
② right Sims.
③ supine.
④ left lateral.

16. When is the Apgar assessment completed?

① within 2 hours of birth.
② at 1 minute and 5 minutes.
③ at 5 minutes and 10 minutes.
④ within first hour of birth.

17. The primigravida client is experiencing Braxton Hicks contractions. What are the characteristics of this contraction?

① contractions increase with ambulation.
② do not increase in intensity or frequency.
③ cause a rapid dilatation and effacement.
④ do not occur with the second pregnancy.

18. A young woman has been prescribed oral contraceptives. What is the priority information to teach her?

① call the clinic if you have nausea, vomiting, or diarrhea.
② take the pill with a glass of milk to increase the effectiveness.
③ if you forget a pill discontinue taking them till the next month.
④ call the clinic if you have a sudden headache or severe leg pain.

19. Which medication is used to suppress contractions?

① oxytocin (Pitocin).
② conjugated estrogen(Premarin)
③ terbutaline (Brethine).
④ ergot alkaloid (Cafergot)

20. During the postpartum assessment, the nurse notes a blood pressure of 98/68, pulse at 110, respirations at 28 and profuse lochia rubra. What is the priority nursing action?

① immediately advise the RN.
② massage the mother's fundus.
③ check her urinary output.
④ change her perineal pad.

Appendix 20-1: CONTRACEPTIVE METHODS

METHODS / DESCRIPTION	NURSING IMPLICATIONS / CLIENT TEACHING
NATURAL METHODS:	
Calendar (rhythm) Basal body temperature (BBT) Ovulation (Billings) Symptothermal Cervical mucus Fertility awareness	Client Teaching: *Calendar (rhythm) method*: calculate the days of fertility; considered to be days 10 to 17 of a 28-day menstrual cycle. *BBT method*: a slight decrease then an increase of about 0.4 to 0.8 degrees in temperature when ovulation occurs; fertile period ends three days after temperature elevation. *Cervical mucus method*: prior to ovulation, mucus becomes clear and stringy; nonfertile period occurs when mucus becomes thick, cloudy, and sticky, or no mucus apparent.
INTRAUTERINE DEVICE: (IUD) Progestasert, Paragard-T 380 A	
	Client Teaching 1. Recommended in women who have had at least one child. 2. May be inserted at any time during the mentstral cycle. 3. Emphasize the need for yearly checkups and Pap smears. 4. Encourage client to check IUD string, especially after each period. 5. At increased risk for pelvic inflammatory disease.
ORAL CONTRACEPTIVES:	
Pill: (combination of estrogen and progesterone) **Minipill:** (progesterone only - 0.35 mg norethindrone)	Client Teaching: 1. Instruct as to the correct use of medication, the need for periodic checkups every six months, and the importance of taking the pill the same time each day. 2. Explain if a pill is forgotten one day, she should take it when she remembers, then take the next pill as scheduled the following day. 3. If two pills are missed, she should take them as above and use some other form of contraception for the remainder of the month. 4. If taking antibiotics, need to use a second method of birth control. 5. Review common side effects, serious complications, and the reporting of any of the following symptoms: abdominal pain, chest pain, shortness of breath, headaches, eye problems, and severe leg pain.
CHEMICAL BARRIERS:	
Spermicides: jellies, creams, foams, suppositories, sponge.	Client Teaching: 1. Instruct as a proper insertions of spermicide. 2. Explain how to wash applicator in warm water with a mild soap, making sure plunger is separated from barrel; do not boil applicator. 3. Advise not to douche for 6 to 8 hours after intercourse. 4. Educate about alternative methods of contraception.

Appendix 20-1:
CONTRACEPTIVE METHODS

METHODS / DESCRIPTION	NURSING IMPLICATIONS / CLIENT TEACHING
MECHANICAL BARRIERS:	
Diaphragm: a dome-shaped rubber device that fits over the cervix. **Condom:** "rubbers" are thin sheaths of rubber which fit over an erect penis.	Client Teaching: Diaphragm: 1. Should be refitted after every pregnancy or when there is a weight gain or loss of 20 lbs. 2. Instruct client to use spermicidal jelly or cream around diaphragm rim and in the dome. 3. Instruct that diaphragm is left in place 6 to 8 hrs. after intercourse. 4. Explain the proper method for cleansing (use Ivory soap only), storing (dry thoroughly and dust with constarch , not baby powder), and checking for defects or holes in the diaphragm. 5. Allow for sufficient practice of insertion/removal techniques. Condom: 1. Advise client to apply condom to erect penis by rolling the sheath along the entire shaft, and leaving enough slack at the end of the penis to receive the semen. 2. Explain importance of holding the condom in place while withdrawing the penis to prevent emptying of sperm into the vagina. 3. Condom should be applied prior to any penetration as the pre-ejaculatory seminal fluid may contain sperm.
UNRELIABLE PRACTICES:	
Withdrawal (coitus interruptus) **Douching** ***Description:*** Coitus interruptus: withdrawal of penis prior to ejaculation. Douching: the act of cleansing/washing the semen out of the vagina.	***Nursing Implications:*** Requires absolute cooperation and control of partner. Associated with high level of sexual frustration. ***Client Teaching:*** Encourage use of a more reliable contraceptive practice.
PERMANENT STERILIZATION:	
Tubal ligation	Client Teaching: 1. Discuss the permanence of the sterilization procedure with the couple. 2. Explain that often after surgery, referred shoulder pain is common due to CO_2 insufflation during laproscopy.
VASECTOMY:	
Action: Surgical ligation and resection bilaterally of the vas deferens.	Client Teaching: 1. Discuss with couple the permanence of vasectomy; even if the vas deferens is reconnected, the fertility varies between 5 percent to 60 percent. 2. Activity level should be moderate for 2 days. 3. Encourage the use of a scrotal support and apply ice for pain or swelling. 4. Follow-up visit for sperm sample is usually done in 4 to 6 weeks. 5. Advise couple to use another form of birth control until ejaculate contains no sperm.

Appendix 20-2:
MAGNESIUM SULFATE

MEDICATIONS	SIDE EFFECTS	NURSING IMPLICATIONS
ANTICONVULSANT: **Magnesium Sulfate** ($MgSO4$)		
IV: Given via an IV pump; preferred route. **IM:** 4 to 5 gm into each buttock (deep IM); 1 percent procaine may be added to decrease pain of injection.	**Maternal**: sweating, flushing, muscle weakness, depressed or absent reflexes, oliguria, respiratory paralysis. **Fetal:** crosses placenta, lethargy, hypotonia, and weakness. **Contraindications:** maternal-impaired renal function.	1. Criteria for administrations: a. Respirations - greater than 12/min. b. Presence of patellar knee-jerk movement. c. Urinary output - greater than 30 cc/hour. 2. Check blood pressure frequently for symptoms of hypotension. 3. Antidote of magnesium sulfate is *calcium gluconate*; should be available at bedside in case of respiratory paralysis. 4. Monitor fetal heart rate. 5. MgSO4 is continued at least 24 hours after delivery to reduce risk of seizure activity postpartum. 6. May be used as a tocolytic agent. 7. IM administration: a. Use deep IM or Z track into ventrogluteal muscle. b. Massage site after injection. c. Apply warm, dry pack to promote absorption and increase comfort. 8. **Uses:** prevention or control of eclampsia.

NCLEX ALERT: *Monitor fetal heart rate, especially when mother is receiving Mg SO_4 and Pitocin.*

Appendix 20-3:
OXYTOCIC MEDICATIONS

MEDICATION	SIDE EFFECTS	NURSING IMPLICATIONS
OXYTOCIC MEDICATIONS: Stimulate contraction of uterine muscle fibers; have a mild antidiuretic effect; stimulate postpartum milk flow, but not amount.		
Oxytocin (PITOCIN, SYNTOCINON): IM, IV, intranasal Ergonovine **(ERGOTRATE)**: PO, IM, IV Methylergonovine **(METHERGINE)**: PO, IM, IV	***Maternal*** - tetanic uterine contractions, hypertension, tachycardia. ***Fetal*** - hypoxia, irregularity and decrease in fetal heart rate, possible hyperbilirubinemia. ***Contraindications:*** Severe preeclampsia or eclampsia. Predisposition to uterine rupture or CPD. Preterm infant, or the presence of fetal distress.	1. Apply fetal monitor - assess fetal heart rate throughout oxytocin administration. 2. *Assess maternal vital signs prior to increasing oxytocin infusion rate. Report any changes to RN.* 3. *If any of the following occurs, report immediately to RN.* a. *Fetal distress* (decreasing FHR). b. *Sustained uterine contractions over 2 minutes.* c. *Insufficient relaxation of the uterus between contractions.* 4. ***Uses***—uterine dystocia; induction of labor for diabetes mellitus, preeclampsia, eclampsia clients; control of hemorrhage and uterine atony; uterine involution.

Appendix 20-4:
TOCOLYTIC AGENTS TO SUPPRESS LABOR

MEDICATIONS	SIDE EFFECTS	NURSING IMPLICATIONS
TOCOLYTIC AGENTS: Relaxes myometrial cells of the uterus, leading to inhibition of labor. Also results in bronchial dilation and cardiac output		
Terbutaline (**Brethine**): IV, SQ, PO	***Maternal:*** tachycardia (very little effect on blood pressure), nervousness and tremors, headache, and possible pulmonary edema. ***Fetal:*** tachycardia, hypoglycemia.	1. Assess maternal and fetal vital signs frequently; fetal monitoring is necessary; *notify RN if maternal pulse is greater than 120 beats/min or FHR is greater than 180 beats/min.* 2. Encourage left lateral position (Sims') to decrease hypotension and increase placental perfusion. 3. Uterine contractions will decrease in frequency and intensity during treatment. 4. ***Use:*** premature labor.
Ritodrine (**Yutopar**): IV, PO	***Maternal:*** altered pulse and blood pressure (dose related), widening pulse pressure, tachycardia, hypotension, nausea and vomiting, hyperglycemia, nervousness and tremors, and skin rash. ***Fetal:*** Altered FHR (dose-related), increased serum glucose, acidosis, hypoxia, and hypotension at birth.	1. Terbutaline usually preferred over ritodrine because of minimal effects on blood pressure. 2. ***Contraindications:*** severe preeclampsia, hypovolemia, cardiac disease; used with caution in diabetic mothers.

Appendix 20-5:
RHOGAM

MEDICATIONS	SIDE EFFECTS	NURSING IMPLICATIONS
Immune globulin human Rho (D): Prevents Rho(D) sensitization in nonsensitized Rh neg mothers following pregnancy or accidental transfusion; "tricks" the body into thinking it has already made antibodies.		
Rhogam: IM	Pain and soreness at site of injection	1. Must be administered within 72 hours of delivery, or after an abortion, miscarriage, or transfusion. 2. Do not administer this to the infant. 3. **Uses:** prevention of hemolytic disease of the newborn. 4. **Contraindications**: sensitized Rh neg person.

Notes

T- 94°F (34.4°C)

low- 92°F (33.3°C)

Newborn 21

NORMAL NEWBORN

NCLEX ALERT: *Provide physical care appropriate to developmental level (e.g., newborn, child, etc.); compare a client's development to norms. Monitor a newborn.*

Data Collection

A. Respiratory system.

1. Respirations are usually established within one minute after birth; often within the first few seconds.
2. Lusty cry usually accompanies good respiratory effort.
3. Newborn respiration should be quiet; no dyspnea or cyanosis.
4. Cyanosis may be apparent in the hands and the feet (acrocyanosis); circumoral cyanosis (around the mouth) may persist for an hour or two after birth, but should subside.
5. Neonate breathes through the nose (obligate nose-breather); consequently nasal obstruction or mucus will lead to respiratory distress.

B. Circulatory system.

1. Closure of the openings in the heart necessary for fetal circulation (ductus arteriosus, foramen ovale, and ductus venosus).
2. Circulatory changes are not always immediate and complete - usually complete in a few days; often this period is called *transitional circulation*.

C. Body temperature and heat production.

***NURSING PRIORITY:** Excessive heat loss occurs because of the newborn's larger surface area when compared to body weight.*

1. Body temperature may drop to 94°F (34.4°C) or even as low as 92°F (33.3°C) after birth unless the infant is adequately protected.
2. Heat generated immediately by *shivering*; infant shivering is characterized by increased muscular activity, restlessness and crying.

D. Head.

1. Molding.
   a. Head may appear elongated at birth; usually molding disappears within 24 to 48 hours.
   b. Occurs due to abnormal fetal posture in utero and pressure during passage through the birth canal.
2. Caput succedaneum.
   a. Edema of the scalp due to the pressure occurring at the time of delivery.
   b. Disappears within 1 to 2 days.
3. Cephalhematoma.
   a. A collection of blood between the periosteum and the skull.
   b. Usually results from trauma during labor and delivery.
   c. Absorbed in a few weeks.
4. Head measurement.
   a. Average circumference of the full-term neonate: 34.2 cm; usual variation ranges between 32 to 36 cm.
   b. Head circumference is approximately 2-3 cm greater than the chest circumference.

***NURSING PRIORITY:** Extremes in size may indicate microcephaly, hydrocephaly or increased intracranial pressure.*

5. Fontanel.
   a. Palpated for size and tension.
   b. Increase in tension may indicate increasing intracranial pressure or hydrocephaly.
   c. Decrease in tension (sunken fontanel) may indicate dehydration or shock.

E. Umbilical cord.

1. Determination of number of blood vessels; two arteries and one vein surrounded by Wharton's jelly.
2. Cord atrophies and sloughs off by day 6 to 10.

F. Nervous system.

1. Nervous system is relatively immature and characterized by the following:
   a. Poor nervous control; easily startled.
   b. Quivering chin.
   c. Tremors of short duration of the lower extremities.
2. Presence of positive Babinski sign.
   a. Considered a normal finding until age one year.
   b. Dorsiflexion of big toe and fanning of the other toes.
3. Reflexes found in infancy (Table 21-1).

Table 21-1: MAJOR NEONATAL REFLEXES

REFLEX	DISAPPEARS	HOW TO ELICIT	RESPONSE
Babinski	1 year	Lightly stroke lateral side of foot from heel to toe across the foot.	Infant's toes fan, with dorsiflexion of great toe.
Extrusion (touch tongue)	3 to 4 months	Touch tongue.	Tongue moves outward.
Grasp:			
Palmar	3 to 4 months	Press a finger against infant's palm	Infant's fingers momentarily close around object.
Plantar	8 to 10 months	Press an object against ball of infant's foot.	Infant's toes curl down and around object.
Moro (Startle)	3 to 4 months	Make a loud noise or suddenly disturb infant's equilibrium.	Infant stiffens, briskly abducts and extends arms with hands open and fingers extended to C-shape. Infant's legs flex and abduct, and arms return to an embracing posture. Crying is usual.
Rooting	3 to 4 months; May persist during sleep until 7 to 8 months	Stroke cheek.	Head turns toward side that is touched.
Stepping (dancing)	7 to 8 weeks	Hold infant so that sole of foot touches flat surface.	Infant makes walking or stepping motion.
Sucking	10 to 12 months	Touch or stroke lips.	Baby sucks.
Tonic neck (Fencer's position)	6 months	Turn supine infant's head over the shoulder to one side.	Infant's arm and leg partially or completely extend on side to which head is turned; opposite arm and leg flex.

***NURSING PRIORITY:** Intactness of the neonate's nervous system is indicated by the state of alertness, resting posture, cry, and quality of muscle tone and motor activity.*

G. Hematologic system.

1. Physiologic jaundice - jaundice occurring on the second or third day of life due to increase in serum bilirubin level.

2. Transitory coagulation defects.

   a. Due to the lack of intestinal synthesis of vitamin K as a result of insufficient bacterial flora in the GI tract.

   b. Administration of vitamin K (0.5 to 1.0 mg IM) is ordered to prevent complications.

H. Gastrointestinal tract.

1. Stools.

***NURSING PRIORITY:** The progression of the newborn's stool is from meconium within the first 8-24 hours followed by transitional stools.*

   a. Meconium - sticky, black, odorless, sterile stool which occurs within the first 24 hours after birth; if no stool is passed, possibility of imperforate anus may exist.

   b. Stools change according to infant feeding.

      (1) Transitional stools - period between second and fourth day; consist of part meconium and part milk; greenish-brown or greenish -yellow in color; loose and often contain mucous.

      (2) Stools of the breast-fed infant are golden yellow in color, a pasty consistency, and occur more frequently than stools of formula-fed infants.

      (3) Formula -fed infant - stools are dryer, more formed, and a paler color.

I. Urinary system.

***NURSING PRIORITY:** Most newborns void within the first 24-48 hours after birth.*

1. 30 to 60 cc voided per day during the first two days of life; followed by 200 cc per day by the end of the first week.

2. Frequency of voiding - average of 2 to 6 times per day, increasing up to 10 to 15 times per day.

J. Integumentary system.

1. Vernix caseosa - a white cheesy-like material; covers the skin at birth; particularly noted in the folds and creases.
2. Petechiae - pinpoint bluish discolorations on the skin, (primarily the face) as a result of pressure from delivery; may see bruising of tissues.
3. Lanugo - downy, fine covering of hair that may be present on the shoulders, back, ear lobes, and forehead; disappears during the first week.
4. Milia - pinpoint white bumps seen over the bridge of the nose and on the cheeks during the first two weeks of life.
5. Erythema toxicum - splotchy, pink, papular rash appearing anywhere on the body; disappears within the first few days of life; no treatment necessary.
6. Mongolian spots - bluish, darkened pigmented areas seen on the back or buttocks of dark-skinned infants (from black, oriental, and Mediterranean countries); disappears usually by school age.
7. Hemangiomatous area "stork bites" - areas on the upper eyelids, between the eyebrows, upper lip, or at the nape of the neck which are light red in appearance; fade and disappear between one and two years of age.

K. Sensory system.

1. All infants' eyes are blue or slate blue at birth; become their permanent color at age 3 months.
2. Tears do not develop until three to four months.
3. Sudden loud noises may elicit startle response.
4. Smell developed at birth.
5. Differentiates between pleasant and unpleasant tastes.
6. Most sensitive area is around the mouth.
7. Searches for food when cheek is touched; begins sucking movement when lips are touched.

L. Musculoskeletal system.

1. Assumes the position of comfort, which is usually the position he/she assumed in utero.
2. Normal palmar crease is present (simian crease indicative of Down's syndrome).
3. Spine is straight and flat when in prone position.

Nursing Intervention

NURSING PRIORITY: *During the admission period (first 4 hours after birth) the priority nursing goals are to: maintain a clear airway, maintain a neutral thermal environment, prevent hemorrhage and infection, and initiate bathing and oral feedings.*

✦ *Goal: to establish and maintain a patent airway and good oxygenation.*

1. Position infant with head slightly lower than chest; may use postural drainage, or side-lying position.
2. Suction nostrils and oral pharynx with bulb syringe or a De Lee Mucus trap.
3. Observe for apnea, cyanosis and mucus collection and report to RN.
4. Use oropharyngeal suctioning, stimulation, oxygen administration, or resuscitative procedures if necessary.

NURSING PRIORITY: *Important to monitor infant closely as apnea, decreased heart rate, gagging, choking, and regurgitation are likely to occur and require nursing intervention.*

✦ *Goal: to protect against heat loss from the body.*

1. Immediately after birth, dry off amniotic fluid from body using a warm blanket.
2. Replace wet blanket with warm dry blanket.
3. Cover wet hair and head with a blanket.
4. Place baby on a warm padded surface; preferably under a radiant heater or in an incubator, or with skin- to-skin contact with the mother's body.
5. In the nursery, place in a heated bassinet until body temperature is stable.
6. Avoid any unnecessary procedures until body temperature is stable.

✦ *Goal: to collect data and assess physical condition and behavior.*

1. Apgar at 1 minute and then 5 minutes (See Table 20-9 for Apgar scoring).

NURSING PRIORITY: *The APGAR at one minute evaluates the status of the neonate's intrauterine oxygenation; at 5 minutes it evaluates the status of transition to extrauterine life.*

2. Monitor vital signs every 15 minutes for one hour, every 30 minutes for one hour, every 1 to 2 hours x 4 until stable; also record incubator temperature.
3. Handle the infant with gloves and follow standard precautions until the infant has been bathed.

4. Weigh and measure infant.
   a. Average length of full-term neonate: 45.2 cm to 55 cm (17.8 inches to 27.7 inches).
   b. Infant is measured by being placed flat on the back and determining the distance from head to heel by using a pencil to mark the distance and then measuring the distance when the infant is removed.
   c. Average birth weight for a full-term neonate: 3,400 grams (7 lb 8 oz).

✦ *Goal: to properly identify infant.*

1. Secure identification bands to wrists, or ankles of infant and wrist mother in the delivery room.
2. Prints of infant's foot, palms or fingers may be obtained according to hospital policy; also mother's palm or fingerprints may be obtained.

✦ *Goal: to promote maternal-infant attachment to parents immediately after birth; if temperature stable allow mother and father to hold child.*

1. Keep infant warm under a heat lamp and permit parents to examine during the first hour or so if possible.
2. Provide opportunities for parents to learn to care for their infant.

✦ *Goal: to protect against infection.*

1. Proper hand washing before handling infant.
2. Administer prophylactic treatment to eyes soon after birth.
   a. 1 to 2 percent silver nitrate solution, penicillin, or erythromycin antibiotic eye ointment in the conjunctival sac.
   b. Prevents ophthalmia neonatorum.

> **NURSING PRIORITY:** *Prophylaxis for eye infection can be delayed for up to one hour after birth in order to promote attachment behavior, i.e., eye-to-eye contact between mother and infant.*

3. Avoid contact by various personnel in nursery area; avoid exposure to people with upper respiratory, skin or gastrointestinal illness.

✦ *Goal: to prevent bleeding problems.*

1. Administration of 0.5 to 1.0 mg of vitamin K (**Aqua Mephyton**) IM into the upper third of the lateral aspect of the thigh.

✦ *Goal: to initiate and evaluate feeding ability and provide nutrition.*

1. First feeding or test feeding - administer 10 to 15 cc of sterile water, followed by a 5 percent or 10 percent glucose solution.
2. *Observe for respiratory problems during feeding and report to RN.*
3. First milk intake.
   a. Breast - three to four minutes sucking time at the breast.
   b. Formula - 25 to 30 cc of formula; usually hungry from four to six hours after birth.

Home Care

✦ *Provide daily general care.*

1. Care of the umbilical cord.
   a. A drying solution of alcohol, triple dye or **Merthiolate** is applied to the cord.
   b. Clean the umbilical cord several times a day, especially after voiding (for a male infant).
   c. To encourage drying of the cord, expose to air frequently and position diaper below umbilicus.
   d. Observe for bleeding, oozing, or foul odor.
2. Circumcision care.
   a. Keep area clean.
   b. Observe for bleeding.
   c. A sterile gauze dressing with petroleum jelly may be applied to the area during the first 24 hours.

> ***NURSING PRIORITY:*** *Teach the parents that a whitish yellow exudate around the glans is granulation tissue and is normal and not indicative of infection. It may be observed for 2-3 days and should not be removed.*

3. Neonate's bath.
   a. Bath is delayed until vital signs and temperature are stabilized.
   b. Mild baby soap and warm water is used.
   c. Apply principles of clean to dirty area - eyes, face, ears, head, body, genitals, buttocks.
   d. Head is an area for significant heat loss.
4. Assess and observe daily weight and record gain or loss.
5. Assess stools.
   a. Meconium stools.
   b. Transitional stools.
6. Although a PKU is drawn while the newborn is in the hospital, explain the importance of returning to the physician's office to get the infant's PKU test done in about 7-10 days after birth.
7. Obtain T_3 and T_4 (usually 3rd day) as indicated to rule out congenital hypothyroidism.

NURSING PRIORITY: *It is important to explain to parents to have tests of both PKU and T_3 and T_4 performed at 7-14 days to insure against a possible false negative result on the first screening.*

8. All infants should receive the first dose of hepatitis B vaccine soon after birth and before hospital discharge; the first dose may also be give by age 2 months if the infant's mother is HBsAg-negative.
9. Explain to parents reportable signs of illness in the newborn: temperature above 38.4°C (101°F) or below 36.1°C (97°F), more than one episode of projectile vomiting, refusal of 2 feedings in a row, cyanosis, and absence of breathing for longer than 15 seconds.
10. Teach about home phototherapy for mild to moderate physiologic jaundice.
    a. Usually started with bilirubin levels between 10-14 mg/dl.
    b. Bili-lights or fiberoptic phototherapy blankets are rented.
    c. Teach parents how to keep a daily record of infant's temperature, weight, intake and output, and stools.

NURSING PRIORITY: *Explain importance of covering infant's eyes and genitalia when under bili lights. Fiberoptic blankets - do not need to cover eyes & genitalia.*

HIGH-RISK NEWBORN

Data Collection

A. Respiratory parameters.
1. Observe respiratory rate, rhythm, and depth.
    a. Initially, rate increases without a change in rhythm.
    b. Flaring of nares and expiratory grunting are early signs of respiratory distress.
2. Increase in apical pulse rate.
3. Subcostal and xiphoid retractions.
4. Color.
    a. Progresses from pink to circumoral pallor to circumoral cyanosis to generalized cyanosis.
    b. Increased intensity of acrocyanosis.
5. Progressive respiratory distress.
    a. Chin tug (chin pulled down and in with mouth opening wider - auxiliary muscles of respiration are used).
    b. Abdominal seesaw breathing patterns.
    c. Increase in apneic episodes.
6. Falling body temperature.
7. Progressing anoxia leading to cardiac decompensation and failure.
8. Increased muscle flaccidity - frog-like position.

B. Nutrition.
1. Determine readiness and ability to feed - swallowing, gag reflexes.
2. Screen for hypoglycemia.
3. Observe for congenital dysfunction and anomalies related.
4. Check amount and frequency of elimination pattern.
5. Assess for vomiting or regurgitation; a pre-term infant's stomach capacity is small, and overfeeding can occur.
6. Check mucous membranes, urine output and skin turgor to recognize fluid and electrolyte imbalance.
    a. Skin turgor over abdomen and inner thighs.
    b. Sunken fontanel.
    c. Urinary output less than 30 cc per day.

C. Temperature regulation.
1. Assess infant's temperature — skin probe is frequently utilized.
2. Check coolness or warmth of body and extremities.
3. Detect early signs of cold stress and report to RN.
    a. Increased physical activity and crying.
    b. Respiratory rate increases.
    c. Increased acrocyanosis or generalized cyanosis along with mottling of the skin (cutis marmorata).
    d. Male with descended testes - presence of cremaster reflex (testes are pulled back up into the inguinal canal upon exposure to cold).
4. Monitor infant's temperature.
    a. Axillary temperature: 36.5°C (97.7°F).
    b. Rectal temperature can be taken; however, it is discouraged as it irritates rectal mucosa, can stimulate bowel movement, and may lead to possible tissue trauma.

Nursing Intervention for the High-Risk Newborn

✦ *Goal: to maintain respiratory functioning.*
1. Provide gentle physical stimulation to encourage infant breathing.
    a. Gently rub the infant's back.

b. Lightly tap the infant's feet.

2. Ensure patency of respiratory tract.
   a. Maintain open airway by nasal, oral, or pharyngeal suctioning.
   b. Position to promote oxygenation.
      (1) Elevate head 10° with neck slightly extended by a small folded towel under the shoulders.
      (2) Flex and abduct infant's arms and place at sides.
      (3) Keep diapers loose to avoid pressure on diaphragm.
      (4) Turn side to side every 1 to 2 hours.
      (5) Do not place in prone position.
3. Assist infant's respiratory efforts.
   a. Monitor oxygen pressure — avoid high concentrations of oxygen for prolonged periods-leads to complications of retrolental fibroplasia and bronchopulmonary dysplasia.
   b. Continuous positive airway pressure (CPAP).

✦ *Goal: to provide adequate nutrition.*

1. Detect hypoglycemia and treat immediately.
   a. Dextrostix done frequently.
   b. IV of D_5W if infant unable to tolerate oral feeding.
2. Oral feeding - initial feeding.
   a. Use sterile water - 1 to 2 cc for a small infant.
   b. Use preemie nipple to conserve infant's energy.
   c. Due to small size of stomach, feedings are small in amount and increased in frequency.

NCLEX ALERT: *Administer a tube feeding.*

---

3. Orogastric tube feedings.
   a. Usually administered by continuous flow of formula with an infusion pump (kangaroo pump) when the infant is:
      (1) Having severe respiratory distress.
      (2) Too immature and weak to suck.
      (3) Tired and fatigues easily using a preemie nipple.
   b. Placement and insertion of orogastric feeding tube.
      (1) Position infant on the back or toward the right side with the head and chest slightly elevated.
      (2) Measure correct length of insertion by marking on the catheter the distance from the tip of the nose to the ear lobe to the tip of the sternum.
      (3) Lubricate tube with sterile water and slowly insert catheter into mouth and down the esophagus into the stomach.
      (4) Test for placement of the tube by aspirating stomach contents or injecting 0.5 to 1.0 cc of air for the premature, up to 5 cc for larger children, and auscultating the abdomen for the sound.
      (5) Prior to instilling feeding by gravity into stomach, may need to check for residual; this is done by aspirating and measuring amount left in stomach from previous feeding; often the residual amount is subtracted from the current feeding so that overfeeding does not occur.
      (6) If feeding is not continuous remove tubing by pinching or clamping it and withdrawing it rapidly.
      (7) Burp infant after feeding by turning head or positioning him or her on the right side.
4. Hyperalimentation (TPN) may be ordered to provide complete nutrition through an indwelling catheter threaded into the vena cava.
5. Detect complications that arise with feeding the pre-term infant as a result of the following:
   a. Weak or absent sucking and swallowing reflexes.
   b. Necessity for high caloric content of food with a very small stomach capacity.
   c. Poor gag reflex, leading to aspiration.
   d. Increased incidence of vomiting, regurgitation, and development of abdominal distention.
   e. Inability to absorb essential nutrients.
   f. Excessive loss of water through evaporation from the skin and respiratory tract.

✦ *Goal: to maintain warmth and temperature control.*

1. Prevent and minimize cold stress.
   a. Dry infant quickly, wrap, and place in warm incubator; may be unwrapped under a radiant heat shield.
   b. All surfaces that touch the infant should be warm.
   c. Oxygen and air should be warmed and humidified.
2. Maintain abdominal skin temperature at 36.1 to 36.7°C (97° to 98°F); axillary temperature 36.5°C (97.8°F).
3. Monitor infant's temperature continuously; make sure that thermostat is set on control panel, probe is in contact with infant's skin, and all safety precautions are maintained.

4. Prevent rapid warming or cooling, as this may cause apnea and acidosis; warming process is increased gradually over a period of 2 to 4 hours.
5. Infant may need extra clothing or need to be wrapped in an extra blanket for additional warmth. A cap or cover will reduce loss of body heat from the head.
6. Kangaroo Care—uses skin-to-skin contact with preterm infant usually wearing only a diaper and small cap; hold infant next to body similar to how a kangaroo keeps its offspring warm in its pouch.

✦ *Goal: to assist in phototherapy treatment for jaundice.*

NCLEX ALERT: *Administer phototherapy treatments to newborn.*

1. Involves the use of intense fluorescent light on the infant's exposed skin.
2. Place infant nude under bili-lights.
3. Expose all areas to the light except for eyes and genitalia - cover infant's eyes with an opaque mask or eye patch.
4. Monitor skin temperature to prevent hyperthermia or hypothermia.
5. Chart pertinent information relating to time phototherapy was started and stopped, maintenance of shielding of the eyes, type and intensity of lamp used, distance of light to infant, whether used in combination with an isolette or an open bassinet, and any side effects.

Disorders Related to Gestational Age

Respiratory Distress Syndrome

Data Collection

❑ **Hyaline membrane disease (HMD), also referred to as respiratory distress syndrome (RDS). Occurs as a result of the deficiency of surfactant which lines the alveoli.**

❑ **Meconium aspiration syndrome occurs when the fetus passes meconium in utero and aspirates the meconium into the lungs,which leads to obstruction in the small airway passages.**

1. Tachypnea - more than 60 respirations per minute.
2. Apneic spells.
3. Abnormal breath sounds - rales and rhonchi.
4. Chest retraction.
5. Chin tug - noticed on inspiration; mouth open, lips apart.
6. Flaring of the nares.
7. Expiratory grunt.

NURSING PRIORITY: *Grunting is an ominous sign and indicates impending need for respiratory resuscitative efforts.*

Complications

1. Retrolental fibroplasia (damage to the retina of the eye) due to high levels of oxygen.
2. Bronchopulmonary dysplasia - loss of lung elasticity.

Treatment

1. Respiratory distress syndrome.
   a. CPAP is the primary treatment.
   b. If fatigue occurs due to breathing, IPPB along with CPAP may be instituted.
2. Meconium aspiration.
   a. Oxygen with humidification.
   b. Postural drainage and percussion.
   c. Antibiotic therapy.
   d. Acid-base imbalance correction if needed.

Nursing Intervention

✦ *Goal: to promote oxygenation and respiratory functioning.*

1. Administer glucocorticoids (**Celestone**) to stimulate surfactant production.
2. Refer to nursing intervention for the high-risk newborn.

Disorders of Development

Cleft Lip and Cleft Palate

❑ **Cleft lip is a fissure or split in the upper lip which may vary from a slight notch to a complete separation extending into the nostril; may be unilateral or bilateral.**

❑ **Cleft palate is a fissure or a split in the roof of the mouth (palate).**

Data Collection

1. Visible at birth as an incompletely formed lip.
2. Sucking difficulties and breathing problems with cleft palate.
3. Increased incidence of upper respiratory infection and otitis media.
4. Later problems related to speech and hearing difficulties with cleft palate.

Treatment

1. Surgical.

Table 21-2: DISORDERS ACQUIRED DURING AND AFTER BIRTH

	TRAUMA	PERIPHERAL NERVE INJURIES	NEONATAL SEPSIS
DATA COLLECTION	Soft tissue injury. Caput succedaneum. Cephalhematoma. Injury to bones.—fractured clavicle is the most common; often occurs with a large-sized infant.	Temporary paralysis of the facial nerve is the most common. Affected side of the face is smooth. Eye may stay open. Mouth droops at the corner. Forehead cannot be wrinkled. Possible difficulty sucking. Brachial palsy - a partial or complete paralysis of the nerve fibers of the brachial plexus. Cannot elevate or abduct the arm. Abnormal arm position or diminished arm movements.	Apathy, lethargy, low-grade temperature. Poor feeding, abdominal distention, diarrhea. Cyanosis, irregular respirations, apnea. Hyperbilirubinemia. Infant often described as "not acting right" Complete blood count, chest x-ray, and viral studies (**TORCH**) — an acronym for **T**oxoplasmosis, **R**ubella, **C**ytomegalovirus, and **Her**pes virus blood screening.
NURSING INTERVENTION	1. Place affected arm against chest wall with hand lying across chest. 2.Position is held by a figure 8 stockinette around the arm and chest. 3. Pick infant up carefully; shoulder should not be pressed toward the middle of the body. 4. Affected side should not be placed in a gown or undershirt.	1. Brachial nerve palsy Arm is kept abducted and externally rotated with elbow flexed Arm is raised to shoulder height, and elbow is flexed 90 degrees.	1. Prenatal prevention, maternal screening for sexually transmitted diseases, and assessing rubella titers. 2. Maintenance of sterile technique. 3. Prophylactic antibiotic treatment. 4. Cesarean birth for mother with genital herpes.

a. Closure of lip defect usually precedes treatment for a cleft palate (which is done in stages).

(1) Extensive orthodontics to correct problems with teeth.

(2) Speech therapy.

(3) Hearing problems related to chronic, recurrent otitis media; varying degrees of hearing loss may occur.

b. "Rule of Tens" applies to the planning of surgical repair of cleft lip - infant must be either 10 lb, 10 weeks old, or have a hemoglobin of at least 10 gm/dl.

c. Long-term care management - speech therapy, orthodontics; frequent occurrences of otitis media.

Nursing Intervention

✦ *Goal: to provide preoperative care.*

1. Maintain nutrition.

a. Use a large-holed nipple, a soft regular cross-cut nipple, lamb's nipple (which is longer and softer), an asepto rubber-tipped syringe, or a Haberman feeder.

b. Feed slowly and while child is sitting up.

c. Bubble and burp frequently (after every 15 to 30 cc).

d. Rinse cleft with water after each feeding, to help prevent infection and irritation of the lip.

2. Prevent infection.

a. Teach parents symptoms of otitis media.

b. Teach about various methods to meet infant's sucking needs.

3. Prepare parents for newborn's surgery.

a. Encourage parent to position infant on back frequently to accustom him or her to the postoperative positioning.

b. Prior to admission, encourage parents to place infant in arm restraints periodically, so that he/she becomes familiar with restriction of arm motion after surgery.

c. Encourage parents to feed infant with the device that will be used postoperatively.

✦ *Goal: to provide postoperative care.*

1. Prevent trauma to suture line.
   a. Position on back or side.
   b. May require a protective device on lip.
   c. Restrain arms and use a jacket restraint on an older child — be certain to provide rest periods to exercise arms.
   d. Avoid use of any objects in the mouth, (e.g., straws, suction catheters, tongue depressors, pacifiers, or spoons).
   e. Avoid crying, if possible, by providing attention and affection or diversional activities if child is older.
2. Maintain a patent airway and facilitate breathing.
   a. Use side-lying position.
   b. *Assess for respiratory distress, swelling of the nose, tongue, and lips and report to RN.*
3. Provide adequate nutrition.
   a. Feed in an upright, sitting position.
   b. Feed slowly and burp/bubble at frequent intervals.
   c. Cleanse lip suture line after each feeding; use cotton-tipped applicator and *roll* along suture line.
   d. Prevent any crust formation on lip and suture line.
   e. Fluids initially after palate repair, then advance to soft diet; milk is avoided.
   f. Older child is not allowed to eat hard items such as cookies, potato chips, toast, etc.
   g. Cleanse palate suture line after each feeding by rinsing mouth with sterile water.

Esophageal Atresia with Tracheoesophageal Fistula

❑ **Proximal end of esophagus ends in a blind pouch and the lower segment connects to the trachea.**

Data Collection

1. Characterized by the classic 3 Cs: choking, coughing, and cyanosis.
2. Excessive mucous secretions and constant drooling.
3. Aspiration is a complication, especially during feeding.

Nursing Intervention

***NURSING PRIORITY:** If there is any suspicion of possible esophageal problems, infant should be placed NPO until further evaluation.*

✦ *Goal: to provide preoperative care.*

1. Maintain patent airway.
   a. Supine position with head elevated on an inclined plane of at least 30 degrees.
   b. Suction nasopharynx.
   c. *Observe for symptoms of respiratory distress (classic 3 Cs) and report to RN.*
2. Prepare parents for infant's surgery.

✦ *Goal: to provide postoperative care.*

1. Maintain respirations and prevent respiratory complications.
   a. Administer oxygen as needed.
   b. Suction secretions and position for optimum ventilation.
   c. Maintain care of chest tubes.
   d. Administer antibiotics as ordered.
   e. Place in warm, high humidity isolette.
2. Provide adequate nutrition.
   a. Gastrostomy feedings are withheld until the second or third postoperative day.
   b. Oral feedings are delayed for two weeks.
   c. Meet oral sucking needs by offering a pacifier.

Imperforate Anus

❑ **Absence of anal opening.**

Data Collection

1. Absence of meconium.
2. No anal opening.
3. Gradual increase in abdominal distention.

Nursing Intervention

✦ *Goal: to identify and detect anal malformation.*

***NURSING PRIORITY:** Record the first passage of meconium stool; if infant does not pass stool within twenty-four hours, further data collection is required.*

1. Detect increasing abdominal distention.
2. Inspect anal area for opening and report to RN if there is absence of opening.

✦ *Goal: to provide postoperative care (abdominal-perineal pull-through surgical procedure).*

1. Prevent infection by maintaining good perineal care and keeping operative site clean and dry, especially after passage of stool and urine.

2. No rectal temperatures.
3. Side-lying prone position with hips elevated to prevent stress on perineal sutures.
4. May have a colostomy.

Spina Bifida

❑ **A congenital malformation leading to defects in closure of the spinal cord. Most common site is lumbosacral area.**

Data Collection

1. Types.
   a. Spina bifida occulta - bony defect (bone of spine does not cover spinal cord).
   b. Spina bifida cystica.
      (1) Meningocele - a sac-like cyst of meninges filled with spinal fluid that protrudes through a defect in the bony part of the spine.
      (2) Myelomeningocele - a sac-like cyst containing meninges, spinal fluid, and a portion of the spinal cord with its nerves that protrudes through a defect in the vertebral column; most frequently associated with hydrocephalus.

> ***NURSING PRIORITY:*** *Closure of defect within twenty-four to forty-eight hours to decrease infection, relieve pressure, repair sac, and possibly insert a shunt.*

Nursing Intervention

> ***NURSING PRIORITY:*** *Correct positioning of the infant is of paramount importance in preventing damage to the sac, as well as in providing nursing care after surgery.*

✦ *Goal: to provide preoperative care.*

1. Protect sac and prevent and from drying, rupturing, and infection.
   a. Position on abdomen.
   b. Avoid touching sac.
   c. Careful cleaning following voiding and bowel movements.
   d. Observe for the development of meningitis.
   e. Sterile, normal saline soaks with antibacterial solution placed over sac to prevent drying.
   f. A barrier drape may be used to prevent contamination from stool.
2. Detect early development of hydrocephalus.
   a. Measure head and check circumference frequently.
   b. Check fontanel for bulging and separation of suture line.
3. Monitor elimination function.
   a. Note whether urine is dripping or is retained.
   b. Use Crede method to empty bladder; apply slight pressure at the umbilical area, downward and under the symphysis pubis toward the anus at least every two to four hours during the day.

✦ *Goal: to provide postoperative care.*

1. Prevent trauma and infection to the surgical site.
   a. Position as stated preoperatively.
   b. Continue to provide skin care as listed under preoperative goals.
2. Assess neurological status frequently for indications of increasing intracranial pressure, the development of hydrocephalus, or early signs of infection.
   a. Continue to measure head circumference daily.
   b. Neuro checks frequently.

Drug-dependent Newborn

❑ **A newborn of a substance-abusing mother, either alcohol or drugs or both. After delivery, the newborn may experience withdrawal symptoms.**

Data Collection

1. Clinical manifestations.
   a. Fetal alcohol syndrome (FAS).
      (1) CNS problems - mental retardation, microcephaly, hyperactivity.
      (2) Growth deficiencies.
      (3) Distinctive facial abnormalities.
      (4) Anomalies of the heart, eyes, kidneys, and skeletal system.
   b. Drug dependent.
      (1) Respiratory distress.
      (2) Jaundice.
      (3) Congenital anomalies and growth retardation - genitourinary and cardiac defects.
      (4) Behavioral anomalies - sleep/wake cycles have problems.
      (5) Withdrawal symptoms - watch for them prior to discharge (24-48 hours).

Nursing Intervention

✦ *Goal: to monitor and identify symptoms and newborns at risk for FAS and drug dependent problems.*

1. FAS newborn - able to tolerate feedings and gain weight, hyperirritability controlled.

2. Drug dependent newborn - temperature regulation, monitoring of VS, small frequent feedings, positioning on right side to avoid aspiration, medications for withdrawal as ordered, monitoring for diarrhea and vomiting.
3. Newborns benefit from being "swaddled" - wrapped in blanket with hands near mouth to minimize injury and calm newborn.

✦ *Goal: to provide referral and community based care for parents.*

1. Counseling about available resources.
2. Follow-up visits, especially for missed appointments.

Isoimmune Hemolytic Disease of the Newborn

❑ **An antigen-antibody response causing destruction of fetal RBC. Two types: ABO incompatibility (milder form) and Rh incompatibility (occurs when an Rh negative mother and an Rh positive father produce an Rh positive fetus.)**

Data Collection

1. Clinical manifestations.
   a. Jaundice within twenty-four hours (pathologic jaundice). Begins in the face and advances downward on the bodyto trunk and extremities and finally to the palms and the soles of the feet.
   b. Anemia.
2. Diagnostics.
   a. Prenatal screening - Indirect Coomb's test (mother's blood).
   b. Post-delivery detection - Direct Coomb's test (infant's blood).

Nursing Intervention

✦ *Goal: to administer preventive treatment.*

1. Prenatal - administration of Rh_o(D) immune globulin (**Rhogam**).
   a. Given within the first 72 hours postpartum.
   b. After every pregnancy, abortion, or blood transfusion - **MicRhogam** (microdose of Rh immune globulin) is administered as a mini-dose.

✦ *Goal: to identify and recognize jaundice from the physiologic type (which occurs within 48 to 72 hrs) versus the pathologic type (occurs within 24 hours)*

1. Prenatal monitoring of maternal-fetal status.
2. Monitor bilirubin levels in the newborn.
3. Refer to Nursing Intervention of the high-risk newborn.

Infant of the Diabetic Mother

Data Collection

1. Clinical manifestations.
   a. Large size for gestational age.
   b. Puffy appearance with round cheeks and stocky neck.
   c. Enlarged heart, liver, and spleen.
   d. Rapid, irregular respirations.
   e. Lethargy.
2. Common complications.
   a. Hypoglycemia.
      (1) Lethargy, irritability, hypocalcemia.
      (2) High-pitched cry.
      (3) Twitching, jitteriness.
      (4) Seizures.
      (5) Apneic spells and abdominal distention.
   b. Hyperbilirubinemia.
   c. Respiratory distress syndrome.
   d. Birth trauma due to excessive size.
   e. Congenital defects, specifically, cardiac.

***NURSING PRIORITY:** Prolonged hypoglycemia can cause irreversible brain damage and report symptoms of hypoglycemia immediately to the RN.*

Nursing Intervention

✦ *Goal: to monitor glucose levels.*

1. Blood glucose levels using glucose strips or glucometer are done frequently, 30 min., 1 hr., 2 hrs., and 4 hrs. after birth.
2. Minimize trauma to heel site by performing heel stick correctly.
   a. Do not use needles; use soft-touch lancet or accujet.
   b. Warm heel for 5-10 minutes prior to stick.
   c. Cleanse site with alcohol and dry before sticking.
   d. The lateral heel is the site of choice; however, the toes can be used if needed.

Cataract – waterfall
Caput – succedaneum – diffuse edema under the scalp.

Study Questions—Newborn

1. What equipment should the nurse have available immediately after birth to assist the infant with his initial respiratory effort?

① stethoscope and suction catheter.
② heated crib and a stocking cap.
③ bulb syringe and oxygen.
④ oxygen and stethoscope.

2. What are the characteristics of the meconium stool?

① well formed and dark in color.
② often passed in the first 4 hours of life.
③ light in color and loose.
④ passed within the first 2 days of life.

3. The nurse is assessing a newborn for the presence of a caput succedaneum. What findings would confirm the presence of this condition?

① swelling confined to the parietal areas of the skull.
② diffuse edema under the scalp.
③ a collection of blood under the scalp.
④ petechial hemorrhages in the conjunctiva.

4. What signs would a nurse observe in a newborn with respiratory distress?

① flaring of the nares, grunting, and chest wall retractions.
② lusty crying, heaving chest wall, and flailing arms.
③ respiratory rate of 50, pulse 166, sneezing, .
④ uncontrolled crying, acrocyanosis, and respiratory rate 60.

5. The nurse is assessing the newborn. What nursing assessment data would cause the most concern?

① has loud crying with periods of light sleep.
② has a blood sugar of 75mg/dl.
③ turns dusky and cyanotic when crying.
④ acrocyanosis is present four hours after birth

6. The newborn is given vitamin K soon after birth. What is the purpose of this medication?

① prophylaxis since the newborn does not have an immediate supply.
② to assist with building iron stores in the blood of the newborn.
③ helps to stabilize the electrolytes in the newborn's system.
④ prevents jaundice by breaking down the newborn's bilirubin.

7. What is a characteristic of the newborn with hypoglycemia?

① acrocyanosis.
② respirations of 50/minute.
③ increased irritability.
④ deceased pulse.

8. What nursing measures are important to decrease the loss of body heat in a newborn?

① keep the infant bundled with a stocking cap on his head.
② regulate the room temperature between 68°- 70°.
③ keep the infant in a warmer for the first 8 hours after birth.
④ assess the core temp and respirations every 3 hours.

9. What is a nursing measure to reduce the possibility of infection in the newborn?

① keep the cribs at least three feet apart in the nursery.
② wash hands before and after care delivered to each newborn.
③ wash hands prior to diaper changes.
④ decrease visiting times to only one hour and groups of 3 people.

10. The nurse is observing a new mother breast feed her infant. To decrease the amount of air the infant swallows, what would the nurse suggest to the mother?

① place the newborn on the back with head turned to the left.
② offer the infant the pacifier after each feeding.
③ burp or bubble the infant after the first few minutes of feeding.
④ limit the infant to only 10 minutes nursing at one feeding.

11. In which situation would the nurse anticipate Rho(D) immune globulin human (Rhogam) to be given?

① when the mother is Rh+ .
② within 48 hours after delivery.
③ after a postpartal hemorrhage.
④ when the mother is Rh-

12. What laboratory test is important to obtain on the newborn in order to detect complications?

① alpha-fetoprotein.
② urinalysis.
③ Phenylketonuria (PKU).
④ serum iron.

Simulated NCLEX-PN Practice Test #1

1. A client is receiving 5 units of U100 regular insulin at 7:30 a.m. daily. Based on this information, when would be the most likely time for an insulin reaction?

① By 8 a.m.
② At 4 p.m.
③ During the night.
④ Around 11 a.m.

2. What is a characteristic symptom of hypoglycemia that would alert the nurse to an early insulin reaction?

① Diaphoresis.
② Drowsiness.
③ Severe thirst.
④ Decreased consciousness.

3. At 9 a.m. a twenty-four-hour urine specimen is started. How should the nurse instruct the client to collect the specimen?

① Place the first voided specimen in the container and continue to collect the urine until 9 a.m. the following day.
② Discard the first morning specimen, collect urine for the next 24 hours making sure to void before the sample is completed at 9 a.m.
③ Discard the first morning specimen because it may contain concentrated abnormal components.
④ Collect all urine from 9 a.m. in separate containers that are labeled for time and amount of voiding.

4. A client received penicillin fifteen minutes ago. How would the nurse know the client is developing an anaphylactic reaction?

① Swelling around the injection site.
② A red raised rash over his trunk.
③ Pupillary dilatation and double vision.
④ Severe respiratory distress.

5. The client calls the nurses' station and reports the area around his IV is hurting. The practical nurse assesses his IV and finds the site pale, cool to the touch and the fluid is not infusing. What is the best interpretation of this observation?

① The IV is out of the vein and the fluid has infiltrated into the tissue.
② Warm packs need to be applied because of the problem with thrombophlebitis.
③ The fluid container needs to be higher in order to infuse at the proper rate.
④ Since there is no blood in the line, the IV is patent and needs no attention at this time.

6. The nurse is teaching the mother of a school age child how to manage pediculosis capitis (head lice). What would be included in the teaching?

① Determine the live nits from the dead ones and remove them with a fine tooth comb.
② Remove all of the nits that are located on the shaft of the hair.
③ Soak hair in hydrogen peroxide to kill lice and help remove the nits.
④ For severe infestation, removal may be facilitated by cutting the hair short.

7. In caring for the postoperative thoracotomy client, frequent coughing and deep-breathing exercises are:

① Not encouraged because of the severe pain and dyspnea.
② Supervised by the PN in order to evaluate the level of pain.
③ Encouraged to promote adequate ventilation in the unaffected lung.
④ Done only if the client's chest x-ray indicates areas of atelectasis.

8. A client has cancer and has lost his hair as a result of chemotherapy. He asks the nurse if it will grow back. What is the nursing response based on?

① The dose and type of drug administered will be the determining factor for hair regrowth.
② The hair loss is permanent regardless of any efforts to prevent it.
③ The hair won't grow back unless special measures were taken during chemotherapy.
④ The color and texture of the new hair may be different but the hair loss is usually not permanent.

9. A geriatric client is extremely agitated on admission to the unit. What would be the best nursing intervention during this time?

① Place him in a private room in a quiet area, away from other clients.
② Encourage him to walk around the unit to increase his physical activity.
③ Tell him he is in the hospital and he is going to have to control himself.
④ Encourage the family to leave so he can begin to adjust to their absence.

10. A cardiac client has a history of dysrhythmias and has been treated with Quinidine for the past 6 months. What information obtained during the nurses data collection would indicate problems with the drug therapy?

① Increased confusion, lethargy with recent memory loss.
② Tinnitus, visual changes, diarrhea.
③ Dry mouth, urinary retention, agitation.
④ Insomnia, joint pain, headache.

11. The nurse must consider Maslow's hierarchy in planning care for the geriatric client. The nurse will assign the highest priority to which group of needs?

① Physiologic.
② Psychologic.
③ Self-esteem.
④ Self-actualization.

12.What is the most important assessment for the nurse to make before a client has a cardiac catheterization?

① Verify whether the client has been NPO since midnight.
② Assess the pulses and temperature of his extremities.
③ Prepare the client for a pre-procedure EKG.
④ Determine if the client understands the procedure.

13. A client has just returned from his cardiac catheterization. His right femoral artery was the insertion site. What is a priority nursing action?

① Maintain continuous cardiac monitoring, anticipate cardioversion.
② Encourage him to ambulate in the hall within 6 hours.
③ Monitor the temperature and pulse of the right lower leg.
④ Monitor the apical pulse hourly, withhold his digitalis if the rate is below 60.

14. A new resident is being admitted to a long term care facility. The nurse is interviewing the client and family. What is an important area for the nurse to evaluate?

① What is the client's routine at home for his activities of daily living.
② Does the client and family understand about the clients diagnosis.
③ Who assisted or administered the clients medications in the home setting.
④ Did the client contribute to or interrupt the family environment.

15. A cardiac client is being discharged. He is started on nitroglycerin sublingual. Which of the following statements indicates that he understands how to take the medication?

① "If I have a chest pain, I'll immediately stop what I am doing, sit down and take the medication."
② "I'll chew the tablet then let is dissolve in my mouth."
③ "I'll take only one dose. If the pain doesn't stop, I'll call the doctor."
④ "If I have chest pain, I'll call the doctor and put two tablets under my tongue."

16. The practical nurse is assigned to care for a client with anginal pain. He is started on a nitroglycerine (Nitro-Dur) patch daily. What nursing observation of the client indicates the medication is achieving the desired effect?

① Chest pain is reduced by the nitroglycerin.
② Performs activities of daily living without chest pain.
③ Able to control pain with frequent patch changes.
④ Tolerates minimal activity without pain.

17. A geriatric client is taking digoxin. Prevention of low serum potassium for this client is particularly important. What effect does low potassium have on digoxin?

① Causes it to become less effective.
② Enhances the side effects.
③ Increases rate of digitalis toxicity.
④ Deactivates the digoxin.

18. A 76 year old man had a transurethral resection of the prostate (TURP) and he is four hours postoperative. He is beginning to complain of bladder spasms. What is the most important nursing assessment at this time?

① Time of his last pain medication.
② Rate of flow of the irrigating fluid.
③ Patency of the catheter.
④ Amount of output since surgery.

19. The nurse is administering a DPT immunization to a four month old infant. The parents are concerned about possible reactions. What is important for the nurse to teach the parents?

① Reactions to DPT are very rare and they should not be worried about it.
② Gastrointestinal problems can be relieved by keeping the child on clear liquids for six hours.
③ Administer acetaminophen if the child has a fever and put ice on the injection site.
④ A rash may occur over the trunk, there should be no problem with itching.

20. An 80-year-old man has a long history of congestive heart failure and is being admitted to the hospital. The admitting nurse would assess the client for which of the following symptoms?

① Increased BUN, confusion and dysphagia.
② Orthopnea, restlessness, and wheezing respirations.
③ Slight dyspnea, cyanosis, pursed lip breathing.
④ Low grade fever, hemoptysis, bilateral rales.

21. A client has been diagnosed and treated for tuberculosis. At discharge, the nurse is discussing with her how to take care of herself at home. What is a critical area to include in this discussion?

① It is important for her to have a job that is not in close contact with people.
② She will need to continue the respiratory isolation procedure at home.
③ She will need to return to the doctor for weekly sputum cultures.
④ It is critical that if the condition is to be cured, she must continue to take all of her medications.

22. Daily weights are ordered for the cardiac clients assigned to the practical nurse. Why are daily weights so important on these clients?

① Weights are critical in evaluating adequacy of nutritional status and healing.
② Changes in the weight are important in determining if the client had a heart attack.
③ A client's fluid retention or fluid loss is reflected in the weight gain or loss.
④ An increase in weight indicates the client is better able to handle the fluid intake.

23. To evaluate a client's apical heart rate, where would the nurse place the stethoscope:

① On the right side at the mid-clavicular line, fourth intercostal space.
② On the left side at the mid-clavicular line, fifth intercostal space.
③ On the sternum, directly over the heart.
④ On the left side, mid axillary level.

24. An 84-year-old client, is discouraged by his inability to have a daily bowel movement as he always had in the past. What principle does the nurse consider in the response to the client?

① Older clients tend to be overly concerned about their bowels.
② The client has probably decreased his food intake as he aged.
③ Constipation occurs in the older individual because of a decreased peristalsis.
④ Chronic diseases of the older individual usually have a negative effect on gastrointestinal function.

25. A 6 years old child is to receive 0.2mg atropine as a preoperative medication. What would be the correct dosage to administer to if the dosage on hand is 0.4 mg in 1 cc?

① 0.05 cc.
② 0.5 cc.
③ 0.25 cc.
④ 0.3 cc.

26. A 10 year old client arrives in the recovery room after her tonsillectomy. Which position should the nurse in the recovery room place her?

① Semi-Fowler's position, with her head turned to the side.
② Supine position, with the head of the bed slightly elevated.
③ On her back, with her head turned to the right side.
④ On her abdomen, with her head turned to the side.

27. Which fluids should the nurse offer first to the pediatric tonsillectomy client?

① Cool water.
② Cranberry juice.
③ Milk.
④ Orange juice.

28. A client is one day postoperative following colostomy surgery. She refuses to look at the stoma and talks about her "surgical incision" rather than the stoma. The nurse determines that she is using denial as a coping strategy. The nurse does not intervene with the client's denial. This nursing decision represents which principles?

① Allows the client some time to develop needed resources.
② Encourages a maladaptive coping strategy.
③ Supports inappropriate adaptation to a short-term problem.
④ Delays the initiation of nursing care designed to help the client adapt.

29. A client is admitted to the hospital for acute Hepatitis A (HAV). What is essential in implementing safe nursing care?

① Teach the client the importance of correct way to use isolation masks and gloves.
② Modify the procedures for handling needles and syringes.
③ Discuss with the client what standard precautions are and how it prevents transmission.
④ Notify the dietary department for utilization of disposable dishes.

30. The nurse is assessing a client with pre-eclampsia. What assessment data would indicate that the condition is getting worse?

① Headaches, facial edema, weight gain.
② Hypotension, decreased weight, ankle edema.
③ Hypoglycemia, proteinuria, tachycardia
④ Diarrhea, gastric reflux, dysuria.

31. A woman is in the clinic for her first prenatal check up. She reports that her last menstrual period was November 10. She asks the practical nurse, "When will my baby be due?" The practical nurse knows that the best answer is:

① July 3.
② August 25.
③ Around the middle of September.
④ The first or second week of August.

32. When teaching clients in a prenatal clinic, all of the following are areas which may be discussed. What is the most important area for clients in their first trimester?

① Diet to promote fetal development and maternal well-being.
② Postpartal care with emphasis on hygiene and breast care.
③ Anticipation and points on how to deal with sibling rivalry.
④ Signs of beginning labor and to come to the hospital as soon as the membranes rupture.

33. A client is admitted for a liver biopsy. Immediately after the procedure is completed, the nurse would place the client in what position?

① Left lateral Sims for 10 hours
② Supine with the head flat for 6 hours.
③ Flat with the legs elevated at about 45 degrees.
④ Right side with a pillow at costovertebral area

34. A postpartum client complains about her "stretch marks." What is the best nursing response?

① Occur in almost every pregnancy.
② Are silvery streaks which appear especially during the last trimester.
③ Can be decreased by a local application of cocoa butter or other types of emollient creams.
④ Will fade from their present reddish appearance.

35. A client returns from surgery with a Foley catheter in place. What nursing care will assist to prevent the development of urinary tract infection secondary to the catheter?

① Thoroughly cleanse the perineal area with Betadine every 4 hours.
② Keep the urine collection container at or above the level of the bed.
③ Disconnect the catheter and drain it every 4 hours to prevent occlusion.
④ Maintain a closed drainage system without any obstruction to urine flow.

36. A client is admitted to the hospital about four hours after a spinal injury. She is paralyzed in both of her lower extremities. The nurse would anticipate and carefully assess for what complications?

① Progression of the extent of the paralysis secondary to swelling and edema of the spinal column.
② Autonomic nerve dysfunction resulting in cerebral edema.
③ Spasticity of the muscles of the affected extremities precipitating an increase in blood pressure.
④ Decrease in the sensation of the affected extremities and development of decubitus.

37. What is important in the immediate care of a client with a thoracic lumbar injury?

① Check for presence of bowel sounds and assess for abdominal distention.
② Perform frequent neuro checks for indications of increased intracranial pressure.
③ Evaluate hourly output and perform glucometer checks.
④ Position in semi-Fowlers to promote respiratory function.

38. When planning initial interactions with a trauma client, what is an important nursing action?

① Repeat information several times.
② Give reassurance about their condition.
③ Utilize silence until client request information.
④ Share other clients' experiences with injuries.

Hurira — RA

39. The preoperative teaching plan for most clients includes deep breathing and coughing procedures. Which statement by the nurse regarding postoperative deep breathing and coughing is most appropriate?

① If you practice, you'll be able to take just as deep a breath right after surgery as you can now.
② Before you take a deep breath, you should breathe out as far as possible.
③ After you take the deep breath, hold it in for several seconds before exhaling.
④ Taking a deep breath will feel good.

40. An elderly client has arthritis and has been taking high doses of aspirin for a year in order to relieve his symptoms. Which actions would the nurse anticipate to be taken prior to surgery?

① Discontinue aspirin at least 48 hours prior to surgery.
② Administer vitamin K preoperatively.
③ Administer the aspirin in suppository form.
④ Evaluation of serum aspirin levels.

41. On the evening prior to a client's scheduled abdominal surgery, the nurse notes that his oral temperature is 101° F. What action by the nurse would be the most appropriate?

① Obtain an order for aspirin.
② Notify the RN or the client's physician immediately.
③ Take the client's temperature in two hours to see if it has gone down.
④ Report the fever to the night shift and have them check his temperature.

42. A client is to begin ambulation after surgery for an abdominal aortic aneurysm resection. What is the best way to evaluate the clients response to activity?

① Check his apical radial pulse before and after ambulation.
② Evaluate his muscle strength and coordination prior to the activity.
③ Take his vital signs before and after ambulating.
④ Determine if he is experiencing any problems with pulse pressures.

43. The nurse asks the client to empty his bladder prior to leaving for surgery. What is the rationale for this request?

① Obtain a preoperative urinalysis.
② Measure the amount of urine.
③ Prevent bladder over distention in surgery.
④ Measure urine output before surgery.

44. The practical nurse is caring for a client who has experienced a brain accident (CVA) resulting in right side paralysis. The nurse is supervising the nursing care provided by a patient care aid. What activity by the patient care aid would the nurse question?

① Performing passive ROM exercises.
② Providing the client with a footboard.
③ Applying warm packs to the right leg.
④ Turning client every 2 hours.

45. The nurse is caring for a client with problems of peripheral vascular disease. His history indicates a problem with intermittent claudication. What is the best interpretation of this information?

① Extensive discoloration of the extremity.
② Bilateral dependent edema
③ Excessive bruising of the lower leg.
④ Pain is associated with activity.

46. A patient's orders read "up ad lib." He has a thoracotomy dressing and a chest tube. He asks if he can walk in the hall. What would be the best nursing response?

① He may get out of bed, but he should not ambulate.
② It is to remain on bed rest as long as he has a chest tube.
③ Walking in the hall with assistance is encouraged.
④ He may get up to the bathroom, but not walk outside his room.

47. The practical nurse is assigned to care for a client with a kidney stone. Which nursing observations would indicate that he is experiencing renal colic?

① Severe flank pain, radiating toward the testicles.
② Stress incontinence with full bladder.
③ Hematuria, severe burning on urination.
④ Enuresis with hyperalbuminuria.

48. What is an important nursing interventions in the care of a client with a kidney stone?

① Force fluids to 3000cc in 24 hours.
② Maintain complete bed rest.
③ Collect a 24-hour urine specimen.
④ Insert a Foley catheter.

49. A client returns to his room after surgery (nephrolithotomy), he has a right nephrostomy tube. What is a priority nursing action?

① Irrigate the tube with 30 cc normal saline qid.
② Clamp the tube if drainage is excessive.
③ Advance the tube ½ inch every 8 hours.
④ Ensure that the tube is draining freely.

50. The nurse instructs her client in measures to prevent kidney stone formation in the future. What response by the client would indicate he understood the teaching plan?

① "I will begin a daily 45-minute jogging program."
② "I should decrease my intake of dairy products."
③ "I will call the doctor when nocturia occurs."
④ "I will increase my supplemental vitamin C and D daily.

51. A low-calcium diet is prescribed for a client with renal stones. What foods would be included on the diet?

① Hot chocolate, oatmeal, whole wheat toast.
② Cream soup, green salad, cheese and crackers.
③ Boiled shrimp, cabbage salad, vanilla milk shake.
④ White toast, orange juice, egg.

52. A client is one day post operative for a cholecystectomy. She is having difficulty taking deep breaths and coughing. Why is this client having difficulty with coughing?

① Nephrostomy tube causes irritation.
② Incision is close to the diaphragm.
③ Renal stone causes internal abrasion.
④ Positioning during surgery results in muscle aches.

53. A 6-month-old child is admitted to the hospital with a closed head injury and a diagnosis of chronic subdural hematoma. What nursing data collection would correlate with this diagnosis?

① Posterior fontanel is closed, anterior fontanel is open.
② Decreased urine output and decreased BP.
③ Increased irritability and vomiting.
④ Diarrhea and regressive behavior.

54. The practical nurse is caring for an infant suspected of being abused. She overhears the mother say, "I'm so sorry, baby, I thought I would be so happy once you were born." What is the nurse's interpretation of the mother's behavior?

① Guilt is always present in these cases.
② It is a very real indication of her remorse.
③ This represents part of the mother's need for mothering.
④ The comment is an attempt to make the nurses feel sorry for her.

55. The nurse is assessing a client prior to administering medications via a nasogastric tube. What is the best nursing action?

① Withdraw fluid from the stomach to determine placement.
② Insert 5cc of water and assess client's tolerance.
③ Position the client flat and listen for breath sounds.
④ Withdraw all fluid from the stomach and measure residual.

56. An elderly client has severe painful osteoarthritis. In taking her health history, what would the nurse expect her to report?

① A gradual onset of the disease with the involvement of weight bearing joints.
② A sudden onset of the disease with involvement of her fingers.
③ No complaints of morning stiffness.
④ Joint pain that is not affected by exercise.

57. A client is admitted with painful osteoarthritis. The treatment regimen includes heat, massage, and exercise. What response will the nurse anticipate from the client?

① Help relax muscles, and relieve pain, and stiffness.
② Restore range of motion that was previously lost.
③ Prevent the inflammatory process.
④ Help keep client's mind off the pain.

58. A client has been on bed rest for the past three days. In the morning report, the nurse is told the client has developed thrombophlebitis in her left leg. The nurse would anticipate what findings on her initial assessment?

① The left leg is cool to touch with decreased pulse.
② Respiratory difficulty secondary to the pulmonary emboli.
③ Decreased blood pressure with increasing pulse pressure.
④ The left leg is warm with red streaks along the calf.

59. The nurse is admitting an elderly client to the long term care facility. What is the most effective question to assist the nurse to determine the client's level of confusion?

① Where are you?
② What day is it?
③ What is your name?
④ Do you feel confused?

60. An elderly client's wife says that he has become increasingly confused, unaware of the presence of others, combative, and he does not remember things she has just told him. What is the assessment priority for this client?

① Determine if his judgment is impaired.
② Evaluate recent changes is his life style.
③ Determine if he has contact with reality.
④ Assess his level of memory impairment.

61. A three month old infant is brought into the emergency clinic. His mother says he has had vomiting and diarrhea for the past 36 hours. The nurse would anticipate what findings on the initial physical examination?

① Weight loss, increased hematocrit, increased lethargy.
② Weight gain, dyspnea, dry mucous membranes.
③ Bradycardia, oliguria, rales and depressed fontanelles.
④ Anuria, bulging fontanel, hypokalemia.

62. A 20-year-old primigravida who is in her third trimester says she is having backaches and some shortness of breath, when she walks in the evening. She has gained one pound for a total of 20 pounds for the pregnancy. There is no pedal edema and her breath sounds are good. What is the nurses interpretation of this information?

① Early signs of cardiac decompensation.
② A normal discomfort of this period of pregnancy
③ Early indications of respiratory distress.
④ She is exercising too much and should stop walking.

63. A 22-year-old pregnant woman comes to the clinic for her monthly check up. She has gained three pounds; her blood pressure is 150/110; and she is complaining of her hands swelling. Based on this information, what is the best nursing action?

① Notify the doctor of the client's status.
② Schedule her to return in two weeks.
③ Teach her how to avoid excessive salt intake.
④ Assess her for changes in her vision.

64. A mother brings her 14-month-old infant to the clinic. He is diagnosed with leukemia. Which of the following symptoms would the practical nurse anticipate finding on her assessment?

① He doesn't walk yet.
② He takes a longer afternoon nap.
③ He has increased bruising.
④ He doesn't eat as much as he used to.

65. A ten-year-old child has cancer and is on several chemotherapy drugs. She is nauseous and an antiemetic drug is prescribed. When is the best time to administer these drugs?

① 30 minutes before chemotherapy.
② With meals.
③ Early in the morning.
④ PRN as requested by her mother.

66. A young mother has a hospitalized child. She works in a factory at night and says if she misses any more work she will be fired. She is worried about leaving her child in the hospital at night because he is so young. What is the nurse's reply based on?

① The child is really too young to suffer any untoward consequences.
② The child will be okay if the mother will just leave a favorite toy.
③ It would be better if mother could stay, however there is adequate staff to care for the child.
④ Hospitals are expensive and the mother needs to go to work to pay the hospital bill.

67. In treating the cancer client, what is the main goal of the chemotherapeutic drugs?

① Prevent all future relapses.
② Assist the client into remission.
③ Decrease intervals between exacerbations.
④ Increase the positive effects of radiation.

68. An adult leukemia client is having a bone marrow aspiration to determine his response to chemotherapy. What site for this procedure would the nurse describe to the client?

① The upper part of the of the leg bone.
② Right or left iliac crest or "hipbone."
③ The sternum, or bone in the middle of the chest.
④ The radius or the larger bone in the arm.

69. A client is diagnosed with rheumatoid arthritis and is started on prednisone. What is a priority nursing intervention for all clients on steroids?

① Increase salt intake.
② Limit activity.
③ Check weight daily.
④ Check vital signs twice a day.

70. When obtaining a health history from an older client, which additional characteristic of the older client must be taken into consideration?

① The older client responds to pain sensation with the same intensity as a young client.
② Hearing is the most common sensory loss in the aged population and it may hinder the interview.
③ The older client requires a lot of repetition because the IQ declines with the aging process.
④ An older client's response time to answering a question is just as quick as a young client.

71. An elderly woman is diagnosed with congestive heart failure. Her treatment includes furosemide (Lasix) and digoxin. What is a priority nursing a evaluation regarding these medications?

① Potassium will be gained.
② Sodium will be lost.
③ Fluid intake needs to be increased.
④ Potassium will be lost.

72. Which of the following would give the most information regarding the progress of a client with congestive heart failure?

① Her medication schedule.
② An accurate intake and output record.
③ Her weight gain or loss.
④ Length of her afternoon nap.

73. The nurse is planning the discharge for a client with left ventricular failure. The nurse discusses with the client the importance of not becoming fatigued. Which statement best reflects this principle?

① An increase in stimulation will increase the cardiac rate.
② Bed rest promotes venous return and increases cardiac output.
③ Frequent rest periods decrease the fluid retention.
④ Fatigue will increase the cardiac workload.

74. A 12-year-old, is being admitted with a tentative diagnosis of appendicitis. The nursing assessment is most likely to reveal what characteristics concerning his pain?

① Rebound tenderness in the right lower quadrant, associated with decreased bowel sounds and vomiting.
② Gnawing pain, radiating through to the lower back, with severe abdominal distention.
③ Sharp pain with severe gastric distention, frequently associated with hemoptysis.
④ Pain on light palpation in mid-epigastric area, chronic low grade fever and diarrhea.

75. In caring for a client with appendicitis, nursing actions to promote comfort prior to surgery would include:

① Ambulate to increase the passage of flatus to decrease the distention prior to surgery.
② Position him on his side, legs flexed to the abdomen with the head slightly elevated.
③ Position him on his left side, apply a warm K-Pad to the abdomen.
④ Administer meperidine(Demerol) and allow to assume the position of comfort.

76. The nurse would question which doctor's order on a preoperative appendectomy client?

① 50 mg meperidine (Demerol) on call.
② Obtain signed consent form from parents.
③ Administer enemas until clear.
④ Bed rest in position of comfort..

77. Postoperative abdominal surgery nursing care includes the observation for peritonitis. If peritonitis were developing, what information would be evident on the nursing assessment?

① Abdominal pain in the area of the incision, pain increases with coughing.
② Temperature increases to 102° F, rigid abdomen, decreased or absent bowel sounds.
③ Purulent drainage from the surgical wound, nausea and vomiting after clear liquid intake.
④ Absent bowel sounds, decreased white cell count, low grade fever.

78. A client has peripheral vascular disease that requires amputation of his right leg. In the immediate postoperative period, what is a priority nursing action?

① Check for bleeding from the incision.
② Keep the stump adducted from the hip.
③ Begin passive exercises to affected leg.
④ Externally rotate the stump to prevent abduction.

79. In the immediate postoperative period following an amputation, the nursing care plan should include which of the following measures to decrease stump edema?

① Apply ice packs to the stump for 72 hours.
② Elevate the stump on pillows for 24 to 48 hours.
③ Wrap the stump with Ace bandages from proximal to distal ends.
④ Administer anti-inflammatory medications.

80. The nurse is teaching a client to care for his stump. What is an indication that he requires further teaching?

① He uses a mirror to examine the stump for skin breakdown.
② He is wearing woolen stump sock to provide comfort.
③ He puts his prosthesis on two hours after arising.
④ He avoids the use of alcohol and creams on his stump.

81. A client is five days postoperative mastectomy. She has expressed an intense dislike for hospital food and her appetite is unusually poor. What is important for the nurse to explain to the client?

① An IV line with sugar water will have to be inserted if she will not eat.
② The lack of food, especially protein, will interfere with her wound healing.
③ When she is discharged she will need to gain back the weight she lost during hospitalization.
④ No one enjoys hospital food, so it is fortunate she is not hungry.

82. The mastectomy client becomes increasingly withdrawn, refuses her food, and asks that the curtains be kept drawn around her bed. What principle will the nurse include in her response to the client?

① Client needs to eat and move around in order to feel better.
② Depressed clients need their privacy, decrease visitors and unnecessary procedures.
③ Acknowledge to the client this is a difficult time and maintain contact with her.
④ Ask the client why she is feeling this way, is their something wrong with her care.

83. A client is admitted for a craniotomy to remove a brain tumor. An important factor in preoperative bowel care for a craniotomy client is to:

① Avoid bowel care.
② Avoid straining at defecation.
③ Utilize enemas only.
④ Avoid use of laxatives.

84. In planning preoperative teaching for a craniotomy client, what is a priority nursing assessment?

① Determine level of consciousness.
② Evaluate his educational background.
③ Determine his weight and vital signs.
④ Perform a complete health history.

85. A 35-year-old client is admitted with cerebral edema. The practical nurse would anticipate what findings on the data collection?

① Nausea and vomiting.
② Increased mental alertness.
③ Decreased output.
④ Increased pulse rate.

86. What is an important nursing intervention after a craniotomy?

① Measure temperature every two hours.
② Maintain safety with a vest restraint.
③ Suction the client every two hours.
④ Maintain the client in semi-Fowler's position.

87. An elderly client is admitted to the hospital with a new diagnosis of Parkinson's disease. When obtaining a health history, what would the nurse expect the client to report?

① Weight loss.
② Slowness of movement.
③ Continual motor tremors.
④ Depression.

88. The practical nurse is assisting the Parkinson's client with an exercise program to maintain his optimal health status. What would be important for the nurse to recommend to this client?

① Perform isometric exercise.
② Participate in aerobic exercise.
③ Pay attention to posture during exercise.
④ Practice deep breathing during exercise.

89. The nurse should be aware of what factors when considering the psychosocial needs of a Parkinson's client?

① Intellectual capabilities may decrease.
② Diversional interests may decrease.
③ Mood fluctuations may occur.
④ Communication skills may fluctuate.

UTI - A20

90. A client is experiencing anorexia, vomiting, and gastrointestinal discomfort since beginning his medication. What should the nurse do?

① Assess his food preferences.
② Monitor his blood pressure.
③ Hold his medication and notify the physician.
④ Administer his medication with food.

91. The nurse admits an elderly woman to the unit for surgery. The nurse discusses the need for safety in the environment and points out the need to use handrails, and call for assistance when getting out of bed. Why is it important for the nurse to give the client these instructions?

① The nurse has stereotypes regarding older individuals.
② The older woman would be more likely to sue the hospital if she fell.
③ Precautions in the environment and geriatric client safety are critical.
④ Medicare regulations require that this information be charted.

92. The practical nurse takes an operative permit (consent form) to the client. What is important for the client to have before he signs the operative permit?

① Be seen by the chaplain and notations on the chart for last rites.
② All surgical procedures and possible complications explained to him by the doctor.
③ His vital signs taken and recorded, history and physical, and all lab reports on the chart.
④ A tour of the operating room and a complete explanation of all equipment.

93. An elderly lady is scheduled for a colon resection at 10 a.m. At 2 a.m. she asks why she cannot have a snack. What would the nurse's response by based on?

① Most hospitals discourage clients eating after midnight.
② A light snack and some clear fluids are okay if taken in moderation.
③ Foods and fluids are with held to avoid aspiration during and after surgery.
④ Any foods or fluids taken before surgery will interfere with the anesthesia during surgery.

94. The practical nurse is performing PM care. After giving the HS medication, what is an important nursing action?

① Put up the side rails.
② Shut the door.
③ Make the client's bed.
④ Shut off all the lights.

95. A geriatric client is 85 years old. Which dietary modification should the nurse consider due to the client's age?

① Increase caloric intake.
② Increase dietary intake of vitamins C and A.
③ Use fewer herbs and spices in food.
④ Omit fluids with meals.

96. After a lengthy hospitalization, a client is moved to a long term care facility. What should be considered when arranging for the decorating of her assigned room?

① Change colors and style to avoid reminding her of home.
② Encourage her to be involved in the room arrangement.
③ Bright, primary colors will assist to stimulate perceptions.
④ She will enjoy furniture that is soft and overstuffed for comfort.

97. Immediately after abdominal surgery, a client was taken to the recovery room. She had received general anesthesia. Her family asks how long she will remain before returning to her room. What will the nurse base her response on?

① Recovery usually takes about an hour.
② The surgeon must discharge her from the recovery room; she'll return after he sees her.
③ Just a little while unless she develops some serious complication.
④ When she has awakened from the anesthetic and it is safe to move her to her room.

98. A client had surgery this morning and she is still drowsy from the anesthetic. She becomes nauseous and begins to vomit. What is the best nursing action?

① Place a pillow under her head.
② Position her on her side.
③ Place a cool cloth on her head.
④ Insert an airway.

99. A client has liver disease and there is an order to administer vitamin K preoperatively. What is the purpose of this medication?

① To increase the digestion and utilization of fats.
② To support the immune system and promote healing.
③ To aid in the emptying of the bile from the gallbladder.
④ To facilitate coagulation activities of the blood.

100. Which position is best for the cholecystectomy client in the immediate postoperative period?

① Side lying, to prevent aspiration.
② Semi-Fowler's position, to facilitate respirations.
③ Supine, to decrease strain on the incision line.
④ Prone, to reduce nausea.

101. A client returns to her room after a cholecystectomy. She has a T-tube in place. What is the purpose of the T-tube?

① Remove bile leaking from the incision.
② Provide a means of wound irrigation.
③ Drain bile from the common bile duct.
④ Prevent rupture of the inflamed gall bladder.

102. In assessing the postoperative client, when would the practical nurse identify as the most common time that urinary retention becomes a problem?

① Within the first 8 hours.
② After the first 24 hours.
③ On the third postoperative day.
④ In the first 48 hours.

103. What is a common cause of nausea and vomiting in the first 24 hours following surgery?

① Paralytic ileus.
② Use of narcotics.
③ Fluid and electrolyte imbalance.
④ Intense pain.

104. When admitting a surgical client to her room, the nurse notes drainage of about 2-3 centimeters on the client's abdominal dressing. What action by the nurse would be the most appropriate?

① Reinforce the dressing.
② Change the dressing before the client is alarmed.
③ Notify the surgeon.
④ Circle the drainage and chart significant observations.

105. A client tells the nurse his incision "feels funny," the nurse observes a small area of bowel protruding through the incisional area. What is the best nursing action?

① With a sterile glove, very gently press the exposed bowel back into the incision.
② Soak a sterile dressing with normal saline and place over exposed bowel.
③ Clean area with Betadine and replace sterile dressing.
④ Apply Vaseline gauze over exposed bowel and cover with saline soaked dressing.

106. A geriatric client in a long term care facility requires an indwelling urinary catheter. The nurse observes the urine to be dark, and very foul smelling, with sediment in the collection bag. What is the best nursing action?

① Provide catheter care using sterile technique.
② Change the catheter and drainage equipment.
③ Encourage increased oral fluid intake.
④ Irrigate the catheter with 30cc of normal saline.

107. The nurse is explaining to a client how to collect a sputum specimen for tuberculosis diagnosis. What priority information should the nurse include in this instruction?

① Drink plenty of fluid so the sputum will be easier to get out.
② Collect the specimen when you wake up in the morning.
③ Save all sputum in the container provided for twenty four hours.
④ Rinse your mouth with an antibacterial mouthwash before collecting specimen.

108. After a cerebral vascular accident, an elderly man is experiencing problems with ataxia. What is the priority nursing considerations?

① Assist him with ambulation to prevent falls.
② Sit him on the side of the bed prior to getting him up.
③ Put him in semi-Fowlers position with legs elevated.
④ Increase oral fluid intake and evaluate potassium levels.

109. The medical record is a legal document. What is important for the nurse to consider when making entries?

① Include any information she thinks is true.
② Thoroughly delete mistakes so that it cannot be misinterpreted.
③ Skip lines so entries may be made later to reflect the current time of activity.
④ Include only facts pertinent to care, only use opinions in assessment area of charting.

110. When the client gives the nurse information, what is important for the nurse to do?

① Share this information with everyone in the unit.
② Share this information with those needing to know for planning care.
③ Write the information only in the chart.
④ Share this information only with other nurses on the unit.

111. Most states have reporting laws which require health care workers to report certain situations and behavior to authorities. Which of the following is not usually a reportable matter?

① Child abuse.
② Communicable disease.
③ Gunshot wounds.
④ Attempted suicide.

112. How should errors on the client's chart be corrected?

① White out error and write over it.
② Recopying information to decrease confusion.
③ Straight line, initials, and date.
④ Obliterating the error so it will not be confusing.

113. Which is not a consideration when providing care to a client receiving internal radiotherapy?

① Time spent with the client.
② The organ that is being irradiated.
③ The distance from the radiation source.
④ Shielding used by the care giver.

114. A client is being discharged after a cholecystectomy. The nurse would determine the client understood the dietary teaching if she selected what foods?

① Broiled fish, green beans, and an apple.
② Avocado salad, whole milk, white bread.
③ Pork chops, gravy, carrots, and grapes.
④ Whole wheat rolls with butter, potatoes, steak.

115. A client is returning from the delivery room after a cesarean section, she has had a spinal anesthesia. What is important nursing care for this client?

① Position her in left lateral Sim's with the head elevated 30 degrees.
② Encourage her to ambulate as soon as sensation has returned.
③ Maintain her in the supine position for 6-8 hours.
④ Place in semi Fowlers position, and maintain bed rest for 12 hours.

116. The nurse is teaching the new mother how to care for her son's penis after circumcision. What instructions would be important for the nurse to include?

① Carefully rinse the penis with sterile water after each diaper change.
② Keep the area protected by dry gauze around the penis until it heals.
③ Place a gauze with petroleum jelly around the penis and change when soiled. .
④ Keep the circumcision area covered with cortisone cream to decrease swelling.

117. A woman asked the nurse how often women over 65 years old should have a mammogram? What is the best response?

① Mammograms are not necessary at this age.
② Women over 65 should have mammograms every five years.
③ Any woman over the age of 50 should have a yearly mammogram.
④ Mammograms are useful only if you had a baseline mammogram done before the age of 40.

118. A group of women, age 60 to 75, asks when they should perform breast self-examination. What is the best response?

① Daily with your shower.
② At the end of your monthly period.
③ Every six months.
④ The same day every month.

119. What nursing action should be included in the care plan of all clients with cancer?

① Monitor the client for infection.
② Increase assessment for pleural effusions.
③ Assist the client to achieve a peaceful death.
④ Modify the environment to eliminate nausea.

120. The nurse is caring for several clients with acquired immuno deficiency syndrome (AIDS). How is this disease transmitted?

① Via airborne infected droplets.
② Through blood or blood products.
③ In saliva shared when kissing.
④ Through all of the above routes.

Bayer
Back & Body

Answers and Rationale for Practice Test #1

1. ④ The most likely time for insulin reaction is at the peak of the insulin, peak time for regular insulin is $2\ ^1/_2$ to 4 hours.

2. ① Diaphoresis and a shaky feeling are early signs of hypoglycemia. Severe thirst is a sign of hyperglycemia while drowsiness and coma are late symptoms of hypoglycemia.

3. ② First urine is concentrated and will falsely influence the test. Timing of the 24 hour specimen collection begins after the first voiding.

4. ④ Bronchospasm and laryngeal edema which are indicative of severe respiratory distress are one of the more severe consequences of anaphylactic reaction that must be addressed immediately.

5. ① Pain and discomfort around the IV site, paleness and coolness to the touch are symptoms of fluid infiltration. The practical nurse should turn the fluid off and immediately notify the RN.

6. ④ It is difficult to manage problems with head lice if the child has thick or long hair. With the hair cut short the problem is easier to control.

7. ③ The unaffected lung is very prone to underinflation, atelectasis, and infection. Coughing and deep-breathing exercises are of priority.

8. ④ The nurse may inform the client that hair will grow back after all chemotherapy is complete but that color and texture might be slightly different.

9. ① To protect the client, he should be moved into a quiet environment away from others. This will help him regain some control and will not produce unneeded stimuli.

10. ② Tinnitus, diarrhea and visual changes are the classic signs of toxicity with quinidine.

11. ① Maslow's hierarchy of needs serves as a useful guide for establishing priorities. The base or first level addresses physiological needs. These needs must be met before the higher levels can be accomplished.

12. ② When a client is scheduled for an arteriogram, it is vital that the pulses and temperature distal to the insertion site be assessed prior to the procedure. The other assessments are important but not the priority.

13. ③ Post-test, the priority again is monitoring the pulses and temperature distal to the insertion site. The client should be on bed rest for 24 hours post-test, and the insertion site should be closely monitored for a hematoma or bleeding.

14. ① Routine repetition and reinforcement are very important when introducing an elderly client to a new living environment. Find out what his routine has been previously and try to change as little as possible.

15. ① Nitroglycerin is a vasodilator and can cause orthostatic hypotension. For safety, the client should take it only while sitting or lying down. In order to decrease the chest pain, the client should stop all activity.

16. ② **Nitro-dur** is used to prevent angina so that the client can perform the normal activities of daily living without chest pain.

17. ③ Hypokalemia increases myocardial sensitivity to digitalis, making toxicity a greater risk even when dosage is maintained within normal ranges.

18. ③ Bladder spasms are caused by many things but one is obstruction of the Foley, usually with clots.

19. ③ A slight fever and discomfort at the injection site is not uncommon reaction, acetaminophen is medication of choice, do not use aspirin and do not tell the child's parents "not to worry."

20. ② The CHF client breathes better in the sitting position, but he is frequently restless from his hypoxia.

21. ④ It is critical in the treatment of TB that the client take all of the medication and at the prescribed times. If medications are not taken as prescribed then it will facilitate the development of a resistant strain of TB.

22. ③ One of the most important facts in determining a client's fluid status is to evaluate the daily weight. Increase in weight indicates the client is retaining fluid, which would thus increase his cardiac workload.

23. ② The apical heart rate is best counted at the point of maximum impulse (PMI). This is at the level of the apex of the left ventricle, which is located at the fifth intercostal space, mid-clavicular line on the left side.

24. ③ Peristalsis decreases and nerve impulses are dulled.

25. ② The calculation is: $\frac{0.2mg}{0.4mg} x\ 1cc = .5cc.$

26. ④ Before the child is fully awake, she should be placed on her abdomen with her head turned to the side to facilitate the drainage of secretions and to prevent aspiration. When alert, she may sit up, but she should remain in bed for the remainder of the day.

27. ① Cool water or synthetic fruit juices are offered first.

28. ① Denial and distancing serve as protective coping mechanisms and allow conservation of the client's energy. The client needs some time after the surgery to adjust and to identify resources and gain support.

29. ③ Enteric precautions are the classic isolation for hepatitis, this usually is covered by universal precautions, however the saliva may also be contaminated and precautions should be taken.

30. ① Headaches indicate increased blood pressure, weight gain and edema occur with increase loss of protein, with these symptoms the client is getting worse.

31. ④ Naegle's rule states that you count back three months from the date of the last menstrual period and add 7 days to determine the EDC. 35 percent of all women deliver within 5 days either before or after this date.

32. ① Ideally, counseling about nutrition begins at the first prenatal visit, starting with the assessment of dietary intake. Labor and postpartal needs are appropriate teaching for the third trimester.

33. ④ This position will put increased pressure on the biopsy site in the liver to decrease bleeding.

34. ④ Striae gravidarum are caused by the stretching, rupture, and atrophy of the deep connective tissue of the skin. They are pink or reddish during pregnancy and become silvery white after delivery.

35. ④ Urinary catheterization is a sterile procedure and a closed system should be maintained. Betadine every four hours will irritate the perineal area and the drainage container should be lower then the bed.

36. ① The nurse should assess for an increase in the level of paralysis due to the edema of the spinal cord and plan appropriate nursing interventions.

37. ① Peristalsis may be affected by the injury site. It is important to prevent gastric distention and vomiting.

38. ① After a traumatic injury, individuals are in shock. It is important to give orienting information repeatedly.

39. ③ With or without incentive spirometry devices, the postoperative deep breathing maneuver is called an SMI - sustained maximal inspiration - the client breathes out normally, takes a deep breath in and holds it.

40. ① Aspirin has anticoagulant effects that can increase the risk of hemorrhage. Gradually discontinue anticoagulants 48 h before surgery.

41. ② Fever (above 101 °F) in an adult could indicate infection or dehydration. Abnormal vital signs may cause the postponement of surgery until the underlying problem is treated and the client's condition is stable.

42. ③ Check the vital signs to determine the client's response to the ambulation and to identify if he has any problems with orthostatic hypotension.

43. ③ Once the client is prepared for surgery, the nurse asks the client to empty his or her bladder to prevent incontinence or over distention, which may prevent exposure of the surgical site.

44. ③ The rehabilitation program for a stroke client includes actions that prevent deformity (passive range of motion and use of the footboard) and complications that may be associated with bed rest (turning client every 2 hours).

45. ④ Pain associated with activity is the definition of intermittent claudication, it occurs when the muscle is working and does not get adequate amount of oxygenated blood.

46. ③ The client may be up as tolerated, he will need assistance with the tubes, especially the chest tubes. Ambulation and activity should be encouraged.

47. ① The most characteristic symptom of renal colic is sudden, severe pain. The client may also exhibit nausea and vomiting, pallor, and be diaphoretic during the acute pain episode.

48. ① Increase fluids to promote a high urine output to decrease risk of infection and to promote passage of the stone. A Foley catheter is not indicated if the client can void, mobility assists to prevent urine stasis.

49. ④ Failure of the tube to drain freely can result in pain, trauma, wound dehiscence, and infection. The nurse does not clamp, irrigate or position the tube.

50. ② Dairy products are a main food source of calcium. Increased calcium intake may precipitate the formation of kidney stones.

51. ④ Most renal calculi are composed of calcium oxalate or calcium phosphate. The avoidance of dairy products reduces the calcium intake, and food such as rhubarb, spinach, and chocolate are high in oxalate.

52. ② The cholecystectomy incision is close to the diaphragm, making coughing and deep breathing difficult.

53. ③ Irritability and vomiting are common signs of increased intracranial pressure in the infant, the symptoms are often delayed in the infant due to the open fontanel.

54. ③ Abusing parents have poor ego strengths and received inadequate mothering as children.

55. ① Correct placement of the naso gastric tube should always be checked prior to putting anything into the tube. This is a reliable method of determining correct placement.

56. ① Osteoarthritis has a gradual onset and affects weight-bearing joints with pain that is more pronounced after exercise and morning stiffness.

57. ① Physical therapy helps relax muscles, and relieves aching and stiffness of the involved joints.

58. ④ Signs of thrombophlebitis are those of inflammation of the vein - redness, pain, edema,⑤ temp.

59. ③ The first question to ask the client is if he knows who he is, if he does not, then the rest of the questions will be unnecessary. #1 and 2 may be disorientation from surroundings and client can be easily reoriented.

60. ① If the clients judgement is impaired, he should not be left alone, as he cannot determine appropriate responses to dangerous situations - hot stove, busy traffic in streets, how to get home, etc.

61. ① These are signs of dehydration on a client of any age, #3 are late signs of severe hypovolemia.

62. ② The client here is experiencing normal physiological discomforts of pregnancy. There would be cause for concern if she experienced these symptoms with minimal activity.

63. ① These are early signs of PIH and the doctor should be advised. The nurse should continue her assessment, but the client will not be put on sodium restriction.

64. ③ The other options can all be within normal limits for a two-year-old. Increased bruising is not normal.

65. ① Antiemetic drugs are administered 30 to 60 minutes before chemotherapy and then at appropriate intervals throughout the expected duration of nausea and vomiting.

66. ③ Try to make the young mother feel as comfortable as possible about leaving her child. It is not easy for her and she needs reassurance that her child will be cared for in her absence.

67. ② The main goal is to get the child into remission. Medications are usually discontinued after 3 years of remission.

68. ② The iliac crest is the most common site used.

69. ③ Weight gain is expected with steroid therapy due to increased sodium retention.

70. ② When interviewing an older client, auditory acuity is the most common age-related aspect to take into consideration.

71. ④ Diuretic therapy increases sodium excretion, and potassium loss. Also, digoxin has a diuretic effect.

72. ③ Weight loss is used to evaluate the success of diuretic therapy in the CHF client.

73. ④ If the cardiac client becomes fatigued, it puts an increased workload on the heart. It is important that cardiac clients avoid fatigue and get plenty of rest.

74. ① Rebound pain is elected by pressing firmly over the area known as McBurney's point. The rebound pain, decreased bowel sounds, fever, rigid abdomen are all characteristic of the clinical picture of appendicitis.

75. ② The characteristic position of comfort for the appendicitis client is on the side with the legs flexed against the abdomen, the head of the bed should remain slightly elevated to decrease the upward spread of infection in case the appendix ruptures.

76. ③ Enemas or laxatives are not administered prior to surgery. If gastric motility is stimulated, there is an increased danger of appendix rupture, all other orders are appropriate preoperatively.

77. ② Peritonitis, or an inflammation of the lining of the peritoneal cavity occurs if the appendix ruptures prior to removal. Symptoms include those associated with an acute infection, plus rigid guarding of the abdomen, shallow respirations, and absent bowel sounds.

78. ① Hemorrhage can be a postoperative complication for clients who are to undergo delayed prosthesis fitting.

79. ② Elevation of the stump in the initial postoperative period is used to prevent edema. Wrapping the stump is done from the distal to proximal areas.

80. ③ The prosthesis should be applied immediately upon arising.

81. ② Protein-calorie malnutrition causes a deficiency in energy in protein synthesis. The usual manifestations include poor wound healing.

82. ③ The nurse must help establish open, honest communication.

83. ② Straining at defecation or the use of the Valsalva maneuver may aggravate increased intracranial pressure.

84. ① Although the client may have impaired cognition, preoperative teaching should be individualized according to the level of consciousness of the client.

85. ① Cerebral edema will precipitate an increase in intracranial pressure. The symptoms of IICP include changes in the level of consciousness, headache, nausea and vomiting, and respiratory problems.

86. ④ Semi-Fowler's position will promote venous drainage and assist to ⊕ increased cranial pressure. Lowering the client's head increases the client's intracranial pressure.

87. ② An early symptom of Parkinson's disease is slowness of movements in all normal activities of daily living.

88. ③ Paying attention to posture is critical to prevent deformities.

89. ③ Due to the emotional stress of Parkinson's disease, mood disturbances often occur.

90. ④ The first side effect to be noticed may be gastrointestinal problems. Taking medication with meals may alleviate these symptoms.

91. ③ Precautions in the environment cannot be over stressed, as serious and crippling injuries can occur from falls, strains, and other accidents.

92. ② This is part of the legal process of informed consent.

93. ③ A client is NPO prior to surgery to avoid aspiration which could compromise their respiratory status.

94. ① Safety is a primary concern in a client who has received a sedative or medication for sleep.

95. ② Increased dietary intake of calcium, vitamin C, and vitamin A is needed because alterations with age disrupt the ability to store, use, and absorb these substances.

96. ② Older people need to participate in deciding how their room and area will be arranged and what they can keep in their environment. It is important for elderly people in long term care facilities to be able to personalize their surroundings.

97. ④ After general surgery, a client needs to be awake a stable period prior to moving back to her room.

98. ② Turning her head to the side will help prevent aspiration of vomitus. Inserting an airway will cause choking.

99. ④ Vitamin K increases blood clotting. Liver disease can lead to potential difficulties with clotting.

100. ② Semi-Fowler's position increases lung expansion. The incision following a cholecystectomy is high and may interfere with respiratory exchange. The other positions would probably interfere with respirations.

101. ③ A T-tube is used after a common bile duct exploration to maintain patency of the duct until healing can occur. A T-tube should never be irrigated by the nurse. The purpose of the tube is to maintain bile drainage.

102. ① Voluntary control of urinary function does not return for six to eight hours after inhalation, intravenous, or spinal anesthesia.

103. ② In addition to general anesthesia, abdominal surgery and narcotics reduce intestinal peristalsis during the first day after surgery and predispose the client to nausea and vomiting.

104. ④ When inspecting the dressing, the nurse checks for drainage and notes the amount, color, consistency, and odor of the drainage fluid and the date and time of the observations on the client's chart.

105. ② When eviscerations occurs, it is important to cover the bowel, and keep it moist. The doctor should be notified immediately.

106. ③ The client's urine is concentrated and he is probably dehydrated, he needs increased fluid intake to dilute the urine and restore hydration.

107. ② Sputum specimens collected in the morning have an increased concentration of bacteria.

108. ① Ataxia is a problem with balance and walking that occurs frequently after a stroke, the client will need assistance.

109. ④ The chart is a legal document which contains accurate notes which honestly record the events that occur during your care of the client. No blank lines should be left in the chart and no information should be obliterated.

110. ② Conversation is confidential. It is covered under invasion of privacy which states that the client has the constitutional right to be free from undesired publicity and exposure to public view.

111. ④ Legal reporting laws are exceptions under the invasion of privacy. Communicable diseases, gunshot, knife wounds, and child abuse are reportable.

112. ③ Errors in charting should never be obliterated, recopied, or covered with "white out." When the erroneous information is not legible, it raises questions as to what the person was trying to "cover up."

113. ② Guidelines for protection are based on three concepts: time, distance, and shielding.

114. ① Client needs to decrease fat intake after surgery, #1 represents healthy low fat foods.

115. ③ After spinal anesthetic, the nurse should increase fluids and the client should be flat to prevent a post spinal headache.

116. ③ Place a moisture protective barrier (petroleum jelly or Vaseline) around the circumcision area to keep urine from the area. It is not necessary to rinse it, and cortisone cream will decrease the healing.

117. ③ A mammography is recommended for the early detection of cancer every year for women aged 50 years and older.

118. ④ If you do not have menstrual periods, BSE should be done on the same day of every month.

119. ① Because clients with cancer frequently have suppressed immune systems and altered physical and mechanical barriers, the nurse is vigilant for signs of infection.

120. ② The HIV is transmitted via sexual contact, via blood or blood products, and from mother to newborn child.

121. A man has been newly diagnosed with adult onset diabetes mellitus. What would be noted by the nurse as an important finding on her data collection?

① Anorexia.
② Polyuria.
③ Weight gain.
④ Nausea and vomiting.

122. A client is receiving NPH insulin 20 units subq at 7 a.m. daily. At 3 p.m. the nurse finds him apparently asleep. How would the nurse know if the client is having an hypoglycemic reaction?

① Feel client and bed for dampness.
② Observe client for Kussmaul respirations.
③ Smell client's breath for acetone odor.
④ Check client's pupils for dilatation.

123. A client is found to be disoriented and a blood sugar of 50 mg%. What is the first nursing action?

① Give him 7 units of regular insulin, sub q.
② Put him in semi-Fowler's to facilitate respirations.
③ Check the client's urine for the presence of sugar and acetone.
④ Assist him to drink a glass of milk and eat some crackers.

124. A client has recently been diagnosed with chronic pulmonary disease (COPD). He finds that after smoking or exercise he experiences difficulty breathing, headaches, and nausea. The nurse recognizes that these are symptoms of what problem?

① Increased levels of carbon dioxide.
② Decreased level of serum potassium.
③ Decreased level of carbon dioxide.
④ Tachypnea and metabolic acidosis.

125. A chronic obstructive lung disease (COPD) client complains of dyspnea after his daily exercises. What is the best nursing response?

① Assist him to bed and put his oxygen on at 3 liter per minute.
② Have him lay down immediately and administer an aerosol treatment.
③ Explain that the dyspnea is an anticipated response to the increased level of activity.
④ Discourage him from further exercising since it is increasing his dyspnea.

126. What should the nurse teach a COPD client regarding proper breathing exercises?

① Encourage pursed lip breathing.
② Inhalation should be two to three times that of exhalation.
③ Encourage high abdominal breathing using the muscles of the diaphragm.
④ Inhale through the mouth and out through the nose.

127. An elderly lady is admitted to the hospital with a possible fractured hip. Prior to surgery, her leg will be maintained in Buck's traction. What is the primary goal of this treatment?

① Reduce the fracture.
② Decrease muscle spasms.
③ Maintain complete bedrest.
④ Set the fracture.

128. In assessing a client in Buck's traction, how can the nurse maintain the counter traction?

① Applying a ten-pound counterweight at the knee.
② Placing shock blocks under the head of the bed.
③ Elevating the knee gatch and elevating the head of the bed about 30°.
④ Elevating the foot of the bed frame and allowing the weights to hang freely.

129. An elderly female client is scheduled for an open reduction internal fixation of her fractured hip. In planning for the postoperative period, what is important for the nurse to consider?

① Blood loss from this procedure is minimal.
② An internally implanted device will require daily pin care.
③ Early mobilization will be important.
④ The neurovascular status of the extremity will not be affected.

130. What is important for the nurse to include in the planning for the postoperative care of a client who has had a fractured hip repair?

① Keep her flat in bed for two days.
② Maintain the Buck's traction with her leg adducted.
③ Get her up in a chair, non-weight bearing, two days post op.
④ Keep her leg slightly bent at the knee to prevent internal rotation.

131. Following surgery for repair of a fractured hip a client is returned to her room. The nurse would plan to put the client in what position?

① Supine with a pillow under the client's knees.
② Supine with several pillows between her legs.
③ Supine with the client's affected leg in a sling.
④ Prone with a pillow under the affected leg's ankle.

132. What is important data collection for the nurse to obtain in a client with a fractured hip?

① Circulation and sensation distal to the fracture.
② Amount of swelling around the fracture site.
③ Degree of bone healing that has occurred.
④ Amount of pain that the fracture is causing.

133. The nurse is caring for a client who has just had a lumbar puncture. What are the nursing measures to be implemented at this time?

① Monitor ability to move lower extremities.
② Encourage increased oral fluid intake.
③ Position the client in high Fowler's position.
④ Apply an occlusive pressure dressing over the site..

134. What is important information for the nurse to determine in a client who is being treated with balanced skin traction?

① Assess the skin under the traction boot every eight hours.
② Check the pin sites at least daily.
③ Check the area around the hip where the traction is applied.
④ Verify that weights are amount ordered and are hanging freely.

135. An immobilized client is at risk for developing deep vein thrombi. What nursing actions are appropriate to help prevent this complication?

① Ambulate in the hall twice a day.
② Massage the legs every four hours and apply warm K-pad for 30 minutes.
③ Encourage the client to perform active ROM on all extremities.
④ Passive ROM every 2 hours on lower extremities.

136. A postoperative client is receiving meperidine (Demerol), 50 mg (IM), along with hydroxyzine (Vistaril) IM q 6 hours PRN for postoperative pain. What is the primary purpose for the use of hydroxyzine (Vistaril)?

① Prevent nausea.
② Increase pain relief.
③ Decrease the incidence of addiction.
④ Maintain GI motility.

137. Considering the side effects of meperidine (Demerol) which nursing actions should be incorporated into the plan of care?

① Assess GI motility and constipation.
② Observe for diarrhea and distention.
③ Monitor for indications of increased bleeding.
④ Evaluate serum potassium levels for hypokalemia.

138. What is the best procedure to obtain an accurate blood pressure on the hospitalized client?

① Obtain a cuff that covers the upper one-third of the client's arm.
② Position the cuff approximately 4" above the antecubital space.
③ Use a cuff that is wide enough to cover the upper two-thirds of the client's arm.
④ Identify the Korotkoff sounds, and take systolic reading at 10mm Hg after the first sound.

139. A hypertensive client is on a diet that is low in salt, cholesterol, and calories. Which client statements indicates the need for further teaching?

① "I can eat frozen fruit and fresh vegetables."
② "I'll buy water-packed, canned tuna."
③ "I'll stop putting catsup on my potatoes."
④ "I'm going to decrease beef to one time a day."

140. Which instructions should be included in the teaching plan of a client who does not like dairy products and rarely eats vegetables?

① Calcium supplements may be necessary.
② Increase the protein intake.
③ Don't exercise until your diet improves.
③ Limit fluids in your diet.

141. What items in the data collection would alert the nurse to consider the possibility of osteoporosis in elderly women who are nursing home residents?

① Sudden weight loss that is not associated with dietary intake.
② Shortened height occurring over a long time period.
③ Decreased appetite and GI distress.
④ Difficulty walking in the morning due to joint stiffness.

142. A newly admitted client appears quite anxious about his upcoming surgery. Which action by the nurse could help reduce his anxiety?

① Ask open-ended questions regarding his feelings about surgery.
② Limit the amount of preoperative teaching.
③ Encourage his family members to cheer him up.
④ Limit the number of visitors.

143.What is important for the nurse to include in the preoperative teaching regarding effective coughing techniques?

① If pain occurs when coughing, do not continue.
② Shallow coughs are just as effective as deep coughs.
③ Coughing is performed with deep breathing exercises.
④ It is important to exhale completely before coughing.

144. The nurse is preparing a client for surgery. The client does not want to remove his wedding band prior to surgery. What is the best nursing action?

① Wrap tape around it to secure it to his finger.
② Tell him that the surgery cannot be done if he does not remove the ring.
③ Place a note on the chart stating that he refused to remove it.
④ Remind him that the hospital will not be liable for any loss.

145. A client returns to his room from the recovery room after extensive surgical resection for colon cancer. He is complaining of nausea. What is a priority nursing action?

① Evaluate his nasogastric tube for patency.
② Notify the physician.
③ Put him in semi-Fowler's so he will not aspirate.
④ Medicate him with a narcotic analgesic.

146. At 2pm, the nurse is assessing a client who had surgery for an aortic femoral bypass graft this morning. The client complains that he is feeling cold. What is the best nursing action?

① Apply a heating pad to his back for warmth.
② Recognize that this is a symptom of shock and notify the physician.
③ Realize that he may be bleeding internally and call the physician.
④ Apply several blankets to help promote maintenance of a normal body temperature.

147. A client has had a gastric resection, on the third postoperative day, the nasogastric tube is draining bile-colored liquid containing coffee ground material. What is the best nursing action?

① Continue to monitor the amount of drainage and correlate it with any change in vital signs.
② Reposition the nasogastric tube and irrigate the tube with normal saline.
③ Notify the RN regarding the possibility that the client is actively bleeding.
④ Irrigate the nasogastric tube with iced saline and attach the tube to gravity drainage.

148. In order to prevent the complications of immobility, the nurse would anticipate which activities on the first postoperative day following abdominal surgery?

① Turn, cough and deep breathe every 30 minutes around the clock.
② Out of bed and ambulate to a bedside chair.
③ Passive range of motion three times a day.
④ It is not necessary to worry about complications of immobility on the first postoperative day.

149. A diabetic woman is admitted for an above-the-knee amputation secondary to an injury. Which emotional response would be most common in the preoperative period?

① Relief that the procedure will remove the source of infection.
② Grieving over the anticipated loss of her limb.
③ Anger at the health-care team for taking away her leg.
④ Improved feelings of self-worth related to the removal of her disfigured limb.

150. Which nursing interventions would best meet the mobility needs of a geriatric client four days after an above-the-knee amputation ?

① Assist him to be out of bed and do full range of motion on the affected side.
② Continuous elevation of the amputated extremity on a pillow.
③ Help him practice lifting weights with his arms to increase mobility.
④ Provide passive range-of-motion exercises to the unaffected leg.

151. A client has had an above-the-knee amputation (AKA) due to osteogenic sarcoma. He is learning to wrap his stump. What will the nurse explain regarding the purpose of the purpose of wrapping the stump?

① Provide range of motion for the upper extremities as well as the residual limb.
② Keep the residual limb clean and dry.
③ Improve the muscle tone in the residual limb.
④ Promote shrinkage and shape the stump for the prosthesis.

152. In considering safety aspects, nursing interventions would include what actions to assist the client with a below-the-knee amputation (BKA) to ambulate?

① Emphasizing to him the importance of always using the walker.
② Encouraging him to use the wheelchair until the prosthesis is comfortable.
③ Assisting him to ambulate by supporting him on his affected side.
④ Teaching him to lie in the supine position whenever he is in bed.

153. A woman reports that her home pregnancy test was positive. A positive pregnancy test is related to the presence of which hormone?

① Chorionic gonadotropin.
② Progesterone.
③ Lactogen.
④ Estrogen.

154. The nurse receives report and is told that her client is having problems with bleeding secondary to a cervical laceration during delivery. What would the nurse expect to find on the initial assessment?

① Vaginal bleeding and a firm uterus.
② Fundus soft and palpable at the level of the pubic bone.
③ Boggy fundus and a hematoma at the episotomy site.
④ Swollen bleeding cervix on vaginal exam.

155. A diabetic client at 35 weeks' gestation has come to the antepartal testing unit for a non-stress test. Which statement is accurate about this test?

① It is a non-invasive test that observes the response of fetal heart rate to the stress of activity.
② It is a test that determines fetal-maternal-placental function.
③ It requires attachment of an electrode to fetal scalp.
④ It locates and identifies placental placement.

156. On admission to the nursery, the nurse puts gentamycin ointment in the eyes of a newborn. The following day, what observation would cause the most concern?

① Eyes have purulent drainage in them.
② No tears are present when the infant is crying.
③ Eyes are reddened and lids are swollen.
④ The infant does not appear to be able to focus.

157. The nurse is checking a postpartum client the day after her delivery and notes the lochia has a foul smell. What is the best nursing intervention?

① Immediately report the foul smelling lochia to the RN.
② Do nothing; this is normal during the first few days after delivery.
③ Begin vaginal irrigations to decrease the odor and increase client comfort.
④ Stop the use of perineal pads for the next few days.

158. What is important for the nurse to do when administering a Fleets enema to a postpartum client?

① Use a small catheter.
② Administer no more than 100 cc of solution.
③ Be careful not to irritate the perineum when inserting the catheter.
④ Encourage the client to administer her own so she will know how to do it at home.

159. A client is receiving total parenteral nutrition (TPN) after extensive abdominal surgery for colon cancer. How will the nurse know the TPN is achieving the desired results?

① The clien's weight is increased by five pounds over three days.
② There is no glucosuria, and the serum glucose is 160mg%.
③ Mucous membranes are moist, and the urine output is 60cc per hour.
④ There is significant increased healing of the abdominal and perineal wounds.

160. An 8-year-old boy is admitted with a green stick fracture of the ulnar. On the nursing assessment the nurse would identify what characteristics of a green stick fracture?

① The bone is broken across the epiphyseal plate.
② There is a splintering of the bone on one side.
③ There is a separation of the bone at the fracture site.
④ The bone is broken into several fragments.

161. A 10 year old boy has a cast on his right arm. He complains of numbness and tingling in his right hand. The nurse's assessment for compartmental syndrome is confirmed. What is the priority nursing action?

① Place ice packs at the fracture site.
② Elevate the arm and recheck in one hour.
③ Encourage increased movement of the arm.
④ Notify the doctor regarding the symptoms.

162. A geriatric client is on bedrest. The nursing assessment reveals redness and tenderness of the sacral area, the area is cool to touch with slight edema. What is the best nursing action?

① Apply warm wet to dry dressings.
② Place a dry heat lamp on the area to facilitate healing.
③ Initiate passive range of motion to increase circulation.
④ Place the client on an air mattress.

163. A client is scheduled for a myelogram. What is important nursing care regarding this test?

① Keep the client flat for 24 hours after the test.
② Insert a Foley catheter and maintain urinary drainage.
③ Encourage fluids prior to and after the test.
④ Encourage him to ambulate after the test.

164. The physician prescribes conservative treatment for a client with a herniated disk. Which intervention would most likely be considered part of this therapy?

① Bedrest in lateral Sims position.
② Bedrest and Robaxin (methocarbamol) to decrease muscle spasms.
③ Small incision in the spinal column to remove the disk.
④ Daily physical therapy and ambulation with crutches.

165. A client returns to his room from a laminectomy surgery. What is important to include in the nursing care for this client?

① Keep the client flat in bed for four days.
② Encourage the client to ambulate around the unit.
③ Evaluate clients ability to control bowel and bladder.
④ Assist client to perform straight leg exercises.

166. A 9 month old infant, has nose drops ordered for nasal congestion. To achieve a therapeutic effect from the nose drops, the nurse should take which of these measures?

① Place him in Trendelenburg position after instillation of the nose drops.
② Suction the secretions in his nasal passages after the drops are instilled.
③ Dilute the medication with saline prior to instilling it in the nose.
④ Give the medication about a half hour before he is to be fed.

167. A 4-year-old is admitted for a myringotomy. What is the primary purpose of this procedure?

① To promote drainage into the eustachian tube.
② To irrigate the eustachian tube.
③ To correct a congenital malformation in the inner ear.
④ To promote drainage from the ear.

168. A mother expresses concern that her one-year-old son refuses solid food and that his diet consists mostly of milk and simple carbohydrates. The nurse should make what recommendation regarding the child's nutrition?

① Exclude milk from the child's diet until he begins to like other foods.
② Offer him small amounts of meat and vegetables before offering him milk.
③ Withhold desserts until he has eaten his vegetables.
④ Mix strained meat and vegetables into the milk.

169. A six-month-old is to receive an immunization intramuscularly. The nurse should administer the intramuscular injection into which muscle?

① Biceps.
② Dorsogluteal.
③ Vastus lateralis.
④ Ventrogluteal.

170. A severely hypoxic client has a tracheotomy and requires periodic suctioning of both the upper and lower airway. Which statement correctly describes proper suctioning technique?

① The catheter is inserted into the artificial airway; intermittent suction is applied until no further secretions are retrieved; the catheter is then withdrawn.

② The catheter is inserted through the nose and the upper airway is suctioned; the catheter is then removed from the upper airway and inserted into the tracheotomy tube to suction the lower airway.

③ With suction applied, the catheter is inserted into the lower airway; when resistance is met, the catheter is slowly withdrawn.

④ The catheter is inserted into the lower airway to a point of resistance, suction is applied during withdrawal.

171. In caring for a client with a tracheotomy, what observations would indicate that his tracheal cuff is leaking?

① Increased respiratory rate

② Client able to speak.

③ Increased swallowing efforts by client.

④ Increased crackles (rales) over left lung field.

172. Which nursing care is important in caring for a 19-month-old child with respiratory syncytial virus (RSV)?

① Maintain humidified oxygen at 60% to prevent hypoxia.

② Carefully evaluate child for increasing inspiratory stridor.

③ Assess child for presence of a sore throat and frequent swallowing.

④ Wear gown and gloves when having direct contact with child.

173. The nurse is assessing a child who has asthma. What data collection would confirm early problems of hypoxia?

① Cyanosis.

② Tachypnea.

③ Confusion.

④ Frequency of cough.

174. A client returns to the clinic for interpretation of a tuberculin skin test. What observations would the nurse identify as a positive test?

① There is a raised area about 15mm in diameter.

② There is an inflammed area about 20mm in diameter.

③ The client complains of increased itching and tenderness around the site.

④ There are streaks of redness up the interior aspect of the arm.

175. What psychosocial data collection would indicate that a 19 month old child is demonstrating a nonadaptive reaction to the hospitalization?

① Cries when mother leaves.

② Ignores mother when she arrives to visit.

③ Eats using fingers rather than utensils.

④ Is afraid of the dark.

176. A client has a chest tube inserted in the right anterior chest. When transporting him to the x-ray department, how should the nurse provide for the chest drainage system?

① Maintain a sealed system and hang the drainage apparatus on the head of the bed.

② Clamp the chest tube and place drainage container on the bed.

③ Keep the water seal bottle below the level of the chest.

④ Disconnect chest tube from drainage apparatus and reconnect it in x-ray.

177. What source of data will provide the practical nurse with the most accurate assessment of the outcome of the chest drainage therapy?

① Volume of fluid drained.

② Breath sounds.

③ Pulmonary function studies.

④ Client's level of shortness of breath.

178. The nurse is completing her data collection of a client who is 12 hours post delivery. Where would the nurse anticipate the level of the fundus?

① Two fingerbreadths above the umbilicus.

② One to two fingerbreadths below the umbilicus.

③ At the level of the umbilicus diverted to the right.

④ Behind the symphysis pubis.

179. A post partum client complains to the nurse of abdominal cramping following breast-feeding. What is the best nursing interpretation of this information?

① All women experience abdominal discomfort during the postpartal period.

② Breast-feeding causes the release of oxytocin which acts on the uterus.

③ Abdominal pain is not normal and may indicate problems of involution.

④ Abdominal discomfort may be an indication of problems with peristalses.

180. The nurse is preparing the new mother for discharge. The client says to the nurse, "I used birth control pills before we decided to have another baby. I guess it's okay to go back to them." What is the best nursing reply?

① "Birth control pills may interfere with milk production while you are breast-feeding."
② "If that was an effective method for you, then you can return to it."
③ "Birth control pills really aren't very good for anyone."
④ "Certainly, you only have to wait until your postpartum checkup to start using them again."

181. On the tenth day after delivery, a client calls the clinic to say that her vaginal discharge is turning white and yellowish. What is the best nursing interpretation of this information?

① The client has an infection.
② The lochia is normal for this period post delivery.
③ Uterine involution is delayed.
④ This is a prolonged time for this type of locia.

182. The nurse is caring for a client who has been diagnosed with AIDS and pneumocysitis carinii pneumonia (PCP). What is the primary goal of nursing care?

① Maintain adequate oxygenation.
② Prevent pulmonary embolism.
③ Maintain metabolic acid base balance.
④ Increase activity to prevent respiratory acidosis.

183. A 15 year old boy has cancer. When he asks, "Will I die?" what is an initial therapeutic response based on the needs of the dying child?

① "Think about getting well instead of dying."
② "Tell me what you are thinking about dying."
③ "You need to ask your doctor."
④ "I really don't know."

184. A cancer client expresses fear regarding dying in pain. Which nursing action is most appropriate?

① Tell the client that worrying about pain makes it worse.
② Reassure the client that good pain control is available
③ Explain pain control theories.
④ Inform the client that pain is a part of illness.

185. An 18-year-old primigravida has a blood type of 0-. In her postpartal care plan, the nurse should include what information concerning RHO immune globulin (RhoGAM)?

① RhoGAM should be administered only if the baby's father is Rh positive.
② Instruct the client that RhoGAM must be received after each pregnancy.
③ Discuss with the client that RhoGAM only needs to be given after this pregnancy.
④ Administer RhoGAM within a month after the birth of the baby.

186. A 65 year old man tells the nurse that he thinks he has gonorrhea. The nurse would identify what finding that would correlate with this infection?

① There is a round raised lesion on the penis.
② The client is having difficulty with urinary dribbling.
③ The client complains of dysuria.
④ There is increased perineal pain on deification.

187. A 75 year old woman has been told that her PAP smear revealed cancer "in situ". She asks you what that means. What is the best nursing response?

① The cancer has spread to the pelvic wall.
② There are metastasis to the bone.
③ It is confined to the epithelial cells of the cervix.
④ The cervical tissue and vaginal mucosa show small lesions.

188. The client is postoperative abdominal perineal resection for colon cancer. The perineal wound is healing by secondary intention. What data collection would support this interpretation of wound healing?

① The wound is well approximated with sutures, no granulation tissue is observed.
② The wound is open and there is evidence of purulent drainage.
③ The wound edges are together and there is evidence of some scar formation.
④ The wound is open and there is granulation tissue present.

189. A client returns from surgery with Jackson-Pratt drains in place. What is appropriate nursing care for this type of drainage tube?

① Empty the drainage container only at the end of the shift and record the drainage.
② Check the drains and empty when about one half filled or at the change of shift.
③ Maintain the client on bedrest until the drains are removed.
④ Irrigate the drains with sterile normal saline to maintain the patency and drainage.

190. In caring for a woman after a vaginal hysterectomy, what is a priority nursing action in the immediate post operative period?

① Assist with sitz baths tid.
② Provide a high-protein diet.
③ Teach the client exercises to strengthen the abdomen.
④ Observe the client for adequate urine output.

191. The practical nurse assesses the postoperative client and determines that his bladder is distended. A Foley catheter is in place. Which action by the nurse is most appropriate?

① Check for kinking of the catheter.
② Remove the catheter.
③ Irrigate the catheter with a warm solution.
④ Evaluate the intake and output for the past eight hours.

192. Considering the complications most likely to occur in the first 48 hours following major surgery, which nursing actions would help to decrease the chances of these particular complications?

① Increase fluid intake and check for urinary tract problems.
② Teach client how to splint the incision to prevent tension on the suture line.
③ Have the client turn, cough, and breathe deeply every two hours.
④ Encourage a high-protein diet to facilitate healing.

193. Which breakfast selections would best meet the postoperative client's nutritional needs once solid food is allowed?

① Pancakes, bacon, and orange juice.
② Poached egg on toast, sausage, and milk.
③ Cereal with milk, banana, and apple juice.
④ Whole wheat toast, cereal and an apple.

194. The discharge teaching plan for a hysterectomy client should include what information?

① Avoid heavy lifting for 2 months.
② Douche daily with a weak vinegar solution.
③ Take hormone replacement therapy.
④ Anticipate heavy vaginal bleeding.

195. A client is being discharged after a mastectomy. Before leaving the hospital, she comments to the nurse, "I'll never get married now. No man would want a disfigured woman." Which response by the nurse would be most appropriate?

① "Why do you say that? You still look like a woman outwardly."
② "You'll feel better about yourself once you're home and things get back to normal."
③ "Has some man rejected you since you had your operation?"
④ "Are you afraid that you won't be attractive to men now?"

196. When doing the admission assessment on a client with hyperthyroidism, the nurse would expect the client to report which symptoms?

① Constipation.
② Lethargy.
③ Obesity.
④ Diaphoresis.

197. What is important to include in the postoperative nursing care for a thyroidectomy client?

① Have the client speak every 5 to 10 minutes if hoarseness is present.
② Provide a low-calcium diet to prevent hypercalcemia.
③ Check the dressing at the back of the neck for bleeding.
④ Apply a soft cervical collar to restrict neck movement.

198. A client is administered a dose of penicillin. He rapidly develops severe itching, wheezing, hypotension and tachycardia. What is the priority nursing action?

① Assist client to lie down and start oxygen.
② Obtain an immediate arterial blood gas analysis.
③ Position the client so that his head is dependent.
④ Stay with the client and provide emotional support.

199. The nurse is assessing a client who sustained multiple injuries. Significant bleeding is noted from the transverse fracture site at the left femur. What action should the nruse take after applying pressure over the area?

① Place the client in the Trendelenburg position.
② Apply direct digital pressure over the femoral artery.
③ Put the extremity in ice.
④ Wrap the leg in an Ace bandage.

200. A client's fracture is being stabilized with balanced suspension traction utilizing a Pearson attachment with a Thomas splint and a Kirschner wire. The nurse would identify this as what type of traction?

① Intermittent skin traction.
② Continuous skeletal traction.
③ Intermittent skeletal traction.
④ Continuous skin traction.

201. Nursing care to maintain effective traction includes what actions?

① Elevate the end of the bed frame to provide counter traction, traction weights should hang free from the end of the bed.
② Elevate the head of the bed, do range of motion on the affected extremity tid, assess for pressure areas from traction.
③ The traction weights should be gently removed every four hours and the client turned to the side to evaluate pressure areas.
④ Place a trochanter roll just below the popliteal space to prevent outward rotation of the lower leg.

202. What is the priority nursing intervention(s) in the care of a client in skeletal traction?

① Increase fluid intake to prevent the development of renal stone due to the stasis of urine in the bladder.
② Frequent pulse checks distal to the affected extremity, cleanse the pin site and apply antibiotic ointment to area.
③ Keep an abduction device between his legs to prevent external rotation of the affected leg.
④ Encourage a diet high in calcium to promote an increase in bone strength and repair.

203. A CVA client, is started on subcutaneous heparin injections, 5000u bid. What is the purpose of this medication for this client?

① Prevent venous stasis that promotes vascular complications associated with immobility.
② Promote vascular perfusion by preventing formation of micro-emboli in the left leg.
③ Prevent thromboemboli resulting in pulmonary emboli associated with immobility.
④ Decrease the incidence of fat emboli associated with long bone fractures.

204. What is a nursing action necessary to administer Heparin safely?

① Check the hemoglobin and hematocrit. Do not administer if they are decreased.
② Utilize a 20 gauge, ½ inch needle, inject into the deltoid muscle and gently massage the area.
③ Use a 20gauge 1½ inch needle, inject into the upper outer quadrant of the hip.
④ Utilize a 25 gauge, ½ inch needle, and inject the medication into the subcutaneous tissue of the abdomen.

205. A client is scheduled for a lumbar laminectomy with bone graft. In preparation for surgery, what should the nurse include in the teaching plan?

① How to get on and off a bedpan by lifting his hips.
② Stretching from the waist when reaching for things.
③ Completing straight leg raises while on bed rest.
④ Logrolling when turning from side to side.

206. What data collection information is important to include in the chart of a client who is going to surgery for a lumbar laminectomy?

① Movement and sensation in the lower extremities.
② Shoulder pain that radiates to the arms.
③ Reflexes in the upper extremities.
④ Pupillary reaction to light.

207. What is important nursing intervention in the immediate postoperative period after a vertebral bone graft?

① Check the dressing for spinal fluid leak.
② Ambulate the client.
③ Change the surgical dressing.
④ Begin an exercise program.

208. Prior to discharge, the nurse teaches proper body mechanics to a client with back problems. What observation indicates the client understood the instructions?

① Bends from the waist to lift a heavy object.
② Carries a heavy object away from his body.
③ Squats down to pick up a heavy object.
④ Leans backward when carrying a heavy object.

209. A cancer client is in the terminal stages of her illness. As the dying process progresses, she is experiencing severe weakness. What is a therapeutic nursing intervention for this response to dying?

① Administer pain medication more frequently.
② Determine her attitude toward death.
③ Place her in a private room.
④ Institute comfort measures.

210. When providing nursing care for the dying client, what the most common nursing priority?

① Physical needs.
② Psychological needs.
③ Spiritual needs.
④ Needs of the family.

211. The family is present as their mother is dying. They need assistance as her death becomes imminent. How can the nurse can best assist the family to begin preparatory grieving?

① Assuring them that she will suffer no intense pain.
② Advising them about ways they can manage after she dies.
③ Supporting them while they share feelings about her impending death.
④ Sympathizing with them as they talk about the meaning of her imminent death.

212. The nurse is preparing to do a dressing change on a client with a large abdominal wound. Nursing assessment reveals the dressing is adhered to the wound and the incisional area. What is the best nursing action?

① Remove the dressing quickly then apply pressure to the incisional area.
② Moisten the dressing with tepid tap water and remove it in a few minutes.
③ Slowly remove as much of the dressing as possible, use bandage scissors and cut remaining dressing.
④ Moisten dressing with sterile normal saline and remove it when it no longer adheres to the wound.

213. An infant chokes, gasps and becomes dusky on his first feeding. Prior to the doctor arriving to assess the infant, what is a priority nursing action?

① Comfort and cuddle infant.
② Start a small amount oral feeding.
③ Keep the child NPO.
④ Isolate the infant.

214. The mother has not seen her premature baby since birth and is very distressed. Upon her first visit to the intensive care nursery, she is concerned about the feeding tube and asks if her baby will be able to eat like a normal baby. What is the best nursing response?

① "You will need to ask your doctor these questions."
② "Don't worry, your baby will be fine."
③ "This type of feeding method is usually only temporary."
④ "He is getting all the nutrition a normal baby needs."

215. The nurse is assessing a craniotomy client. What information on the data collection would cause the most concern?

① Restlessness, bradycardia, vomiting.
② Photophobia and complaints of a headache.
③ Presence of nystagmus, pupils pinpoint, and equal.
④ Blood pressure 108/80 and a temperature of 101 degrees.

216. A client has genital herpes type II. When is the time this client is most contagious?

① Vesicles rupture, releasing exudate.
② Superficial, painful ulcers appear.
③ Yellow vaginal drainage is present.
④ Pustules become inflamed and erythematous.

217. When the lesions are present, what is a nursing measure to prevent the spread of genital herpes II?

① Careful hand washing by client and staff.
② Private room and bath for the client.
③ Needle precautions.
④ Respiratory isolation.

218. The nurse is assisting the CVA client to get out of bed and into the wheelchair. He is experiencing right sided weakness and cannot support his weight on his right side. What is the correct movement of this client?

① Get the client out of bed on his left side to provide stability and pivot with his left leg to the chair.

② Assist the client to get out of bed on his right side so support can be maintained initially.

③ Put the wheel chair at the foot of the bed and assist the client out of bed on his right side.

④ He should not have weight bearing on either side so obtain assistance for a total lift into the chair

219. The nurse has been caring for pulmonary clients and her tuberculin skin test is positive. What is the recommended course of action?

① Get a chest x-ray and begin prophylactic medication.

② Repeat the skin test in two weeks, if still positive begin treatment.

③ Nothing is necessary now as this just means exposure to the bacilli.

④ Respiratory isolation until sputum can be evaluated for tubercle bacilli.

220. When assisting the doctor to do a pelvic examination on a female client, what is an important nursing action?

① Instruct the client to douche prior to the exam.

② Explain to the client that she will not feel any pain.

③ Have the client empty her bladder before the examination begins.

④ Lubricate the speculum well before handing it to the doctor.

221. The doctor informs a client that she has *Trichomonas* vaginitis and her sexual partner should use condoms during sexual intercourse. What is important for the nurse to explain to the client regarding the condoms?

① Enhances sexual arousal for the client.

② Decreases the client's complaint of dyspareunia.

③ Decreases the partner's exposure to infective organisms.

④ Reduces irritation of the client's inflamed vaginal mucosa.

222. The client with a vaginal infection is given a prescription for metronidazole (Flagyl) 250 mg PO tid for 10 days. The teaching plan would include informing her to avoid which activities while taking this medication?

① Drinking alcoholic beverages.

② Driving a car.

③ Taking vaginal douches.

④ Taking tub baths.

223. A client has a diagnosis of gastroesophageal reflux disease (GERD). What would the nurse teach him in order to decrease his distress?

① Increase intake of fluids with meals.

② Lie down for about an hour after meals.

③ Drink warm liquids prior to going to bed.

④ Avoid eating or drinking for 30 minutes before bedtime.

224. A man is admitted with a diagnosis of a myocardial infarction (MI). The nurse would question which orders?

① Clear liquid diet, bedrest with bathroom privileges.

② 5 L O_2 per nasal cannula, monitor per telemetry.

③ General diet and progressive ambulation.

④ Furosamide (Lasix) 10mg PO, serial enzyme studies.

225. The practical nurse is caring for a client with congestive heart failure. How would the nurse accurately evaluate the fluid balance in this client?

① Weigh the client daily before breakfast.

② Take the BP with the client sitting and lying down.

③ Place a Foley catheter in the bladder for an accurate output.

④ Evaluate the client's sputum for amount and color.

226. An teenage boy is in a left hip spica cast. The nursing care plan would include which measures to check the circulation under the cast?

① Palpate the left brachial artery and compare it to the right.

② Check cast for tightness by inserting fingers between skin and cast.

③ Blanch the skin of areas proximal to the casted left leg.

④ Evaluate lower extremities for swelling and discoloration.

227. In caring for a child with a damp cast, which nursing actions should be appropriate?

① Use only the fingertips when moving the cast.
② Keep the child and cast covered with blankets.
③ Support the cast on plastic covered pillows.
④ Place a heat lamp directly over the cast.

228. The nurse is assigned to care for a client who is becoming weaker and difficult to arouse. He is dyspneic and has difficulty with secretions, there is a current do not resuscitate order (DNR). What is the best position for this client?

① Supine on his back
② Out of bed in a chair.
③ On his side with head slightly elevated.
④ Sitting up in bed leaning over a bedside table.

229. The family of a dying client should be given what information regarding noise in the client's room:

① Attempt to get the client to talk.
② Avoid making any noise when you are with them.
③ They probably will not be able to hear you or anything in the room.
④ Talk softly to the client whenever you are with him.

230. A client is admitted for dehydration. On admission, which measurements should the nurse obtain in order that fluid needs of the client can be accurately calculated and hydration evaluated?

① Height and weight.
② Blood pressure.
③ Skin turgor.
④ Previous 24-hour intake.

231. During a physical assessment, what cardiovascular changes might the nurse expect to identify as a result of dehydration?

① Widening pulse pressure.
② Increased heart rate.
③ Hypertension.
④ Increased pulse deficit.

232. The RN formulates the following nursing diagnosis for the client with a diagnosis of dehydration: Altered oral mucous membrane related to inadequate oral secretions. Which nursing actions should the practical nurse use in the care plan in relation to this diagnosis?

① Swab mouth frequently with glycerin swab.
② Rinse mouth with dilute solution of hydrogen peroxide every hour.
③ Gently brush teeth with a soft brush..
④ Rinse mouth every hour with diluted commercial mouth wash.

233. The nurse is performing range of motion (ROM) exercises on an immobilized client. What is the minimum number of times per day these exercises should be done?

① Once.
② Twice.
③ Three times.
④ Five times.

234. The client is too weak to assist the nurse with range of motion (ROM) exercises. The nurse performs the exercises. What type of notation should be made in the record?

① Passive ROM performed.
② Assisted ROM done for the client.
③ Resistive exercises accomplished.
④ Client refused ROM.

235. A client is admitted to the hospital with a diagnosis of immunodeficiency syndrome. What is important for the nurse to consider for this client?

① Has probably not had a normal immune system since birth.
② Is experiencing the early symptoms of the AIDS syndrome.
③ Has a problem with immune function, not infection at this time.
④ Has a severe decrease in resistance and will require reverse isolation for protection.

236. The nurse is caring for a tonsillectomy client. What measures can the nurse take to decrease the discomfort?

① Put an ice collar to the neck to decrease the swelling.
② Assist the client with range of motion to prevent stiffness and contractures.
③ Omit oral hygiene on the operative day.
④ Spray the oral pharyngeal area with antiseptic analgesic spray.

237. The nurse is caring for an alcoholic client who is beginning to experience delirium tremors. What is important to include in care of this client?

① Plan to administer a CNS depressnant and keep down environmental stimuli.
② Keep the room dark to decrease stimuli and risk of seizures.
③ Explain to the client where he is and how important it is for him to cooperate.
④ Assist client to determine alternative coping mechanisms rather then alcohol.

238. A confused client in a long term care facility is found walking the halls in his underware. He keeps staggering and stumbling as he tries to walk. What is the best nursing action?

① Assist him to put his clothes on and return to his room.

② Assist him back to his room and conduct a thorough physical assessment.

③ Sit down with him in the hall and determine his level of orientation and why he is in the hall.

④ When he is back in his room, attempt to determine why he was in the hall.

239. A client had a transurethral resection of his prostate (TURP) for benign prostatic hyperplasia yesterday. The nurse observes the drainage from the catheter to be increasingly bloody when he stands at the beside. What is the best nursing action?

① Check the continuous irrigation flow rate and the patency of the catheter drainage.

② Notify the RN, keep the head of the clients bed flat, evaluate the vital signs.

③ Irrigate the catheter with approximately 100cc of normal saline to remove the clots.

④ Assess the client for increased pain and determine source of bleeding.

240. A four month old infant has a rectal temperature of 103.6°F. What is the most appropriate nursing action to decrease his temperature?

① Place him in a cool mist croupette with compressed air.

② Sponge his trunk and extremities with tepid water.

③ Encourage him to take clear liquids such as apple juice.

④ Sponge him with a solution containing half water and half alcohol.

241. A child you are caring for has a grand mal seizure. As the seizure ends, which nursing intervention should receive the highest priority?

① Loosen or remove constricting clothing and protect him from injuring himself.

② Maintain a patent airway by turning the child's head to the side and suctioning him if necessary.

③ Remain with the child and administer anticonvulsant medications as ordered by the physician.

④ Describe and record events before the onset of the seizure, during the seizure, and after the seizure.

242. A young woman is being admitted for acute leukemia. The nurse would anticipate what findings on her data collection?

① Diarrhea, hypertension, and restlessness.

② Fatigue, fever, and bleeding.

③ Dehydration, paresthesia, and chills.

④ Tremors, blurred vision, and headache.

243. A chronic renal failure client is on hemodialysis. He has a shunt in his left forearm. What are the nursing actions to maintain patency of the graft?

① Daily irrigations with 25 gauge needle and sterile normal saline.

② Note on Kardex and on the bed regarding no blood pressure or needle sticks on the left arm.

③ Frequent assessment of the left arm and compare to size to the right arm.

④ Assist client with active exercises to increase muscle tone in left arm.

244. What is the correct method for obtaining a urine specimen for a culture and sensitivity from a closed drainage system?

① Disconnect the catheter and allow it to drain into the sterile urine container.

② Drain approximately 50cc of urine from the urine collection bag into the sterile container.

③ Empty the urine collection bag and allow it to fill again and collect sample in sterile container.

④ Withdraw a sample of urine with a sterile syringe from the entry port of the catheter.

245. An elderly client is 2 days postoperative abdominal aortic aneurysm repair. Morphine 8 mg IM q 4 hrs PRN is ordered. Her respiratory rate is 20; pulse rate is 100; and blood pressure is elevated slightly above her normal level. She is complaining of severe pain. What is the best nursing intervention?

① Question the physician regarding the size of the dose for a client of this age.

② Turn her and then reevaluate her need for narcotic analgesia.

③ Administer the medication as ordered.

④ Assist hcr to cough and breathe deeply.

246. A client has developed acute renal failure. During the oliguric phase, the plan of care would include which nursing measures?

① Observation for signs of secondary infection.

② Provision of a high-protein, low-carbohydrate diet.

③ Encouraging progressive ambulation.

④ Forcing fluids to 2,000 ml in 24 hours.

247. Which illness places the elderly client at increased risk for sensory deprivation?

① Gallbladder disease.
② Cataract surgery.
③ Hypertension.
④ Coronary artery disease.

248. The nurse's goal for a client who recently experienced a right-sided CVA, is to prevent complications resulting from immobility. Which measure is most likely to achieve this objective?

① Force fluids.
② Encourage activity.
③ Apply splints.
④ Increase fiber in the diet.

249. Which client is at the highest risk of developing a pressure ulcer?

① An elderly man who is one day post operative.
② A client with a spinal cord injury who refuses to eat.
③ A man convalescing from a colon resection 3 days ago.
④ A young woman receiving total parenteral nutrition.

250. What is the most effective measure to prevent the development of a pressure ulcer?

① Frequent position changes.
② Turning the client every three hours.
③ Limiting fluids.
④ ROM exercises.

251. Which finding in the nurse's data collection would be classified as a pre-ulcer?

① A reddened area that does not fade within thirty minutes.
② Pallor over a bony prominence immediately after moving.
③ An area of the skin that has impaired pain perception.
④ A slight break in the skin over an area of pressure.

252. What is the most appropriate nursing intervention to prevent the development of a pressure ulcer in areas that are red and do not blanche with digital pressure?

① Vigorously massage the skin.
② Relieve pressure on the area.
③ Apply an occlusive dressing.
④ Provide ROM to the affective extremity.

253. Within the hospital setting, what is the most effective means of preventing the spread of nosocomial infections?

① Washing surfaces with an antiseptic cleaning solution.
② Using only sterile equipment for client contact.
③ Effective hand washing between caring for different clients.
④ Using sterile gloves during client care.

254. A client is to take an antibiotic for the treatment of a urinary tract infection. She asks the nurse why she has to take all of the medication. The nurse's response would be based on what principle?

① Urinary tract infections are from multiple bacteria and are difficult to treat.
② Urinary tract infections frequently return and it may become more difficult to treat.
③ In order to be effective all antibiotics should be taken for the full length of time ordered.
④ If the full length of antibiotics are not taken there is increased risk of bladder abscess.

255. In the elderly client, what is an early symptoms of an infection?

① Enlarged lymph nodes.
② Dizziness.
③ Bradycardia.
④ Change in mental status.

256. A post operative client has patient-controlled analgesia (PCA) prescribed. What is the major advantage of this method of pain control?

① Pain relief is improved.
② Nursing time is saved.
③ Pain is not blamed on the staff.
④ Respiratory depression is avoided.

257. An insulin-dependent diabetic, has been receiving insulin every morning during his hospitalization. On the morning of his surgery, no specific changes have been made regarding his insulin. Which actions by the nurse is most appropriate?

① Give his regularly scheduled insulin dosage.
② Hold his insulin until after the surgery.
③ Check with the charge nurse or physician about the insulin order.
④ Give the insulin only if it is long acting.

121. ② The osmotic pressure of glucose in the urine prevents the kidney tubules from reabsorbing water; thus, it is excreted and excess urine results.

122. ① When clients are sleeping, the only observable symptom of hypoglycemia is diaphoresis. Kussmaul respirations and acetone breath are seen in hyperglycemia.

123. ④ The hypoglycemic client needs immediate glucose intake, this can be from a complex carbohydrate. Complex carbohydrate will prevent the sudden decrease in bloodsugar experienced from simple carbohydrates.

124. ① Hypercapnia or increased blood carbon dioxide will result from smoking or exercise in this client. The symptoms of hypercapnia include: increased respiratory rate, headache, confusion, lethargy, nausea, and vomiting.

125. ③ The COPD client is always dyspneic. It is important that he exercise to prevent the detrimental effects of immobility.

126. ① Pursed lip breathing slows or retards the flow rate of exhaled air; this keeps airways open and prevents alveolar collapse.

127. ② Buck's traction is used to decrease pain by reducing muscle spasms.

128. ④ Countertraction is best applied by using the client's own weight as the counter pull. This is best achieved by elevating the end of the bed frame to maintain the countertraction.

129. ③ Open reduction allows the surgeon direct visualization and repair of the fracture site and permits early client mobilization.

130. ③ When the hip is pinned, early mobility is possible. There is no reason to keep the client flat.

131. ② On return from the post-anesthesia care unit, the client is placed in a supine position with the head slightly elevated. An abduction pillow with or without straps is usually placed between the client's legs to prevent adduction beyond the body's midline. Some hospitals no longer use this device because it is uncomfortable for the client; several regular pillows are used instead.

132. ① Circulation and sensation are the priority assessments that must be made after any fracture because of the possibility of nerve or circulatory involvement.

133. ② Increased fluid intake is needed to replace the fluid drawn out of the spinal column. Most often the client is kept flat and a banded may be placed over the puncture site. Nerve damage that would affect the lower extremities is not a problem with an LP.

134. ④ In any client in traction, a nursing priority is to determine the correct amount of weight, and to assess for effectiveness of countertraction. Weights must hang freely for countertraction to be effective.

135. ③ Leg exercises commence in the immediate post-operative period and include plantar flexion and dorsiflexion (heel pumping), circumduction of the feet, gluteal and quadriceps setting, and straight leg raises.

136. ② A relatively common practice in the treatment of chronic pain is the administration of narcotic potentiator, drugs which potentiate the action or effect of narcotics.

137. ① Demerol can cause respiratory depression, hypotension, and an increase in constipation and urinary retention.

138. ③ To obtain an accurate reading in an adult, the blood pressure cuff should cover the upper two-thirds of the client's arm, it should be positioned approximately 2" above the antecubital space. The systolic reading is obtained with the first of the Karotkoff sounds.

139. ④ The client is on a low cholesterol diet, beef should be eaten only two to three times a week, not every day. Options 1, 2, & 3 will decrease sodium intake.

140. ① If an individual cannot ingest sufficient quantities of calcium in the diet, calcium supplements are used.

141. ② The client often states that height has been shortened, perhaps as much as 2 to 3 inches within the previous 20 years.

142. ① Verbalization of feelings, fears, and concerns is an appropriate way to reduce anxiety.

143. ③ Coughing is performed in conjunction with deep breathing every 1 to 2 hours postoperatively. Coughing may be uncomfortable for the client, but when performed correctly, it does not harm the surgical area.

144. ① Dislodging his wedding band during surgery is the primary risk. If a client refuses to remove a band, it must be safely and securely held in place with tape.

145. ① Evaluate the nasogastric tube patency; it is very important to assess the client and determine the source of the nausea prior to calling the doctor.

146. ④ Chilling is normal after surgery because the temperature of the operating room is cool. Simply apply blankets to maintain the client's body temperature.

147. ① Coffee ground material is old blood. This is a normal occurrence on the third postoperative day.

148. ② Weightbearing increases the vascular tone and decreases the venous stasis, thereby preventing

thrombi from developing; the increase in activity increases the respiratory expansion and quality of breathing.

149. ② Clients undergoing amputation experience grief and a sense of loss.

150. ① It is very important to prevent a flexion contracture in the right hip. If a flexion contracture occurs, it will be very difficult to have a functioning prosthesis.

151. ④ Wrapping the stump with an Ace bandage in a figure eight style helps to control edema and maintain the stump in a tapered shape that can more easily be fitted for a prosthesis.

152. ③ The center of gravity changes when a lower limb is amputated. Assist the client from the affected side while letting him move his unaffected side.

153. ① Chorionic gonadotropin is a placental hormone which, when present, indicates the presence of pregnancy.

154. ① The fundus should be around the level of the umbilicus on the first day after delivery. Since the laceration was on the cervix, the fundus will remain firm.

155. ① A non-stress test is a non-invasive test conducted with a fetal monitor and designed to evaluate the response of fetal heart rate to the stress of activity. It is reported as reactive or non-reactive.

156. ① The presence of purulent drainage is indicative of an infection. The other observations are within the normal findings for a neonate.

157. ① Foul odor may indicate the presence of an infection and should be reported to the RN. She can call the physician to start antibiotics.

158. ③ It is important to be gentle since the episiotomy is easily irritated and hemorrhoids are quite common.

159. ④ Hyperalimentation is done to replace protein and amino acids to facilitate healing. Just because the client is gaining weight does not mean he is healing.

160. ② Greenstick fracture occurs most often in children as a result of the flexibility of the bone. The bone bends and splinters on one side, there is no separation or fragmentation of the bone.

161. ④ Compartmental syndrome rapidly causes injury to the nerves in the radial area, the doctor must be notified and the pressure is going to have to be released or there will be permanent damage in a short time.

162. ④ This is early sign of pressure and development of decubitus ulcer, place the client on an air mattress to decrease the pressure.

163. ③ Increasing fluids promotes the excretion of the dye and also promotes formation of spinal fluid.

164. ② Conservative treatment means without surgical intervention. The most common conservative therapy includes bedrest and a muscle relaxant.

165. ③ The urinary bladder receives innervation from the sacral area of the spine. If there edema in this area, the client may experience a loss of control for bowel and for bladder. He may also retain urine.

166. ④ Because children naturally breathe through the nose, administration of nose drops before feeding promotes clearance of the nasal passages.

167. ④ The goal of a myringotomy is to promote drainage by making a surgical incision into the tympanic membrane which also relieves the pressure and prevents ear drum perforation and reduces pain.

168. ② Children at this age are prone to anemia especially when milk is offered frequently. Therefore, holding liquids till after solid food is offered prevents the child from "filling up" on the liquid.

169. ③ Until the child walks or is one year of age, the vastus lateralis is the preferred muscle group site.

170. ④ The catheter must be advanced to an adequate depth (to prevent secretion buildup at the end of the tube and to clear the airway as much as possible); to minimize trauma, suction is only applied during catheter withdrawal.

171. ② A leak in the cuff would allow air to pass through the cords, allowing the patient to make a noise and to speak.

172. ④ The RSV virus is very contageous. A gown and gloves should be worn when having direct contact with the child. Inspiratory stridor is not a common problem with RSV, and oxygen levels are maintained according to the arterial blood gas levels.

173. ② Studies have shown that the respiratory rate correlates with the degree of hypoxemia; cyanosis and confusion would be late signs of hypoxemia.

174. ① The interpretation is made from the area of induration or raised area not the area of inflammation.

175. ② Usually the toddler clings to the mother; as separation anxiety becomes intolerable the child ignores the parent at this stage the child relates better to the staff and doesn't mind the absence of the parent.

176. ③ The bottle must be kept below the level of the chest to prevent drainage from flowing back into the pleural space; the incorrect options would inhibit the drainage of air and fluid from the pleural space. Drainage container should never be clamped or raised above the client's chest.

177. ② The presence of and characteristics of breath sounds are critical information necessary to determine if the lung has reinflated.

178. ② Immediately after delivery, the fundus is at the level of the umbilicus, midline. Each day after that it descends 1 to 2 cm.

179. ② The release of oxytocin from the posterior pituitary during the infant's suckling increases the contractions of the uterus and gives rise to afterpains.

180. ① Oral contraceptives should be avoided when a woman is lactating since the increased estrogen and progesterone tend to interfere with the peripheral action of prolactin, thus decreasing the supply of milk.

181. ② The changes in the amount and color of lochia are indicative of the normal process of involution.

182. ① Maintaining oxygenation with good pulmonary hygiene is primary goal at this time. He is not immobilized, and there is no acid base problem.

183. ② The child usually has a fairly accurate evaluation of a situation and the nurse needs to respond to his questions about dying in a way that allows him a chance to express his concerns.

184. ② Many people fear dying in unbearable pain. Clients can be reassured that we now have very sophisticated treatments for pain control. The most effective pain regimen possible will be utilized for the client's comfort.

185. ② RhoGAM, Rh(D) immune globulin, must be given after each delivery or abortion of an Rh-positive fetus. The globulin will remain for several months, and during the period, the mother will have positive titers which will gradually decrease in potency.

186. ③ Dysuria and purulent urethral discharge are classic symptoms of gonorrhea. Lesions are seen in syphilis, dribbling and pain on defecation in BPH.

187. ③ Stage O or preinvasive cancer is defined as carcinoma in situ; it is limited to the epithelial cells of the cervix.

188. ④ Secondary intention means the wound heals from the inside out without sutures. Granulation tissue is fragile new tissue in the wound.

189. ② The drains should be monitored, if they are more the one half full then the negative pressure may not be effective.

190. ④ Low back pain and decreased urine output are serious symptoms that may indicate accidental intraoperative cutting of the ureter.

191. ① A common cause of bladder distention is kinking of the urinary catheter.

192. ③ During the first 72 hours postoperatively, the client is at greatest risk of developing respiratory complications such as atelectasis and pneumonia.

193. ② A diet that is high in protein and calories promotes wound healing.

194. ① Prior to discharge, the client should be told to avoid lifting heavy objects for about 2 months.

195. ④ The client should be encouraged to express her feelings and fears.

196. ④ Increased levels of circulating thyroid hormone cause the bodily processes to increase; one resulting symptom is diaphoresis.

197. ③ If bleeding occurs, the blood will drain posteriorly.

198. ① In an anaphylactic reaction, airway and breathing is the primary concern, other options do not address the respiratory problem

199. ② Apply direct pressure on the area if there is bleeding and pressure over the proximal artery nearest the fracture.

200. ② The placement of a Kirschner wire through the affected femur constitutes skeletal traction. Skeletal traction is continuous.

201. ① Elevation of the end of the bed increases the countertraction and prevents the client from sliding toward the pull of the traction. If the traction weights do not hang free, then there is no counter pull at the fracture site and it negates the affect of the traction. Traction weights should remain constant, they should not be removed.

202. ② Pulse checks distal to a fracture are priority concerns whether the client is in traction or in a cast. The area around the pin insertion should be cleansed and closely observed for the development of an infection that could lead to osteomyelitis.

203. ③ Heparin is administered prophylactically to prevent thromboembolic complications in clients who are immobilized for prolonged periods of time.

204. ④ Medication should be administered with a small gauge needle (25 gauge) into the subcutaneous tissue, without aspirating or massaging the area. Partial thromboplastin time (PTT) is utilized to monitor heparin.

205. ④ The client should be taught the log rolling manner of turning preoperatively to avoid twisting his spine postoperatively.

206. ① Preoperative assessment of lower extremity movement and sensation allows for comparison with postoperative findings.

207. ① Anytime the spinal column has been entered, the nurse needs to observe for leakage of spinal fluid. The RN should be notified if there is any evidence of a spinal fluid leak.

208. ③ The client should be taught to pick something up from the floor by squatting down rather than bending over.

209. ④ When the client's condition weakens, there is decreased sensation and need for pain medication,

however, other measures need to be instituted to keep the client as comfortable as possible.

210. ① Because of the nurse's discomfort and the need to increase her distance from the dying person, she is likely to focus first on physical needs of the person.

211. ③ If family members can share their feelings during their time of grieving, the impending separation can be dealt with more realistically and the family can come to a state of acceptance.

212. ④ Soften the dressing with saline to prevent further disruption or damage to the incisional area..

213. ③ Any further attempts to feed the child will increasingly compromise his oxygen supply. The remaining actions can await a physician's order.

214. ③ Inform the mother very succinctly that once the baby is older and has more strength, he will be able to eat normally.

215. ① The nurse is observing for signs of increased intracranial pressure, first option is most representative of signs of this complication.

216. ① The herpes virus type II is present in the vesicles, and therefore the infection is highly contagious when this fluid is released.

217. ① A highly contagious exudate is released when the vesicles rupture. Therefore, the client and others in contact with the client should be advised to wash their hands carefully.

218. ① The client should be assisted out of be on his unaffected side so he can assist in stabilizing himself.

219. ① People with a positive skin test need to have a chest x-ray and receive prophylactic treatment, most often with INH. They do not have active disease, but they have been exposed.

220. ③ Having the client void before the examination will make the procedure less painful and more accurate.

221. ③ Use of condoms will help prevent the sexual partner from contracting the infecting organism.

222. ① FLAGYL and alcohol consumed together may cause GI upset, resulting in vomiting.

223. ① to decrease the reflux an increase in fluids will assist the food to move more rapidly out of the stomach. Lying down will delay it, client should not drink liquids for 3-4 hours prior to bedtime.

224. ③ Options 1, 2, and 4 are all appropriate for the newly admitted MI client. The nurse would question the general diet and ambulation because both activities would ⌠ the cardiac workload.

225. ① The most accurate way to determine if a client is retaining fluid is by evaluating changes in daily weight. A weight gain of 2 pounds overnight would indicate fluid retention.

226. ② There should be enough room to insert fingers between the cast and skin beneath it.

227. ③ Supporting a wet cast on pillows covered with plastic prevents indentations which could result in pressure areas.

228. ③ He may be made more comfortable by being placed on his side, with the head slightly elevated and firmly supported on a pillow.

229. ④ Caretakers should be encouraged to talk softly to the client, to touch and to gently stroke him or her.

230. ① Height and weight are important measurements for calculating approximate fluid needs. Because weight and liquid measurements are related, changes in weight are good indicators of fluid losses or excesses.

231. ② The heart rates increases with vascular volume deficits. Blood pressure decreases, as does the pulse pressure, with a greater decrease being present in the systolic blood pressure.

232. ③ Brushing the teeth assists to cleanse the mouth and relieve the discomfort. Commercial mouthwashes should be avoided. These products tend to dry the oral mucosa further and may cause increased discomfort. Rinsing the mouth with dilute solutions of hydrogen peroxide two to three times per day is a good form of oral hygiene; however, when used more frequently, this treatment can increase oral dryness.

233. ③ For ROM exercises to be effective, the entire process should be completed at least three times daily.

234. ① Passive exercises are performed by the nurse for the client.

235. ③ Client has a problem with immune function, can be from steroids, cancer, or HIV +, there is no indication of infection, however he will be at high risk.

236. ① A ice collar will decrease the inflammation, other options are not effective or recommended.

237. ① Physiological needs are the priority at this time. A CNS depressant (Librium, Valium) is frequently given to decrease the agitation.

238. ② It is important to focus on possible physiological problems associated with his disorientation. A thorough nursing assessment should be done and compared it to previous assessment data.

239. ① Bloody drainage increases with client activity and is normal for this time frame, need to make sure the irrigation is running smoothly and there is adequate outflow for drainage.

240. ② Tepid sponge baths reduce temperature by promoting evaporation. Ice or alcohol baths may reduce temperature too rapidly, leading to vascular collapse or vasoconstriction, which defeats the purpose of the cool applications. Do not allow the

child to become chilled as this will increase heat production and raise the temperature.

241. ② The priority after a grand mal seizure is to maintain a patent airway.

242. ② Typical symptoms of leukemia include an increase in abnormal white cells, bleeding (decreasing RBC) and fatigue.

243. ② Protect the shunt by not allowing blood pressures or needle sticks in the arm. Irrigations are not done, and other options are not appropriate to shunt care.

244. ① It is important to maintain the closed system to prevent introducing bacteria. The urine should be collected in a sterile syringe from the entry port of the catheter.

245. ③ The stress of pain, anxiety, and insomnia are detrimental to the body's homeostatic mechanisms. Narcotic analgesics should be administered in their optimal doses if the client's physiological status is stable.

246. ① Secondary infections are the cause of death in 50 percent to 90 percent of clients with acute renal failure.

247. ② Clients who have had eye surgery are at high risk of becoming deprived of stimulation if an eye patch is used, which reduces visual ability and causes limitations in activity levels.

248. ② The mainstay of prevention of the numerous and systemic complications of inactivity is increasing the client's mobility.

249. ② Clients with inadequate nutrition and decreasing mobility are at the greatest risk for developing pressure ulcers.

250. ① The cornerstone of prevention of pressure ulcers is frequent position changes in combination with adequate skin care and sufficient nutritional intake.

251. ① If a reddened area does not fade within thirty minutes after pressure relief, it may be classified as a pre-ulcer area. A break in the skin is a stage 2.

252. ② If pre-ulcer areas are noted, the nurse does not rub these areas, because this causes more extensive damage to the already fragile capillary system. Rather, the nurse maintains careful observation of the pre-ulcer areas for further breakdown and relieves pressure on the areas as much as possible.

253. ③ Hand washing is the single most effective mechanism for preventing the spread of infection.

254. ③ Perhaps the most obvious complication of inadequate therapy is relapse. Incomplete compliance with the regimen may expose the bacterial flora to sub-inhibitory concentrations of antimicrobial agents, thereby facilitating the emergence of strains resistant to the antibiotic.

255. ④ In the elderly, a change in mental status may be the first, if not the only, presenting symptom.

256. ① PCA utilizes pain medication more effectively. This approach to pain control can improve pain relief and increase client satisfaction.

257. ③ The nurse consults the charge nurse or client's physician for clarification regarding insulin coverage. If the client is NPO, there is no carbohydrate coverage for the insulin. Frequently insulin is held the morning of surgery.

Chapter Study Questions: Answers & Rationales

Chapter 2: Health Implications Across The Lifespan

1. ① Whenever there is dislodgement of a radiation implant, there should always be a lead container and tongs in the room to place the radiation source.
2. ② DPT, polio, hepatitis-B as will as the influenzae vaccination are required immunizations by age 6 months. Varicella and MMR are not given until the infant is a year old.
3. ④ Recommendations are for the infant to be kept on formula until age 6 months, if tolerated. This decreases the incidence of allergies. Rice cereal should be the first solid offered.
4. ① A 9-month-old infant should be able to sit alone without support. The other options are expected at this stage of growth.
5. ① Chemotherapy is the treatment of a malignancy by medications. Palliative is the relief of pain and providing comfort to a terminal client. Immunotherapy is for the client who has received a transplanted organ.
6. ① Gastrostomy is a tube into the stomach for tube feedings when a client cannot eat. This is done with the cancer client as well as with the elderly client who cannot swallow.
7. ③ Nausea, vomiting, and bone marrow suppression are common problems with the chemotherapy medications.
8. ② The skin in the area of radiation is sensitive to sunlight, it is important to leave the markings on the skin so the radiologist will know the boundaries of the treatment.
9. ① Physiological needs must be addressed first. The other options may be used for this client, however the emesis and dehydration must be addressed first.
10. ③ Recognition of familiar faces begins around age 4 months, especially recognition of mother's face.
11. ① Girls typically begin the physiological changes of puberty about 2 years earlier then boys.
12. ④ Peer groups, or other adolescents are very important in the developmental phase of the adolescent.
13. ② The fluid balance needs to be carefully monitored in order to determine changes in output as well as fluid retention. Baseline fluid balance should be determined when client is begun on the chemotherapy.
14. ② The client should be encouraged to eat fresh fruits, fruit juices, tomatoes, etc., to increase his intake of potassium that he is losing due to the diuretic.
15. ③ The hepatitis-B vaccine is started at birth or shortly thereafter. The DPT is started at 2 months.
16. ④ The MMR is not started until the child is 1-year-old, the immune system cannot respond effectively to the vaccination until this age.
17. ① The rash from varicella typically contains vesicles with clear fluid. They are not filled with pus unless there is a secondary infection present.
18. ① The wound should be cleansed to prevent infection. The client may need a tetanus, however that can wait until later.
19. ① Animal products are limited on a low cholesterol diet. This includes milk products, meat, cheese, and eggs.
20. ② Eggs contain fat, however the non fat milk is a source of protein and not fat.

Chapter 3: Concepts of Nursing Practice

1. ② The assessment phase of the nursing process is where information that relates to clients needs is categorized.
2. ③ The collection of data in the role of the practical nurse is to assist in the development of a data base for client information.
3. ④ Objective information can be seen and concretely validated. Subjective data is information that the client, or client's family tell the nurse.
4. ① The semi-Fowler's position increases the ability of the client to deep breath.
5. ④ Do not obliterate any information on the client's chart and always initial entries. It is recommended not to write the word "error". You cannot recopy anyone else's notes, so recopying the page is not recommended.
6. ④ By placing a client NPO, it decreases the incidence of nausea and vomiting, regardless of the client's initial problems.
7. ③ These are common medications to be used preoperatively. Cardiac medications, antidepressants, diuretics, anticonvulsants are not typically preoperative medications.

8. ③ Since the client does not have control of their body needs during surgery, basic needs need to be addressed prior to and during the surgery.

9. ② Most often the shock that occurs postoperatively is due to hemorrhage, which causes a decrease in blood volume.

10. ④ If there is too much strain on the suture line, the area will pull apart, which is dehiscence. Evisceration is extrusion of the intestine through the incision.

11. ② A paralytic ileus is the absence of bowel sounds and the lack of movement of waste products through the bowel.

12. ② Healing by first intention is when the wound edges are together and are healing well. Secondary intention is when the wound heals from the inside out by formation of granulation tissue.

13. ④ If an incision is dehisced or open, there is an increased risk of an evisceration, or extrusion of intestine.

14. ① The primary purpose of turn, cough, and deep breath is to prevent respiratory complications.

15. ④ The informed consent means that the client understands the surgery and the risk involved. It is the doctors responsibility to initially discuss with the client.

16. ③ It is important to relieve pain around the clock and before the client experiences severe pain. If the nurse depends on it to be PRN, frequently the client is already in severe pain before they call to request the medication.

17. ① The geriatric client has decreased respiratory reserve and does not breath as deeply as younger adults.

18. ③ The knee is another area of pressure when the client is prone, or on his abdomen.

Chapter 4: Pharmacology

1. ① Frequently the elderly client is receiving several different medications. The client does not excrete them differently it is still primarily the liver and the kidney, however the organs are not as effective.

2. ③ The client will receive two tablets in the morning and two at noon for a total of 4 tablets for the day.

3. ③ If the order is for 300mg, and 500mg is on hand, then divide the 300 by 500 = 0.6cc .

4. ① If there are 40mg per cc, the desired dose is 60mg, divide 60 by 40 = 1.5cc.

5. ③ It is important to make sure the medication administration record and the doctors order correlate. Checking the client's ID band is making sure you have the correct client.

6. ③ The dose should be recorded as "not taken" and the nurse should waste the poured dose. If the dose is a controlled substance the wasted dose must be witnessed by another nurse. Checking the medication order for changes before accessing the medication helps to eliminate waste.

7. ② Liquid oral medications are already in solution and are thus absorbed more rapidly.

8. ④ Medications are absorbed. Elimination is when the body excretes the medication.

9. ④ The drug must be ordered for a nurse to administer it to a client.

10. ③ By drawing up 0.3cc of air you will be able to clear the total amount of drug from the needle and seal the site from leakage.

11. ① Intradermal is under the skin, if it is injected further it becomes a subcutaneous injection. A 25-28 gauge needle is used.

12. ④ The tip of the applicator should not touch the eye, and the medication should be placed in the middle of the lower conjunctival sac.

13. ④ IM injections are given in the vastus lateralis of the thigh prior to the infant walking. Most infants do not walk prior to 12 months of age.

14. ① The desired dose is 2.5 mg which is half of the dose on hand, which is 5mg in 1cc. Therefore, 0.5 or ½ cc provides the correct dose.

15. ④ Topical medications can be absorbed through the nurses skin also, the medication should not be rubbed in, and the site should be rotated with each application.

16. ④ Both liver and renal function are decreased in the geriatric client.

17. ③ Z track is used for IM injections The skin is pulled to the side when the needle is injected to prevent the medication from leaking back through the needle track.

Chapter 5: Homeostasis

1. ③ It is important for the client to continue the medication schedule, and the medication should be taken with food. A side effect is fluid retention, therefore the client needs to watch his fluid intake.

2. ① An anaphylactic reaction is the most severe type of reaction, whether it is to a medication such as penicillin, or to an insect bite. It can be fatal if medication is not available to reverse the reaction.

3. ④ Autoimmune is the term used for diseases that alter the body's immune system where the body has difficulty recognizing itself. Therefore, these diseases are call autoimmune diseases.

4. ② Corticosteroids are anti-inflammatory medications. These medications decrease the ability of the body to fight infection.

5. ① Immune depressed clients do not have an intact immune system and cannot defend the body against invading bacteria.

6. ④ Active acquired is a vaccination. Natural active is when the client has the disease. An example of passive immunity is the immunity that is transferred from the mother to the infant.

7. ④ The body produces antibodies in response to an invasion of pathological organisms or antigens.

8. ② Dehydration frequently precedes the development of hypovolemia. When hypovolemia occurs, there is an increased risk of the client developing low blood pressure and consequences of poor cardiac output.

9. ② The best way to determine the adequacy of body fluids is to measure the daily weight at the same time each day. Sudden increases or loss of body weight is most often due to fluid loss or retention.

10. ④ 1+ edema is lowest level, with 4+ being severe pitting edema.

11. ① The kidney is responsible for maintaining the fluid and electrolyte balance in the body.

12. ① Fever increases the body loss of fluid. The body attempts to decrease the temperature by cooling the skin, which increases fluid loss.

13. ③ Dry, flushed skin is typically of a client who is experiencing fluid loss, or beginning of dehydration. Further evaluation regarding fluid balance should be done.

14. ③ Dry mucous membranes and confusion are cardinal signs of dehydration in a geriatric client. Skin turgor is not a reliable sign of dehydration in the geriatric client.

15. ② The very young and the elderly are more susceptible to fluid changes. These two clients do not have adequate compensatory mechanisms to deal with sudden changes in fluid balance.

16. ④ Anytime there is a risk of body fluids being splattered, the nurse should wear protective eye gear.

17. ④ Respiratory acidosis is caused most often when the client is not breathing adequately and there is an increase in the retention of carbon dioxide. It is important to increase the quality of the client's respirations.

18. ① The human immunodeficiency is most often transmitted via unprotected sexual contact. The other options are methods of transfer, however, the most common is via sexual transmission.

19. ② A priority problem with the HIV positive client is the development of infections. The client does not have an intact immune system to resist the infection. The other options are important, but not as important as preventing infection.

20. ② The aminoglycoside classification of antibiotics causes neurotoxicity resulting in ototoxicity, as well as nephrotoxicity resulting in renal problems.

Chapter 6: Psychiatric Nursing Concepts and Care

1. ③ The following are elder abuse/neglect indicators—poor hygiene, poor nutrition, poor skin integrity, contractures, urine burns/excoriation, pressure ulcers, dehydration, bruising on inner surfaces of extremities.

2. ② Physiological needs are a priority for a confused client. They often will forget to eat and not remember when and where to go eat or bathe, etc. After the physiological needs are meet, then safety and security would be the next level.

3. ① Placing locks on doors in new areas that a client with dementia might wander into would be an excellent safety precaution. It is not necessary and is restrictive to keep the client confined to two rooms.

4. ② The client's background and history of drug abuse bring up historical issues in the nurse's past which she may not have dealt with. The derogatory comments are a defense mechanism to help her avoid the unresolved family issues she has.

5. ④ It is very important to be direct, honest, and not too overly friendly with a paranoid client. Touching should be avoided as it may be misinterpreted as a threat (delusion of persecution).

6. ① It is important to determine where the anxiety is coming from and then intervene to prevent it from escalating.

7. ② During a depressive episode, there is a general slowing down of bodily systems and behavior, i.e., anorexia, sad affect, psychomotor retardation, lack of social interaction, and poor grooming.

8. ④ An elated sense of well-being, euphoria, and speeded up psychomotor behavior are common signs of manic type behavior noted in bipolar disorder.

9. ① Classic symptoms of schizophrenia include disturbances in perception which are characterized by hallucinations, delusions, and illusions. Other symptoms include inappropriate affect, thought disorder, difficulty relating to others, and disorganized purposeless activity, etc.

10. ③ Symptoms of Parkinson's disease (shuffling gait, cogwheel rigidity, pill-rolling tremor, etc.) are characteristic of some of the extrapyramidal side ③ effects of antipsychotic medications, such as chloropromazine (Thorazine).

11. ② Safety is a concern when a client experiences an auditory hallucination, as the he may hear a voice

that tells him to do something harmful or inappropriate.

12. ② When a client hears an auditory hallucination, they often look preoccupied and turn their head to a side to better "hear" what is being said to them.

13. ③ It is helpful and supportive to the family who may feel overwhelmed with the care of a family member with Alzheimer's disease. Prioritizing care and supporting them for their efforts along with providing respite care are important nursing measures.

14. ④ Safety and security are enhanced with a familiar environment characterized by routine, repetition, and reinforcement.

15. ④ Careful documentation and reporting to proper authorities are the legal responsibility of the practical nurse when she suspects child or elder abuse.

16. ① This is a characteristic behavioral sign (feeling humiliated, ashamed, and defensive about the abusive experience) of an abused elder client along with the physical signs of: poor hygiene, poor nutrition, poor skin integrity, contractures, urine burns/excoriation, pressure ulcers, dehydration, bruising on inner surfaces of extremities

17. ② Cardiac arrhythmias are a complication of cocaine use. Pulse and blood pressure need to be monitored closely along with placing the client on telemetry.

18. ③ A support group for the family of an alcoholic is Al-Anon. Alcoholics Anonymous is a support group for the alcoholic.

19. ③ The classic defense mechanism used by clients who abuse alcohol and drugs is denial of their problem.

20. ② Establishing trust is paramount for the nurse to attain to work with the schizophrenic client. Their disturbed interpersonal relationships make this a difficult task for the nurse.

21. ④ Lithium toxicity is a serious problem for bipolar clients. Symptoms include: diarrhea, confusion, ataxia, slurred speech, hypotension, seizures, oliguria, coma, and death.

Chapter 7: Sensory

1. ② The important action is to provide artificial tears as the edema has prevented the eyelid from closing. Also, placing an eye patch on the eye will reduce excessive eye movement which would be further irritating and painful.

2. ④ Clients with glaucoma experience an increase in intraocular pressure which is controlled by miotic eye medications, such as **Timoptic**.

3. ① Ménière's disease is characterized by vertigo, tinnitus, and sensorineural hearing loss. Attacks may occur, lasting 10 minutes or up to several hours. There is no pain or loss of consciousness.

4. ② Mydriatric (remember "d" in word for dilate) eye medications cause pupillary dilatation and are contraindicated in the care of the glaucoma client.

5. ④ It is important to decrease the risk of otitis media recurrence by preventing milk from pooling around the eustachian tube by holding or elevating the infant's head while feeding, not propping a bottle and allowing the infant to fall asleep, and encouraging juice or water prior to sleeping.

6. ② Asepsis should be maintained on the applicator tip. There is no need for him to blow his nose. He should be in the supine position, but prevent solution from flowing into opposite eye. The medication should be placed in the lower conjunctival sac.

7. ② Glaucoma is a condition characterized by an increase in intraocular pressure and progressive loss of peripheral vision. It is a chronic disease and a leading cause of blindness.

8. ③ Penicillin and cephalosporin medications are not ototoxic. Aminoglycosides are ototoxic. The other three options all are risk factors for hearing loss.

9. ① As the hearing impaired depend readily on their hearing aids, it is important to teach them to have a extra set of batteries on hand. They should not be soaked in alcohol and turned off when not in the client's ear. It is not necessary to wear the hearing aid while sleeping and may in fact be uncomfortable to the client.

10. ① Mydriatic medications, such as atropine (Atropisol), are contraindicated in the care of the glaucoma client. Pilocarpine (**Pilocar**) is a miotic and is used to reduce intraocular pressure. **Demerol** and **Duragesic** can be administered to a glaucoma client.

11. ② The use of an ophthalmic anesthetic agent in the eye would necessitate the nurse to teach the client not to rub his eye until the "feeling" has returned (usually in 30min) to avoid additional trauma.

12. ② The use of a warm normal saline irrigation along with instillation of mineral oil would soften the wax to assist in the removal of the cerumen from the ear canal.

13. ③ It is not necessary to use short sentences with frequent pauses for the hearing impaired. Helpful strategies are to stand in front of client at eye level to speak with light on your face helps with speech reading, (i.e., reading lips), get client's attention by raising your hand or arm, do not walk back and forth in front of client while speaking, and speak clearly and in an even tone; do not shout.

14. ② The hearing aid amplifies sound, but does not change the overall ability to hear. It is used for conductive hearing loss clients.

15. ④ Nursing management of a client with Ménière's disease includes: maintain bed rest in a quiet, dimly lit room, client may assume a position of comfort, move the client only when necessary, and avoid unnecessary nursing procedures.

16. ③ A stapedectomy is the procedure used to correct otosclerosis which is removal of the stapes.

17. ③ Age related macular degeneration is found mostly in adults older than age 65 and accounts for a large percentage of diminished central vision in the older adult. Glaucoma results in a loss of peripheral vision. Retinal detachment is a separation of retinal layers that leads to areas of blank vision. Cataract is an opacity of the lens leading to blurred vision.

Chapter 8: Endocrine System

1. ① Kussmaul's respirations, which are deep, and rapid are typically seen in ketoacidosis. This occurs when the client's blood sugar is high.

2. ④ Hypoglycemia occurs with insulin shock, therefore the client will need glucagon. This is a high concentration of glucose that can be given IV.

3. ② Regular insulin is the only type that is given with sliding scale dosing.

4. ① The fruity breath is a symptom of a high blood sugar, the serum blood sugar should be checked immediately..

5. ① Glycosolated hemoglobin reflects the level of blood glucose control over the past 120 days. The fasting blood glucose is the measurement of the current blood sugar level.

6. ② Rotating sites helps to maintain healthy subcutaneous tissue and promote equal distribution of the injected insulin.

7. ④ The rapid deep ventilations, tachycardia and confusion occur in diabetic ketoacidosis.

8. ④ Insulin dependent diabetes most often has an onset prior to age 15 years. These clients require insulin. Adult onset diabetes may be controlled with diet, exercise and frequently oral hypoglycemics.

9. ② Airway is critical post operative thyroidectomy. A tracheotomy set should be easily available in case of respiratory distress. If swelling occurs at the operative site, an oral airway will not be effective.

10. ② During surgery, thyroid hormone can enter the blood as the surgeon attempts to remove the gland. This will cause an increase in all of the symptoms the client was experiencing preoperatively.

11. ④ The characteristics symptoms of hyperthyroidism are those of hyperactivity. Pulse rate, respiratory rate, blood pressure and temperature all will increase. The client may have difficulty sleeping and has a high energy level.

12. ③ When bleeding occurs at the incision, the blood will run down the client's neck and back. It is frequently not visible from the front. Increasing voice hoarseness should be evaluated, however not every 5-10m minutes.

13. ② The Cushing's client will be at increased risk for infection due to the decreased inflammatory response. He will tend to retain fluid and gain weight. They are most often on a low sodium diet, and their hydration is carefully evaluated.

14. ① It is important to give the hyperthyroid client proteins and carbohydrates to help her body maintain her energy level. When the condition is corrected, then the dietary intake can be decreased. The increased fibers assist to help control the diarrhea.

15. ① The parathyroid gland controls the calcium levels in the body. The client is at increased risk for hypocalcemia which may result in tetany.

16. ④ Nausea, vomiting, severe abdominal pain, and low grade fever are classic symptoms of pancreatitis. The nurse should limit po intake to clear fluids and carefully assess his tolerance.

17. ② The protrusion of the eyes causes them to dry out easily. Moisture drops or artificial tears are used to maintain the eye moisture. An ointment may be used at night because it will maintain moisture for a longer time.

18. ① The client with Addison's disease has difficulty controlling his blood pressure. He may have significant decrease in blood pressure with activity. The other options are not common complications associated with Addison's disease.

Chapter 9: Hematologic System

1. ④ The abnormal white cells from the leukemia affects the ability of the immune system to protect the body from infection. Infections are often the cause of death.

2. ① The cause of pernicious anemia is the inability of the client to utilize the vitamin B12 in his food, therefore it is necessary for the client to have injections of B12.

3. ④ To utilize Vitamin K it is necessary to have E-coli bacteria in the intestinal tract. The newborn does not have the bacteria at birth, therefore Vitamin K is administered to prevent hemorrhagic episodes.

4. ④ Aplastic anemia is the anemia that results as a serious side effect to some medications. Pernicious anemia is caused by lack of the intrinsic factor in the stomach order to utilize vitamin B12.

5. ① The sickled red cells are characteristic of sickle cell anemia. The cells tend to clump together causing small emboli, and impair circulation.

6. ③ Platelets begin the coagulation process. A client with low platelets or thrombocytopenia will have problems with bleeding gums, epistaxis, hematuria and easy bruising.

7. ② The characteristics of hemophilia are those of bleeding, whether the bleeding is internal or external. The large joints of the body are a common area of bleeding.

8. ③ The primary use of Epogen is to stimulate bone marrow to increase production of red cells, regardless of the cause of the decreased cell production. It is commonly used in the renal failure client.

9. ② The client has a low hemoglobin, therefore activity should be limited. The client frequently is cold, and tachycardia is not an uncommon problem.

10. ① One of the primary measures to prevent another sickle cell crisis is to maintain adequate hydration. Normal growth and development and routine immunizations are encouraged.

11. ③ Pallor, fatigue, tachycardia, and lethargy are common symptoms of problems with anemias. These symptoms frequently occur regardless of the cause of the anemia.

12. ② Pressure at the site is the first step to stop bleeding. The ice bag can be obtained after the pressure has been applied, and pressure should be applied to the radial artery.

13. ② Encourage the client to wear shoes all the time to prevent injury to his feet. Soft toothbrushes, no flossing, and frequent mouth rinses are encouraged for oral hygiene.

14. ④ The complete blood count (CBC) is a very common test to determine the red cells, platelets, white count and hemoglobin and hematocrit.

Chapter 10: Respiratory System

1. ① Pulse oximetry does not require any invasive procedure, it is a clip that is placed on the client's finger or ear lobe and is an estimate of the oxygen concentration in the blood. Spirometry measures capacity of the lungs, it does not measure the oxygen levels.

2. ③ The COPD client is dependent on his level of oxygen for his stimulus to breath, to increase his oxygen level too much will decrease his stimulus to breath and he will begin to hypoventilate or even develop apnea.

3. ② The client needs to be in an upright position leaning over a bedside table for easier access to the thoracic cavity. Another position may be with the client on his side and the head of the bed elevated.

4 . ① There is a decrease in breath sounds over the area of consolidation. The use of accessory muscles indicates difficulty breathing, not necessarily pneumonia.

5. ② Mucolytics decrease the surface tension of the mucus and allow it to become more liquid. By making the mucus more liquid, it is easier to cough up. Antihistamines dry up the mucus and make it difficult to remove by coughing.

6. ③ The decongestants cause vasoconstriction which will cause an increase in the blood pressure. This will increase the difficulty in maintaining control of the client's hypertension.

7. ① The respiratory rate is within normal limits. The increased pulse rate and the low oximetry levels correlate with respiratory difficulty and are not indicative of an improvement in the client. Secretions should mobilize as client improves.

8. ④ Pulmonary embolus is the common complication of immobility (venous pooling of blood), estrogen therapy (increased incidence of embolism on high doses), and long bone fracture (fat embolus).

9. ③ Dyspnea and fatigue are characteristic in the progression of chronic pulmonary disorders. Production of sputum and cough are common and not indicative of progression of the disease, temperature and headache may be indicative of an infection. An infection would be a complication, not progression of the condition.

10. ① Hypoxemia is the condition of decreased oxygen in the blood. Septicemia is a systemic infection, hypercapnia is the increase of carbon dioxide in the blood, and hyperventilation is rapid respirations.

11. ② In a total laryngectomy the client will have a permanent tracheotomy and will have lost his normal voice. The tracheotomy should be suctioned as necessary. He may or may not experience respiratory fatigue with activity.

12. ① Three days after surgery the lung should be expanded, which means there will be a minimum amount of dark drainage and no fluctuation of the fluid level in the tubing. 300 cc of serosanguineous drainage is not expected, and there should be no bubbling in the collection chamber.

13. ③ The wheezing is due to broncho spasm and narrowing of the bronchial airways. The mucus plugs the airways and causes trapping of distal air.

14. ④ The catheter is advanced till slight resistance is met, and suction is applied intermittently on withdrawal of the catheter. Suctioning on withdrawal will help to decrease trauma during suctioning. Suction is applied only about 15-20 seconds to prevent precipitation of hypoxia.

15. ③ Bronchospasm is a medical emergency that can rapidly develop into a respiratory arrest. Respiratory acidosis is the most common acid base imbalance with this condition.

16. ② The ineffective clearing of secretions with resultant pooling can lead to an increased risk of infection. Their appetite is usually decreased and they have an increased A-P diameter of the chest. Dehydration and immobility would contribute to the pooling of the secretions.

17. ① Symptoms of tuberculosis include fatigue, cough, low grade fever, night sweats, shortness of breath, and weight loss. They usually do not have problems with rash, pleural edema, or oliguria.

18. ④ When interpreting a tuberculosis skin test for a non-high risk individual a 15mm raised area indicates the person has been exposed to the TB bacillus. A 16mm induration is positive and he should have a chest x-ray, and possibly follow up with a sputum study.

19. ① On the first postoperative day, the fluid level in the chest tubes should be fluctuating with each ventilation due to the pressure changes in the thoracic cavity. If the lungs are re-expanded breath sounds should be present.

20 ② The culture and sensitivity should be started prior to the beginning of the antibiotic. The early morning sputum may have a better concentration of the bacteria, but frequently it is not feasible to postpone the beginning of the antibiotic until the next morning.

Chapter 11: Vascular System

1. ① Hypertension puts an increased workload on the left ventricle. The compensatory mechanism is an increase in the size of the left ventricle, when the left ventricle can no longer compensate, congestive failure occurs.

2. ③ Hypertension accelerates the development of atherosclerosis and damage to the vessels in the brain. Transient ischemic attacks frequently precede the occurrence of a brain attacks.

3. ① Orthostatic hypotension occurs when the client has been lying down and suddenly assumes an upright position. This commonly occurs in clients who are starting antihypertensive medications, who are hypovolemic, or who have a severe bradycardia.

4. ④ The activated partial thromboplastin (APTT) time is checked prior to the administration of heparin. The medication is injected subcutaneously with the smallest gauge needle and the area is not rubbed after the injection.

5. ④ These are considered to be modifiable risk factors for the development of atherosclerosis which predisposes a client to the development of cardiac disease and hyper tension.

6. ③ To maintain effective control, the hypertensive client is frequently on medication indefinitely. If the client begins a regular exercise routine and loses excess weight, it will impact the medication dosage.

7. ④ Peripheral vascular disease decreases the delivery of oxygenated blood to the tissue, the goal of therapy is to increase the arterial circulation thus increasing oxygen to the tissue.

8. ③ With arterial occlusion there is a decrease in quality of the pulse, the feet are pale and cool to touch. Healing ability is significantly diminished.

9. ① The surgery puts the client at an increased risk for renal complications as well an aortic aneurysm is commonly in the area of the renal arteries. A urinary output of 110 cc over 12 hours is too low and the doctor should be contacted immediately.

10. ③ It is critical that the client be on bed rest to prevent the dislodgement of a thrombus. The client will also be on an anticoagulant.

11. ② The classic findings of thrombophlebitis is pain in the leg with dorsiflexion of the foot, which is also known as Homan's sign. The affected area will be warm, inflamed, and tender.

12. ③ Intermittent claudication is the term used to describe pain in the legs that is relieved by resting the muscle.

13. ① Diabetes puts the client at significant risk for development of PVD, hypertension increases the risk as well.

14. ④ The typical symptoms of deep vein thrombosis is that of venous pooling, pain on dorsiflexion of the foot, swelling and tenderness over the affected area.

15. ④ The most common oral anticoagulant is Coumadin, Heparin cannot be taken by mouth, the other medications are not anticoagulants.

16. ① The only option that indicates a decrease in tissue perfusion is the decrease in urine output. Jugular vein distention is present with an increase in venous pressure. The chest output is expected and the vital signs can be within normal limits.

17. ③ Caffeine, amphetamines, and nicotine all cause an increase in blood pressure and would affect the control of the client's blood pressure. This option is more of a risk then the option with chocolate, tea, and caffeine.

18. ① The fruits are commonly high in potassium, especially the dried fruits.

19. ① The geriatric client's vascular system does not respond as rapidly to changes in position as the younger client.

20. ② Postural hypotension is the same as orthostatic hypotension. This occurs when a person suddenly moves from sitting or lying to a standing position, their blood pressure decreases.

Chapter 12: Cardiac System

1. ① After the cardiac catheterization, the client will be required to lie flat. The client is usually awake and alert, and pain is not a problem. He will not be allowed out of bed for several hours, however a urinary catheter is not used, unless he cannot void.

2. ③ An allergy to shellfish may be indicative of an allergy to iodine. The dye used in the catheterization is an iodine based dye.

3. ① The isoenzymes are indicative of cardiac tissue damage. The isoenzyme CPK-MB is a specific indicator of damage to the cardiac muscle.

4. ② The apex of the heart is located at the fifth intercostal space in the mid-clavicular line on the left side. This is the area to count an apical pulse.

5. ③ With bacterial endocarditis, the client will be on long term antibiotics. It is important that he maintain the dosing schedule.

6. ① Sodium increases the client's retention of fluid. An increase in fluid retention puts an increased workload on the heart. Therefore when there is a decreased sodium intake, it will assist to improve cardiac function.

7. ④ The primary action of nitroglycerine is vasodilatation of the arteries. This may precipitate a headache as the cerebral arteries are dilated as well as the coronary arteries.

8. ④ High Fowler's position with the legs dependent will assist to decrease venous return, this will decrease the workload of the heart and increases cardiac efficiency. Increasing cardiac efficiency will assist to improve the quality of ventilation.

9. ④ Nitroglycerin should be taken at the first sign of any chest pain, if the pain is not relieved within five minutes, then another tablet should be taken. A total of three tablets can be taken five minutes apart, if the chest pain continues, the EMS should be notified.

10. ① The action of digitalis is to strengthen and slow cardiac rate which will improve cardiac output. As cardiac output is improved, so is renal perfusion which increases in urinary output.

11. ④ As edema is reduced, the fluid moves back into the vascular system. With increased vascular volume, the kidney will excrete more water thereby increasing the urinary output.

12. ③ The cardiac client should not do isometric exercises because it puts an increased workload on the heart. Walking and stationary bikes are good examples of exercise for this client.

13. ③ Right sided heart failure causes an increase in pressure within the venous system and the right side of the heart. The increased venous pressure causes jugular vein distention.

14. ④ Tachycardia in the cardiac client increases cardiac workload and oxygen utilization. The development of pedal edema is a late sign of digitalis toxicity. First degree block can only be determined via a monitor or EKG.

15. ④ Because of the vasodilatation effect of the medication, there may be orthostatic or postural hypotension.

16. ② Morphine sulfate is the pain medication of choice for a client with chest pain. especially in the client with a history of cardiac problems.

17. ③ The dietary intake is the only one that the client has any control over. Non-modifiable risk factors are the ones in which the client has no control.

18. ④ A cardiac catheterization requires the insertion of a catheter into the femoral artery with the injection of a dye in order to visualize the coronary arteries. The insertion of the catheter makes it an invasive procedure.

19. ② The early side effects of digitalis are those of the GI system. Bradycardia is a late sign of digitalis toxicity. First degree block can only be determined via a monitor or EKG.

20. ① During CPR, the heart is compressed between the sternum and the spine to push the blood out of the ventricles. It is this pumping motion that produces cardiac output. Compressions should be done on a hard surface to be most effective.

Chapter 13: Gastrointestinal System

1. ① Normal saline is non-irritating to the suture line in the mouth. The sutures should be rinsed off every time the client eats. Peroxide and strong mouth washes should not be used. If the client is eating, they can have cool or warm foods, but no temperature extremes.

2. ① Nasogastric tubes are put into the stomach to decrease the gastric distention in the client with a bowel obstruction. It will not eliminate nausea and vomiting, however it will make vomiting less likely.

3. ④ The lower in the colon the colostomy is performed, the more formed the stool will be. Black and bloody stools are indicative of disease process. An ileostomy client will have a liquid stool.

4. ② Immediately after removing the tube, offer/provide oral hygine. The client is most often on clear liquid initially, abdominal distention and bowel sounds will need to be evaluated later to determine client's toleratnce of removal of the tube..

5. ③ This is only the day after surgery therefore the area around the stoma has not had time to heal. The stoma should be pinkish red, moist and often there is some swelling present.

6. ② It is important to know if the client is experiencing problems with diarrhea and constipation. This has

implications on the client's fluid and electrolyte balance.

7. ① Sometimes it is difficult to hear bowel sounds, especially in the postoperative client after abdominal surgery. The nurse should listen for at least 2 minutes before noting that bowel sounds are not heard.

8. ③ It is the client's right to refuse treatment or to refuse to have a diagnostic procedure done. The physician should be notified.

9. ③ Prior to an appendectomy, the client is usually maintained in a position of comfort, kept NPO, and no heat is applied to the abdomen. Narcotics are used sparingly. It is important to be able to identify changes in the character of the client's pain.

10. ④ The nasogastric tube should not be repositioned on this client without first talking with the physician. The positioning of the tube was done during surgery. The tube is not irrigated except with specific orders, it is not clamped, and the gastric output is measured at the end of the shift, unless it appears to be excessive.

11. ④ Concentrated formula given too rapidly will cause problems with cramping, distention and diarrhea. The optimum method of tube feeding is the continuous drip method. Intermittent via a drip rate is the next preferred method.

12. ④ Clients who experience problems with GERD should not lie down after they eat, or within three hours of going to bed. They should rest in the sitting position after eating, and maintain an adequate amount of fluid intake with their meals. Antacids will not relieve the problem.

13. ③ Positioning the client on his side will facilitate the client spitting out the vomitus. High Fowler's position is also a good position to assist in preventing aspiration.

14. ④ The histamine antagonist medications actually decrease the production of gastric acid. The antacids such as Maalox and Mylanta coat the stomach to neutralize the acid that is present.

15. ② Old blood that has been disintegrated by the digestive juices has the appearance of coffee grounds. This does not reflect any active bleeding, however the source of the old bleeding should be identified.

16. ① When the stomach is removed, the intrinsic factor is removed. The intrinsic factor is necessary for the body to utilize the vitamin B12 in the food. Therefore, the client will require B12 injections.

17. ② The client with a tendency toward the development of a peptic ulcers should not take any medication that causes gastric irritation and bleeding tendencies. This would include any aspirin products as well as corticosteroid medications.

18. ③ These medications are all stool softeners and do not cause any bowel irritation. This is the type of medication recommended to elderly clients to prevent constipation.

19. ① The initial treatment is directed toward relieving the gastric distention and decreased the potential for vomiting. The client is NPO, and most often on bed rest initially.

20. ① Dehydration is a serious problem in the client with IBD. The bloody stool and distended abdomen are common symptoms associated with this condition. Hyperglycemia is not a common problem.

Chapter 14: Hepatic and Biliary System

1. ④ The primary method of transmitting Hepatitis A is via contamination food and poor hygiene. Shell fish caught in contaminated water, improper handling of food, improper hygiene practices, and oral-anal sexual activity are the primary methods of transmission.

2. ④ Direct contact with blood to mucous membrans or splashed in the eyes carries a higher riske than other activities listed.

3. ① Acetaminophen products are hepatotoxic. Any client with liver problems should not take products that contain acetaminophen. The vitamins are okay, and there is usually no problem with cough medications.

4. ① It is important for the health care worker to be immunized against hepatitis B, it is transmitted by serum and body fluids. Hepatitis A is most often controlled by good hand washing, and there is no vaccination for HIV. The varicella vaccination is important but it is usually a community based problem, not a hospital based problem.

5. ④ Hepatitis A is also known as an infectious hepatitis. It is transmitted primarily by the fecal oral route and is the less severe type of hepatitis.

6. ① There are many medications that are detoxified by the liver. If the liver is not functioning normally these toxins are not eliminated from the body and become hepatotoxic.

7. ① The client with liver disease will have problems with bruising, petechia, and spider angiomas. There is a characteristic yellowing or jaundice color of the skin due to the increased bilirubin. There should be not be a problem with hypoxia, or changes in LOC until the final stages of the disease.

8. ④ When the bilirubin levels increase in the client with liver problems, a yellowish tinge occurs in the skin and sclera of the eyes. This is known as jaundice and is commonly seen in clients with liver disease.

9. ③ Fresh fruits and vegetables have the lowest sodium content. The client should avoid breads, pastries dairy products and all processed meats.

10. ④ The client with liver disease has a problem with portal hypertension which causes the problem of ascites. This is a collection of fluid in the abdominal cavity of the client with liver problems. Melena or bloody stool may occur with the bleeding problems, but ascites is characteristic.

11. ② The best position for the client is semi-Fowlers. Frequently the diaphragm is irritated by the surgery and the client has increased difficulty taking a deep breath.

12. ② The increased blood ammonia will cross the blood brain barrier and cause problems with altered or decreased levels of consciousness. The other options are common in clients with liver problems, but are not due to the blood ammonia level.

13. ④ Demerol is a more effective drug of choice. Morphine can cause problems with pancreatic and bile duct spasms thus causing an increased pain problem.

14. ① The client with liver problems will have a problem with the utilization of Vitamin K which is necessary for normal clotting factors.

Chapter 15: Neurological System

1. ① L-dopa is the most common medication for treatment of Parkinson's disease. The desired effect is to reduce the tremors. These tremors most often occur in the upper extremities. They are usually present at rest and decrease with purposeful movement.

2. ② To promote safety, the client should always be assisted out of bed on the unaffected side. The wheelchair should be placed on the unaffected side. This option is specific to the situation. The client should be placed near the edge of the bed, but the option does not state which side of the bed.

3. ① Even thought CP is not evident at birth, it is usually traced back to some incident a birth that is related to hypoxia. The other options are not associated with an infant at birth.

4. ② Anytime a client experiences neurological damage whether by an accident or by surgery, they are at an increased risk for seizures. A TIA occurs in clients with hypertension and frequently precedes a brain accident. The other options do not have anything to do with neurological problems.

5. ④ The client with MS has a progressive deterioration of the neurons in the spinal cord and the brain (CNS). The neurons from the spinal cord to the extremities are intact. The upper motor neurons (CNS) have to be intact in order for the muscle to respond. As the disease progresses, there is total destruction of the nerve with resulting motor problems.

6. ④ The removal of cerebral spinal can cause a headache. To decrease the incidence of headache, the client is kept supine for 6-12 hours to prevent further leakage of spinal fluid. P O fluids are encouraged during this time to assist in replacing the spinal fluid.

7. ① The hypothalamus is responsible for temperature control. A client who experiences increased intracranial pressure, for whatever reason, is at an increased risk for problem with temperature control due to pressure on the hypothalamus.

8. ④ In order to perform a spinal puncture, the spine needs to be flexed in order to provide as much space between the vertebrae as possible. The client may also lean across a bedside table to achieve the same effect. The other options are conducted from a supine position.

9. ① Bradycardia is a characteristic occurrence in clients with increased intracranial pressure. The other options are complications, however they are not specific to the neurological status.

10. ④ Reality checks assist the nurse to determine confusion and disorientation early. The other options do not determine the presence of confusion. Reality checks are more specific to the mental status then the level of consciousness. A person can be lethargic, but oriented.

11. ③ Initially with increased intracranial pressure, one eye may be larger and have a decreased or sluggish reaction as compared to the other eye. As ICP becomes established, there is pressure on the optic nerve and both eyes will dilate with no reaction to direct light stimulus.

12. ② The immobility occurring as a result of the brain accident makes the client more prone to constipation. The paralysis that occurs is not of the bowel but of the motor function of the body.

13. ④ The client is at increased risk of pneumonia due to the pooling of secretions as well as the decreased ability to cough them up. Cardiac, renal and liver problems are not uncommon in the elderly client due to other chronic conditions. Pneumonia is a common problem in all stroke clients.

14. ③ An increase in lethargy, increase in temperature, and tachycardia are symptoms expected on admission of the meningitis client. The presence of a purple appearing rash is suggestive of meningococcal meningitis, which is very serious and contagious.

15. ① The client needs to be positioned where the head and neck can be maintained in an extended state to maintain the open airway, this will also allow for drainage of oral secretions. The side lying position best meets these needs.

16. ② The airway is the most critical physiological need at this time. The other options are important to implement, but at a later time when life threatening problems with the airway have been addressed.

17. ① Mannitol (Osmitrol) is given to reduce intracranial pressure by pulling fluid across the cell membrane. However it is also a diuretic and I&O have to be carefully maintained to assist to evaluate the adequacy of hydration.

18. ② Recurrent seizures are frequently due to the client not taking the medication as directed. The other options are not common factors for reoccurrence of seizures.

19. ④ The term quadriplegia refers to an injury involving the cervical vertebrae and involves all four extremities. Depending on the severity of the damage as to what responses or movement the client will be able to achieve.

20. ④ Anytime a client is immobilized there is increased risk for skin breakdown. Spinal cord injury clients have also suffered damage to the nerves and cannot tell if there is pain in the area or not. These clients should always be visually checked for redness and skin breakdown. It is not adequate to ask the client if the area is uncomfortable.

Chapter 16: Musculoskeletal System

1. ① The sitting position keeps the hip and most often the knee in a flexed position. The flexed position contributes to the development of contractures. Passive and active range of motion help to prevent contractures, and the wedge pillow is most often used to maintain abduction following hip surgery.

2. ③ Bright red bleeding should not be occurring this late postoperative. A small amount of bleeding may be expected immediately postoperative. Serosanguineous drainage is normal, however purulent drainage would be indicative of an infection.

3. ④ In any client in traction, a nursing priority is to make sure the feet are not touching the end of the bed. This eliminates the pull of the traction on the affected extremity. The weights must also be hanging freely for counter traction to be effective.

4. ② The normal capillary refill is 2-3 seconds, increased time may be due to poor peripheral circulation due to arterial constriction, edema, or cold temperature.

5. ③ The sensation of phantom limb pain is not uncommon in the amputee. The client feels the amputated extremity, the nerve endings do not accurately reflect the area of the pain. The client needs to be medicated and the pain is usually self-limiting.

6. ② The casted extremity should be supported on a pillow that will not absorb the moisture and keep the cast moist. The client needs to be turned frequently to allow for air circulation around the cast for drying. The cast should be handled with the palm of the hand to prevent indentations in the cast. Heat should not be applied, however a fan will increase movement of air and drying of the cast.

7. ① When a pin is inserted, the periosteum of the bone is broken and there is an increased risk of infection. The skeletal traction and pin insertion help to maintain an effective realignment of the bone. There is no reason to suspect a flexion contraction. Compartmental syndrome occurs when there is a circulatory problem, most often with a cast.

8. ② This amount of drainage is within normal limits immediately after surgery. The operative record is going to be of no benefit and it will not help to put pressure on the incisional area because the drainage is coming from deep within the wound.

9. ① The increase in pain and warmth over the cast are indicative of an infection under the cast. The capillary refill and decreased movement are problems with circulation or nerve compression. Itching and general discomfort are expected.

10. ② Increasing pain unrelieved by medication often is indicative of compartmental syndrome. This is more likely to be the problem then a thrombosis. Compartmental syndrome should always be considered when there is significant increase in the level of pain.

11. ③ "Petaling" of the cast is done by taking pieces of tape and applying them around the edges of the cast to keep it from crumbling and to decrease skin irritation from the edges of the cast. It is important to assess the problem precipitating the discomfort and utilize other methods to relieve the pain as appropriate.

12. ③ Osteoporosis is the most common reason for hip fractures. It causes a degeneration and decalcification of the bone. When the bones are weaker, they are at increased risk of fracture. Geriatric women are at highest risk for osteoporosis, and are most common client with hip fractures as well.

13. ② When a joint is acutely involved with rheumatoid arthritis, the joint should be at rest, and cold packs are used to decrease the inflammation. To apply heat and exercise the joint will increase the inflammation. Heat and exercises should be done to prevent acute problems, and to decrease stiffness.

14. ② The client will most likely be placed in Buck's traction to maintain immobility and alignment of the fracture site. Circulating air mattress, or cast are not being used to treat this client.

15. ④ For healing to occur there has to be an adequate amount of protein. The client does not need an in-

crease in his calcium due to his fracture and bed rest. The parathyroid will regulate the necessary amount of calcium needed for healing, it is not dependent on intake of calcium. Since he is on strict bed rest, he is not utilizing as many calories and does not need high carbohydrates.

16. ④ In the postoperative laminectomy client it is important to assess for any indication of pressure against the spinal column. This may be caused by swelling or by a hematoma. Numbness and tingling, inability to move the extremity are common indicators of the problem. The surgery does not cause any circulatory compromise, and the pain is to be expected immediately postoperative.

17. ④ Balanced suspension traction does not use the boot for traction. Weights should not be taken off, but the weights should always hang free on any type of traction.

18. ④ The crutch should not put any pressure in the axillary area. The client's arms should be at a 30 degree angle in order to support the client's weight. When going up the stairs, the unaffected leg is advanced first.

19. ① The pain from a fracture is most often described as sharp and piercing.

20. ① Vitamin B is a necessary diet, however, estrogen replacement and increased calcium in the diet helps to prevent bone deterioration. The client is encouraged to participate in weight bearing exercises

Chapter 17: Reproductive System

1. ① A small amount of bleeding is expected after this surgery. Postoperatively for a suprapubic prostatectomy a bladder irrigation system is most often not used.

2. ② The herpes virus type II is concentrated in the vesicles, and therefore the infection is highly contagious. The virus can be transferred to another area of the body by direct contact.

3. ② The Center for Disease Control studies the profile of the STD's and develops programs to decrease the incidence, identify areas of higher concentration of problems, and to establish protocols for treatment. Each state has responsibility for establishing what conditions are reportable. Most states adhere to guidelines from the CDC.

4. ④ The VDRL, ELISA, and cultures are most commonly used for the screening of STD's. The VDRL is for syphilis, and it is inexpensive. The ELISA will identify presence of HIV antibodies, but not the virus. The culture will identify specific pathogenic organisms and assist to select treatment.

5. ① A painless sore is characteristic of the chancre lesion of syphilis. Gonorrhea is characterized by urethral discharge, and herpes simplex (HVH II) has a characteristic painful lesion. The human papillomavirus is a genital wart.

6. ④ It is important for the bladder to be empty. This will promote the comfort for the client and allow the doctor to examine the pelvic contents easier. A cleansing enema is not done. The client may be anywhere in her cycle, however clients usually do not schedule an exam during their period. Pregnancy is a consideration, however an empty bladder is more important immediately prior to the examination.

7. ③ It is important to observe the arm on the affected side of the client who has had a mastectomy. If the lymph drainage in the arm has been compromised, there is an increased risk of swelling and edema on the affected arm. The arm should be protected from needle sticks, blood pressure, etc. The temperature, and slight increase in blood sugar are normal for first day postoperative.

8. ② The itching and burning may be caused by drying of the vaginal walls. The estrogen cream will help to decrease the problem. The client should not douche, and soap may further irritate the area. A water based lubricant as in petroleum jelly may improve lubrication during sexual activity, but will not resolve the problem.

9. ② Frequency, urgency, difficulty starting the urinary stream, and hematuria are common findings with BPH. The bladder may have residual, but should not be distended. There may be a burning pain present if the client has a UTI.

10. ③ The doctor will evaluate the client's prostate by doing a digital rectal examination. No special equipment is needed other then gloves and lubricant.

11. ① Clots in the urinary drainage system are common problems in the immediate postoperative period. The doctor should be notified immediately if the nurse cannot easily reestablish catheter patency. The catheter placed postoperatively is an irrigation catheter that is specific for use with a bladder irrigation. If a new one is placed, the doctor will do it.

12. ④ This is a malignancy that occurs in young men. The self examination is important in identifying the problem and getting treatment started as soon as possible. Frequently the only symptom is a mass that can be palpated in the scrotum.

13. ① An increase in prostatic specific antigen (PSA) is suggestive of a malignant process. When the serum acid phosphatase is elevated, the cancer is most often extensive. The urine specific gravity is to evaluate renal function and the culture is for infections.

14. ③ Parotitis (mumps) may cause the orchitis and epididymitis, especially if the virus occurs after puberty. It is important to determine if the boy had his MMR that is recommended at 12 months of age, then again at 4-5 years. A urinary tract infection, and a streptococcal infection (sore throat) are not of significance here. The sexual activity should be discussed with the boy without the mother present.

15 ① Simple vaginitis is common in geriatric women. A douche will cause an increase in the problem as the normal flora of the vaginal area are removed. Frequently feminine hygiene products will irritate the area. A wet mount prep and serum lab work should be done to determine if she needs further testing for STD.

16 ④ The question does not state the client was menopausal, therefore if she is menstruating the best time to perform the examination is the week after her period. This is a time the breast are less tender.

17 ① The lithotomy position provides exposure to the pelvic area. Semi-Fowler's is sitting up, Trendelenburg is with the head down and Sim's is flat with the client on their side.

18 ② The affected arm should be elevated to decrease the development of edema. Nothing should be put on the incision, and the diuretics are not part of the routine post operative care for this client.

19 ① This early postoperative and with the bladder irrigation running, there should be more drainage. The catheter may be occluded with tissue or clots causing urine to collect in the bladder, which causes pain. The other options are expected occurrence at this time.

20 ① This medication is also used for treatment of hypertension. The client needs to have his blood pressure monitored and observed for the development of postural hypotension.

Chapter 18: Urinary-Renal System

1. ③ The nurse should encourage the client to void whenever she feels the urge. Refraining from voiding increases the concentration of urine in the bladder and increases the irritation.

2. ④ Dysuria, or painful urination is a common complaint of clients with UTI. Low back pain occurs with upper UTI, and painless hematuria is not a characteristic of lower UTI.

3. ② First specimen is discarded, all urine is saved for next 24 hours. The client is asked to void again and that specimen is added to the container to complete the 24 hour collection.

4. ① To promote continence, a schedule for toileting should be established. P O fluids should be encouraged, except immediately prior to bedtime. Assessing for distention is important, however the question asked methods to establish continence.

5. ③ The shunt should be lightly palpated for presence of a "thrill" or vibration. Shunt may also be auscultated for bruits or sounds of blood passing through the shunt.

6. ③ Circumcision is usually delayed until the repair of the urethral opening can be completed. This is usually somewhere between 3 to 6 months of age.

7. ③ Injections would actually be discouraged. All other options are important in preventing infections in the client who has a compromised immune system.

8. ① These are classic symptoms in the GI system that occur with the development of uremia. Other changes occur throughout the body which may also include confusion, bleeding, hypertension, and an increase in serum potassium.

9. ① The most common cause of acute renal failure is the client who has experienced an episode of low blood pressure. Of all of these clients, the one with placenta previa is at highest risk for a period of low blood pressure. The diabetic client is at risk for development of chronic renal failure.

10. ② Erythropoietin is produced by the kidney and is responsible for the production of red blood cells. Anemia is a common problem in the chronic renal failure client.

11. ③ Nitrofurantoin is a common urinary tract antiseptic. The other medications are not for urinary tract problems.

12. ① The pain is described as sharp and severe as the calculi or stone progresses down the ureter. It frequently will radiate down the leg or to the groin area.

13. ③ The perineal area should be cleansed from the front to back to avoid contaminating the urethra with e-coli. All other options are encouraged.

14. ① This is the best description for the cystoscopy examination. The client is most often in lithotomy position and conscious sedation may be utilized. It is important to explain to the client he should not experience severe pain.

15. ④ The skin is typically dry and frequently the client complains of itching. The bruising occurs due to the effect of the renal failure on coagulation.

16 . ③ Congestive heart failure is the only option listed that is associated with an increase in fluids. The other options are problem of renal failure, but are not associated with the increase in fluid volume.

17. ④ The classic sign of oliguria is urine output between 100-400cc over 24 hours. The potassium is increased, hematuria is not common, and the specific gravity usually is at a fixed level.

18. ④ When urine is not present on a catheterization, the most common reason is the catheter is not in the bladder. On a female, it is most often in the vagina.

19. ② Anytime the catheter is contaminated it should not ever be reused. A new catheter should be obtained. It is not necessary to get a new setup if the current setup is still sterile. Take an extra catheter, or have a co-worker bring an additional catheter.

Chapter 19: Integumentary System

1. ④ Most pressure ulcers or decubitus are caused from pressure on an area that interferes with adequate blood supply to the area. Poor nutrition decreases the healing, and also puts the client at an increased risk, but it does not cause it initially.

2. ③ The first stage of a pressure ulcer is a reddened area that does not blanche with slight digital pressure. When this occurs damage has already occurred in the capillary bed of the tissue under the skin.

3. ③ This best describes the stage 3 of the decubitus ulcer. The area is not infected and does not extend past the subcutaneous tissue.

4. ② The first action is to keep the client off the area to decrease pressure at the site. Once the skin is broken, the transparent plastic dressings are common to protect the area from contamination.

5. ① There are many commercial moisture creams available. Showering will increase the dryness, and protective pads will not help decrease the problem. The cotton clothing helps, but frequently the problem occurs in areas not covered by clothing.

6. ④ The impetigo is caused by a streptococcal infection. Ringworm is a fungal skin infection, and herpes zoster is more common in elderly clients.

7. ③ Impetigo is a very contagious skin lesion that is common in children. Any irritation or open lesion is at risk of being infected with the bacteria.

8. ④ Herpes zoster in the elderly is accompanied by nerve pain or neuralgia. There is not vaccination, all clients are on standard precautions, and the antifungal cream is not effective with this client.

9. ② This is the characteristic description of the lesion found in the client with basal cell carcinoma.

10. ① Steroids are frequently the first line of treatment for the psoriasis client. The moisture and ice packs are not effective, and debridement irritates the area.

11. ② Topical application of a scabicide is the best way to kill the mite. Due to the tunneling effect of the mite and the burrowed eggs it is important to leave the scabicide on for 8-12 hours before washing it off. All family members should be treated.

12. ② Tachypnea may be the first indication of impending respiratory difficulties secondary to the inhalation of smoke or heat. Symptoms of hypoxia will be progressive.

13. ④ The lesions of psoriasis are classically reddened, scaley plaques that slough.

14. ③ The lesions of impetigo are moist vesicles that crust over. Removing the crust and applying antibiotic cream has not been particularly effective. The treatment of choice is oral antibiotics and it is important for the parent to administer all of the medication.

15. ③ It is important to keep the lesions moist to assist in decreasing the itching. Child may have other allergies, especially asthma as an older child. It is recommended that sunlight be avoided.

Chapter 20: Maternal Care

1. ④ Iron needs during pregnancy can most readily be met by taking iron supplements. Iron supplements should be taken with additional Vitamin C to increase absorption.

2. ① Gravida refers to the number of times the woman has been pregnant - two live births, history of one miscarriage, and she is pregnant now for a total of 4 pregnancies. She has two living children for para 2.

3. ③ Positive signs of pregnancy are those that are diagnostic. These signs demonstrate without a doubt there is a fetus in the uterus.

4. ④ Suggest to the woman that she eat smaller meals. Fluids and protein are good to increase in the pregnancy, but will not assist in decreasing the nausea and vomiting. Over the counter medications should not be recommended.

5. ① Elevating the feet and legs assists to decrease venous stasis. When the client is standing, the pregnant uterus exerts increased pressure on the large pelvic veins. It is not recommended that the pregnant client restrict sodium intake, and an increased fluid intake is okay, however it does not assist to decrease the venous stasis.

6. ③ During the pregnancy the woman becomes introverted and begins to work on acceptance of herself as a mother. During the first few days postpartum, there is physical contact with infant. Attachment behaviors include touching and eye-to-eye contact.

7. ③ Stretch marks cannot be prevented with any type of lotions or oils. They will gradually fade and become silvery streaks during the months after delivery. There is nothing that can be done to prevent them, however a positive answer that they will fade is a better approach.

8. ① Regardless of the length of the contractions, whether the membranes have ruptured, or if a bloody show is present, if the woman is not having any effacement or dilatation she is not considered to truly be in labor.

9. ① The duration of the contraction is the length of the contraction -from the beginning of the contraction to the end of it. The frequency of the contractions is from the beginning of one contraction to the beginning of another.

10. ③ Green leafy vegetables, citrus fruit, and yeast products are good sources for folic acid. Folic acid is necessary for DNA synthesis.

11. ④ During pregnancy, the woman needs to increase her caloric intake by 300 calories per day, during lactation the calories need to be increased by 500 calories per day. The infant usually has adequate iron stores from mother, but needs the protein for growth.

12. ② The recommended weight gain during pregnancy for a woman of average weight is 25-35 pounds. There is considerable variation, but this is the average amount that is consistently recommended.

13. ④ Weight gain, edema, proteinuria and increased blood pressure are the classic indications of the development of early problems with pregnancy induced hypertension.

14. ① During the time of labor and delivery (intrapartal) placenta previa would cause problems with bleeding and potentially severe hemorrhage. This is the only condition listed that is associated with severe bleeding problems during the intrapartum period.

15. ④ Left lateral position increases the delivery of blood to the placenta, as well as preventing the problems of vena caval syndrome.

16. ② The Apgar is completed at one minutes to assist in to identifying any intrauterine problems and to evaluate the current status. The Apgar is again done at 5 minutes to determine any problems in transition to extrauterine life.

17. ② Braxton Hicks or false labor contractions usually decrease when walking, are not concentrated in one part of the uterus, and do not increase in intensity and frequency. These contractions do not result in cervical effacement and dilatation..

18. ④ The serious side effects of oral birth control pills include problems with hypertension and clotting. If the woman develops a headache or leg pain, she report it to the doctor immediately.

19. ③ Terbutaline (Brethine) is most commonly used to suppress contractions. Another medication used to suppress contractions is magnesium sulfate.

20. ② The postpartum vital signs are indicative of hemorrhaging. The quickest way to stop a uterine hemorrhage in a postpartum client is to message the uterus (fundus). The nurse should stay with the client, keep the fundus firm, and have someone else call the doctor.

Chapter 21: Newborn

1. ③ Immediately after birth the infant frequently has mucous in his upper airway. He needs to be suctioned and occasionally will need additional oxygen. A bulb syringe to suction the upper airways should be kept in the infant's crib.

2. ② The meconium stool is often passed within the first few hours after birth. It is thick, black and sticky. It will gradually become lighter and more of a stool consistency.

3. ② This is the characteristic description of the caput. It is a collection of fluid under the scalp and it crosses the suture line on the cranium. It will gradually be absorbed and does not require treatment.

4. ① These three factors, grunting, flaring nares, and sternal retractions are classic symptoms of respiratory distress in infants.

5. ③ There is frequently a concern with cardiac output when the infant turns dusky with crying. The other options are within the normal range of findings for a newborn.

6. ① E-coli is necessary for the utilization of vitamin K. Since the newborn's bowels are sterile at birth he has difficulty with the syntheses of vitamin K. An injection is given to provide enough vitamin K until his system begins to function.

7. ② Problems with hypoglycemia may range from increased irritability to generalized seizures. Acrocyanosis is normal in the newborn, the respiratory rate is around 40-60 immediately after birth and levels off to 30-50 after the first 24 hours.

8. ① Keep the head covered to decrease convection heal loss. It is important to promote bonding during the first 8 hours therefore the infant is not kept in the warmer. Bathing is delayed until the infant's vital signs and temperature have stabilized.

9. ② Hand washing between clients is just as critical in the nursery as it is on other patient care units. This is the most effective way to decrease transmission of infection.

10. ③ The infant should be burped or bubbled after the first few minutes of feeding. The first few minutes of feeding is when the air is more likely to enter the infant's stomach. If the air is not removed, the infant tends to "burp up" a large amount of feeding. This occurs in breast and bottle fed infants.

11. ④ Rhogam is administered when the mother is Rh -. If she is carrying an Rh+ infant, she will begin to build up antibodies that will affect the next pregnancy. Rhogam prevents the buildup of the antibodies.

12. ③ The PKU test can be done from the blood on a heel stick. It will identify a complication in the ability of the infant to convert phenylalanine. It can be handled by dietary management.

Index

A

B

C

D

E

F

G

H

Actonel helps. prevent osteoporosis

I

J

K

L

M

N

O

P

R

S